MUSCLE BIOPSY

Commissioning Editor: Michael J Houston
Development Editor: Louise Cook
Project Manager: Glenys Norquay
Senior Designer: Sarah Russell
Illustration Manager: Bruce Hogarth
Illustrator: Richard Tibbitts
Marketing Manager(s) (UK/USA): Leontine Treur/Kathleen Neely

MUSCLE BIOPSY
A Practical Approach

Third Edition

Victor Dubowitz MD PhD FRCP FRCPCH

Emeritus Professor of Paediatrics
Dubowitz Neuromuscular Centre
Faculty of Medicine
Imperial College London
Hammersmith Campus
London, UK

Caroline A Sewry BSc PhD FRCPath

Professor of Muscle Pathology
Dubowitz Neuromuscular Centre
Faculty of Medicine
Imperial College London
Hammersmith Campus
London, UK
and
Centre for Inherited Neuromuscular Disorders and
Department of Musculoskeletal Pathology
Robert Jones and Agnes Hunt Orthopaedic Hospital
Oswestry, UK

With a contribution on Toxic and Drug-Induced Myopathies by:

Russell Lane BSc MD FRCP

Consultant Neurologist and Honorary Senior Lecturer in Neurology
Faculty of Medicine, Imperial College London
Charing Cross Campus, London, UK

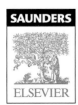

SAUNDERS
ELSEVIER

An Imprint of Elsevier Limited

© 2007, Elsevier Limited. All rights reserved.

First edition 1973
Second edition 1985
Third edition 2007

ISBN-10: 1–4160–2593–6
ISBN-13: 978–1–4160–2593–1
    Reprinted 2007

British Library Cataloguing in Publication Data
A catalogue record for this book is available from the British Library

Library of Congress Cataloging in Publication Data
A catalog record for this book is available from the Library of Congress

Notice
Medical knowledge is constantly changing. Standard safety precautions must be followed, but as new research and clinical experience broaden our knowledge, changes in treatment and drug therapy may become necessary or appropriate. Readers are advised to check the most current product information provided by the manufacturer of each drug to be administered to verify the recommended dose, the method and duration of administration, and contraindications. It is the responsibility of the practitioner, relying on experience and knowledge of the patient, to determine dosages and the best treatment for each individual patient. Neither the Publisher nor the authors assume any liability for any injury and/or damage to persons or property arising from this publication.
The Publisher

Printed in China

Last digit is the print number: 9   8   7   6   5   4   3   2

Contents

SECTION 1

The biopsy: normal and diseased muscle

SECTION 2

Pathological muscle: individual diseases

Preface to the third edition

When Mike Brooke and I did the first edition of Muscle Biopsy in 1973, our main objective was to bring the application of the newly established enzyme histochemical techniques on rapidly frozen samples, as well as electron microscopy, to the routine study of muscle biopsies. This was rapidly achieved and within a few years most laboratories processing muscle biopsies were routinely identifying the basic fibre types and selective pathology in relation to them.

By the time of the second edition in 1985, there had been further major developments, particularly in relation to the introduction of immunohistochemistry and the use of specific antibodies. I was fortunate to have the contribution of a chapter dedicated to this early application of the technique to muscle pathology from Caroline Sewry and Robin Fitzsimmons.

Over the past two decades, there has been a tremendous advance in relation to the molecular genetic identification of many individual muscle disorders. Thus, for example, limb-girdle muscular dystrophy, which was initially looked upon as a single recessive disorder, now has 18 different genetic entities and, similarly, congenital muscular dystrophy has at least 10. This was also associated with a further quantum leap in immunohistochemistry and development of individual antibodies to specific proteins related to these genetic disorders.

This has now become a major player in the armamentarium of diagnosing neuromuscular disorders and I am extremely pleased that Caroline Sewry has agreed to come on board as a full co-author of this new edition, which has been totally revised and restructured. Caroline has been closely associated with the diagnostic and research activities of the Neuromuscular Unit at Hammersmith Hospital ever since its inception soon after my appointment to the Chair of Paediatrics in 1973.

We have retained a basic structure of the text, as in the earlier editions, with a fully comprehensive review of both normal and diseased muscle, using standard techniques of histology and electron microscopy and also the specific contributions of enzyme histochemistry, and protein specific immunohistochemistry.

The majority of illustrations are now in colour, compared to the black and white of the previous edition, and the immunohistochemistry is a major component of the book.

The molecular genetic advances have brought new clarity to the neuromuscular disorders but have also created complexity and some confusion. The same pathology may be related to different genetic disorders and, conversely, some genetic disorders may be associated with different clinical syndromes and different pathological features. This has raised controversy as to the appropriate nomenclature, with the geneticists and biochemists on one hand wanting to relate the diagnosis to the underlying abnormality, and the pathologists and clinicians on the other hand, wanting to retain some handle of diagnosis still based on the clinical presentation and pathological picture, which may be the initial diagnostic features following the patient's presentation.

The wider use of immunohistochemistry has thrown further light on the fibre types within muscle and the use of antibodies specific to different isoforms of fast and slow myosin, as well as neonatal and fetal isoforms, has opened the way for more specific designation of the fibre type profile within pathological muscle. This is also providing some insight into the pathogenesis of some of the disorders.

This is still a rapidly growing and expanding field and the coming years will undoubtedly see further major advances. Our current aim has been to provide an up-to-date and comprehensive overview of muscle pathology and to include clinical and molecular details that are relevant to the pathologist, in order to provide sufficient understanding and background into the various neuromuscular disorders.

Victor Dubowitz

Acknowledgements

The major component of the clinical material has come from our muscle clinic at Hammersmith and we are grateful to our current clinical colleagues, Francesco Muntoni and Adnan Manzur for the continuing flow.

Following a change of domicile in 1998, Caroline has divided her time between the Hammersmith unit and the Centre for Inherited Neuromuscular Disorders at Oswestry, where the diagnostic muscle biopsy service she established is an integral part of the clinical service and active research programme. We are grateful to her clinical colleague there, Ros Quinlivan, and to Glenn Morris, the Research Director, for further material. We are also grateful to the colleagues who have referred biopsy material that we have used for illustrations, including Natalie Costin-Kelly, Janice Holton, Jim Neal, and Waney Squier. The occasional illustrations we have obtained from outside colleagues are acknowledged in the captions to individual illustrations.

We are particularly appreciative of the contribution of our laboratory colleagues at Hammersmith over the years, including in earlier years Lesley Wilson, Carol Lovegrove, Rhoda McDouall, Christine Heinzmann, and currently Frederico Roncaroli, Sue Brown, Cecilia Jimenez-Mallebrera, and Lucy Feng, and also to Karen Davidson, for her help with the photographic work.

At the laboratory in Oswestry we are particulary grateful to Pat Evans, Nigel Harness and Martin Pritchard, and to Ellen Harrison for secretarial help.

Finally, a word of appreciation to Louise Cook and Glenys Norquay and their teams at Elsevier for the very friendly and productive working relationship we have had with them and also to our commissioning editor, Michael J Houston.

List of abbreviations

ABC	avidin–biotin complex
ADP	adenosine diphosphate
ALS	amyotrophic lateral sclerosis
AMP	adenosine-5-monophosphoric acid
ATP	adenosine triphosphate
ATPase	adenosine triphosphatase
AZT	azidothymidine
BAF	barrier-to-autointegration factor
BDMA	benzyl dimethylamine
BMD	Becker muscular dystrophy
BSA	bovine serum albumin
CD	cluster of differentiation
CK	creatine kinase
CMD	congenital muscular dystrophy
CoA	coenzyme A
CoQ	coenzyme Q
COX	cytochrome oxidase
CPT	carnitine palmitoyl transferase
CSF	cerebrospinal fluid
CT	computed tomography
DAB	3,3′-diaminobenzidine tetrahydrochloride
DAG	dystrophin-associated glycoprotein
DAPI	4′6-diamidino-2-phenylindole
DDSA	dodecenyl succinic anhydride
DM	myotonic dystrophy
DMD	Duchenne muscular dystrophy
DMP	dimethoxypropane
DMPK	myotonic dystrophy (DM) protein kinase
EACA	epsilon aminocaproic acid
ECG	electrocardiogram

EMG	electromyogram
ENMC	European Neuromuscular Centre
ESR	erythrocyte sedimentation rate
FCMD	Fukuyama CMD
FF	fast twitch, fatigue sensitive
FG	fast twitch, glycolytic
FITC	fluorescein isothiocyanate
FKRP	fukutin-related protein
FMN	flavin mononucleotide
FOG	fast twitch, oxidative glycolytic
FR	fast twitch, fatigue resistant
FSHD	facioscapulohumeral muscular dystrophy
GNE	UDP-N-acetylglucosamine 2-epimerase/N-acetylmannosamine kinase
H&E	haematoxylin and eosin
HIV	human immunodeficiency virus
HMG-CoA	3-hydroxy-3-methylglutaryl-coenzyme A
HMSN	hereditary motor and sensory neuropathy
IgG	immunoglobulin G
IGHMBP	immunoglobulin microbinding protein 2
KSS	Kearns–Sayre syndrome
LAMP	lysosomal associated membrane protein
LDH	lactate dehydrogenase
LDL	low density lipoprotein
LEM	LAP2-Emerin-Man 1
LGMD	limb-girdle muscular dystrophy
LHON	Leber hereditary optic neuroretinopathy
MAC	membrane attack complex
MDC1A	congenital muscular dystrophy type 1A
MEB	muscle-eye-brain
MELAS	mitochondrial encephalopathy, lactic acidosis and stroke-like episodes
MERRF	myoclonic epilepsy with ragged-red fibres
MH	malignant hyperthermia
MHC	major histocompatibility complex
MHCf	myosin heavy chain fast
MHCn	myosin heavy chain neonatal
MHCs	myosin heavy chain slow
MILS	maternally inherited Leigh syndrome
MNGIE	myoneurogastrointestinal disorder and encephalopathy
MRF	myogenic regulator factors
MRI	magnetic resonance imaging
mtDNA	mitochondrial DNA
NAD	nicotinamide adenine dinucleotide
NADH-TR	reduced nicotinamide adenine dinucleotide-tetrazolium reductase
NAIP	neuronal apoptosis inhibitory protein

NARP	neuropathy, ataxia and retinitis pigmentosa
NBT	nitroblue tetrazolium
N-CAM	neural cell adhesion molecule
NFAT	nuclear factor of activated T cells
nNOS	neuronal nitric oxide synthase
OMIM	Online Mendelian Inheritance in Man database
OPMD	oculopharyngeal muscular dystrophy
ORO	oil red O
PABPN1	polyadenylate-binding protein nuclear 1
PAS	periodic acid-Schiff reaction
PCP	phencyclidine
PCR	polymerase chain reaction
PDHC	pyruvate dehydrogenase complex
PEO	progressive external ophthalmoplegia
PFK	phosphofructokinase
POLIP	polyneuropathy, ophthalmoplegia, leucoencephalopathy and intestinal pseudo-obstruction
PROMM	proximal myotonic myopathy
PTAH	phosphotungstic acid haematoxylin
rRNA	ribosomal RNA
RSMD	rigid spine muscular dystrophy
RYR1	ryanodine receptor 1
SCARMD	severe childhood autosomal recessive muscular dystrophy
SDH	succinic dehydrogenase
SEPN1	selenoprotein N1
SERCA	sarcoendoplasmic reticulum calcium ATPase
SMA	spinal muscular atrophy
SMARD	spinal muscular atrophy with respiratory distress
SMN	survival motor neurone
SO	slow twitch, oxidative
SR	sarcoplasmic reticulum
tRNA	transfer RNA
UCMD	Ullrich congenital muscular dystrophy
VCLAD	very long-chain acyl-CoA dehydrogenase
VVG	Verhoeff–van Gieson
WWB	Walker–Warburg syndrome
XMEA	X-linked myopathy with excess autophagic vacuoles
ZASP	Z line alternatively spliced PDZ protein

The biopsy: normal and diseased muscle

CHAPTER 1

The procedure of muscle biopsy

Muscle biopsy is a relatively simple procedure; yet in the past it was frequently poorly done. The pathologist who receives a small fragment of an unnamed muscle, coiled into a disorientated ball after being dropped into formalin, is unlikely to get any meaningful information from it, no matter how careful the processing. With the upsurge of interest in neuromuscular disorders, clinicians and surgeons are now better informed on the handling of samples. The following are some guidelines worth following when planning a muscle biopsy.

Selection of the patient

A full clinical assessment of the patient is essential. Diagnosis should always be based on a detailed clinical and family history, and clinical examination, in conjunction with any special investigations such as serum enzymes, muscle imaging and electromyography, and the biopsy looked upon as an additional confirmatory test of an underlying muscle and/or neural disorder. In general, the main indication for muscle biopsy is some evidence of neuromuscular disease such as muscle weakness, muscle cramps or discomfort (especially on exercise) and muscle fatigue with activity. Pathological change may be found in some conditions in the absence of any apparent neuromuscular signs, for example collagen vascular diseases. On the other hand, the muscle biopsy may show no apparent morphological abnormalities in conditions such as myasthenia gravis or myotonia congenita in which the clinical diagnosis is more readily confirmed with electrodiagnostic methods.

With the spectacular advances in the identification of molecular defects, many clinicians question the need for a muscle biopsy if a defect in a gene can be identified. In some conditions such as spinal muscular atrophy, myotonic dystrophy and facioscapulohumeral dystrophy molecular analysis is so reliable that it can provide a direct confirmation of diagnosis without the need for a biopsy. Genotype and the results of DNA analysis, however, cannot always be related to phenotype and there are exceptions to every rule. This is well demonstrated in Duchenne muscular dystrophy, in which the molecular defect may not always correlate with the protein expression seen in the muscle. More importantly, clinical severity cannot be judged by molecular analysis alone. We therefore feel that assessment of muscle pathology, with modern techniques, is an important component of patient assessment.

Selection of the muscle

This should be based on the distribution of the muscle weakness, as judged by detailed clinical assessment. In selecting the muscle for biopsy, it is important not to choose either a muscle which is so severely involved by the disease process that it will be largely replaced by fat or connective tissue and show little recognizable trace of the underlying disease process or, on the other hand, a muscle which is so little affected that it does not show sufficient change. Differential involvement of muscle occurs in several disorders and ultrasound imaging is a simple, quick technique for assessing this (Heckmatt et al 1982, Dubowitz 1995a) and can help in the selection of the biopsy site. Magnetic resonance imaging (MRI) of muscle gives superior quality, and patterns associated with individual diseases are now emerging (Mercuri et al 2005, Jungbluth et al 2004a,b, Pichiecchio et al 2004) but ultrasound is a rapid and practical method to apply before a biopsy and can be done in the outpatient clinic.

In general, where the distribution of the weakness is proximal, we select a moderately affected proximal muscle which is also reasonably accessible, such as the quadriceps (rectus femoris or vastus lateralis) in the leg or the biceps in the arm. In other circumstances, the deltoid or gastrocnemius are also suitable muscles for biopsy. Where weakness is mainly distal, a more distal limb muscle may be selected, but even in these circumstances biopsy of a proximal muscle may reveal the underlying pathological process adequately.

In a chronic disease such as muscular dystrophy, a muscle with only moderate weakness may be the ideal site for biopsy. In an acute disease, on the other hand, because the process has not had time to progress to extensive destruction, a more severely involved muscle may be chosen. In addition, the biopsy technique (see below) may influence the choice of muscle. For example with a needle technique the quadriceps is often considered relatively safe as the muscle is readily accessible and major nerves and blood vessels lie close to the femur and are unlikely to be damaged.

There are advantages in trying to limit the biopsies to certain muscles so as to be familiar with the normal pattern in that particular muscle. It is important to be aware of anatomical differences between muscles, and be familiar with possible age-related changes. Thus, the distribution of fibre types and fibre sizes is well recognized in the biceps and the quadriceps but the pattern may be unfamiliar in such muscles as the intercostals, the abdominal muscles or the hand or foot muscles. In certain circumstances, for example when studying motor endplates, the muscle selected will be determined by the particular line of investigation. In this instance a motor-point sample is required, but in most institutes this is rarely performed and for diagnostic analysis of most muscle disorders it is not necessary. For any quantitative studies, adequate control determinations of the same muscle are essential. Sampling at the site of either electromyography or any form of injection should also be avoided as needling of any kind can produce changes in the muscle (Engel 1967; see Ch. 23). Similarly, sports injuries or other traumas, the use or disuse of the muscle and any possible effect of contractures, should also be taken into account.

For certain immunohistochemical studies, skin or buccal cells may be useful and for prenatal diagnosis chorionic villus samples can be used (see Ch. 6).

Technique of biopsy

We have always performed all our muscle biopsies in adults as well as infants under local anaesthesia and there seems to be no justification for submitting patients who may already be at risk of respiratory deficit to general anaesthesia. In addition, there is a particular hazard of general anaesthesia and relaxant drugs in several conditions such as myotonic dystrophy, central core disease and malignant hyperthermia. Under local anaesthesia, the risks of muscle biopsy, as with other minor procedures, are negligible. In our own unit we have always done the biopsies ourselves and not required the services of our surgical colleagues. There is always merit, however, in alerting a surgeon to the need for a muscle sample if a patient is undergoing some other surgical procedure under general anaesthesia. In these cases, particular note should be taken of the site sampled as this may influence the pathology. For example, a biopsy taken near the tendon when the Achilles tendon is being lengthened may be very fibrous and difficult to interpret.

Over the past two decades we have used exclusively a needle biopsy technique for obtaining muscle samples, both for diagnostic as well as research purposes, and it is no longer necessary to subject patients to more extensive open biopsy procedures with the resultant larger and more unsightly scarring. Needle biopsy is a safe procedure, singularly free of any complications, and the scar is often almost invisible. Open biopsies provide a larger sample, which may be useful for biochemical studies, but in most situations we find the same diagnostic conclusion can be reached in a needle sample. Developments in the sensitivity of biochemical and immunoblotting techniques have also reduced the need for large samples.

Needle biopsy

Although a needle for muscle biopsy was introduced more than 100 years ago by Duchenne (1861), the technique did not find wide application until relatively recent times. Bergström (1962) introduced a percutaneous needle with similar features to those of Duchenne's, mainly for the study of normal muscle in relation to various physiological changes. Edwards and colleagues (Edwards 1971, Edwards et al 1973, 1983) applied the Bergström needle for routine muscle biopsy mainly in adult patients and over the past 25 years we have found it to be suitable and satisfactory for infants and children, right down to the newborn period. We use mainly a 5 mm diameter needle and occasionally a smaller 4 mm one in newborn infants. Refinements to the prototype instrument have been made but we have continued to use the original Bergström type. Edwards et al (1983) reviewed their experience in 1000 cases and we reviewed 670, mainly childhood, needle biopsies (Heckmatt et al 1984). Other types of needles have been applied but do not produce adequate samples, with the exception of the conchotome, alligator-type forceps (Henriksson 1979). The major advantages of the needle biopsy procedure over open biopsy are its simplicity, its speed, and the fact that it can readily be done (by physicians) as an outpatient procedure in a clinic without any special theatre facilities.

In infants under 6 months sedation is not normally used although chloral hydrate may be used (100 mg/kg), following discussion with a senior member of the clinical team, especially if there are concerns about breathing difficulties and thin ribs have been seen on the chest X-ray. In children between 6 months and 10 years, we usually use chloral hydrate (80 mg/kg, maximum 1000 mg) if their weight is less than 15 kg and diazepam orally (0.2–0.4 mg/kg, maximum 10 mg) if their weight is above 15 kg. In our experience children heavier than 15 kg tend not to be well sedated with chloral hydrate, occasionally becoming hyperactive. If no sedation is achieved within 45 minutes we administer midazolam 0.1 mg/kg intranasally or orally (maximum 10 mg). The patient has to be connected to a saturation monitor and flumazenil (10 mg/kg) readily available in case the effect of midazolam has to be reversed (although we have never had a case in which this has been necessary). In older children and adults the procedure can be performed without sedation. Most of our biopsies have been from the quadriceps (vastus lateralis) (Figs 1.1a–d, 1.2). The skin is prepared in the usual way with antiseptic and draped. The skin and subcutaneous tissue down to the muscle sheath are infiltrated with 1% lignocaine (Xylocaine). It is important not to infiltrate the muscle as this can cause artefacts. A small incision is made with a scalpel blade down into the muscle sheath, at approximately mid-thigh level in the midline. Pressure is applied with a swab until any bleeding has completely stopped. The Bergström needle with the sliding cannula assembled and the window closed is then inserted into the muscle while the other hand steadies the thigh. The window is opened by sliding the cannula and the muscle gently squeezed so it goes into the window of the needle and ensures a reasonably-sized specimen. After a quick to and fro movement of the cannula with the palm of the hand, the needle is withdrawn and the muscle sample removed. Sampling is rapid and takes only a few seconds. The sensation is of pressure within the muscle rather than pain. The needle can be reintroduced and multiple samples obtained through the same incision, if necessary, to produce an adequate quantity of muscle. The quality of the sample, and whether it is adequate, should be assessed immediately under a dissecting microscope and it

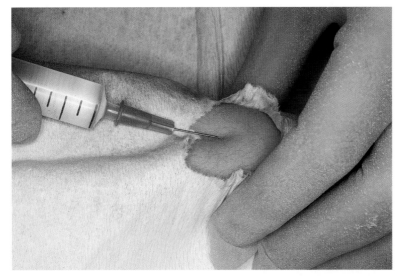

a

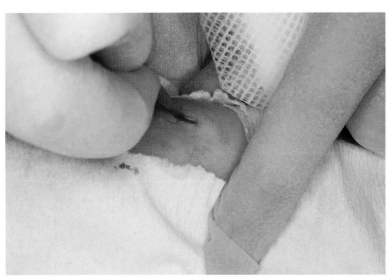

b

FIG. 1.1(a) *After appropriate cleansing and draping, the site is infiltrated with local anaesthetic.*
FIG. 1.1(b) *A small incision is made in the skin with a pointed scalpel blade.*

is therefore advantageous to have a member of the laboratory staff close at hand, and not rely on samples being assessed sometime later in the laboratory. An average needle biopsy is approximately 3 mm^3 in size and weighs about 20 mg.

After completion of the biopsy, sustained finger pressure is applied to the site with a swab until bleeding has stopped. This prevents any haematoma formation or other complications. A butterfly dressing is then applied to approximate the skin edges. No sutures are necessary and the small 4–5 mm scar fades

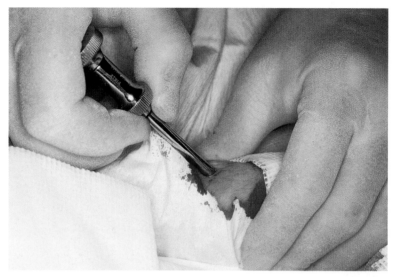

c

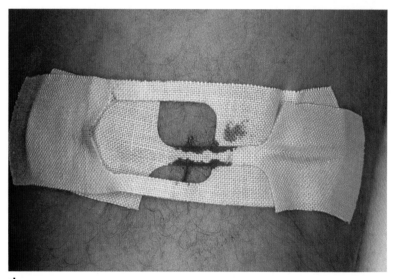

d

FIG. 1.1(c) *The biopsy needle (with cannula in and the window closed) is inserted.*
FIG. 1.1(d) *After withdrawal of the needle and firm pressure on site applied for a few minutes, the incision is closed with a butterfly dressing. No sutures are required.*

with time. The limb can be used normally after the procedure and any slight sensation of stiffness around the biopsy site recedes after about 24 hours. Numbness around the incision is also felt for a few weeks until the sensory nerves have grown back.

After removal from the muscle, the biopsy specimens should be kept moist on a piece of gauze *lightly* moistened with isotonic saline prior to further process-

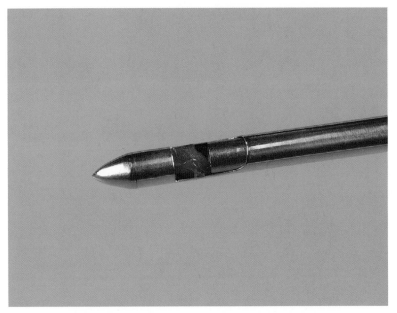

FIG. 1.2 *The biopsy sample lies in the window of the needle and is removed.*

ing. Multiple samples can be mounted collectively on a cork disc. Orientation under a dissecting microscope in a transverse plane in order to obtain true transverse sections is essential (Fig. 1.3a). The easiest way to do this orientation is to line up all pieces and fibres in a longitudinal plane first and then turn the sample on its end. The cut transverse ends can usually be seen under the dissecting microscope, particularly if the light is placed at an angle to shine through the sample. In this way, over 1000 fibres per single section can be readily obtained (Fig. 1.3b). To prevent the samples drying, a 'cold' fibre-optic light source should be used, if possible. Care should also be taken to handle the specimens gently with fine forceps, or syringe needles, in order not to traumatize them. If drying-out occurs and the sample adheres to the forceps, OCT mountant can be placed on top, but the orientation is then less clear and any fat in the sample may appear as droplets on the surface.

A separate small sample of muscle is prepared for electron microscopy (see below). As the importance of biochemical analysis such as immunoblotting, metabolic studies or RNA extraction, has increased over recent years, a separate frozen sample should also be taken whenever possible. These are frozen in screw-topped cryovials in liquid nitrogen as soon as possible after taking the sample, to avoid degradation, and stored at −40°C or lower, until required. If very rapid freezing is required for a biochemical study, the whole Bergström needle with the sample in the window can be plunged straight into liquid nitrogen.

The quadriceps is our favoured site for needle biopsy but the same technique can also be used for other muscles such as gastrocnemius, deltoid and biceps,

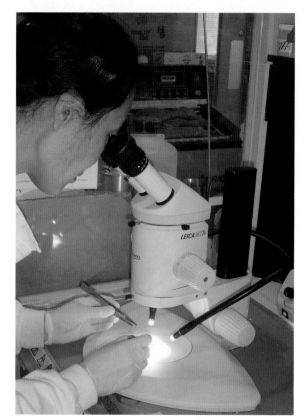

a

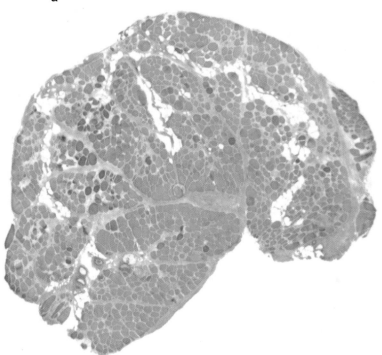

b

FIG. 1.3 (a) *The sample(s) is placed on a cork disc and the fibres orientated transversely under a dissecting microscope using a 'cold' fibre-optic light source to prevent drying.* **(b)** *Low power view of a whole needle biopsy from a patient with Duchenne muscular dystrophy, showing the quality that can routinely be obtained with the Bergström needle.*

but particular care is necessary to avoid any vital structures such as major vessels or nerves.

Open biopsy

We no longer practise this and details can be found in earlier editions of this book. Centres where this is practised each have their own particular method. One advantage of an open biopsy used to be clamping of the specimen to prevent contraction of the muscle fibres but this requires a large incision and its use has declined. The use of needle biopsies illustrates that clamping is not necessary for satisfactory results.

Preparation of specimen

All histological, histochemical and immunohistochemical studies are performed on frozen material. Fixation and wax-embedding distort the fibre architecture and enzyme and metabolic studies are not possible on such material. Some immunohistochemistry is possible on archival wax-embedded material, depending on the antibody, but a full panel of studies is not possible. Transverse sections yield much more information than longitudinal sections for light microscopy.

Ideally the specimen should be frozen as soon as possible after removal, particularly if biochemical studies are to be performed; but adequate morphological studies can be performed on samples transported from another site, if necessary, provided they are wrapped in *lightly* dampened gauze to prevent drying and the delay is not more than a couple of hours. Degradation may affect some biochemical studies in samples that have to be transported. We have not found any of the commercial transporting media to be of any advantage. Some meaningful information can be obtained from postmortem material but enzyme histochemistry is rarely possible. Immunohistochemistry of some proteins, such as laminins and myosins, are possible on postmortem material but dystrophin and plasma membrane proteins are not always detectable, depending on the time from death to freezing the sample.

Instead of direct immersion of the specimen into liquid nitrogen, which causes some gaseous nitrogen to surround the specimen and slows the cooling process, more rapid freezing and better preservation of structure is achieved by freezing in isopentane, cooled in liquid nitrogen to −160°C (see Fig. 1.6). The isopentane is first frozen in a container immersed in liquid nitrogen until it is completely solid. It is then allowed to warm to a point when there is solid and liquid together.

We usually mount the specimens on cork discs which can be labelled with the sample identity and easily removed from the cryostat chuck for storage. The sample is held in place on the cork by a small amount of OCT mounting medium (Merck) around the base of the specimen (Figs 1.4 and 1.5). The cork with its specimen is then inverted into the liquid phase of the isopentane (Fig. 1.6). The

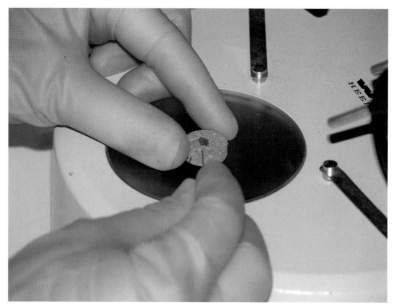

FIG. 1.4 *Close-up view of a biopsy ready for orientation under a dissecting microscope.*

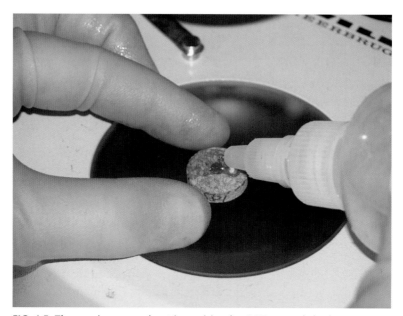

FIG. 1.5 *The specimens are kept in position by OCT around the base.*

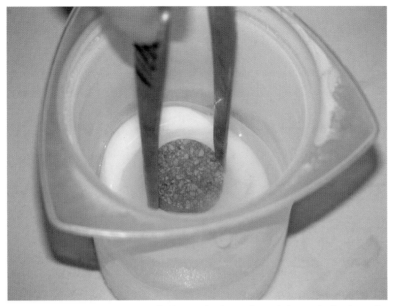

FIG. 1.6 *The specimen is rapidly frozen by inversion of the cork disc into the liquid phase of isopentane previously cooled in liquid nitrogen.*

duration of cooling must be judged by experience and partly depends on the size of the specimen; usually 10–20 seconds is sufficient. Too short a period may give artefact with ice crystal formation in the fibres, whereas too long may lead to cracking of the block. Frozen blocks can be stored at −40°C or lower until ready for sectioning. For long-term storage liquid nitrogen is advisable, in case of electrical disasters. Prior to sectioning, the cork is frozen onto a microtome chuck with OCT. After sectioning, the specimen may be removed by cleavage of the cork from the chuck and stored for future use. Wrapping the specimen in foil and using airtight containers may help to prevent freeze drying, but this is less of a problem if specimens are stored in liquid nitrogen.

Cutting the sections

A suitable section thickness for histology and histochemistry is 8–10 μm, cut in a cryostat at −23 to −25°C (Fig. 1.7a). For immunohistochemistry 5 μm is suitable. If sections are too thick they may come off the slide during subsequent procedures. If specimens have a lot of adipose tissue, a lower temperature facilitates cutting and cooling sprays are available to cool the knife and specimen further. Specimens stored at low temperatures must be given sufficient time to equilibrate with the temperature of the cryostat before sectioning, to avoid shattering of the tissue. Sections can be readily picked up on coverslips or slides (Fig. 1.7b) and a battery of histological, histochemical and immunohistochemical methods carried out on them; these will be discussed in subsequent chapters. Sections on slides can be stored frozen, if wrapped in cling-film and allowed to dry fully

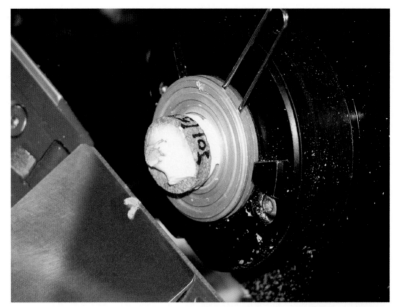

a

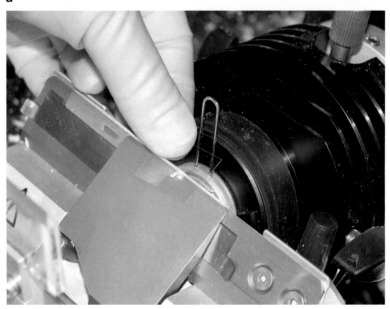

b

FIG. 1.7(a),(b) *Sections are cut in a cryostat and are mounted directly onto coverslips or slides.*

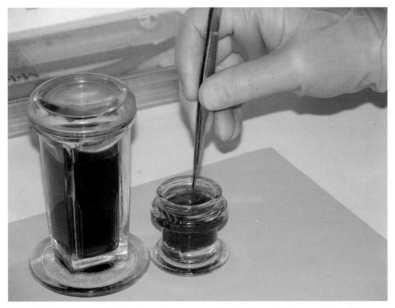

FIG. 1.8 *The coverslip is placed in a coverslip jar for staining or the slide placed in a 50 mL coplin jar.*

before use. Sections on coverslips can be placed in racks and these wrapped in foil. When only a few slides or coverslips are removed for staining it is important that the remaining sections are not allowed to thaw, as artefacts may occur if re-freezing occurs. Sections for some histological and histochemical stains can be kept dry at room temperature, at least overnight, sometimes longer. Sections adhere well to coverslips and do not require coating. A variety of slides with improved adhering properties (e.g. *Superfrost plus*) are also now commercially available and are particularly useful for histochemistry and immunohistochemistry. Alternatively slides can be coated with poly-L-lysine or silane, but the extra cost of *Superfrost* slides is offset by convenience. Storage of sections enables batches of several biopsies to be stained simultaneously, which is useful for controlling for technical problems as well as being time/cost effective. Staining may be done either by immersing the coverslips or slides in special containers (10 mL Columbia jars, or 50 mL coplin jars) (Fig. 1.8), or by adding the incubating solution on top of individual sections in a moisturized container such as a Petri dish with moistened filter paper to prevent drying (Fig. 1.9). Commercial staining trays are also available (e.g. from CellPath plc; Fig. 1.10). Staining sections flat in a Petri dish is necessary in some reactions such as for reduced nicotinamide adenine dinucleotide-tetrazolium reductase (NADH-TR) and phosphofructokinase, as the tetrazolium reaction product may diffuse out into the medium if done vertically in a jar. This method is also suitable for other histochemical reactions and for all immunohistochemical labelling, for economy of reagents.

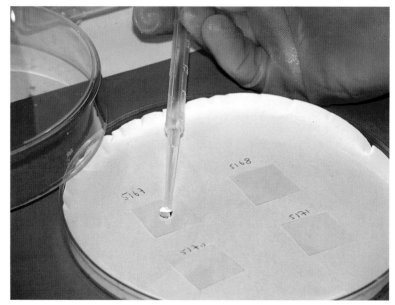

FIG. 1.9 *Substrate solution, or antibody, is pipetted directly onto individual sections on a coverslip for incubation in a closed Petri dish with a moist atmosphere.*

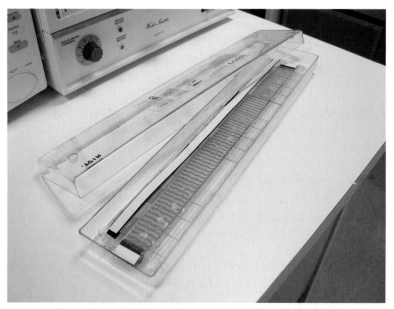

FIG. 1.10 *Slides placed flat in a staining tray above moistened gauze are held in place by a magnetic strip for easy rinsing. Shown here with the lid to one side which is used to cover the slides and maintain a moist atmosphere during staining or immunolabelling.*

Electron microscopy

Electron microscopy is a time-consuming technique but it can provide useful information (see Ch. 5). It is worthwhile and good practice to always have a sample available for electron microscopy, and then being selective about the cases that are examined in detail. Studies of semi-thin sections which are quicker to prepare can be very informative (see below).

Specimen preparation

Biopsies obtained by open or needle techniques are both suitable for electron microscopy. Ideally the specimen should be fixed at resting length to avoid contraction artefacts. With open biopsies this can be achieved by placing a suture at each end of a small strip of muscle and removing this with the sutures. The sutures can then be secured to a tongue depressor or applicator stick so that the muscle is slightly stretched. Care must be taken to avoid overstretching. The sample is then placed in fixative for several hours before being cut further.

With needle biopsies it is not possible to suture the sample and some contraction is then inevitable. Similarly, open biopsies obtained through a small incision cannot be sutured. We find, however, that the contraction does not interfere with diagnostic interpretation and good longitudinal sections can be obtained from most samples. A short delay of about 10 minutes before fixation reduces some of the contraction and has no detrimental effect on the ultrastructure. In practice, this short delay occurs while the biopsy is brought to the laboratory from the theatre, ward or outpatient department and a suitable sample separated for electron microscopy. This sample is orientated longitudinally and then immediately fixed by placing a drop of fixative over it. Once in fixative the sample is too firm to manipulate the fibres any further. The sample is then cut into small pieces under a dissecting microscope. With the dissecting microscope, it is possible to see the orientation of the fibres and to cut the samples accordingly. Unwanted fat can also be removed. The pieces of muscle should be approximately 1 mm³, but if they are made slightly longer than this down the long axis of the fibres, it aids orientation at later stages of preparation. The blocks of tissue are fixed for 1.5–2 hours at room temperature and then washed in buffer. They can then be stored in buffer at 4°C or processed further immediately. Samples can, if necessary, be stored in buffer at 4°C for several days, and even weeks if necessary, enabling several biopsies to be processed at once.

A variety of fixatives and buffers have been used for electron microscopy over the years, but glutaraldehyde is considered to give the best ultrastructural preservation and is the most widely used primary fixative. If a variety of electron microscopic studies, as well as immunohistochemistry or histochemical techniques, are required on the same specimen, the choice of fixative must be considered carefully because antigenicity and enzyme activity are often destroyed by glutaraldehyde. It is then necessary to compromise between acceptable ultrastructural preservation and retention of biochemical activity, and to use a milder fixative such as formaldehyde.

For routine morphological ultrastructural studies, concentrations of glutaraldehyde of between 2 and 6% are recommended using either 0.1 M phosphate or 0.1 M cacodylate as the buffer at a neutral pH of 7.2. Osmium tetroxide is used as the secondary fixative to enhance contrast. A typical processing protocol is shown below:

1. Fix in 4% glutaraldehyde in 0.1 M cacodylate buffer, pH 7.2, for 1.5–2 hours at room temperature.
2. Wash in several changes of 0.1 M cacodylate buffer for at least 30 minutes. At this stage the tissue can be stored overnight or for several days at 4°C.
3. Post-fix in 1% osmium tetroxide in 0.1 M cacodylate buffer for 1 hour at room temperature.
4. Rinse in buffer.
5. Dehydrate in graded ethanols – 50%, 70%, 90% and two changes of 100% – 10 minutes each.
6. Propylene oxide, one change, 5 minutes in each.
7. 1:1 propylene oxide:Araldite I for 1 hour.
8. Araldite I, overnight at 40°C.
9. Araldite II, 2 hours at room temperature, followed by 2 hours at 40°C with one change of resin.
10. Embed in fresh Araldite II in polypropylene or gelatin capsules.
11. Harden at 60°C for 36–48 hours.

Resins

Several resins are commercially available (e.g. Araldite, Epon, Spurr, LR White) and the choice is one of personal preference. The majority of electron micrographs shown in this book have been obtained from Araldite embedded material. If difficulties are encountered, for example in staining contrast or stability of the sections in the electron beam, it is worth experimenting with a different resin. It is also worth remembering that manufacturers may change the specification of a product without informing the customer! LR white is often used for immunohistochemical studies.

Resin quantities
Araldite I
  Araldite CY 212 10 mL
  Dodecenyl succinic anhydride (DDSA) (hardener) 10 mL
  Dibutylphthalate 0.25 mL
  Araldite II
  Araldite I as above + 0.5 mL benzyl dimethylamine (BDMA) (accelerator).

Variations of this procedure can be made using other dehydrating agents such as acetone or dimethoxypropane (DMP) and the other embedding

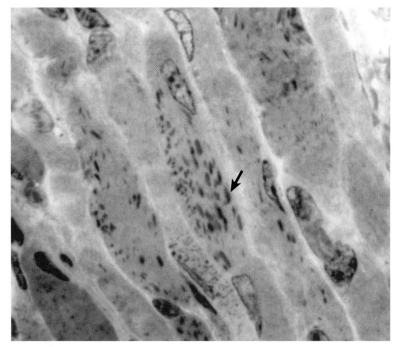

FIG. 1.11 *A 1 μm resin section stained with toluidine blue and viewed under oil immersion from a case of nemaline myopathy showing dark staining rods (arrow).*

media mentioned above. Similarly, a wide variety of embedding moulds and capsules are commercially available and the choice is a matter of personal preference.

Having obtained a block of embedded muscle, semi-thin sections about 1–2-μm thick are cut and stained for a few seconds with toluidine blue (1% in saturated borax, filtered before use). These sections are then examined under oil immersion and areas selected for ultrathin sectioning. Considerable information can be obtained from these sections, in particular in relation to the myofibrils or the presence of some structural abnormalities, such as nemaline rods (Fig. 1.11). Sections for electron microscopy are about 50–60 nm thick, floated on water and collected on 3 mm metal grids. Grids with various types of mesh are available and we find a 100 hexagonal type gives sufficient support to the section whilst giving a suitable size viewing area. The contrast in the section is enhanced by staining with heavy metal salts, usually uranyl acetate, followed by lead citrate. Alcoholic uranyl acetate penetrates more rapidly and the staining time of grids can then be reduced to a few minutes. It is also possible to stain the whole block of tissue with uranyl acetate, before dehydration and embedding. Various staining times in lead citrate can be used but we find adequate contrast can be obtained in 2–3 minutes. Details of staining procedures can be found in standard books on electron microscopy.

Immunohistochemistry

Sections (approximately 5–7 μm) are cut at the same time as those for histology and histochemistry, so they are in series with them, and can be compared. As for histochemistry, sections can be collected on either coverslips or slides, and after drying can be stored frozen. Further details of immunohistochemical methods can be found in Chapter 6.

CHAPTER 2

Histological and histochemical stains and reactions

Just as every pathologist has particular preferences for routine stains, so muscle histochemists have tended to develop preferences for particular reactions, especially in the interpretation of fibre types.

In the early days of the application of histochemical techniques to the study of muscle, large batteries of enzymes were routinely studied in muscle biopsies (see Dubowitz and Pearse 1961). While these many enzyme reactions were of special interest and value in a research context, it became apparent that much of the information required in the assessment of diseased muscle could be obtained from a small number of these procedures, and additional methods were only necessary in specific circumstances.

In this chapter, we discuss the histological and histochemical methods which we routinely use on biopsies (see Table 2.1). General application and illustration of the techniques are discussed in Chapters 3 and 4. The theoretical background of the techniques can be found in standard text books or earlier editions of this book.

Histological stains

The most important stain used routinely is haematoxylin and eosin (H&E), which clearly shows the overall structure of the tissue in relation to the fibres, nuclei, fibrous and adipose tissue, the presence of inflammatory cells, and vascular and neural components. In addition, the distribution of mitochondria may be distinguished, depending on the specific haematoxylin used. With the H&E stain nuclei stain blue, the muscle fibres pink and the connective tissue a lighter pink. Basophilic fibres may be recognized by their blue stain. If Harris' haematoxylin is used the mitochondria can be seen as small dots. Cross-striations are not usually visible in unfixed frozen material. Particularly red, eosinophilic areas may be visible within fibres and may correspond to abnormal accumulations of myofibrillar material or to cytoplasmic bodies (see Ch. 4).

TABLE 2.1 *Panel of histological and histochemical methods for routine analysis of muscle biopsies (This should be read in conjunction with Chapters 3, 4 and 7)*

Stain	Major Use
Haematoxylin & eosin (H&E)	General structure of the sample: fibre size and contours, position of nuclei, fibrosis, inflammation, nerves, blood vessels
Gomori trichrome	Mitochondria red (type 1 fibres darker) Nemaline rods red Membranous whorls of rimmed vacuoles red
Verhoeff–van Gieson (VVG)	Highlights connective tissue (red) and elastin and myelin (black)
Oil Red O (ORO)	Intracellular lipid seen as red dots Lipid of adipose tissue red (may spread over the section)
Sudan black	As for ORO but a black end product
Periodic acid-Schiff	Checkerboard pattern of fibre types; fibres with excess glycogen heavily stained; fibres with loss of glycogen white
Reduced nicotinamide adenine dinucleotide-tetrazolium reductase (NADH-TR)	Fibre type pattern; distribution of mitochondria; myofibrillar disruption
Succinic dehydrogenase (SDH)	Fibre type pattern; fibres with abnormal mitochondria
Cytochrome oxidase (COX)	Fibre type pattern; fibres devoid of activity
Combined COX and SDH	Fibres devoid of cytochrome oxidase activity appear blue
ATPase or myosin isoforms	Distribution and involvement of fibre types and their subtypes
Optional techniques that may be useful, depending on the results of the above and phenotype	
Phosphorylase	Absent in type V glycogenosis (McArdle's disease)
Phosphofructokinase	Absent in type VII glycogenosis
Adenylate deaminase	Absent/deficient in exertional myalgia (significance uncertain)
Acid phosphatase	High in lysosomal storage disorders and vacuolar myopathies
Alkaline phosphatase	High in blood vessels in some inflammatory myopathies
Menadione-linked α-glycerophosphate dehydrogenase	Stains reducing bodies
Congo red	Shows presence of β-amyloid

It is sometimes easier to observe subtle increases in endomysial connective with the modified Gomori trichrome technique (Engel and Cunningham 1963), in which the muscle fibres stain a greenish-blue colour, and the collagen is a lighter but clearly distinguishable blue–green colour. Nuclei stain red with the Gomori stain and the myelin of the nerve stains a foamy red colour. Nerves may appear poorly stained in the absence of myelin. Abnormal accumulations of myofibrillar material may appear to be a paler green–blue colour and cytoplasmic bodies may appear more intensely stained. A major application of the modified Gomori technique is the identification of red staining structures such as rods, abnormal mitochondria and the membranous myelin-like whorls of rimmed vacuoles. Mitochondrial accumulations appear as red aggregates of stain and the intermyofibrillar mitochondria appear as a series of fine dots throughout the fibre. Normal muscle fibres frequently show peripheral aggregates of mitochondria and care is needed not to over interpret their significance. Connective tissue can also readily be revealed with stains such as van Gieson or picrosirius, both of which stain collagen bright red in contrast to the yellow–green of the fibres. As excess connective tissue is visible with H&E and the Gomori trichrome an additional stain for connective tissue is a matter of personal choice. There is some advantage, however, in using the Verhoeff–van Gieson combination, as it also demonstrates the presence of myelin (black) in the peripheral nerves and elastin (black) in the blood vessels. Mitochondria and the intermyofibrillar network are also visible in cross-sections of the fibres as fine dark dots. These histological techniques therefore also reveal a difference between fibre types (see below) with the higher mitochondria content of type 1 fibres giving a darker colour to the fibre. Details of all staining techniques are given at the end of this chapter.

Additional stains which may prove helpful in particular instances are various techniques for nucleic acids (DNA and RNA), cresyl fast violet or toluidine blue for metachromatic material, alizarin red for calcium, phosphotungstic acid haematoxylin (PTAH) which may demonstrate such structures as the rods in nemaline myopathy, and Congo red to show amyloid in inclusion body myositis, but these are not necessary as part of a routine panel.

Histochemical reactions

Histochemical techniques are essential for the study of muscle biopsies for four main reasons. First, they demonstrate the non-uniform nature of the tissue by demonstrating the different biochemical properties of specific fibre types and their selective involvement in certain disease processes. Second, they may show an absence of a particular enzyme (for example, phosphorylase in McArdle's disease). Third, an excess of a particular substrate can be demonstrated (e.g. glycogen in glycogen storage disease or fat in carnitine deficiency). Fourth, they may show structural changes in the muscle which would not be apparent with routine histological stains, such as the enzyme-deficient cores in central core disease, 'moth-eaten' fibres, and abnormalities in the distribution of mitochondria.

The number of histochemical techniques for routine use has diminished over the years; the most important are summarized in Table 2.1. Enzyme histochemistry has become firmly established as a link between the morphology and biochemistry of tissues. The indispensable value of enzyme histochemistry to the study of muscle highlights the need to freeze a biopsy, as fixation destroys the activity of many enzymes. With histochemical and immunohistochemical techniques it is now possible to demonstrate many enzymes. It is clearly beyond the scope of this book to cover the whole range but the following section highlights the application of those of particular importance to the diagnostic pathology of muscle. Minimal biochemical background of the enzyme reactions is given here, but further reference can be made to the excellent manual on enzyme histochemistry of Lojda et al (1979) and to standard biochemistry text books.

Oxidative enzymes

The most useful oxidative enzymes studied in muscle are reduced nicotinamide adenine dinucleotide dehydrogenase-tetrazolium reductase (NADH-TR), succinic dehydrogenase (SDH) and cytochrome oxidase (COX).

The principle of the histochemical technique for NADH-TR and SDH is to employ a colourless, soluble, tetrazolium salt as an electron acceptor which is reduced to a deeply coloured, insoluble formazan product at the site of the enzyme activity. The commonly used tetrazolium salt is nitroblue tetrazolium (NBT) [2,2'-di-p-nitrophenyl- 5,5'-diphenyl-3,3'-(3,3'-dimethoxy-4,4'-biphenylene) ditetrazolium chloride] which gives a bluish final end product. Thus the intensity of the formazan reaction product is a reflection of the number of mitochondria within a fibre and reveals the characteristic checkerboard pattern of fibre types. Some caution in interpretation, however, is needed with regard to specificity with the techniques for NADH-TR and SDH because tetrazolium salts have a strong affinity for phospholipids and with the reaction for NADH-TR the sarcoplasmic reticulum is also revealed. This can, however, be advantageous as the technique for NADH-TR is useful for showing disruption and distortion of myofibrils and the internal structure of whorled fibres (see Ch. 4). The technique for SDH, in contrast, is specific for mitochondria, as is the technique for COX.

COX is very sensitive to fixation and is inhibited by cyanide and azide. Even brief fixation in formaldehyde, glutaraldehyde or alcohol can produce negative results in the histochemical reaction, emphasizing the need for frozen sections. It is an integral component of the mitochondrial membrane and is encoded by mitochondrial DNA. Succinic dehydrogenase, in contrast, is encoded by nuclear DNA. The method commonly used to demonstrate COX activity uses diaminobenzidine as an electron donor and produces a brown end product that can be enhanced by osmium. The reaction for COX reveals differences in mitochondrial number and their distribution in different fibre types (see Ch. 3). It is also an important method for demonstrating fibres devoid of activity caused by certain mutations in mitochondrial DNA. A combination of the technique for COX and SDH provides a clear method for identifying fibres that are deficient in COX but retain SDH activity, as they appear blue in contrast to the brownish-blue/grey of normal fibres.

Transferases

Phosphorylase

In vivo, phosphorylase is a cytoplasmic enzyme concerned with the degradation of glycogen by destruction of α-1,4'-glycosidic linkages. The histochemical method (see Takeuchi and Kuriaki 1955, Eränkö and Palkama 1961, Godlewski 1963) relies on the conversion of the inactive *b* form of the enzyme to the active *a* form, followed by staining of the polysaccharide that is formed with iodine. The purple colour is unstable and fades but can be made permanent using Schiff reagent. Dehydration in alcohol and mounting in synthetic resin also preserves the end product but the colour may be slightly altered. Phosphorylase activity varies with fibre type and is another technique that shows the checkerboard pattern of fibre types. Absence of phosphorylase from muscle fibres only occurs in McArdle's disease and it is therefore questionable if this technique needs to be performed routinely if there is no clinical indication of a glycogenosis, but it should always be checked in a patient with a history of cramps.

Hydrolases

Adenosine triphosphatase (ATPase)

Myosin ATPase, which is calcium activated, is the most important enzyme for revealing fibre types. The method for its localization relies on the release of phosphate, the capture of this by calcium and the substitution of the calcium by cobalt. The phosphate is then replaced by sulphide and the end product is a black precipitate of cobalt sulphide. The reaction is carried out at a non-physiological pH of 9.4 and preincubation at different acid pHs of 4.3 and 4.6 is used to demonstrate the reciprocal pattern and subdivision of fibre types (see section on fibre types in Ch. 3).

In considering the validity of this reaction, it should be borne in mind that it takes place at a very alkaline pH which may not occur *in vivo*. Furthermore, there is a physical alteration of the tissue at some stage during the reaction. When muscle tissue is air dried and exposed to calcium, the intermyofibrillar network is in some way altered so that later in the reaction it disintegrates. Thus with the reaction for ATPase at pH 9.4, the intermyofibrillar network is dissolved out of the section and no ATPase can be demonstrated in this location even though the enzyme may be present there. The reaction thus becomes essentially a myosin ATPase reaction.

The ATPase method has historically been accepted as the standard method for demonstrating fibre types but the advent of immunohistochemistry and the application of antibodies to myosin is equally reliable and has certain advantages (Sewry and Dubowitz 2001, Behan et al 2002). This is discussed in more detail in subsequent chapters. A considerable amount of data has accumulated over the years from ATPase-stained sections, particularly with regard to morphometric analysis (see Ch. 4) and it may be some time before myosin immunolabelling completely replaces the ATPase method. The ATPase can be a difficult method with which to get consistently good results, and in our laboratory we now rarely perform it and usually rely on myosin immunolabelling.

Additional enzymes studies

Additional methods may be useful in association with certain clinical features, and are included in the list of methods. Although several of these formed part of a routine set of procedures in early years of muscle pathology, they only add additional diagnostic information in rare situations. *Acid phosphatase* is localized mainly in lysosomes and may thus be used to indicate foci of degeneration and necrosis within muscle fibres. Very little is apparent in normal muscle fibres, except in perinuclear regions where it is seen as focal deposits associated with lipofuscin. Lipofuscin is more abundant in muscle from adults than from children and therefore there may appear to be more perinuclear acid phosphatase activity in adults. In type II glycogenosis and lysosomal disorders, acid phosphatase is useful as it demonstrates the activity associated with the vacuoles. It also highlights the presence of macrophages. Acid phosphatase activity is also abundant in vitamin E deficiency and Batten's disease and the deposits are autofluorescent. The colour of the autofluorescence can be used to distinguish the two types of deposit as in vitamin E deficiency they are orange–yellow but yellow in Batten's disease.

Alkaline phosphatase is found primarily in cell membranes where active transport processes occur, such as the endothelium of arterioles and the arterial part of capillaries, and also in endoplasmic reticulum, Golgi apparatus and pinocytotic vesicles. The reaction is usually negative in muscle fibres but may be positive in focal necrotic fibres in various disease situations, in some regenerating or non-innervated fibres. Its major use is in the assessment of inflammatory myopathies when perimysial areas may be intensely stained.

Phosphofructokinase may be useful to study if a glycogenosis is suspected, but only a result of total absence can be relied on. A deficiency is difficult to assess histochemically and requires biochemical analysis.

Menadione-linked α-glycerophosphate dehydrogenase reveals a fibre type pattern with type 2 fibres more intensely stained than type 1, but is only of diagnostic value in distinguishing reducing bodies. These are the only abnormal structures to stain with this technique and as the occurrence of these structures is very rare this technique is not included in a routine panel.

Staining for *myoadenylate deaminase* is favoured by some as a deficiency may be the only feature of note in some patients. Interpretation of the significance of a deficiency is hampered, however, by the presence of a common mutation in the normal population which obliterates the enzyme. A secondary reduction in enzyme activity may also occur for unknown reasons. Abundant tubular aggregates are also revealed by the reaction.

Glycogen

The periodic acid-Schiff (PAS) stain, which has a very long history in histochemistry, is frequently used to demonstrate glycogen in muscle. It is worth bearing in mind, however, that not only glycogen but other polysaccharides as well as neutral mucopolysaccharides, muco- and glycoproteins, glycolipids and some unsaturated lipids and phospholipids are stained with this reaction. The glycogen is demonstrated with Schiff reagent (fuchsin-sulphurous acid) which produces a reddish-purple stain and shows a fibre typing pattern. The specificity of the PAS reaction for glycogen may be checked by using α-amylase digestion and the use of celloidin helps to retain the glycogen. Although glycogen storage may be rare, the PAS technique is also useful in revealing damaged and some denervated fibres in several disorders as these may be devoid of glycogen.

Neutral lipid

Neutral lipid can be demonstrated in normal muscle and takes the form of small droplets with a distribution similar to that of mitochondria. It can be demonstrated with the Sudan black or oil red O technique. The concentration and size of the droplets varies with the fibre type and this must be taken into consideration in interpretation. In disorders affecting lipid metabolism, the excessive accumulation of lipid shows up as larger and more extensive droplets. As these disorders are rare, however, the routine inclusion of a stain for lipid is a matter of choice which can be driven by clinical information.

Proliferation of adipose tissue is a common feature of muscular dystrophies but also occurs in spinal atrophies and other disorders. The unstained content of fat cells is readily apparent on routine histological stains but it can also be strikingly demonstrated with lipid stains. Stains for lipid in the presence of adipose tissue may, however, lead to diffuse spread of reaction product over large areas of the section.

Amyloid

It has been found useful to look for the deposition of amyloid in inclusion body myositis (Askanas and Engel 2001). In sporadic forms many of the characteristic rimmed vacuolated fibres contain amyloid but those that occur in various hereditary myopathies do not. These myopathies are often referred to as hereditary inclusion body myopathies and have several pathological features in common with sporadic inclusion body myositis but rarely show lymphocytic inflammation. Amyloid is composed of protein in a β-pleated sheet conformation.

Ultrastructurally it appears as tangled masses of unbranched double filaments of variable length. Each filament is 2.5–3.5 nm in diameter and separated by a 2.5 nm space, giving a total diameter of 8–10 nm. The most common method for demonstrating amyloid uses Congo red and one at high alkaline pH was recommended by Mendell et al (1991). Amyloid stained with Congo red is visible as a red deposit with normal bright field optics but also shows 'apple-green' birefringence with polarized light, and is most easily seen using fluorescence with an excitation filter suitable for fluorochromes such as Texas Red (Askanas et al 1993).

Histological and histochemical methods

In this section we list the methods of the techniques that form our routine panel of tests and that we consider to be the minimum for diagnosis. We also include additional methods used when clinical features are indicative. We have not attempted to produce a fully comprehensive list of techniques, nor included a wide selection of alternative methods which are available for some of the stains or enzymes. For such further information reference should be made to one of the standard histochemical texts (Barka and Anderson 1963, Pearse 1968, 1972, Filipe and Lake 1990).

All histological and histochemical techniques are performed on frozen sections (10-μm) mounted on coverslips or slides, as described in Chapter 1. Sections can be stored frozen until required and should be thoroughly air dried before use. If sections are stained flat a circle around each section, drawn with a hydrophobic pen, prevents the spread of solutions. Several histological stains are now commercially available as ready made solutions (e.g. haematoxylin). Methods for making them from the individual constituents are given here for those who may prefer them. The synthetic mountant that we routinely use is DPX, and when an aqueous mountant is required we now use hydromount (National Diagnostics) as this is also useful for immunofluorescence (see Ch. 6). Glycerin jelly can also be used and sections rarely dry out when mounted in this. DNA could, in theory, be extracted from such sections.

Haematoxylin and eosin (H&E)

1. Place sections in Harris' haematoxylin for 3 minutes.
2. Blue in Scott's tap water substitute or Tris buffer (pH 10.5) if tap water is acid. Otherwise run in tap water for 2 minutes.
3. Differentiate in 0.2% acid alcohol (HCl–alcohol) until pink – if needed.
4. Re-blue as appropriate (step 2).
5. Place in 1% eosin for 15–20 seconds (or longer).
6. Wash quickly in distilled water.
7. Dehydrate rapidly in ascending alcohol series.
8. Clear, and mount in synthetic resin (DPX).

(Continued)

Harris' haematoxylin
Harris' haematoxylin powder   *21.5-g*
Absolute alcohol   *10-mL*
Distilled water   *200-mL*

Add 4% glacial acetic acid just before use. This increases the precision of the nuclear staining. Solution will keep for years in a tightly closed bottle.

Eosin
5-g Eosin/100-mL distilled water

Dilute to 1% for use.

Alkaline solution (Scott's tap water)
Potassium bicarbonate   *2-g*
Magnesium sulphate   *20-g*
Distilled water   *1-L*

RESULTS
Nuclei blue; fibres red with mitochondria as dark dots; connective tissue pink. If staining in haematoxylin is too long the fibres may appear too basophilic. Mayer's haematoxylin is a good alternative if less basophilia is preferred but the mitochondria will not be visible.

Verhoeff–van Gieson (VVG)

1. Stain in Verhoeff's stain for 20 minutes (until black).
2. Wash in distilled water.
3. Differentiate in 2% ferric chloride for a few seconds.
4. Wash in three changes of distilled water.
5. Rinse in 70% alcohol for 1 minute.
6. Wash in three changes of distilled water.
7. Counterstain with van Gieson mixture for 2 minutes.
8. Dehydrate in ascending alcohol series, clear and mount in synthetic resin.

Verhoeff stain
Dissolve 1-g haematoxylin in hot 100% ethyl alcohol – 20-mL.
Add 8-mL Lugol's solution containing 2% iodine and 4% potassium iodide.
Add 8-mL of 10% ferric chloride solution.

NB. This solution is good for 4–6 weeks at 4°C.

van Gieson mixture
1% Aqueous acid fuchsin   *10-mL*
Saturated aqueous solution picric acid *90-mL*

Dilute with an equal volume of distilled water. Boil for 3 minutes to ripen.
NB. Fuchsin is removed by water and picric acid is removed by alcohol.

RESULTS
Connective tissue red; nuclei blue; fibres green–yellow; nerves and reticulin black.

Modified Gomori trichrome

1. Stain in Harris' haematoxylin for 5 minutes.
2. Rinse in distilled water.
3. Stain in Gomori trichrome mixture for 10 minutes (until green).
4. Rinse in tap water.
   (If results are too red differentiation in 0.2% acetic acid can be included at this stage, followed by a rinse in water.)
5. Dehydrate rapidly in ascending alcohol series.
6. Clear, and mount in synthetic resin.

Gomori mixture	
Chromotrope 2R	*0.6-g*
Fast green	*0.3-g*
Phosphotungstic acid	*0.6-g*
Glacial acetic acid	*1.0-mL*
Distilled water	*100-mL*

Adjust pH to 3.4
This mixture should be made up fresh when staining becomes pale. The chemicals used for the mixture should be very pure. If the stain deteriorates, change the first two ingredients.

RESULTS
Nuclei red; fibres green–blue with mitochondria as red dots; connective tissue pale green–blue; nemaline rods red; membranous whorls of rimmed vacuoles red; myelin of nerves red.

Periodic acid-Schiff technique (PAS) for glycogen

1. Fix sections in acetic ethanol or formol calcium for 5 minutes.
2. Wash in distilled water.
3. Place in 0.5% periodic acid for 2–5 minutes to oxidize.
4. Wash in distilled water.
5. Place in Schiff's reagent for 10–15 minutes.
6. Wash in running tap water for 5–10 minutes.
7. Counterstain in Mayer's haematoxylin for 1 minute
8. Dehydrate in ascending alcohol series.
9. Clear, and mount in synthetic resin.

Periodic acid solution
0.5-g periodic acid crystals dissolved in 100-mL distilled water.

Schiff's reagent

Basic fuchsin	*1-g*
Distilled water	*200-mL*
Sodium metabisulphite	*2-g*
Concentrated HCl	*2-mL*
Decolourizing charcoal	*2-g*

Boil the water and carefully add basic fuchsin. When dissolved, cool to 50°C and add sodium metabisulphite. Dissolve and allow to cool to room temperature. Add the HCl. Leave in a dark cupboard overnight. Add charcoal and shake for two minutes. Filter and store in a dark bottle at +4°C.

PAS control
Incubate control sections in 0.5% α-amylase solution at 37°C for 1 hour. Proceed with PAS stain as in preceding method.

Celloidin coating
As glycogen can leach out of sections during staining, sections can be coated with a film of 0.5–1% celloidin, air drying this and then performing PAS as above from stage 3.

RESULTS
Nuclei blue; checkerboard pattern of pink stained fibres, type 2 fibres darker; blood vessels pink; areas of glycogen accumulation intense pink.

Oil red O (ORO) stain for lipid

1. Rinse sections in water.
2. Rinse in 60% isopropyl alcohol.
3. Transfer to ORO stain for 10–30 minutes.
4. Differentiate in 60% isopropyl alcohol.
5. Wash in distilled water.
6. Counterstain in Harris' haematoxylin for 1 minute.
7. Rinse in tap water to blue.
8. Mount in aqueous mountant.

Stock stain
Saturated solution of ORO in isopropyl alcohol (0.5%)

For use
Dilute 6-mL stock with 4-mL distilled water. Stand for 10 minutes and filter.

RESULTS
Nuclei blue; lipid red; more droplets in type 1 fibres.

Sudan black B

1. Stain in saturated Sudan black in 70% alcohol, freshly filtered, for 20 minutes. Keep well covered to prevent evaporation.
2. Wash in water.
3. Stain in filtered haematoxylin for 2 minutes.
4. Wash in tap water for 10 minutes.
5. Mount in aqueous mountant

RESULTS
As for ORO but end product black.

Congo red

1. Counterstain nuclei in haematoxylin, differentiate and blue.
2. Immerse sections in saturated sodium chloride in 80% ethanol for 1 hour.
3. Transfer to Congo red solution for 1 hour.
4. Rinse in 70% alcohol, dehydrate through graded alcohols, clear and mount in synthetic resin.

Congo red solution
0.2-g Congo red in 100-mL of 80% ethanol with saturated sodium chloride adjusted to pH 10.5–11.0 with sodium hydroxide.

RESULTS
Nuclei blue; amyloid red (more easily seen as red fluorescence using an excitation filter in the range 545–580 nm, as for Texas Red).

Reduced nicotinamide adenine dinucleotide dehydrogenase-tetrazolium reductase (NADH-TR)

1. Place fresh sections flat in a Petri dish or staining tray in a *damp* atmosphere.
2. Place one to two drops of incubating solution on the section ensuring that it is completely covered. (A circle round the section drawn with a hydrophobic pen helps to stop the spread of the incubating medium.)
3. Incubate for 30 minutes at 37°C.
4. Rinse in distilled water.
5. Fix in 15–20% formalin solution for 10 minutes.
6. Rinse in distilled water.
7. Mount in aqueous mountant.

Nitroblue tetrazolium (NBT) stock solution
20 mg/20-mL distilled water
Store in aliquots at −20°C.

NADH stock solution

NBT stock	*6.25-mL*
0.2 M Tris buffer pH 7.4	*6.25-mL*
Cobalt chloride 0.5 M (11.9-g/100-mL)	*1.25-mL*
Distilled water	*8.75-mL*

Store in aliquots at −20°C.

Incubating solution

NADH stock solution	*1-mL*
NADH	*1-mg*

RESULTS
Blue–grey end product, higher activity in type 1 fibres and in areas with mitochondrial aggregates. Type 2B fibres weakest; 2A intermediate intensity.

Succinate dehydrogenase

1. Incubate sections flat in damp atmosphere as for NADH-TR at 37°C for 90 minutes.
2. Drain and place in formal calcium for 15 minutes.
3. Wash in distilled water.
4. Mount in aqueous mountant.

Stock succinate medium

Sodium succinate	*4.05-g*
Distilled water	*20-mL*
1 M hydrochloric acid	*0.13-mL*

Adjust to pH 7.0 and make up to a total volume of 25-mL.
Store at −20°C in aliquots.

Tetrazolium solution

NBT solution (4 mg/mL)	*7.5-mL*
0.2 M Tris buffer (pH 7.4)	*7.5-mL*
Distilled water	*10.5-mL*

Adjust pH to 7.0, store at −20°C in aliquots.

Incubating solution
0.1-mL stock succinate solution plus 0.9-mL tetrazolium solution

RESULT
Blue–grey end product, higher activity in type 1 fibres and areas with mitochondrial aggregates. Type 2B weakest; 2A intermediate intensity.

Cytochrome oxidase (COX)

1. Incubate fresh frozen sections for 3 hours at 37°C.
2. Rinse quickly in distilled water.
3. Fix in formol calcium for 15 minutes.
4. Rinse in water.
5. Dehydrate in ascending alcohol series, clear, and mount in synthetic resin.

Instead of fixation in formol calcium optional enhancement can be done by placing the sections in osmium tetroxide (1% stock solution diluted 1 in 100) for 30 minutes.

Incubation medium

3,3'-Diaminobenzidine tetrahydrochloride (DAB)	*7.5 mg*
0.1 M phosphate buffer (pH 7.4)	*9-mL*

Mix together then add:

Catalase C solution (4 mg/mL)	*1-mL*
Cytochrome c	*10 mg*
Sucrose	*750 mg*

0.1 M phosphate buffer pH 7.4

0.1 M sodium dihydrogen orthophosphate	*2-mL*
0.1 M disodium hydrogen orthophosphate	*8-mL*

DAB is carcinogenic and careful handling is required. DAB in tablet and liquid form is commercially available and can be used instead.

RESULTS

Fine brown stain at sites of cytochrome oxidase activity (osmium enhancement gives a darker colour) type 1 fibres darkest, type 2B weakest; 2A intermediate. Fibres with all mitochondria carrying a mutation in cytochrome oxidase appear pure white.

Combined cytochrome oxidase and succinic dehydrogenase (SDH)

1. Incubate fresh frozen sections at 37°C for 1 hour in cytochrome oxidase incubating medium.
2. Wash in distilled water.
3. Incubate in SDH incubating medium at 37°C for 45 minutes.
4. Drain and fix in 10% formalin for 15 minutes.
5. Wash well in tap water.
6. Mount in aqueous mountant.

Always do the cytochrome oxidase activity first.

Cytochrome oxidase incubating medium	
3,3'-Diaminobenzidine tetrahydrochloride (DAB)	*15 mg*
0.05 M Sodium phosphate buffer pH 7.4	*27-mL*
Sucrose	*2.25-g*

Store in aliquots at −20°C.

Incubating medium	
DAB solution	*0.9-mL*
Cytochrome c	*1 mg*
Catalase	*0.1 mg*

Succinic dehydrogenase	
0.2 M sodium succinate	*0.5-mL*
0.2 M phosphate buffer	*0.5-mL*
Store as aliquots at −20°C	

Just before use add 1 mg NBT to 1-mL aliquot.

RESULT
Fine brown/blue–grey fibre type pattern; fibres devoid of cytochrome oxidase activity blue.

Menadione-linked α-glycerophosphate dehydrogenase

1. Incubate at 37°C for 60 minutes.
2. Extract with acetone, 30, 60, 90, 60, 30% in that sequence.
3. Wash in water.
4. Mount in aqueous mountant.

Incubating solution	
α-Glycerophosphate	*30 mg*
0.2 M Tris buffer	*10-mL*
Nitroblue tetrazolium	*10 mg*
Menadione (vitamin K$_3$)	*2 mg*

Menadione is difficult to dissolve in an aqueous medium so a small amount of acetone (0.2-mL) may be used to dissolve it. Alternatively, the menadione may be added to the aqueous solution and mixed well. Although it is not all dissolved, enough will be in the medium to produce the desired effect.

RESULT
Blue–grey end product, higher activity in type 2 fibres; reducing bodies stained.

Phosphorylase

1. Incubate sections for 1 hour at 37°C.
2. Rinse rapidly in distilled water.
3. Transfer to Lugol's iodine.
4. Rinse in distilled water.
5. Mount in aqueous mountant (reaction product fades rapidly) or dehydrate in alcohols, clear and mount in synthetic resin.

Incubation medium

Glucose-1-phosphate	50 mg
AMP (adenosine-5-monophosphoric acid)	10 mg
EDTA	25 mg
Sodium fluoride	20 mg
Dextran	1-g
0.1 M acetate buffer, pH 5.9	6-mL
Absolute ethanol	1-mL

Adjust to pH 5.9 before use.

Lugol's iodine

Iodine	1-g
Potassium iodide	2-g
Distilled water	100-mL

Dissolve the potassium iodide in a small quantity of distilled water, then dissolve the iodine and add the remainder of the water.

RESULT
Checkerboard pattern of purple stained fibres. Type 2 fibres darker.

Phosphofructokinase

1. Incubate sections at 37°C for 1 hour in a Petri dish or staining tray.
2. Wash in distilled water.
3. Mount in aqueous mountant.

Incubating medium

20-mM sodium arsenate pH 7.0	8.0-mL
10-mM fructose-6-phosphate	3.2-mL
10-mM NAD	1.6-mL
10-mM adenosine triphosphate	1.6-mL
40-mM magnesium sulphate	0.4-mL
Nitroblue tetrazolium	6.4-mL
Distilled water	1.2-mL

Adjust to pH 7.0.

RESULTS
Blue–grey checkerboard pattern of fibre types; type 2 fibres darker.

Adenylate deaminase

1. Incubate cryostat sections for 1 hour at room temperature.
2. Drain and fix in formal calcium for 15 minutes.
3. Mount in aqueous mounting medium.

Incubating medium

p-Nitroblue tetrazolium	*20 mg*
Distilled water	*18-mL*
Filter.	
Add AMP–3H$_2$O.	*8 mg*
Add 3 M potassium chloride (slowly whilst stirring).	*1.4-mL*

Adjust pH to 6.1.
Dissolve 10 mg of dithiothreitol in 0.6-mL distilled water. Add drop wise whilst stirring to above medium. (Do not adjust pH again as dithiothreitol damages the electrodes.)

RESULTS
Checkerboard pattern. Type 1 fibres darker with a blue stippled pattern; type 2 fibres have a reticular pattern with a pink/purple background. Tubular aggregates intensely stained.

Adenosine triphosphatase (ATPase)

A number of different methods for demonstrating ATPase have been applied over the years (see Brooke and Kaiser 1970, Padykula and Hermann 1955). The following was published by Round et al (1980).

Method at pH 9.4

1. Incubate sections at 37°C for 30 minutes
2. Rinse well in distilled water.
3. Immerse in 2% cobalt chloride for three rinses, 1 minute each.
4. Rinse well in distilled water.
5. Immerse in dilute (1:10) ammonium sulphide solution for 30 seconds.
6. Rinse well in running tap water.
7. (Optional) stain in Harris' haematoxylin for 1 minute and blue in tap water.
8. Dehydrate in ascending alcohol series, clear and mount.

Method at pH 4.6 and 4.3

1. Pre-incubate at 4°C in 0.1 M sodium acetate buffer with 10-mM EDTA added, for 10 minutes at pH 4.6 or 4.3.
2. Rinse in distilled water.
3. Proceed as for pH 9.4 method.

Incubating medium
5 mg ATP dissolved in a few drops of distilled water
Add 10-mL of 0.1 M glycine/NaCl buffer with 0.75 M CaCl₂.

Adjust to pH 9.4. Add 0.0309 g/10-mL (20 mM) dithiothreitol solution. (Do not recheck pH as this damages electrode.)

0.1 M glycine buffer
0.75-g Glycine + 0.585-g NaCl
100-mL with distilled water

0.1 M glycine/NaCl buffer with CaCl₂
50-mL 0.1 M glycine buffer
10-mL 0.75 M CaCl₂

Add approximately 22-mL 0.1 M NaOH until pH 9.4.

RESULT
Checkerboard pattern of black and white fibres:
pH 9.4 – type 1 white, type 2 black (type 2A may show an intermediate intensity), 2C black;
pH 4.6 – type 1 black , 2A white, 2B intermediate, 2C black;
pH 4.3 – type 1 black, 2A and 2B white, 2C black or intermediate.

Acid phosphatase

1. Incubate sections at 37°C for 1 hour.
2. Wash in distilled water.
3. Counterstain in 2% methyl green (chloroform extracted) for 1 minute.
4. Wash in running tap water.
5. Mount in aqueous mountant.

Incubating medium	
Solution 1	*0.5-mL*
Solution 2	*2.5-mL*
Solution 3	*0.4-mL*
Solution 4	*0.4-mL*

Mix solution 3 with solution 4 until bubbles cease (approx. 2 minutes).
Mix solution 1 and 2 with 6.5-mL distilled water.
Add combined solution 3 and 4
Adjust with 0.1 N sodium hydroxide to pH 4.7–5.0.

Solution 1 (substrate)	
Naphthol AS-B1 phosphate	*5 mg*
Dimethylformamide	*0.5-mL*

Solution 2 (buffer solution)
Veronal acetate buffer stock A
(1.17-g Sodium acetate + 2.94-g sodium barbitone made up to 100-mL with distilled water.)

Solution 3 (must be freshly made)
Sodium nitrite	*40 mg*
Distilled water	*1-mL*

Solution 4 (pararosaniline–HCl stock)
Pararosaniline hydrochloride	*2-g*
2 N hydrochloric acid	*50-mL*

Heat gently, cool to room temperature and filter (store at 4°C).

RESULTS
Acid phosphatase activity red; nuclei green (over counterstaining gives a helpful pale green colour to the muscle fibres).

Alkaline phosphatase

1. Fix in formal calcium at 4°C for 60 minutes.
2. Incubate at room temperature for 60 minutes in the following solution:
Sodium α-naphthyl acid phosphate	10 mg
Fast blue RR	10 mg
0.1 M barbiturate buffer	10-mL
Adjust to pH 9.2.	
3. Wash 3 minutes in distilled water.
4. Wash 2 minutes in 1% acetic acid.
5. Rinse in distilled water.
6 Mount in aqueous mountant.

RESULTS
Alkaline phosphatase activity reddish brown

CHAPTER 3

Normal muscle

In this chapter, the composition and appearance of normal muscle will be discussed. The first part will be concerned with the anatomical constituents of normal muscle at the light microscope level, followed by histochemical aspects of the different types of muscle fibres and ultrastructural details of muscle. We then discuss myogenesis and the development of muscle.

Histological structure

The word muscle is derived from the Latin *mus* (= mouse) and refers to the resemblance of the muscle belly to a mouse. Muscles vary in size, shape and form, according to their function. For example the biceps is a fusiform muscle in which the fibres are all arranged in parallel for quick activity. The deltoid is a penniform, feather-shaped muscle with a septum at an angle to the line of action which allows for maximum strength. Each muscle is enclosed in a connective tissue sheath, the *epimysium*, composed of extracellular matrix proteins including collagen, and merging at either end with a tendon, an aponeurosis or the periosteum of bone. Extensions of extracellular matrix from the epimysium subdivide the muscle into individual bundles or fascicles each surrounded by a well-defined layer, the *perimysium* (Figs 3.1 and 3.2). The width of the perimysium varies with age and is relatively wider in neonates than in infants and adults. The diameter of individual muscle fibres that constitute the muscle bundles varies with age and with the muscle. In adult males fibres of the quadriceps muscle are usually between 40 and 80 µm and may reach a length of up to 10 cm. They are closely packed to each other and in transverse section are polygonal in shape. In some muscles the fibres stretch from tendon to tendon; they also insert into the perimysial fascia. The endomysium, a network of fine collagen fibres and other extracellular matrix proteins, separates the fibres from each other. Although barely visible under normal circumstances, this extracellular matrix may proliferate in pathological muscles and become very striking.

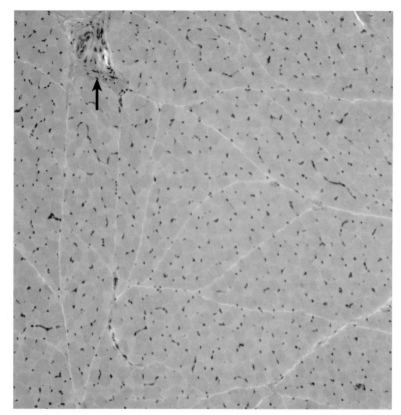

FIG. 3.1 *A low magnification view of a biopsy from a 4-year-old child showing individual fascicles of fibres, each surrounded by perimysium. The arrow indicates a perimysial blood vessel. Mean fibre size is approximately 24 μm (H&E).*

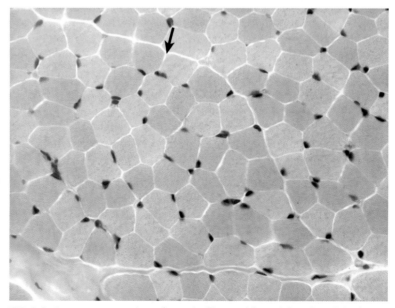

FIG. 3.2 *A transverse section of muscle fibres with peripheral nuclei. The arrow indicates perimysium. Note also the slight variation in colour of different fibre types. Mean fibre diameter is approximately 24 μm (H&E).*

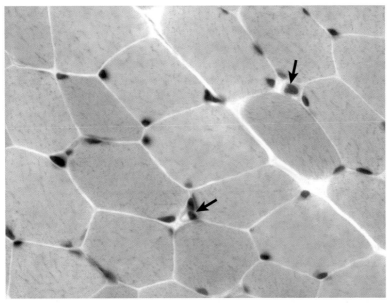

FIG. 3.3 *At high power the intermyofibrillar network is visible and capillaries between the fibres can be distinguished (arrows). Mean fibre diameter approximately 36 μm (H&E).*

Individual muscle fibres, formed by the fusion of single cells, are multinucleated syncytia surrounded by a plasma membrane and basal lamina, the sarcolemma. The *nuclei* are elliptical in shape in longitudinal section and have dense peripheral heterochromatin and may have a prominent nucleolus and finely stippled nucleoplasm (Figs 3.3 and 3.4), although this is less easy to see in unfixed, frozen sections. In normal muscle most nuclei are located under the sarcolemma and in transverse section several per fibre may be visible. Nuclei of muscle fibres, except those of satellite cells (see below), do not divide. They stain blue with haematoxylin, and red with the Gomori trichrome. With both these stains variability in intensity of the fibres can be seen which correlates with differences between fibre types (Fig. 3.5; see below). The mitochondria appear as small dots, red with the trichrome stain and blue with Harris' haematoxylin.

The muscle fibre is composed of many *myofibrils* separated from each other by the intermyofibrillar space. Under light microscopy, particularly with the use of various histochemical reactions, it is possible to distinguish the individual myofibrils, whereas the intermyofibrillar space appears as a continuous network (see below). Within the intermyofibrillar space are various subcellular constituents, which are readily recognized under higher magnification with electron microscopy.

Various other structures can be recognized in a muscle biopsy at the light microscope level.

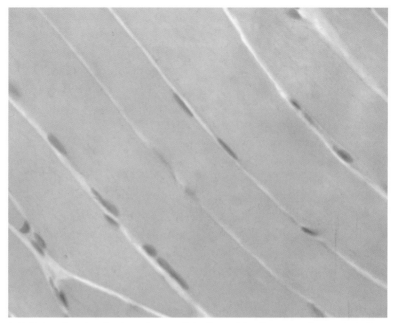

FIG. 3.4 *In longitudinal section nuclei elliptical in shape can be seen at the sarcolemma of each fibre. Cross-striations are not easily distinguished in unfixed frozen sections but can be faintly seen. Mean fibre diameter approximately 50 μm (H&E).*

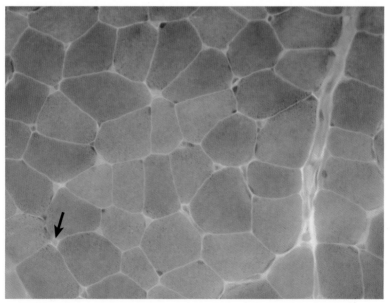

FIG. 3.5 *Transverse section stained with Gomori trichrome in which the intensity of stain varies in individual fibres; nuclei are stained red and capillaries (arrow) can be distinguished between fibres. Mean fibre diameter approximately 40 μm.*

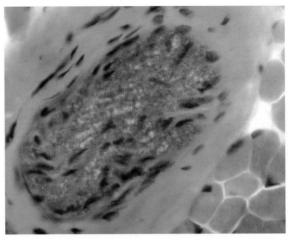

FIG. 3.6 *A myelinated nerve 58 μm in diameter surrounded by the perineurium (Gomori trichrome).*

Blood vessels

The vascular supply of muscle is readily apparent on routine stains and with stains such as periodic acid-Schiff (PAS), especially after diastase digestion. Medium size arterioles and veins run between the fascicles (Fig. 3.1), while within the fascicles there is a capillary network in close relation to individual fibres (Figs 3.3 and 3.5). Type 1 fibres have more capillaries than type 2 and a smaller network is apparent in muscle from neonates.

Nerves

Nerves can be demonstrated between and within muscle bundles, but they are not seen in all biopsies. The junctions of the nerves with the fibre, the neuromuscular junctions, are not easily visible with routine histological stains but can be demonstrated with certain histochemical stains, with specific antibodies and fluorescently labelled bungarotoxin, a snake venom that specifically binds to the acetylcholine receptors. With the Verhoeff–van Gieson stain, the individual axons and the myelin sheath stain black and can be readily visualized, and with the Gomori trichrome stain the myelin of individual axons stains red (Fig. 3.6). The perineurium encasing the axons is also clearly seen. Each fibre is innervated by one nerve, although fibres are polyinnervated at early embryonic stages. In most muscles the motor end plates form a band across the mid-belly of the muscle.

Spindles

Spindles are specialized structures consisting of striated, intrafusal fibres within a fibrous connective tissue capsule (Fig. 3.7). The number of spindle fibres varies but is usually between 4 and 16. The spindles are located between the muscle

MUSCLE BIOPSY

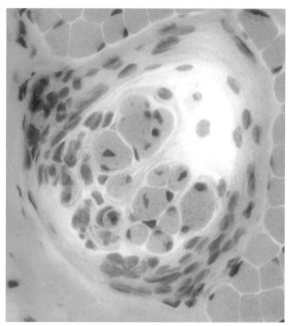

FIG. 3.7 *A muscle spindle. The intrafusal muscle fibres ranging in size from 11 to 17 μm are surrounded by a connective tissue sheath (H&E).*

fascicles in the perimysial connective tissue, usually adjacent to nerves or vessels. The fibres of spindles have their own specialized motor nerve supply (the gamma efferent fibres) as well as sensory nerves. The muscle spindle acts as a sensory organ and is associated with the coordination of muscle activity and stretch, and the maintenance of muscle tone. They are found in all muscles except those of the face. For details of the physiology and anatomy of the muscle spindle see Barker and Banks (1986) and Swash (1992).

Muscle fibres within the spindles are of two kinds: nuclear bag fibres, with a large collection of nuclei in the central area of the fibre, and the smaller nuclear chain fibres, with chains of nuclei throughout much of their length. With the various histochemical reactions, intrafusal fibres vary in their enzyme activities, much as the extrafusal fibres do, and attempts have been made to recognize fibre types among them (see below). Immature isoforms of myosin are present in some normal spindle fibres even though the extrafusal are fully mature, and other isoforms associated with immaturity, such as those of phosphorylase, occur in spindle fibres (see Ch. 16). It is important when assessing muscle biopsies that the intrafusal fibres of the spindles are not mistaken for abnormal extrafusal fibres.

The muscle spindles may be affected in certain circumstances, including sensory and motor denervation, some muscular dystrophies and ageing (see Swash 1992).

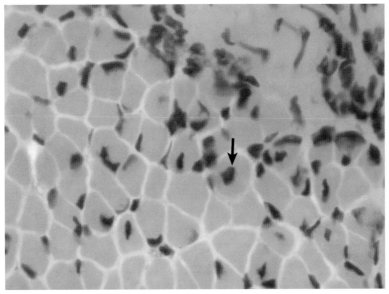

FIG. 3.8 *An area of fascia with myotendinous junctions. Internal nuclei (arrow) are common in such regions (H&E).*

Myotendinous junction

Occasionally a myotendinous area may be encountered in a biopsy. This is a folded zone of the outer fibre surface where the fibre tapers towards the tendon and the epimysial fascia. Finger-like projections interdigitate with collagenous projections and subdivide the fibre, increasing the surface area. Internal nuclei are common at these sites (Fig. 3.8) and a number of proteins are abundant, such as vinculin, talin, tenascin C, dystrophin and certain integrins. Acetylcholine receptors are also present at myotendinous junctions but the reason is unknown.

Muscle fibre types

The application of enzyme histochemical techniques has had a major impact on the interpretation of muscle biopsies. Most skeletal muscles are composed of a mixture of fibres which differ in their physiological and biochemical properties. A major aspect of muscle pathology is concerned with the identification of the fibre types and the way in which these are affected by various pathological processes. Early workers distinguished muscles by their colour, red and white. In animal and avian muscle this distinction can be clearly seen. For example in chicken muscle the pectoral muscle is white compared to the darker red muscles of the thigh. Physiologists tried to characterize this colour difference on the basis of contraction, slow versus fast (see Table 3.1). With the advent of histochemistry it became possible to localize enzyme systems and other chemical constituents at a cellular level. This opened the way for a direct correlation of the functional activity of individual fibres with their morphology.

TABLE 3.1 *Main characteristics of the different fibre types in human muscle*

	Type 1	Type 2A	Type 2B	Type 2C
Colour	Red	White		
Twitch speed	Slow	Fast	Fast	
Fatigability	Resistant	Resistant	Sensitive	
Twitch + oxidative and glycolytic capacity	SO	FOG	FG	
ATPase pH 9.4	+	+++	+++	+++
ATPase pH 4.6	+++	−	++	+++
ATPase pH 4.3	+++	±	−	++ or +++
NADH-TR	+++	++	+	++ or +++
Cytochrome oxidase	+++	++	+	+
Succinic dehydrogenase	+++	++	+	++
Phosphorylase	− or +	+++	+++	+++
PAS	+ or ++	+++	++	++
Lipid droplets	+++	++ or +++	+	
Antibodies to fast myosin heavy chain	−	+++	+++	++ or +++
Antibodies to slow myosin heavy chain	+++	−	−	−, + or ++

FG, fast glycolytic; FOG, fast oxidative glycolytic; NADH-TR, reduced nicotinamide adenine dinucleotide-tetrazolium reductase; PAS, periodic acid-Schiff; SO, slow oxidative
−, +, ++, +++ represent increasing intensity of stain

Enzyme histochemistry identifies two main fibre types and a reciprocal relationship between glycolytic and oxidative enzyme activity in individual muscle fibres (Dubowitz and Pearse 1960a, b). Type 1 fibres have high oxidative and low glycolytic activity, and type 2 fibres have low oxidative and high glycolytic activity, although there is a subtype of type 2 fibres that has a moderate oxidative capacity (see below). The most widespread nomenclature for fibre types is based on the appearance following staining for adenosine triphosphatase (ATPase), with and without preincubation at acid pH (Brooke and Kaiser 1970). Three fibre types can be identified in normal muscle (type 1, 2A, 2B) with an additional subtype of 2C that is an immature fibre type (Fig. 3.9a–c).

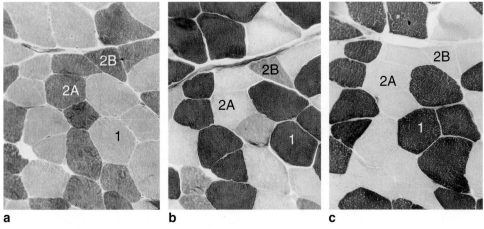

FIG. 3.9 *Serial sections stained with (a) ATPase pH 9.4 and following preincubation at (b) pH 4.6 and (c) pH 4.3 showing a checkerboard pattern of type 1 fibres and the subdivision of type 2 fibres into 2A and 2B.*

The concept of the ***motor unit*** is fundamental to the understanding of fibre types and is important in the interpretation of pathology. The nerves innervating muscle fibres have their origin in the cell body in the anterior horn of the spinal cord. The neurone from the cell body branches to supply a variable number of muscle fibres, which in most muscles is several hundred. The anterior horn, its axon and the muscle fibres supplied constitute the motor unit, all of which are functionally dependent on each other. Muscle fibres of one motor unit are of a uniform type and, although confined to a limited area, they are randomly scattered and not clustered. Motor units are classified by their speed of contraction and resistance to fatigue (Schiaffino et al 1970). Physiologists have identified three main types: FF (fast twitch, fatigue sensitive), FR (fast twitch, fatigue resistant) and S (slow twitch, fatigue resistant). Fatigue resistance correlates with oxidative capacity and mitochondrial content and fibres have therefore also been classified as slow twitch, oxidative (SO) which correspond to histochemical type 1 fibres, fast twitch, glycolytic (FG) that correspond to 2B and fast twitch, oxidative glycolytic (FOG) that correspond to 2A (Burke et al 1973). This classification was based on studies of animal muscle but evidence suggests that human muscle is similar. Most muscles in humans, in contrast to other species, are of mixed type and show a checkerboard pattern of light and dark fibres with ATPase staining. The proportion of each fibre type, however, varies considerably between muscles and even in different regions of the same muscle (Johnson et al 1973). Knowledge of the site from which a biopsy has been taken is therefore important when assessing the proportion of each fibre type. The tibialis anterior, for example, has a higher proportion of type 1 fibres than muscles of the quadriceps. The different enzyme profiles of each fibre type are accompanied by a multitude of fibre type-specific isoforms of structural proteins. In particular, the ***myosin heavy chain isoforms*** have been used to classify fibre types and antibodies to specific isoforms are having an increasing role in muscle pathology. Four main

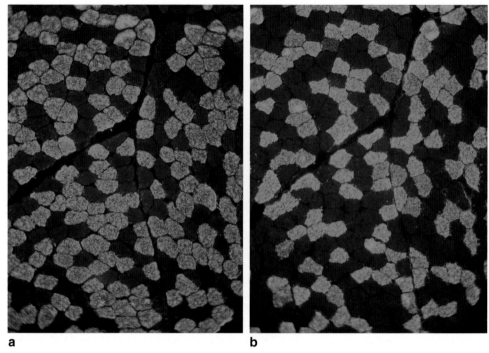

a   b

FIG. 3.10 *Serial sections of normal muscle labelled with antibodies to (a) slow and (b) fast myosin showing most fibres have either slow or fast myosin.*

isoforms have been identified in mammalian skeletal muscle, slow, fast 2A, fast 2B and fast 2X (also referred to as 2D). In addition, facial and ocular muscles express unique isoforms in addition to those that are only found during the development of other muscles. Most fibres in normal mature muscle express only one heavy chain isoform (Fig. 3.10a, b) but co-expression of more that one isoform can occur (hybrid fibres). This frequently occurs in pathological muscle and is an important aspect to assess. This is an advantage of immunohistochemistry compared with the histochemical methods for ATPase which cannot detect this co-expression.

Confusion in nomenclature, however, has now arisen because of this co-expression and also because myosin isoforms have a similar Arabic letter suffix to that based on the use of ATPase. The two, however, are not equivalent. In general type 1 fibres have slow myosin but human fibres do not have fast 2B myosin (see Pette and Staron 2000). Thus an ATPase 2B fibre in human muscle does not have fast 2B myosin but predominantly 2X myosin. There are no specific antibodies to human fast 2X myosin and fibres expressing only 2X are identified by exclusion and the histochemical equivalents in human muscle have not been fully elucidated. Confusion in nomenclature also arises with fibres in pathological muscle that coexpress both fast and slow myosin isoforms, as these may not give a clear distinction with ATPase.

Many laboratories use the ATPase method as a standard technique for classifying fibre types and there is a wealth of information on pathological samples based on it. With the increasing use of immunohistochemistry, however, it is likely that the use of myosin antibodies will soon have a wider acceptance. Their importance will be stressed in later chapters that discuss immunohistochemistry in detail. The advantages of using myosin antibodies are:

- hybrid fibres with more than one isoform can be identified and this co-expression makes good differentiation of fibre types with ATPase difficult to achieve, particularly without acid preincubation;
- immature and regenerating fibres are easily identified with the appropriate myosin antibodies, and different patterns of fibres expressing immature isoforms of myosin can be seen in different neuromuscular disorders;
- fibre typing in postmortem muscle can be assessed with antibodies whereas ATPase activity may be lost.

The equivalent of the histochemical 2B fibre with intermediate staining for ATPase at pH 4.6 cannot be identified with myosin antibodies but the identification of these fibres is now of limited diagnostic value. In practice, the most important distinction is that between type 1 and all type 2 fibres (slow versus fast myosin fibres). A comparison of nomenclature and fibre type properties is given in Table 3.1. Ultrastructural differences in fibre types are discussed below.

Plasticity of fibre types

Many factors can influence fibre typing such as innervation, hormones, exercise, disuse, drugs, age and neuromuscular disorders (see Pette and Staron 2000, 2001).

Early experiments on cross-innervation demonstrated the pivotal role of innervation in controlling twitch characteristics of muscle (Buller et al 1960). In particular, the speed at which the impulse passes down the nerve was shown to be crucial and that altering the innervation could change the histochemical and biochemical profile of a fibre (see Pette and Vrbova 1999). This effect is now known to involve calcium pathways and calcineurin and nuclear factor of active T cells (NFAT) signalling (Michel et al 2004). Several different physiological and pathological factors may influence fibre types. For example, spinal cord injury induces a predominantly fast fibre profile. In myopathic disorders, however, slow myosin often predominates and fibres are consequently more fatigue resistant. Testosterone and thyroid hormone have a profound influence on fibre typing in normal and pathological situations. Hypothyroidism tends to cause a shift from fast to slow myosin whilst hyperthyroidism has the opposite effect (see Pette and Staron 1997). Endurance exercise training programmes increase oxidative enzyme capacity and can also influence myosin heavy chains (Booth and Baldwin 1996). The effects of training on muscle have led to the development of sport science as a discipline. It has been known for many years that endurance athletes have a predominance of slow/type 1 fibres whereas sprinters have a predominance of fast/type 2 fibres. Different exercise protocols have also been developed for therapeutic benefit, for example following prolonged bed rest (see Thompson 2002).

Histochemical identification of muscle fibre types

This section will discuss in further detail the histochemical profile of normal muscle as it appears with the reactions most commonly used for the assessment of pathological samples. There may be some inevitable repetition of material discussed in previous chapters but it was felt it would be more useful to include it here rather than to refer back to previous sections.

Adenosine triphosphatase reactions

The reaction for adenosine triphosphatase (ATPase) is carried out at a pH of 9.4 (see Ch. 2) although minor adjustments may have to be made to achieve optimal results. Under these conditions, the reaction develops in the myofibrils; the inter-myofibrillar network seems to dissolve out of the tissue section at some stage during the reaction. Thus, on examining an individual fibre, the myofibrils can be seen separated by an unstained intermyofibrillar network. On longitudinal section, the stain develops in the region of the bands occupied by myosin. The reaction has therefore been termed the 'myosin ATPase' reaction.

In examining the muscle as a whole, there is a clear differentiation into two fibre types. The type 1 fibres are more lightly stained and the type 2 fibres more heavily. Intermediate fibres are usually not seen with this reaction. Following preincubation at pH 4.3, the reverse pattern is seen, with the type 1 fibres darkly stained and the type 2 fibres lightly. This reciprocal pattern is useful as dark areas are more noticeable than light. Occasionally, type 2 fibres may still retain reactivity at pH 4.3; these are the type 2C fibres. They are rare in normal human muscle but are present in developing muscle and may appear under pathological circumstances. Basophilic, regenerating fibres are usually 2C fibres. Following preincubation at pH 4.6, the type 1 fibres are strongly reactive, as at pH 4.3, but the type 2 fibres can be subdivided. Some will be inhibited and stain lightly (2A) whereas others will still stain with an intermediate intensity (2B) giving a three fibre pattern. 2C fibres at this pH also stain darkly (see Fig. 3.9 a–c and Table 3.1). With the acid preincubation ATPase reactions, the intermyofibrillar network pattern is well demonstrated, as well as the myofibrils. The intermyofibrillar network can be removed by preincubation with calcium, which will not affect the relative staining characteristics of the various fibre types.

If the pH is increased up to 10 a three-fibre pattern can also be obtained. The precise pH for preincubation required to give a good differentiation pattern may have to be determined empirically and conditions for human muscle are not suitable for all species. As discussed previously, the subdivision of type 2 fibres is often, but not always, of limited diagnostic value and the most important distinction is between type 1 and type 2 fibres. A detailed description is included here, however, as the technique is performed and favoured in many laboratories and it is relevant to the interpretation of several stains.

Oxidative enzymes

The various oxidative enzyme reactions show some similarity in the appearance of the sections. Therefore, they will be discussed together and the minor variations will be pointed out.

Reduced nicotinamide adenine dinucleotide-tetrazolium reductase

With this reaction, two fibre types can generally be recognized, sometimes three types (Fig. 3.11a,b). Type 1 fibres show a darker blue colour than the type 2 fibres and some type 2 fibres are of intermediate intensity. The myofibrils are unstained, but the intermyofibrillar network, comprising the mitochondria and sarcoplasmic reticulum, is well demonstrated (Fig. 3.11b). This network pattern is slightly different in the two fibre types. Correlation of the reduced nicotinamide adenine dinucleotide-tetrazolium reductase (NADH-TR) reaction with ATPase activity of fibres on serial section shows that, in human muscle, type 1 fibres (weak with ATPase at pH 9.4) react most intensely to NADH-TR, type 2B fibres show the least reaction with NADH-TR, and the type 2A fibres have an intermediate activity (see Table 3.1).

Succinic dehydrogenase and cytochrome oxidase

These enzymes are purely mitochondrial and both show differentiation of fibre types. In longitudinal section, the mitochondria appear as pairs of dots at the A–I junction (see section on electron microscopy), giving a striated appearance to the muscle. In transverse section, the intermyofibrillar network may have a rather particulate appearance, which has been interpreted as representing mitochondrial distribution. Sections stained for succinic dehydrogenase (SDH) have a bluish colour, as with the NADH-TR technique, because of the use of a tetrazolium salt, and staining for cytochrome oxidase (COX) gives a brown end product (Fig. 3.12a,b). Fibre type distribution is similar to that seen with the technique for NADH-TR. With staining for COX, some type 2B fibres may appear to be very pale and it is important not to interpret these as the negative fibres associated with mitochondrial abnormalities. Careful focusing in and out of the plane of section, however, will reveal small numbers of brown dots. With many of the oxidative enzymes there are additional points to be noted. The region next to the nuclei is very often the site of more intense staining. At times when central nuclei are seen, this may appear as an area of increased stain within the fibre. It is usually either triangular or diamond-shaped on cross-section and the nucleus may be seen as an unstained area within it. Additionally, there is often an area

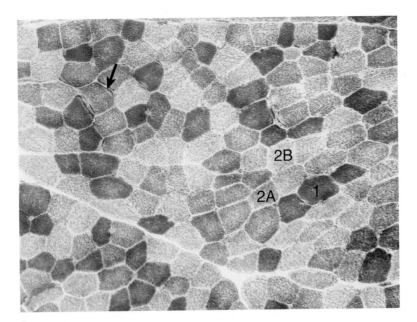

a

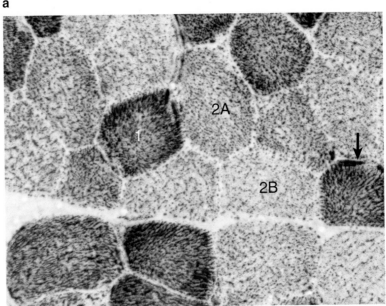

b

FIG. 3.11 *(a) Transverse section stained for NADH-TR showing highest intensity of stain in type 1 fibres, pale staining of 2B fibres and an intermediate intensity of 2A fibres. Note also the darker peripheral areas of clustered mitochondria (arrow). Mean fibre diameter is approximately 36 μm. (b) High power of the same section showing the mitochondria and intermyofibrillar network and peripheral clusters of mitochondria (arrow).*

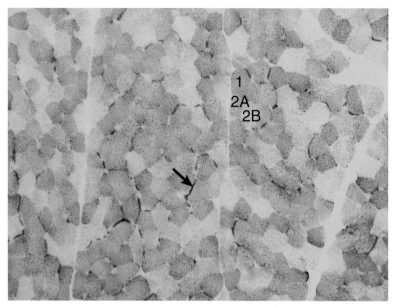

a

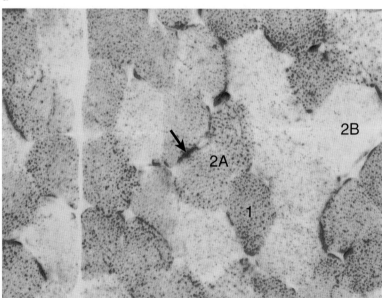

b

FIG. 3.12 *(a) Transverse section stained for cytochrome oxidase showing highest intensity of stain in type 1 fibres, pale staining of 2B fibres and an intermediate intensity of 2A fibres. Note also the darker peripheral areas of clustered mitochondria as with NADH-TR (arrow). Mean fibre diameter is approximately 28 μm. (b) High power of the same section showing the brown dots of the mitochondria which are most numerous in type 1 fibres, least in 2B fibres and intermediate in 2A fibres and peripheral clusters of mitochondria (arrow).*

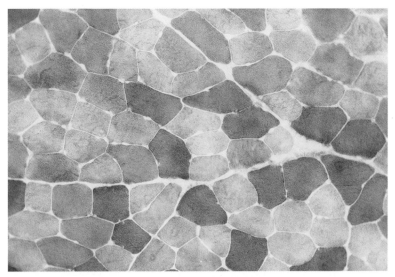

FIG. 3.13 *Fibre type pattern following staining for phosphorylase with higher activity in type 2 than type 1 fibres.*

of increased staining at the periphery of fibres, sometimes near capillaries. This is due to clusters of peripheral mitochondria (Figs 3.11 and 3.12).

Phosphorylase

Phosphorylase is present in the aqueous sarcoplasm and the phosphorylase reaction will thus show up the intermyofibrillar pattern in transverse section. In longitudinal section the enzyme activity is concentrated at the level of the I bands (see section on electron microscopy). In the earlier methods for phosphorylase a clear-cut division into a two-fibre type pattern was obtained; one group of fibres (type 2) giving an intense blue–black or dark-purple colour, while the other group (type 1) was practically negative, with a yellow stain from the iodine. Subsequent modifications and improvements in the technique resulted in the demonstration of intermediate fibres between the two extremes of reaction. As the colour product is dependent on the chain length of the polysaccharide units, gradations of colours are seen. It is thus not possible to define a uniform, single, intermediate fibre type and this has made the reaction more difficult to use for fibre typing. The end product fades rapidly when mounted in aqueous mountants but survives if the section is dehydrated in alcohols and a synthetic resinous mountant is used, although the purple colour may take on a brown/yellow tinge (Fig. 3.13).

Periodic acid-Schiff stain and oil red O

The periodic acid-Schiff (PAS) method stains glycogen and polysaccharides a deep-pink colour and highlights the intermyofibrillar network pattern. Counter

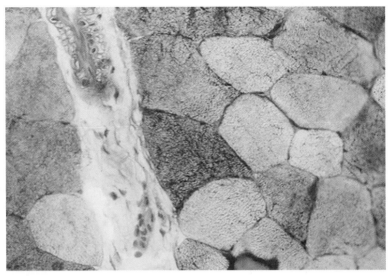

FIG. 3.14 *Section stained with PAS showing a fibre type pattern with more glycogen in type 2 fibres.*

staining with haematoxylin shows the position of the nuclei. Type 2 fibres are more intensely stained than type 1 and intermediate fibres are also demonstrated (Fig. 3.14). The specificity of the stain for glycogen can be checked by digestion with α-amylase prior to PAS staining. In normal muscle this clearly reveals the polysaccharides of the sarcolemma and capillaries.

Oil red O (ORO) stains lipid red and again differences between fibre types can be seen (Fig. 3.15). The intracellular lipid droplets of the fibres appear as fine red dots of variable size and they are more abundant in type 1 fibres than in type 2. Lipid in any adipocytes can spread over the section and make interpretation difficult.

Ultrastructure of the myofibre
Muscle cell surface

Each multinucleated muscle fibre is enveloped and separated from the extracellular environment by the *sarcolemma* (Fig. 3.16). This is composed of a plasma membrane, the plasmalemma, on the inner surface and the basal lamina on the outer surface. The plasmalemma and basal lamina are closely applied and contract in parallel with one another. Most myonuclei lie just beneath the plasmalemma.

The *basal lamina* is the external coat of the muscle fibre and is secreted by the muscle cell itself. It appears as an amorphous or finely granular layer and is about 20–30 nm thick. Components of the basal lamina (also referred to as the lamina densa) include glycoproteins, collagens, laminins, perlecan and nidogen (entactin). Beneath the lamina densa is the lamina lucida which appears as a

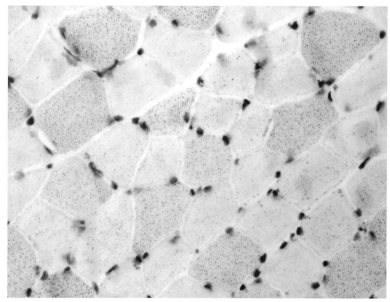

FIG. 3.15 *Section stained with oil red O showing more lipid droplets in type 1 fibres. Mean fibre diameter is approximately 38 μm.*

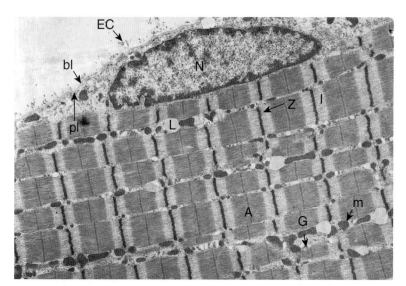

FIG. 3.16 *Electron micrograph of normal human muscle from a needle biopsy showing the major components of each fibre in longitudinal section. The nucleus (N) is beneath the plasma membrane (pl) of the sarcolemma and the basal lamina (bl) with the reticular layer of extracellular collagen (EC) adjacent to basal lamina. The myofibrils show a clear striation pattern of A and I bands (A and I) and Z lines (Z). Mitochondria (m), lipid (L) and glycogen (G) are present between the myofibrils. The A band is 1.5–1.6 μm in length.*

10–15 nm translucent gap between the plasma membrane and lamina lucida and is traversed by fine bridges. It is probably these bridges that ensure that the plasma membrane and lamina densa move in harmony with each other. External to these two regions is the reticular layer composed of collagens, including types III, V and VI, proteoglycans and fibronectin. In pathological muscle the reticular layer may become thickened and prominent. The distribution of the various extracellular matrix proteins, at the ultrastructural level, in relation to each other and to the basement membrane is not yet clear.

The term 'basal lamina' is often used synonymously with 'basement membrane' and the exact structure being referred to is then unclear. The basement membrane described by early histologists (Bowman 1840) refers to the lamina densa and the reticular layer. Throughout this book the term 'basal lamina' is used to describe the lamina densa (the fine granular layer) and the term 'basement membrane' when the reticular layer is also included.

The *plasmalemma* is the electrically excitable membrane of the fibre and is composed of a lipid bilayer and a variety of ion channels and structural, receptor and metabolically active proteins. A number of proteins of pathological significance are located at the plasmalemma and have transmembrane domains. These include proteins of the dystrophin-associated complexes, which link the extracellular matrix with the actin cytoskeleton beneath the sarcolemma, and dysferlin (Bashir et al 1998, Liu et al 1998, Cohn and Campbell 2000, Michele and Campbell 2003). The plasmalemma extends into the muscle fibre in the form of the transverse tubular system (see below) and carries the action potential deep into the fibre. Although the plasmalemma and T system are continuous their protein composition is different. Intermediate filaments, 10 nm in diameter, intermediate between actin and myosin, are associated with the plasmalemma. They surround and link the myofibrils at the level of the Z line to the sarcolemma and to each other, keeping them in register.

The *cytoskeleton* beneath the plasmalemma has a growing number of proteins associated with it, many of which have been studied in diseased muscle, such as β-spectrin, dystrophin, vimentin, vinculin, plectin, desmin (skeletin), nestin and syncoilin. Many of these proteins have been shown to have a costameric periodicity and are concentrated over the Z line and I bands. It has been suggested that the costameres are physically coupled with the underlying myofibrils and are thought to be involved in the lateral transmission of force along the muscle fibre (Pardo et al 1983, Porter et al 1992).

Our understanding of the full macromolecular structure of the plasmalemma is still developing but the distribution of proteins spanning the lipid bilayer can be studied by freeze fracture techniques. Freeze fracture and etching techniques reveal the integral proteins as intramembrane particles or pits on both faces of the membrane. Variations in these distributions have been studied in relation to development, physiological function and disease. Freeze fracture of the plasmalemma also reveals caveolae or small invaginations, particularly on the protoplasmic (P) face. Although their function is not fully known, proteins associated with them such as caveolin-3 are of pathological importance (McNally

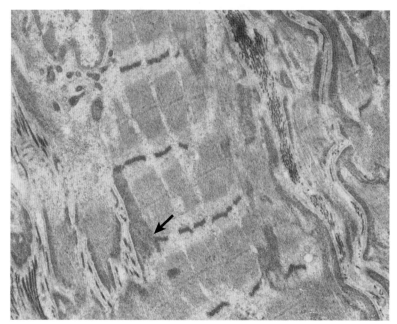

FIG. 3.17 *Electron micrograph of a fibre near a myotendinous junction. The sarcolemma is very folded and the plasmalemma shows an electron dense layer that merges with the Z line (arrow).*

et al 1998). With conventional transmission electron microscopy, the caveolae are seen as numerous small vesicles along the internal surface of the plasma membrane. They are continuous with the plasma membrane and open to the extracellular space. They tend to be more common over the I band regions.

The morphology of the sarcolemma shows variations from the description above at specialized regions of the muscle cell surface. One such region is the myotendinous junction where the surface becomes ridged and folded. The plasmalemma at these points shows a marked layer of electron-dense material which merges with the Z line of the myofibrils (Fig. 3.17; see also Fig. 3.8).

Another specialized region of the sarcolemma is the neuromuscular junction (see below) where the plasmalemma is thrown into post-synaptic clefts. Basal lamina separates the myofibre sole-plate from the axon terminal and extends into the clefts (see Fig. 3.25). The plasmalemma also shows indentations at the site of satellite cells (Fig. 3.18). These mononucleated cells have their own plasma membrane and lie beneath the basal lamina. They are a population of undifferentiated cells that are capable of differentiating into myoblasts and subsequently giving rise to new myotubes. Satellite cells have nuclei with dense peripheral heterochromatin and a small volume of cytoplasm that contains few organelles, free ribosomes, rough endoplasmic reticulum, glycogen, microtubules and intermediate filaments. Organized contractile myofilaments are characteristically absent. Satellite cells are often found near peripheral myonuclei and their

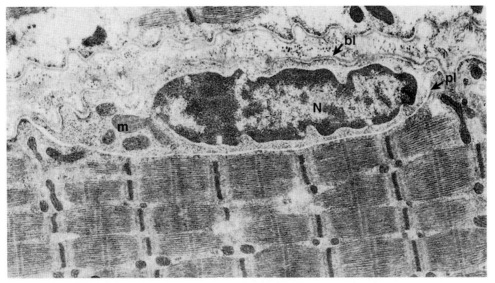

FIG. 3.18 *Satellite cell in normal human muscle between the basal lamina (bl) and plasma membrane (pl) of the fibre. The nucleus (N) is heterochromatic and occupies a large volume of the cell. The cytoplasm contains mitochondria (m), ribosomes and glycogen.*

frequency declines with age. Increased numbers have been found near neuro-muscular junctions and in diseased situations, including denervation, and in regeneration.

Nuclei

In normal muscle the myonuclei lie beneath the sarcolemma, although an occasional one located internally in the fibre may be seen (see Fig. 3.16). Each nucleus has a domain for gene expression, the size of which varies with the gene. Nuclei are elongated structures aligned parallel to the myofibrils and are about 5 μm in length. The nuclear membrane is indented in many places and nuclear pores fenestrate it allowing the trafficking of RNA and proteins in both directions. It is continuous with the endoplasmic reticulum which is in continuity with the sarcoplasmic reticulum (see below). The nuclear membrane has the pathologically important proteins associated with it, emerin and lamin A/C (see Ch. 13). Emerin is a component of the nuclear membrane itself whilst lamin A/C, along with other lamins and related proteins, is localized to the nuclear lamina beneath the nuclear membrane. Chromatin, containing the DNA and histones, is condensed in normal muscle nuclei and is granular in appearance. It is known as heterochromatin and is anchored to the nuclear membrane. Metabolically active chromatin (euchromatin) is in the pale internal areas along with the nuclear matrix which cannot be distinguished by electron microscopy. Each nucleus has one or two nucleoli where ribosomal transcription occurs.

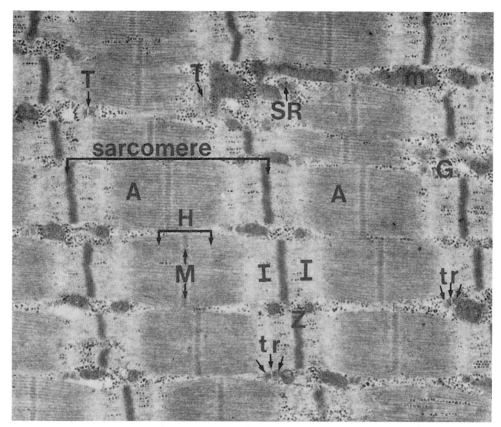

FIG. 3.19 *High power electron micrograph of normal muscle showing the myofibrillar structure and intracellular organelles. Each sarcomere is defined as the area between two Z lines (Z). The I band (I) is bisected by the dense Z line and the band of cross-bridges in the centre of the A band (A) forms the M line (M). The slightly paler H zone (H) in the A bands is delimited by the ends of the interdigitating thin filaments and contains no myosin heads. Triads (tr) are present near the A/I band junction with a pale T tubule (T) and dense lateral sacs. Sarcoplasmic reticulum (SR) and mitochondria (m) lie between the myofibrils and glycogen granules (G) are present between the myofibrils and within the I band. The A band is 1.5–1.6 µm in length.*

Myofibrils

The myofibrils are the major cellular constituent of the fibre and occupy 85–90% of its volume. Each myofibril is composed of a bundle of myofilaments regularly aligned to form repeating structures known as sarcomeres. The regular alternation of different proteins within each sarcomere gives rise to the characteristic striated pattern of skeletal muscle (Fig. 3.19). Each sarcomere is composed of a dark anisotropic band (A band) flanked on either side by a light isotropic band (I band). The central region of the A band is traversed by a narrow dense line, the M line, and is adjoined on either side by the slightly paler H zone. The filaments of the I band are attached to the narrow, dense Z line (Z disc) which marks the longitudinal boundary of each sarcomere (Fig. 3.19). At rest, each sarcomere is 2.5–3.0 µm in length. Contraction of the myofibre occurs by shortening of the sarcomere and is accomplished by the I filaments sliding towards the centre of the A band. During this the I band and H zone shorten but the A band remains at a constant length of 1.5–1.6 µm.

The *A band* consists of a hexagonal lattice of thick myosin filaments 15–18 nm in diameter and 1.5–1.6 µm in length. The myosin molecules of the A band are double-stranded helices with a rod-shaped flexible shaft of light meromyosin joined to two pear-shaped heads of heavy meromyosin. The molecules are arranged so that the light meromyosin molecules oppose one another and the heads point towards the end of the filament and lie on the surface. The region of overlap of the light meromyosin tails with no myosin heads gives rise to the central pale *H zone* in the centre of the A band. In the middle of the H zone is the *M line*, which appears as three to five lines across the thick filaments, the number being fibre-type dependent. The M line is believed to have a role in connecting the myosin filaments and giving stability to the A band. Proteins localized to the M lines include myomesin, skelemin, M protein and a fraction of creatine kinase.

The *I band* filaments are chiefly composed of thin actin polymers of filamentous (F) actin arranged in a double helix and 6–7 nm in diameter. In the grooves of the actin helix is a helix of tropomyosin, to which it is attached at regular intervals. The tropomyosin spiral also has globular troponin complexes regularly attached to it. The actin filaments are anchored at one end to the Z line. The other end interdigitates with myosin filaments to form a lattice in such a manner that each myosin filament is surrounded by six actin filaments (Fig. 3.20). The region of the A band between two sets of I filaments is pale, contains no myosin heads and forms the H zone (see Fig. 3.19). The length of both the I band and H zone is dependent on the state of contraction of the muscle. Similarly the prominence of the M line that traverses the I band varies with the state of contraction.

At the surface of the Z line, the actin filaments are organized into a square lattice and although this is similar to the pattern of tropomyosin crystals, this protein has only been shown in very small amounts in the Z line. The major proteins of the Z line are α-actinin and actin. There is increasing interest in proteins that interact with α-actinin as Z line abnormalities occur in a number of neuromuscular disorders and mutations in some of the corresponding genes have been identified (see Ch. 6). The proteins studied include telethonin (cap protein), myozenin, zeugmentin, syncoilin (see below), vinculin, γ-filamin, obscurin and myotilin (Stromer 1995, Takada et al 2001, Selcen and Engel 2004). Also attached to the Z line are two very large proteins, titin and nebulin, both of which are of pathological importance. A single molecule of titin stretches from the Z line to the M line with its entire N-terminus in the Z line. Titin molecules of adjacent sarcomeres overlap in the Z line and M line. The portion of titin in the I band is believed to be elastic and to act as a molecular ruler, having a role in passive tension during stretching of the myofibrils. Three to six titin molecules are associated with each myosin filament and there may be lateral associations with actin. It has a binding site for calpain-3. Nebulin is specific to skeletal

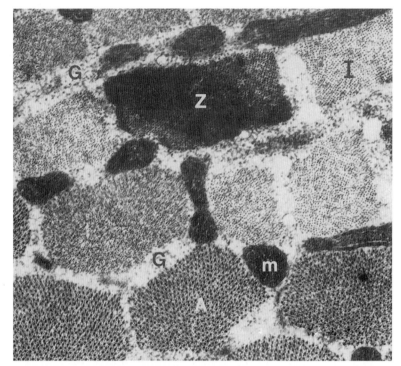

FIG. 3.20 *Electron micrograph from a transversely orientated fibre. Some areas are sectioned slightly obliquely and the myofibrils are not quite in phase with one another, making it possible to see the different myofibrillar regions. The Z line (Z) is dense but components of the lattice are visible. I band (I) actin filaments are adjacent to this. The A band (A) is sectioned in the region where I band filaments are present and the thin actin filaments can be seen around the thick myosin filaments. Mitochondria (m) and glycogen (G) are seen between the myofibrils.*

muscle and is orientated in reverse with its C-terminus anchored in the Z line and extending into the I band. It makes side to side contact with titin and may have a role in regulating the length of the actin filaments. It is now apparent that sarcomeric proteins not only have a structural role but are also involved in signalling pathways (Bönnemann and Laing 2004). A diagrammatic representation of the structure of a sarcomere showing proteins of pathological significance is shown in Figure 3.21.

Sarcoplasm

Each myofibril with its repetitive sequence of sarcomeres is surrounded by the cytoplasm of the fibre, the sarcoplasm. This contains several organelles, including mitochondria, the sarcoplasmic reticulum and T tubule membrane systems, Golgi apparatus and a cytoskeleton of microtubules, intermediate filaments and microfilaments of actin, as well as glycogen, free ribosomes, lipid droplets and lipofuscin. The glycogen granules are 15–30 nm in size and, although not limited

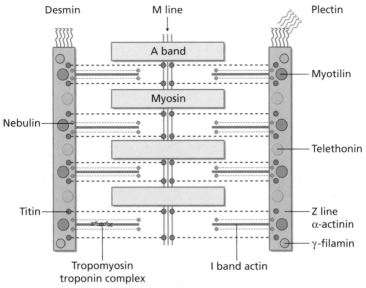

FIG. 3.21 *Diagrammatic representation of the major protein components of a sarcomere. The actin filaments are anchored to the Z line and overlap with the myosin filaments. The N-terminus of titin is in the Z line and it stretches to and spans the M line. The C-terminus of nebulin inserts into the Z line but does not fully span it. The N-terminus of nebulin is located near the ends of the actin filaments. The tropomyosin–tropinin complex is the grooves of each actin filament. Several proteins interact with α-actinin in the Z line; some of known pathological significance are depicted here. Desmin is at the periphery of the Z line and links the myofibrils to each other and to the sarcolemma. Plectin interacts with desmin.*

to any one part of the fibre, are more numerous at the level of the I band than the A band (see Fig. 3.19). Free ribosomes are seen in the subsarcolemmal region and increased numbers are often found in the perinuclear zones, along with Golgi membranes, intermediate filaments and microtubules. Golgi are not often observed, however. Microtubules are cylindrical tubes several micrometers long and 18–25 nm in diameter. Their major protein is tubulin.

Several of the intermediate filament proteins of the sarcoplasmic cytoskeleton are more abundant in immature muscle. Desmin, as previously stated, surrounds the myofibrils and links them to each other and to the plasmalemma. It is prominent in developing fibres and in certain disease situations. It is not, however, morphologically conspicuous in normal adult skeletal muscle, although it is often prominent at the sarcolemma in immunolabelled sections. Vimentin and nestin are also abundant in developing fibres but are down-regulated as fibres mature. Vimentin, however, persists in blood vessels and nestin is abundant at neuromuscular and myotendinous junctions. Syncoilin and desmuslin are recently identified intermediate filament proteins in muscle (Blake and Martin-Rendon 2002) that bind α-dystrobrevin, a component of the dystrophin-associated protein complex, and may act to tether the intermediate network to

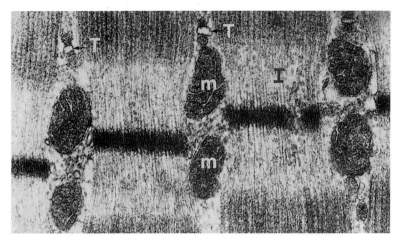

FIG. 3.22 *Electron micrograph showing triads at the A–I band junction. The pale T tubule (T) has on either side a lateral sac filled with amorphous material. Mitochondria (m) are shown at the level of the I band.*

this complex. Similar to desmin, syncoilin is found at the neuromuscular junction, and throughout the sarcolemma at the level of the Z lines and recent data suggest they interact (Poon et al 2002).

Mitochondria

Mitochondria are membranous structures concerned with the energy supply of the fibre and with the intracellular regulation of calcium. Although the size and shape of the mitochondria can be variable, they are usually small and ovoid (Fig. 3.22). They have a single outer membrane and an inner membrane with deep folds known as cristae. The central region is occupied by amorphous material which often contains small, dense granules of calcium deposits.

Mitochondria are found in intermyofibrillar regions adjacent to the I bands (Fig. 3.22) and also in subsarcolemmal clusters (see histochemical stains in Figs 3.11 and 3.12). They tend to occur in greater numbers in type 1 fibres, but in human muscle differences in mitochondrial volume are not a consistent feature distinguishing type 1 from type 2 fibres (see below).

Internal membrane systems

The internal membrane systems, the transverse tubular system (T system) and the sarcoplasmic reticulum, are interrelated membrane systems concerned with the excitation of the fibre during contraction and relaxation.

The *T system* is a branched network of tubules that runs transversely across the fibre. It is developed from and continuous with the plasma membrane of the sarcolemma, allowing the rapid passage of depolarization into the interior of the fibre. In conventional electron microscopic preparations the lumen of the tubules appears empty but it is easily penetrated by fixatives and substances such as lanthanum, horseradish peroxidase and ferritin. In man each sarcomere has two tubular networks at the level of the junction between the A and I bands (Fig. 3.22).

The *sarcoplasmic reticulum* is a fenestrated sheath of membranes between and around each myofibril and is responsible for the release and uptake of calcium ions during contraction and relaxation. At the level of the A/I band interface the sarcoplasmic reticulum forms continuous lateral sacs or terminal cisternae. Two terminal cisternae are in close contact with, but separate from, a T system tubule and collectively these form a *triad* (Fig. 3.22). The repetitive arrangement of triads gives a regular pattern at the A/I band junction along and across the length of the fibre. The lateral sacs of the triads can be distinguished from the T tubules by their amorphous or granular electron-dense material. Other parts of the sarcoplasmic reticulum network do not contain this dense matrix and their smaller size makes them more difficult to distinguish in normal muscle (see Fig. 3.19). The T tubule of the triad is the site of the voltage-gated calcium channel, the dihydropyridine receptor, which is activated by the action potential and induces the ryanodine receptor of the lateral sacs to release calcium. At high magnifications the ryanodine receptors can be seen as dense 'feet' bridging the junction of the lateral sacs and T tubules.

Ultrastructure of fibre types

There are several differences in fibre types at the ultrastructural level and attempts have been made to correlate these features with the histochemical and physiological properties, both in man and other vertebrates. The use of ultrathin frozen sections greatly improved the ultrastructural identification of different fibre types (Sjöström and Squire 1977). The organelles analysed include the Z line, M line, number and distribution of mitochondria, volume and surface area of sarcoplasmic reticulum, T system and triads, glycogen and lipid content.

In animals correlative studies are easier because muscles composed of a single type can be examined. In general, type 1 fibres tend to have wider Z lines and more mitochondria and lipid, but smaller amounts of sarcoplasmic reticulum, T system, triads and glycogen. In addition, studies of ultrathin frozen sections have shown that the M line appearance is characteristic of the fibre type, muscle and species from which the section has been taken.

In human muscle ultrastructural differences between fibre types are less easy to identify because most muscles are of mixed fibre type and no single feature can accurately be used to define the fibre type (Cullen and Weightman 1975, Prince et al 1981). However, a combination of two or more parameters greatly enhances the success rate. Sjöström et al (1982) showed that the Z line and M line are good indicators of fibre type and even when using the M line alone, 95% of fibres could be accurately identified. Type 1 fibres have broad Z lines and five strong M bridge lines; type 2A fibres have intermediate Z lines, and three strong M bridge lines and two weak ones; and type 2B fibres have

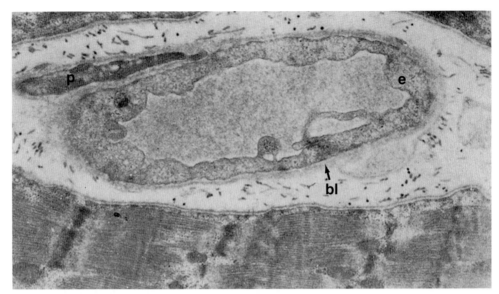

FIG. 3.23 *Electron micrograph of a muscle capillary. Endothelial cells (e) contain numerous pinocytotic vesicles and pericytes (p) are closely applied to the external surface. Basal lamina (bl) covers the external surface and pericytes.*

narrow Z lines and three strong M bridge lines, with the two outer ones very weak or absent.

Ultrastructure of other components in muscle

Muscle capillaries

Muscle capillaries are frequently seen in ultrathin sections and often lie in indentations of the sarcolemma. The endothelial cells contain numerous pinocytotic vesicles but they lack tight junctions (Fig. 3.23). Pericytes are closely applied to the external surface of the endothelial cells and the capillary basal lamina covers the external surface.

Intramuscular nerves

Occasionally an intramuscular nerve is encountered in a biopsy. Schwann cells and both myelinated and unmyelinated axons can be seen and these are surrounded by layers of perineural cells and basal lamina. Within the endoneural space the axons are surrounded by collagen (Fig. 3.24). Pathological changes in peripheral nerves are usually assessed in biopsies of the sural nerve, a sensory nerve. Artefacts in intramuscular peripheral nerves can easily occur and caution in the interpretation of morphological features is therefore needed.

Neuromuscular junction

The point of contact between the nerve terminal and the muscle fibre, the neuromuscular synapse, is a specialized region designed to allow the rapid

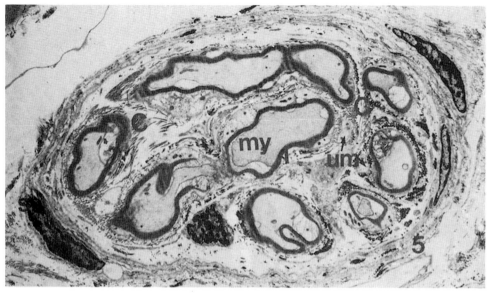

FIG. 3.24 *Electron micrograph of an intramuscular nerve. Myelinated (my) and unmyelinated (um) axons are present and surrounded by layers of perineural cells and basal lamina. Within the endoneural space the axons are surrounded by collagen (C).*

transmission of the impulse from the nerve to the fibre (Fig. 3.25). It is a complex structure, consisting of deep post-synaptic clefts and a pre-synaptic unmyelinated portion of the nerve that is covered by Schwann cell processes. A double layer of basal lamina extends into the folds and anchors neuromuscular junction-specific proteins such as acetylcholine esterase, agrin and neuregulins. With immunohistochemistry a number of proteins, for example dystrophin, can be seen to be concentrated at the neuromuscular junction. This is often a reflection of the membrane folding. In normal mature muscle fibres, proteins such as neural cell adhesion molecule (N-CAM) and utrophin are localized only to the neuromuscular junction and not to extrajunctional regions. The distribution of some proteins within the folds is known, for example utrophin is at the crest with the acetylcholine receptors whereas dystrophin is localized at the bottom with the voltage-gated sodium channels. The complexity of the post-synaptic folds differs with fibre type and in fast-twitch fibres they are usually deeper and more branched. Under the electron microscope the post-synaptic membrane of the nerve terminal may appear darker than the extrajunctional regions because of the aggregation of the acetylcholine receptors (Fig. 3.25). The pre-synaptic nerve terminal contains numerous synaptic vesicles and organelles, in particular mitochondria. The myonuclei around neuromuscular junctions are specialized and have a role in the transcription of the specific proteins of the neuromuscular junction. Alterations in nerve axons and neuromuscular junctions occur in a variety of disorders.

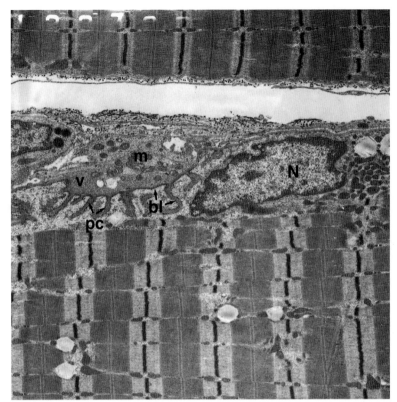

FIG. 3.25 *Electron micrograph of a neuromuscular junction. Basal lamina (bl) extends into the postsynaptic clefts (pc). The pre-synaptic axon contains numerous vesicles (v) and mitochondria (m). A subsarcolemmal nucleus (N) is seen on the right of the micrograph.*

Development of human muscle

An understanding of the salient aspects of myogenesis and the maturation of muscle is important to the understanding of muscle pathology. Muscle fibre regeneration is a common feature of pathological muscle, particularly in the muscular dystrophies, and examination of neonatal muscle to exclude a neuromuscular disorder or in congenital myopathies may be required. Many muscle proteins are developmentally regulated and this is relevant to the interpretation of immunohistochemical data and will be discussed in Chapter 6. Here we will discuss the basic development of muscle and the properties of fetal muscle. Muscle forms from somitic myoblasts, the determination of which is controlled by a family of basic helix–loop–helix transcription factors, the myogenic regulator factors (MRF family). The limb and trunk muscles develop from the mesoderm of the somites, whereas the facial and cervical muscles develop from the branchial arches. From about 7 weeks of gestation, post-mitotic myoblasts fuse

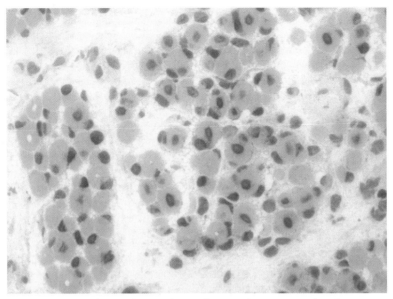

FIG. 3.26 *Muscle from a human fetus of 14 weeks gestation showing primary and secondary myotubes ranging from 5 to 18 μm in diameter (H&E).*

synchronously to form primary myotubes, which express a number of muscle specific proteins such as desmin, titin and nebulin. These myotubes have large central nuclei with a prominent nucleolus, and scattered myofibrils. Early primary myotubes are clustered within a common basal lamina and as differentiation continues they become separated by undifferentiated, mononucleated cells, and basal lamina is deposited round each one. Secondary myotubes then arise from successive waves of fusion of post-mitotic myoblasts along the surface of the primary myotubes (Fig. 3.26). These are initially encased within the same basal lamina as the parent primary myotube but they later separate and each develops its own basal lamina. In small animals the number of fibres of a muscle is set by birth, or soon after, and only fibre growth occurs postnatally, whereas in humans some fibre formation is thought to occur up to 4 months of age. Alterations in fibre number per muscle, however, can occur as a result of pathological processes and of ageing. Fibres increase in length by the addition of sarcomeres to the end of the fibres.

Histochemically there appears to be three phases in the maturation of human fetal muscle (Dubowitz 1965, 1966):

- up to about 18 weeks' gestation, where the muscle is uniform and undifferentiated and the fibres cannot readily be categorized as type 1 or type 2 on the basis of the reciprocal activity of oxidative enzymes and phosphorylase and ATPase;
- from about 20 to 28 weeks' gestation, where a small proportion of larger type 1 fibres, strong in oxidative enzymes and weak in phosphorylase and

ATPase, are readily recognized whilst the remainder are still undifferentiated;

● after about 28 weeks, where a checkerboard pattern of type 1 and type 2 fibres can be distinguished.

At birth, in both full-term and preterm infants, muscle appears histochemically to be differentiated into fibre types but the intensity of staining is not as strong as in mature muscle.

Using variable preincubation pH for the ATPase reaction 2C fibres can be distinguished in immature muscle and Brooke et al (1971) suggested that the 2C fibres were a precursor of the type 1 as well as the 2A and 2B fibres. This was later confirmed by the detailed histochemical studies of developing human muscle by Farkas-Bargeton et al (1977) and Colling-Saltin (1978) who showed that the undifferentiated fibres during the first phase of development were 2C fibres, and that after about 20 weeks' gestation type 1 fibres begin to appear, and after about 30 weeks' gestation type 2A and 2B. At birth, the process of differentiation is not yet complete and there are still about 15–20% of undifferentiated type 2C fibres, and the proportion of 2A fibres is still higher than 2B. In the course of the first year of life the proportion of type 1 fibres gradually increases at the expense of the undifferentiated 2C fibres; by 1 year of age the type 1 fibres comprise about 60–65% and type 2 fibres about 30–35%, with the 2A fibres still predominant and the 2C fibres only about 3–5%. At birth and during the neonatal period some fibres with a particularly large diameter stain intensely with histological stains and have properties of type 1 fibres. These are considered to be the B fibres described in the 1930s by Wohlfart ('Wohlfart B fibres').

This histochemical profile can now be interpreted in the light of myosin heavy chain expression and the developmental expression of different isoforms. There has been considerable debate as to whether the different fibre types arise from different populations of myoblasts and different studies have produced variable results. However, work from the group of Butler-Browne (Bonavaud et al 2001), using single fibres in tissue culture, suggests that satellite cells from a single fibre of human muscle, in contrast to other species, can give rise to either a fast or slow fibre. This, however, has to be interpreted in the knowledge that some cells from a single fibre may be stem cells and be multipotential. Myosin heavy chain isoforms are expressed sequentially. Early primary myotubes express only an embryonic isoform. This is then replaced by a fetal/neonatal form and myotubes then take on the profile of a fast or slow myotube. Innervation and hormones have an important role in this differentiation. Most primary myotubes take on the profile of slow fibres and express only slow myosin. These survive into the neonatal period. Secondary myotubes, however, are hybrid fibres and can express variable combinations of fetal/neonatal, fast and slow myosin (Fig. 3.27a–c). In human fetal quadriceps muscle a population of secondary myotubes, sometimes referred to as tertiary myotubes (Draeger et al 1987), appears as a population of very small myotubes that only express fast and neonatal myosin, never slow myosin (Fig. 3.27c). Neonatal myosin is frequently

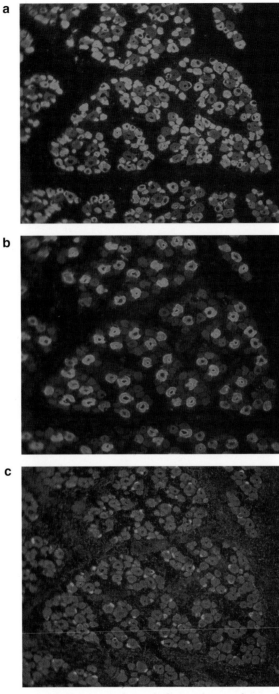

FIG. 3.27 *Serial areas of muscle from a human fetus of 14 weeks gestation immunolabelled with antibodies to (a) neonatal, (b) slow and (c) fast isoforms of myosin heavy chains showing only slow myosin in the large primary myotubes, co-expression of various isoforms in secondary myotubes and very small tertiary myotubes with only fast myosin.*

co-expressed with fast myosin and at birth many fibres will label with antibodies to both fetal/neonatal and fast myosin. The stage at which this immature fetal/neonatal isoform is switched off in human muscle is not clear as samples from most neonates have been taken for a medical reason and cannot necessarily be classified as normal. In our experience many fibres from neonates express fetal/neonatal myosin and even at 6 months of age an appreciable number may be present and a few remain even up to 1 year.

CHAPTER 4

Definition of pathological changes seen in muscle biopsies

This section will deal with the various changes which may occur in a muscle under pathological conditions. As will be seen, very few abnormalities are in themselves pathognomonic of a particular disease. However, by evaluating the constellation of different changes that are present within a given biopsy, and assessing these in the context of clinical features of the patient, one can usually obtain a fairly accurate diagnosis.

In order to describe the abnormalities seen in various muscle diseases, a vocabulary of pathological changes is needed. These are the building blocks of muscle pathology. We shall try to define what we mean by various terms such as internal nuclei, fibre splitting, 'moth-eaten' fibres, and to assess their significance in relation to specific muscle pathology.

The various abnormalities will be considered under the following headings:

Changes in fibre shape and size
Changes in fibre type patterns
Changes in sarcolemmal nuclei
Degeneration and regeneration
Fibrosis and adipose tissue
Cellular reactions
Changes in fibre architecture and structural abnormalities
Deficiency of enzymes
Accumulation of glycogen or lipid
Common artefacts in muscle biopsies

Changes in fibre shape and size

In normal muscle fibres have a polygonal shape but in pathological situations they may become rounded, as in muscular dystrophies (Fig. 4.1), or very angulated, as may be seen in denervating disorders (Fig. 4.2). The observer must also

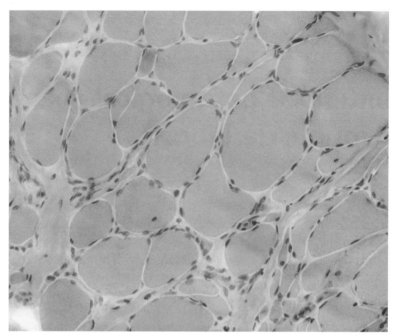

FIG. 4.1 *H&E stained section from a 5-year-old boy with Duchenne muscular dystrophy showing a wide range of fibre sizes (15–125 μm) many of which have a round shape and are separated by excess endomysial connective tissue.*

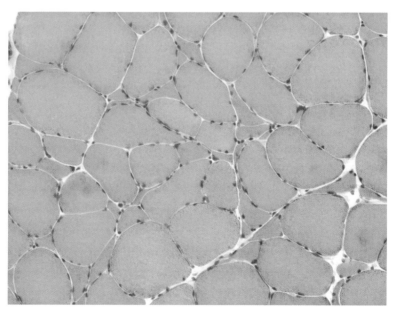

FIG. 4.2 *A small cluster of atrophic fibres (size range 10–17 μm) surrounded by normal sized fibres and hypertrophied fibres up to 135 μm in an adult male with motor neurone disease. Note the angular shape of some atrophic fibres (H&E).*

be aware of artefacts induced by poor handling of the specimen or problems with the staining procedures (see end of this chapter). Assessment of changes in fibre size is fundamental to interpretation and this has a physiological as well as a pathological basis. Fibre size is regulated and influenced by innervation, a number of growth factors such as hormones, insulin-like growth factor, myostatin and other members of the transforming growth factor family, and the amount of work the muscle is subjected to. All of these aspects have a role in pathological muscle. Excessive load on a muscle induces an increase in fibre size (hypertrophy) while disuse causes a decrease in size (atrophy). Fibres will also atrophy when deprived of the trophic influence of their nerve. Longitudinal splitting and branching of fibres occurs under certain pathological circumstances and also results in the appearance of small fibres in cross-section. Some small fibres in a biopsy may be regenerating and must be distinguished from atrophic fibres (see later).

The distribution of large and small fibres is one of the most important criteria for differentiating the myopathies, or so-called 'primary' disorders of muscle, from the neurogenic changes secondary to a denervating process. In myopathies the distribution of the enlarged and small fibres is random and diffuse, whereas in denervation, both occur in clusters or large groups.

It is usually possible to get an impression of the variability and change in fibre size by simple inspection of a biopsy under the microscope. At times the change may be quite clear-cut and unequivocal, but this is not always the case and measurement of fibre diameter is then helpful. This may be done by a simple measurement of the diameter of the smallest and largest fibres with an eyepiece micrometer to establish the range of sizes, and if this is appropriate for the age and sex. A more detailed and accurate appraisal may be made by preparing a histogram of fibre diameters (see below) and comparing it with the data for normal muscle of similar sex and age. There have been a number of attempts to automate and computerize the quantification of fibre sizes, based either on fibre diameter or fibre area in cross-section, but this is time consuming and all methods require a degree of manual involvement. As some workers find this type of assessment useful we have retained aspects of quantification in this section in relation to each fibre type. In practice we now rarely perform detailed studies and rely on measuring the range of fibre diameters within the whole sample. This will determine if the variability of fibre sizes is appropriate for age and will ensure that a pathological process that uniformly affects all fibres does not give a misleading impression.

Atrophy and hypertrophy

A common occurrence is atrophy of only some of the fibres in a biopsy, either singly or in small clusters. When this occurs, the small fibres are usually obvious in comparison to the remaining large fibres. This *small group atrophy* is characteristic, but not diagnostic, of denervation (Fig. 4.2), and in some neurogenic disorders there is *large group atrophy* (Fig. 4.3). This is accompanied by diffuse

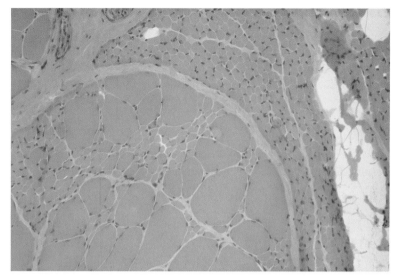

FIG. 4.3 *Distinct groups of atrophic and hypertrophic fibres in a child with spinal muscular atrophy (H&E). Hypertrophic fibres up to 100 μm.*

hypertrophy (Fig. 4.2) or *group hypertrophy* (Fig. 4.3). It should be noted that splitting of a larger fibre may produce an apparent group of small fibres and branching of fibres will also contribute to the impression of fibre size variability (see Fig. 4.27). For this reason caution should be exercised in interpreting small group atrophy in the presence of fibre splitting, or other pathological changes suggestive of a myopathy. Serial sections may be necessary to track a splitting or branched fibre.

In some disorders, such as some congenital myopathies, very small fibres may be difficult to identify with routine stains as they may be hardly larger than a single nucleus. These very small fibres are scattered through the biopsy and can be seen clearly with immunohistochemistry using antibodies to neonatal myosin (see Ch. 6, Fig. 6.25). It is important to remember that not all small fibres are atrophic as some may be regenerating fibres. In myopathic conditions the atrophic and hypertrophic fibres are randomly distributed through the sample (Fig. 4.4). Sometimes, as in congenital myopathies, two distinct populations of fibres of different sizes are apparent but they are not grouped (Fig. 4.5) as seen in denervating disorders (see Fig. 4.3).

In dermatomyositis fibres at the periphery of the fascicles may be small. Some of these are atrophic and some are regenerating. This appearance is called *perifascicular atrophy* and is thought to reflect ischaemic changes secondary to disease of the vessels. It is only seen in dermatomyositis, but not universally (Fig. 4.6).

Aspects of atrophy and hypertrophy relating to each fibre type are discussed in the next section.

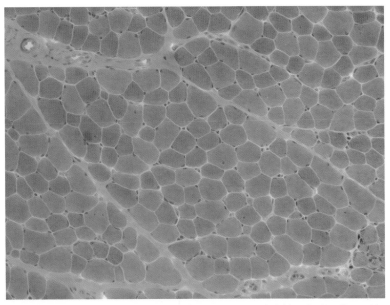

FIG. 4.4 *Fibres of various diameters (range 5–45 μm) diffusely distributed in a boy with Becker muscular dystrophy (Gomori trichrome).*

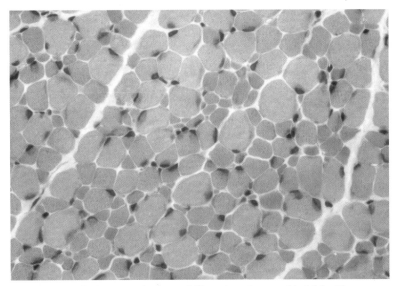

FIG. 4.5 *Two distinct populations of fibres in a 5-year-old child with a congenital myopathy. One population is within the normal range for age (25–30 μm) but appears smaller because of the hypertrophied adjacent fibres up to 65 μm.*

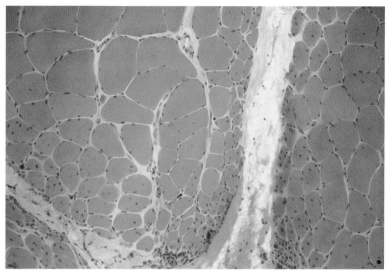

FIG. 4.6 *Small fibres restricted to perifascicular areas in a case of dermatomyositis (H&E).*

Changes in fibre type patterns

Changes in fibre size may specifically affect one or other fibre type, or it may affect both types. In normal muscle, as shown in Chapter 3, there is a checkerboard, mosaic pattern of type 1 and type 2 fibres. In most myopathic conditions a random pattern of atrophic and hypertrophic fibres of both types is seen (Fig. 4.7). In neurogenic disorders, such as spinal muscular atrophy, the groups of atrophic fibres are of both fibres while the groups of hypertrophic fibres are type 1 (Fig. 4.8). The grouping results from collateral sprouting of surviving nerves that reinnervate the denervated fibres. It is important to distinguish fibre type grouping from fibre type predominance (see below). Only groups of both fibre types should be used as evidence of denervation/reinnervation.

Atrophy of type 2 fibres is a non-specific finding that can occur in a number of myopathic situations, not all of which can be defined. It appears in almost any disease in which muscle strength is impaired secondary to problems remote from the muscle. It can be induced by disuse and by corticosteroid therapy (Fig. 4.9). When type 2 subtypes are considered, both 2A and 2B may be affected but specific involvement of type 2B fibres is the most common. Selective type 2A fibre atrophy is very unusual.

Selective *type 1 atrophy* occurs in several congenital myopathies and myotonic dystrophy (Fig. 4.10). Type-specific hypertrophy is much less frequent. However, as mentioned previously the grouped hypertrophic fibres in spinal muscular atrophy are frequently type 1. The hypertrophy of fibres associated with exercise is usually of type 2 fibre and this enlargement of type 2 fibres may account for the normal difference between male muscle (in which type 2 fibres

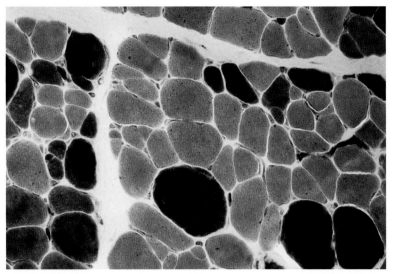

FIG. 4.7 *Variation in size (range 15–80 μm) affecting both fibre types in a case of Becker muscular dystrophy stained for ATPase at pH 9.4. The light fibres are type 1 and the dark type 2. Note also the predominance of the lightly stained type 1 fibres.*

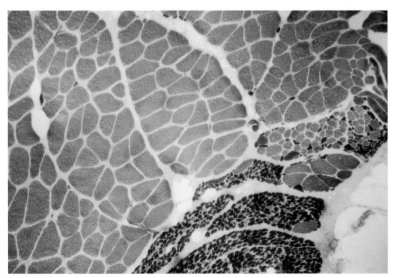

FIG. 4.8 *Fibre type uniformity in a case of spinal muscular atrophy stained for ATPase at pH 9.4. The grouped hypertrophied fibres are all type 1 but the atrophic fibres are of both types.*

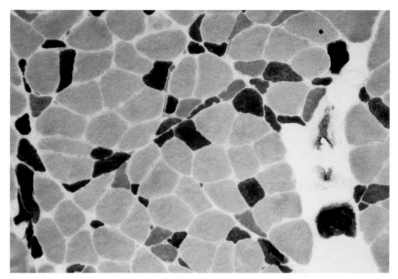

FIG. 4.9 *Atrophy restricted to the darkly stained type 2 fibres, induced by steroid therapy (ATPase reaction preincubated at pH 9.9 and revealing three fibre types; fibres of intermediate intensity are 2A fibres).*

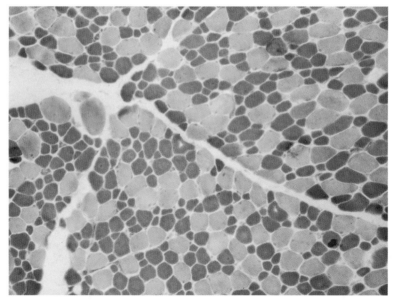

FIG. 4.10 *ATPase staining following preincubation at pH 4.3 showing atrophy selectively affecting the darkly stained type 1 fibres in a case of myotubular myopathy. Note also the hypertrophy of the pale type 2 fibres.*

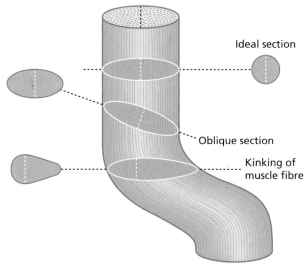

Ideal section

Oblique section

Kinking of
muscle fibre

FIG. 4.11 *This diagram demonstrates the importance of measuring the lesser diameter of each fibre. This is the only measurement not altered by either oblique sectioning or kinking of the fibres, both common occurrences in muscle biopsies.*

are larger than type 1) and female muscle (in which they are roughly equal in size).

Quantification

This section describes the main methods used to quantify the degree of change of fibre sizes and illustrates typical histograms that can be obtained, in relation to fibre types.

The starting point is measurement of the 'lesser diameter' which combines simplicity and speed with reasonable accuracy. This is defined as the maximum diameter across the lesser aspect of the muscle fibre (Fig. 4.11). This measurement is designed to overcome the distortion which occurs when a muscle fibre is cut obliquely, producing an oval appearance in the fibre. Unless the lesser diameter is measured, an erroneously large measurement will result, as Figure 4.11 shows.

Measurements are done on adenosine triphosphatase (ATPase) stained sections so that involvement of each fibre type can be calculated. These can be performed with an eyepiece micrometer or by projecting the imaging on a suitable surface. Several computerized systems are also available but full automation can rarely be achieved as most systems are unable to accurately define two closely adjacent fibres, and this has to be done manually. Computerized systems, however, are useful for calculating cross-sectional area of each fibre type, if the section is perfectly orientated in the transverse plane. A total of at least 100 fibres of each is measured and a histogram of the diameters of each fibre type plotted. This number of fibres has been shown to be representative. A mean fibre diameter and standard deviation is calculated and compared with normal values. Ideally, each laboratory should establish their own normal values but many workers rely on published data (e.g. Brooke and Engel 1969 a–d). A limitation of this is that biopsies used for establishing this normal data in old publications were taken for a clinical reason and, although the samples apparently showed no defects, this cannot be established beyond doubt.

In addition to mean fibre diameter it is important to assess variability. A useful figure is the variability coefficient which is calculated as follows:

$$\frac{\text{Standard deviation} \times 1000}{\text{Mean fibre diameter}}$$

In normal muscle the variability coefficient is less than 250 and any sample with a variability coefficient greater than this is considered to demonstrate abnormal variability in the size of fibres. In children the gradual increase in size with age has to be taken into account.

Atrophy and hypertrophy factors

In an effort to quantify the degree of change of fibre size in a biopsy, atrophy and hypertrophy factors were devised by Brooke and Engel (1969b). These factors are calculated from the histograms of the muscle fibres and are an expression of the number of abnormally small or large fibres in the biopsy. In normal adult muscle most fibres in the histogram are between 40 and 80 μm in diameter in males and 30–70 μm in females. Considering first the abnormally small fibres, a few fibres in the 30–40 μm range in a histogram from a male biopsy would have less significance than the same number of fibres in the range of 10–20 μm or than a larger number of fibres in the same (30–40 μm) range. This is taken into account by multiplying the number of fibres in the histogram with a diameter between 30 and 40 μm by 1, the number of fibres with a diameter between 20 and 30 μm by 2, the number of those from 10 to 20 μm by 3, and the number in the group less than 10 μm by 4. These products are then added together and divided by the total number of fibres in the histogram to put the result on a proportional basis. The resulting number is then multiplied by 1000 and this is the *'atrophy factor'*. The **hypertrophy factor** is similarly derived to express the proportion of fibres larger than 80 μm in the male. A diagrammatic calculation from a histogram is shown in Figure 4.12. In addition to making the calculations for the muscle biopsy as a whole, one can also consider each fibre type separately. Thus, for each histochemical fibre type there are two numbers: the atrophy and hypertrophy factors (abbreviated A or H factors). The histogram for a given biopsy may then be expressed as a series of four numbers for A1, H1, A2 and H2 (atrophy and hypertrophy of type 1 and type 2 fibres, respectively). If fibre subtypes are considered, there will be six numbers: A1, H1, A2A, H2A, A2B and H2B. In adult females the limits 30–70 μm and not 40–80 μm are used to calculate atrophy and hypertrophy factors in a similar way (Table 4.1).

This statistical approach, although somewhat laborious, is useful in detecting the presence of atrophy or hypertrophy that may not be apparent on

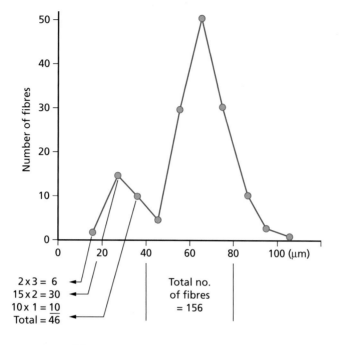

Calculation of A and H Factors

2 x 3 = 6
15 x 2 = 30
10 x 1 = 10
Total = 46

Total no.
of fibres
= 156

A factor = $\dfrac{46}{156}$ = 0.295

H factor = $\dfrac{19}{156}$ = 0.122

FIG. 4.12 *Calculation of atrophy (A) and hypertrophy (H) factors from a histogram. From Brooke and Engel (1969b) with kind permission of the authors and the editor of Neurology.*

TABLE 4.1 *Upper limits for the value of atrophy and hypertrophy factors for normal adult male and female muscles*

	Type 1		Type 2A and type 2B	
	Atrophy	**Hypertrophy**	**Atrophy**	**Hypertrophy**
Biceps				
Male	150	300	150	500
Female	100	200	150	150
Vastus				
Male	150	150	150	400
Female	100	400	200	150

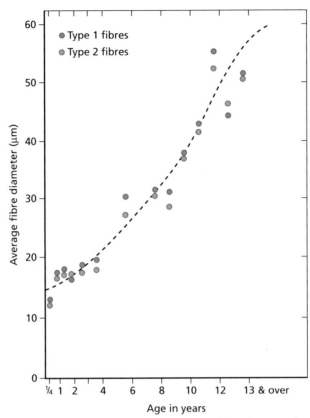

Standard values for average fibre diameters in children

FIG. 4.13 *This graph represents the mean fibre diameter for children at various ages taken from biopsies classified as normal. Each circle represents an arithmetical mean of muscle fibre diameters at each age. From Brooke and Engel (1969d) with kind permission of the authors and the editor of Neurology.*

routine inspection of a muscle biopsy, and for demonstrating the presence of selective atrophy of one fibre type in association with hypertrophy of another type.

Using the atrophy and hypertrophy factors, selective atrophy of fibre types can be readily confirmed. If, in a biopsy, only the atrophy factor for type 1 fibres is above the normal limits the biopsy is said to show selective type 1 fibre atrophy. Similarly, selective hypertrophy may be seen in some biopsies. This type of analysis is a practical way of recognizing atrophy of one fibre type in the presence of hypertrophy of the other. It should be stressed that these atrophy and hypertrophy factors are used only in biopsies from adult muscle and are most useful only when the change is not obvious on inspection. Table 4.1 shows a summary of data obtained from normal muscle using this method. In children under the age of 14, the relative sizes of the type 1 and type 2 fibres are smaller and this has to be taken into account (Fig. 4.13). Mean diameters of type 1 and

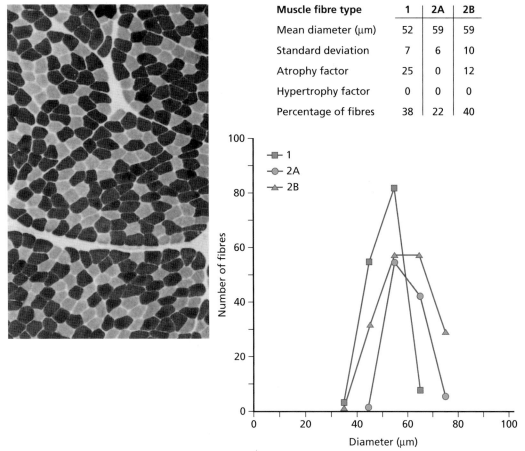

Muscle fibre type	1	2A	2B
Mean diameter (μm)	52	59	59
Standard deviation	7	6	10
Atrophy factor	25	0	12
Hypertrophy factor	0	0	0
Percentage of fibres	38	22	40

FIG. 4.14 *Biopsy from a normal adult male to demonstrate the sizes of lightly stained type 1 and darkly stained 2 fibres (ATPase 9.4). The table and histogram show a summary of data from this biopsy for type 1, 2A and 2B fibres.*

type 2 fibres should not differ by more than 12% of the largest diameter of the largest fibre type. The variability coefficient is again less than 250. Fibre type disproportion, a characteristic of congenital myopathies, is said to occur if the type 1 fibres are at least 12% smaller than type 2 fibres. Illustration of typical histograms from normal biopsies and classical pathological situations are shown in Figures 4.14–4.18.

Fibre type proportions

Another important aspect to assess is the proportion of each fibre type (Table 4.2). As pointed out in previous chapters the number of each fibre type varies between muscles and is influenced by several factors. The percentage of each type is calculated by projecting or printing the image of an ATPase stained section or one labelled with myosin antibodies. A computerized system can also be used but, as with calculating fibre sizes, a limitation of such systems is that they cannot automatically segregate two closely adjacent fibres.

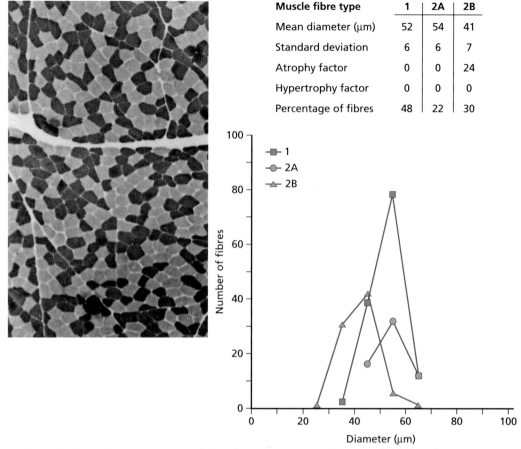

Muscle fibre type	1	2A	2B
Mean diameter (µm)	52	54	41
Standard deviation	6	6	7
Atrophy factor	0	0	24
Hypertrophy factor	0	0	0
Percentage of fibres	48	22	30

FIG. 4.15 *Biopsy from a normal adult female to demonstrate the sizes of lightly stained type 1 and darkly stained type 2 fibres (ATPase 9.4). The table and histogram show a summary of data from this biopsy for type 1, 2A and 2B fibres. Comparison with Figure 4.14 shows that both have a diffuse distribution of type 1 and 2 fibres and that type 1 fibres are similar in size but type 2 fibres are a little smaller in the female than in the male.*

TABLE 4.2 *The mean diameter and proportion of various fibre types in normal adult quadriceps muscle*

	Type 1		Type 2A		Type 2B	
	Male	Female	Male	Female	Male	Female
Average diameter of fibres (µm)	61	53	69	52	62	42
Percentage of fibres in total	36	39	24	29	40	32

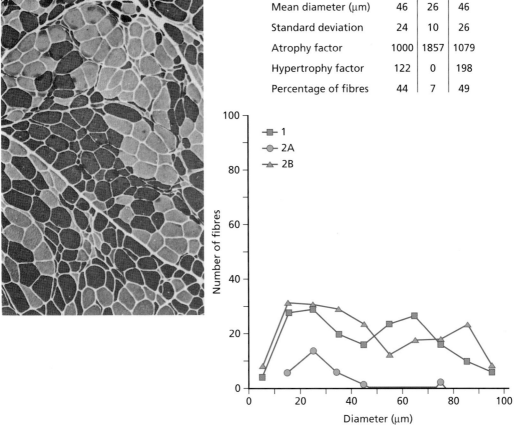

Muscle fibre type	1	2A	2B
Mean diameter (μm)	46	26	46
Standard deviation	24	10	26
Atrophy factor	1000	1857	1079
Hypertrophy factor	122	0	198
Percentage of fibres	44	7	49

FIG. 4.16 *Biopsy from a patient with denervation (ATPase 9.4). The histogram shows a twin-peaked character, especially for type 1 and type 2B fibres.*

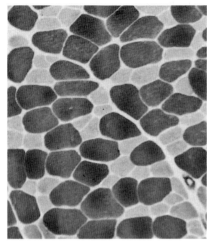

Muscle fibre type	1	2A	2B
Mean diameter (µm)	25	42	41
Standard deviation	8	6	6
Atrophy factor	1013	0	0
Hypertrophy factor	0	0	0
Percentage of fibres	48	31	21

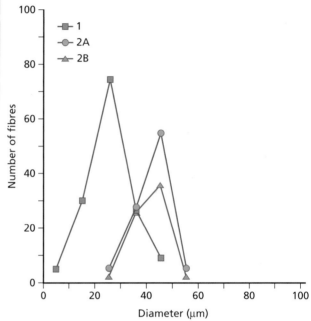

FIG. 4.17 *Atrophy of the lightly stained type 1 fibres (ATPase 9.4). This biopsy demonstrates selective atrophy of type 1 fibres.*

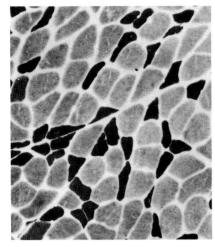

Muscle fibre type	1	2A	2B
Mean diameter (μm)	41	25	28
Standard deviation	7	7	7
Atrophy factor	81	963	714
Hypertrophy factor	0	0	0
Percentage of fibres	67	16	17

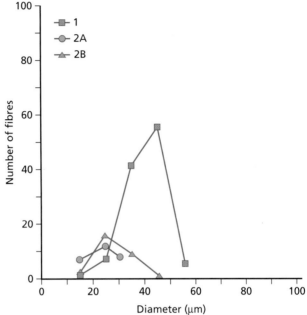

FIG. 4.18 *Atrophy of the darkly stained type 2 fibres (ATPase 9.4). The small size of the type 2 fibres, particularly 2B fibres, and the relatively normal size of type 1 fibres is apparent in the table and histogram.*

Fibre type predominance

Type predominance is an excess of one fibre type (Fig. 4.19). In the interpretation of fibre type predominance, it is important to make careful comparison with controls from the same muscle of similar age and sex. In the quadriceps the normal ratio of type 1 to 2 fibres is approximately 1:2. If the type fibres are sub-divided then type 1, 2A and 2B comprise approximately one-third each. There is, however, some variation within the normal population around these figures. From our experience type 1 predominance is said to occur when more than 55% of the fibres are type 1, and type 2 fibre predominance when more than 80% of the fibres are type 2.

Fibre type predominance may reflect type grouping if the biopsy has been taken from the centre of a very large group of a uniform fibre type. However, some disorders are associated with fibre type predominance in a sufficient number of biopsies to make this explanation unlikely. Type 1 fibre predominance

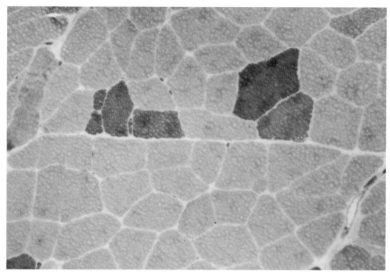

FIG. 4.19 *Pronounced predominance of lightly stained type 1 fibres (ATPase 9.4).*

is a common feature of myopathic conditions, for example the muscular dystrophies and congenital myopathies (Fig. 4.19; see also Fig. 4.7). Type 2 fibre predominance, on the other hand, is associated with motor neurone diseases.

Changes in sarcolemmal nuclei

The changes which occur in sarcolemmal nuclei relate to their position and their appearance. They may be internal within the fibre, rather than in their normal peripheral position. Secondly, the appearance of the individual nuclei may change and may form the so-called *tigroid nuclei* or *vesicular nuclei*. These are not always clear in unfixed frozen sections.

Internal nuclei

When more than 3% of the fibres in transverse section contain a nucleus which is in the substance of the muscle fibre and not at its periphery the biopsy is said to demonstrate internal nuclei (Greenfield et al 1957). In our experience, however, this is probably an overestimate and even a few internal nuclei in paediatric muscle are probably significant. In normal adults they are more common, particularly in individuals involved in sporting activities. In some conditions the nuclei may be central within the fibre, and in longitudinal section they may form a chain down the centre of the fibre. Central nuclei are a characteristic feature of myotubular myopathy but we are now aware that they can also occur in central core disease associated with defects in the ryanodine receptor (see Ch. 15). In other situations (Fig. 4.20), they are scattered within the myofibrils and

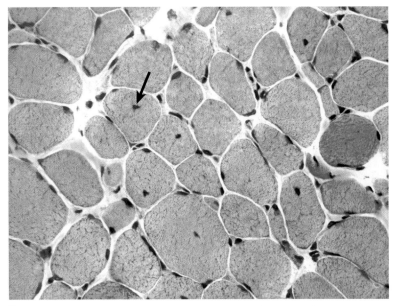

a

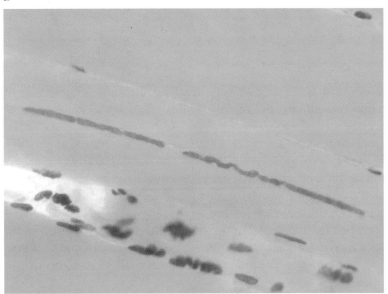

b

FIG. 4.20(a) *Internal nuclei (arrow) within fibres of varying size from a case of Duchenne muscular dystrophy (H&E). Fibre diameter range 15–60 μm. (b) A chain of internal nuclei in a longitudinally sectioned fibre 48 μm in diameter (H&E).*

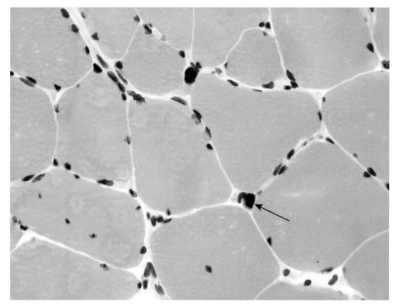

FIG. 4.21 *Clumps of nuclei (arrow) indicating chronic atrophy. Note also the multiple internal nuclei in one fibre (H&E). Fibre diameter range 45–90 μm.*

more than one per fibre may be seen (Fig. 4.21). Internal nuclei are often seen along the fibrous septa in split fibres (see Fig. 4.28); some of these relate to nuclei of the capillary endothelial cells.

It is important when assessing the presence of internal nuclei to examine the transverse sections of muscle and not the longitudinal, since in a longitudinal section (which may be up to 10 μm in thickness) a peripherally placed nucleus may be seen through the overlying myofibrillar tissue and may give the appearance of being within the muscle fibre.

The significance of internal nuclei may be summarized by saying that a great profusion of internal nuclei would be suggestive of a myopathy. They are particularly abundant in myotonic dystrophy but they also occur in chronic neuropathies.

Nuclear chains

The occurrence of nuclei close to one another in chains throughout the length of the fibre probably has the same significance as internal nuclei. Indeed, the two changes usually coexist. Thus, in myotonic dystrophy in which internal nuclei are profuse, chains of nuclei are also seen. In contrast, the central nuclei in myotubular myopathy tend to be spaced out and not in continuous chains. Regenerating fibres may show nuclear chains in longitudinal orientation.

Vesicular nuclei

Sarcolemmal nuclei may undergo a characteristic change, resulting in the formation of vesicular nuclei. The nucleus becomes swollen and rounded, the nucleoplasm transparent, and the nucleolus very prominent. These vesicular nuclei are frequently associated with basophilic fibres, and are thought to be evidence of regeneration. In general, the more numerous the vesicular nuclei the more likely it is that the biopsy represents a myopathy.

Tigroid nuclei

The sarcolemmal nuclei are said to be tigroid when the chromatin material, which is usually finely dispersed throughout the nucleus, becomes granular and clumped. Although the significance of these nuclei is not certain, their presence is usually associated with neuropathies rather than myopathies, and they have also been noted in myotonic dystrophy.

Nuclear clumps

Nuclei may become darkly stained and shrunken. Frequently, these nuclei occur in small groups (Fig. 4.21), and may be pyknotic. This change represents severe atrophy and is commonly seen in longstanding denervation. It also occurs in limb-girdle and other chronic dystrophies.

Degeneration and regeneration

We consider under this heading those changes which may be seen with the routine haematoxylin and eosin (H&E) or trichrome stains, and which represent either degeneration or regeneration of individual fibres.

The simplest change is that of the pale staining 'liquefied' or hyaline fibre. With any of the routine stains, these fibres are only faintly coloured (Fig. 4.22). This represents *necrosis* and such a fibre frequently becomes filled with phagocytes (Fig. 4.23). These fibres are strikingly highlighted with the stain for acid phosphatase. Simple necrosis is usually associated with myopathies but is occasionally also seen in biopsies from either fairly acute neuropathy, such as amyotrophic lateral sclerosis, or chronic peripheral neuropathy, such as peroneal muscular atrophy, the so-called 'myopathic change' in neuropathy. Necrosis is often segmental and only part of a fibre will be affected. In longitudinal section or at a different transverse level parts of a fibre may appear normal while another region is necrotic.

Phagocytosis (Fig. 4.23) is similarly a feature of myopathies, and less commonly occurs in other circumstances, such as chronic or acute denervation. As mentioned above, necrosis and phagocytosis may at times be limited to a portion of the fibre.

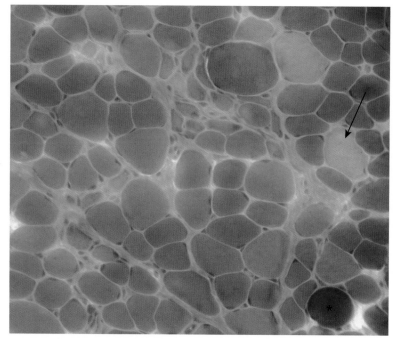

FIG. 4.22 *Pale necrotic fibres about 40–50 μm in diameter (arrow) in a case of Duchenne muscular dystrophy. Note also the dark staining hypercontracted fibre (*) (Gomori trichrome).*

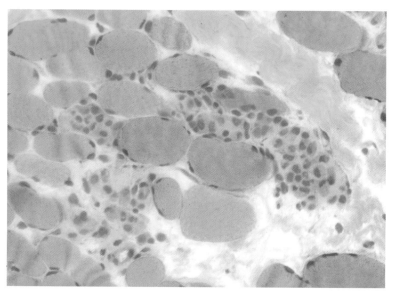

FIG. 4.23 *Phagocytes invading necrotic fibres in a case of Duchenne muscular dystrophy (H&E). Fibre diameter range 30–50 μm.*

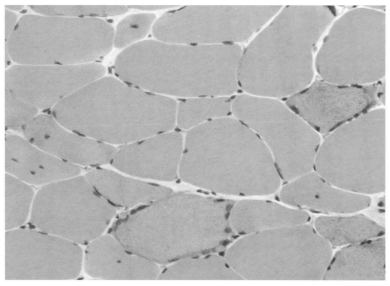

FIG. 4.24 *Two granular, slightly basophilic fibres with abnormal mitochondria in a case of mitochondrial myopathy (H&E). Fibre diameter range 25–85 μm.*

Hypercontracted fibres are also thought to be a form of degenerating fibre, prior to phagocytosis. They are often round in shape and the myofibrils become very contracted and intensely stained with most stains. They are prominent in H&E sections and easily seen with the trichrome stain (see Fig. 4.22). They are common in Duchenne and Becker muscular dystrophy but can occur in other conditions. The Wohlfart B fibres seen in normal neonatal muscle are also intensely stained but whether they are hypercontracted is not known. It is important not to interpret intensely stained damaged fibres at the periphery of a sample as pathological. This is an artefact.

A second type of degeneration, readily seen with routine stains, is a coarsely *granular fibre*, which stains bluish with H&E and red with the modified Gomori trichrome stain (Figs 4.24 and 4.25); hence the name *'ragged-red fibres'* (Engel 1971). They may occur as an incidental feature in dystrophic and other biopsies, but when they occur as a relatively prominent feature they are particularly associated with Kearns–Sayre syndrome and other mitochondrial myopathies and contain structurally abnormal mitochondria (see below and Ch. 18). It is important to distinguish the normal peripheral aggregations of mitochondria that stain red with Gomori trichrome from ragged-red fibres which often also show the abnormal basophilic granularity (Fig. 4.24).

Basophilic fibres, in which the cytoplasm takes on a uniformly bluish colour with H&E, because of a high RNA content, are thought to represent attempts at fibre regeneration, particularly when they are associated with vesicular nuclei (Fig. 4.26). Basophilia is common in many myopathies, particularly in the early stages of Duchenne dystrophy and clusters of basophilic fibres may be seen. They

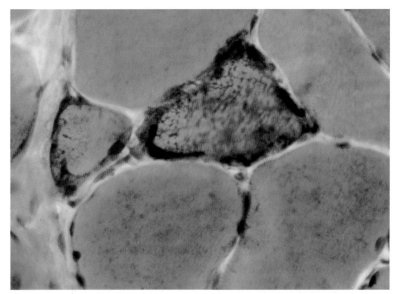

FIG. 4.25 *Prominent peripheral accumulations of abnormal mitochondria in fibres often referred to as 'ragged-red' in the same case as Figure 4.24. In addition to the peripheral staining red stain throughout the fibre is also seen in ragged-red fibres (Gomori trichrome).*

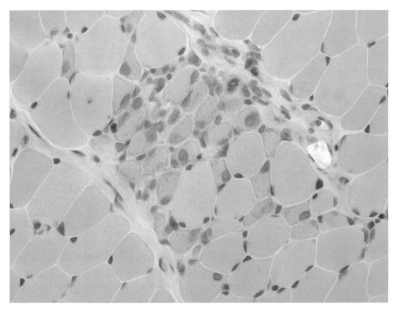

FIG. 4.26 *Cluster of small basophilic fibres (5–15 μm) in a case of Duchenne muscular dystrophy that are slightly more blue than surrounding fibres and have large prominent nuclei (H&E).*

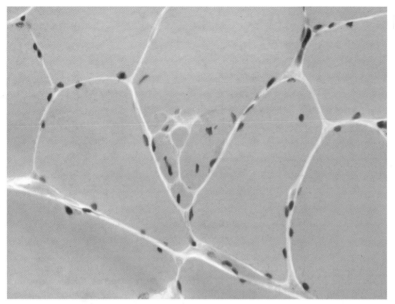

FIG. 4.27 *An area of multiple splitting that resembles a cluster of small fibres (H&E). Fibre diameter range 5–30 μm.*

can also be produced experimentally by trauma or ischaemia of the muscle, and may be very striking during the recovery phase after acute rhabdomyolysis. Regenerating fibres conform to type 2C in their histochemical profile and express neonatal myosin (see Ch. 6). Split fibres can sometimes appear basophilic which may relate to myofibrillar disruption rather than to regeneration.

Fibre splitting may be present in three forms. In transverse section, a large number of small fibres may be clustered (Fig. 4.27); a fibre may show a partial division either in transverse or longitudinal section; or there may be fibrous septa within the body of the fibre. Nuclei are frequently seen alongside these splits or septa (Fig. 4.28).

Fibre splitting is seen under normal circumstances at the myotendinous junction, when it is often associated with a profusion of internal nuclei. Care should be exercised in interpreting pathological changes in this region (see Chapters 3 and 6).

Fibre splitting is common in most muscular dystrophies, but may also be seen in chronic neuropathies such as peroneal muscular atrophy (Charcot–Marie–Tooth disease).

Another reaction of a damaged fibre is loss of glycogen. This appears as white fibres with the periodic acid-Schiff (PAS) stain in contrast to the variable pink colour of the other fibres (Fig. 4.29). These fibres are non-specific but a variable number are quite common in Duchenne dystrophy. When present they suggest fibre damage but loss of glycogen may also occur if there is long delay before freezing. It can also occur in denervation and this loss of glycogen was originally used to map motor units.

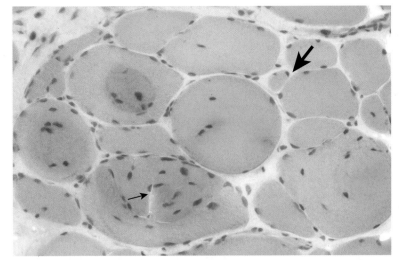

FIG. 4.28 *Hypertrophic fibres (up to 115 μm) with multiple internal splits from a case of Duchenne muscular dystrophy. Note also the nuclei along the splits (small arrow). Some of the variation in fibre size is probably due to branching of the fibres (large arrow) (H&E).*

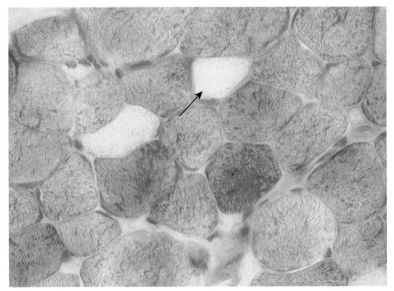

FIG. 4.29 *An isolated fibre (arrow) that has lost glycogen and appears white with the PAS stain (fibre diameter range 35–70 μm).*

Fibrosis and adipose tissue

Fibrosis is common in a number of situations and varying amounts of adipose tissue may accompany it (Fig. 4.30). Proliferation of both the endomysial or perimysial connective tissue may occur but perimysial fibrosis is of less significance than endomysial fibrosis, since wide bands of fibrous tissue separating fascicles are not uncommon in normal muscle, particularly in children. A variety of extracellular matrix proteins, especially various types of collagen, can be identified in the perimysium and endomysium (see Ch. 6). Endomysial proliferation leads to a clear separation of individual muscle fibres. It is more commonly seen in myopathies than neuropathies, and is a prominent feature of Duchenne and Becker dystrophy, the limb-girdle dystrophies and some congenital dystrophies. It is sometimes also seen in facioscapulohumeral muscular dystrophy and can occur in some cases of central core disease. Fibrosis may occur in neurogenic atrophies but endomysial proliferation is not usually a feature of severe infantile spinal muscular atrophies. Connective tissue proliferation is considered to be secondary to the basic disease process, but from time to time it has been invoked as the primary process in muscular dystrophy (Duchenne 1868, Bourne and Golarz 1959).

Excess fat cells and adipose tissue often accompany the fibrosis. In some conditions the fat may be particularly prolific and only islands of fibres are present in a sea of adipose tissue (Fig. 4.30). Although this is a particular feature of some congenital muscular dystrophies, we have also observed it in cases of

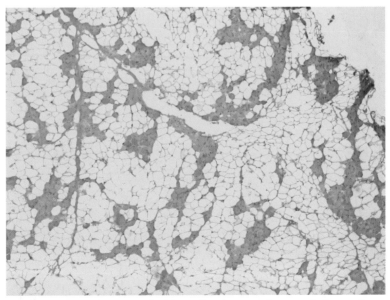

FIG. 4.30 *Low power view of a biopsy from a case of congenital muscular dystrophy showing only islands of fibres (red) in a vast amount of adipose tissue (H&E).*

central core disease (see Ch. 15). The presence of large amounts of connective tissue and fat are therefore not restricted to the severe muscular dystrophies.

Cellular reactions

Under pathological conditions various forms of *cellular reaction* are frequently seen in skeletal muscle (Fig. 4.31). These may occur within the fibres (as discussed above) or in the supporting tissues. In frozen sections, the type of cell is usually more difficult to identify than in fixed material but with specific cell markers immunohistochemistry can accurately identify the cell types. The commonest response is either histiocytes or lymphocytes or, under certain circumstances, other inflammatory cells such as polymorphonuclear leukocytes or plasma cells.

In addition to the phagocytosis within necrotic fibres themselves, there is frequently a marked cellular reaction of histiocytes or macrophages around damaged or necrotic fibres.

Cellular reactions are non-specific. They are common in Duchenne dystrophy, where they may be misinterpreted as representing an inflammatory myopathy. They are less marked in the more slowly progressive forms of dystrophy. In polymyositis and dermatomyositis the reaction may vary from very extensive to a slight and focal change. The cells may be predominantly in perivascular regions or be endomysial. The cell type may also vary, depending on the acuteness of

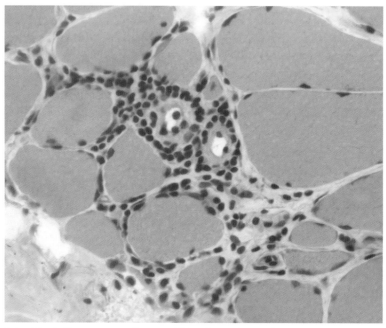

FIG. 4.31 *Inflammatory cells round blood vessels and fibres in a case of inclusion body myositis (H&E). Fibre diameter range 10–50 μm.*

the condition. Extensive cellular reactions are also common in some cases of the facioscapulohumeral dystrophy and the limb-girdle dystrophy with a defect in dysferlin [limb-girdle muscular dystrophy type 2B (LGMD2B)]. Care should be taken in the identification of cellular aggregates as it is easy to mistake clusters of regenerative fibres as apparent increased cellularity in myositis. Neurovascular bundles in relation to muscle fibres or a section through a blood vessel wall may also superficially resemble a cellular response because of the profuse number of nuclei.

Cellular reaction is less common in the neurogenic atrophies but does occur on occasion, particularly in some of the more chronic neuropathies.

Lymphorrhages are tightly packed aggregates of small round cells, which may occur in association with focal abnormal fibres or with otherwise normal-looking muscle. They are seen in myasthenia gravis and also in polymyositis and some of the collagen group of disorders. We have not found the presence of lymphorrhages of particular diagnostic help, in contrast to the presence of cellular reactions generally.

Changes in fibre architecture and structural abnormalities

Several techniques, such as the oxidative enzyme reactions and the Gomori trichrome stain, reveal a number of structural changes within the cytochemical architecture of individual muscle fibres. Some of these changes reflect a specific underlying pathological entity, whereas others are non-specific and incidental, either to other forms of pathology or indeed to otherwise normal muscle. Electron microscopy has helped to define and delineate these structural abnormalities.

Myofibrillar disturbances

Central cores were first recognized by Magee and Shy (1956). Although a more compact zone of myofibrils is seen with the Gomori trichrome stain, they are much more readily identified with the oxidative enzyme reactions. The core zone is devoid of mitochondria and oxidative enzyme activity, in striking contrast to the normal peripheral zone (Dubowitz and Pearse 1960b, Fig. 4.32). The periphery of the core may have enhanced staining, resembling a target or targetoid fibre (see below). In longitudinal section the cores run a considerable length of the fibre. Although often single and central, they may also be eccentric and multiple. They are also devoid of other enzymes, such as phosphorylase, and of glycogen, although often rimmed by PAS stain (Fig. 4.33). They usually retain their sarcomeric structure, although the myofibrils are contracted, and still stain for ATPase. Some may lose their ATPase staining because of the unstructured, disorganized nature of the myofibrils (Neville and Brooke 1973). The cores

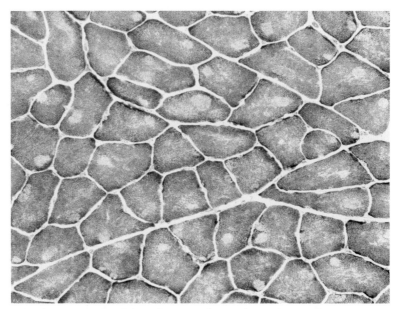

FIG. 4.32 *NADH-TR staining of a case of central core disease showing cores devoid of enzyme activity in many fibres. Note also the lack of fibre type differentiation (fibre diameter range 30–80 μm).*

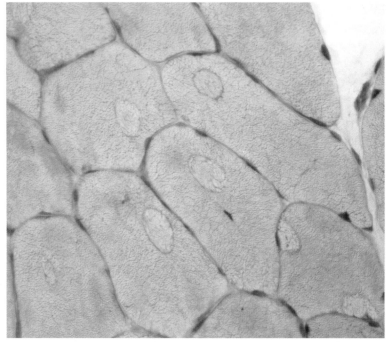

FIG. 4.33 *Cores in a case of central core disease rimmed by PAS staining (fibre diameter range 50–90 μm).*

have a predilection for type 1 fibres and there is often also a predominance of type 1 fibres in the biopsy.

The presence of large cores in many fibres is usually associated with central core disease, but the size of the cores and spectrum of pathological changes in patients with central core disease is now known to be wide (see Ch. 15), even within members of the same family with the same mutation in the *ryanodine receptor 1* gene (Sewry et al 2002). Core-like areas have also been reported in patients with a cardiomyopathy and a mutation in the β-myosin heavy chain gene (*MYH7*) (Seidman and Seidman 2001) and in cases with a mutation in the gene encoding skeletal actin, *ACTA1* (Kaindl et al 2004). Some biopsies may have sporadic cores in occasional fibres, for example some muscular dystrophies. In some biopsies multiple small *minicores* are seen with the oxidative enzyme reactions but, in contrast to the central cores, they are small both in transverse and longitudinal section (Fig. 4.34). The myofibrillar structure within the minicores is usually disrupted and they may show up as weaker staining areas with the ATPase reactions. They are a non-specific feature but are a particular feature of some cases with a mutation in the ryanodine receptor 1 gene (Jungbluth et al 2002, Monnier et al 2003), responsible for central core disease, and of cases with a mutation in the *SEPN1* gene. The latter were previously described as 'minicore myopathy' (Ferreiro et al 2002). They may also occur in the Ullrich form of congenital muscular dystrophy. Marked unevenness of oxidative enzyme stains and myofibrillar disruption resembling minicores have also been observed in a rare dominant disorder caused by a mutation in the myosin heavy chain IIA gene (Martinsson et al 2000). In this disorder the disruption was seen to be more marked in 2A fibres, although older cases showed involvement of all fibre types.

Target fibres bear some resemblance to central cores but are characterized by three distinct zones: a clear central zone devoid of oxidative enzyme activity, a densely staining intermediate zone with increased oxidative enzyme activity and a relatively normal peripheral zone of intermediate activity (Fig. 4.35). This gives the appearance of a three-zone target. The vast majority of target fibres occur in type 1 fibres. If the intermediate zone is not clearly defined they are called *targetoid fibres.*

Target fibres are usually associated with denervating disorders and are most commonly seen in chronic peripheral neuropathies or more acute recovering neuropathies. In some cases the distinction between a core and a target fibre is not always clear. Experimental studies suggest that they may occur during reinnervation (Dubowitz 1967) and they have also been seen in association with tenotomy (Engel et al 1966).

The *intermyofibrillar network*, when seen with the oxidative enzyme reaction, is usually a regular ordered network with a uniform appearance throughout the individual fibre (see Ch. 3). A common change, occurring particularly in type 1 fibres, is disruption of the intermyofibrillar network with a resultant patchy staining giving a *'moth-eaten'* appearance (Fig. 4.36). The distinction between this and minicores is not always clear but the disruption in moth-eaten

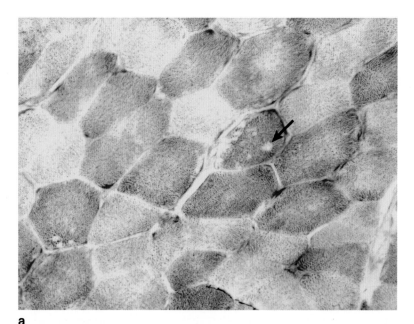

a

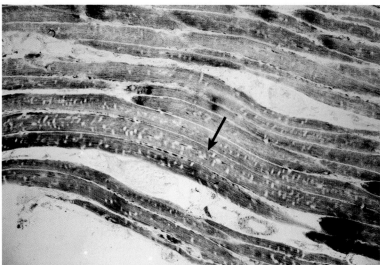

b

FIG. 4.34 *Fibres sectioned (a) transversely and (b) longitudinally showing minicores (arrows) (NADH-TR).*

fibres is often more irregular. The occurrence of moth-eaten fibres is non-specific and is particularly seen in various myopathies, including congenital dystrophy and dermatomyositis. It may also occur in various other disorders as widely ranging as polymyalgia rheumatica and Parkinson's disease. Sometimes the moth-eaten, unevenness of oxidative enzyme stains may be a marked feature and is accompanied by larger areas devoid of stain, resembling cores (Fig. 4.37).

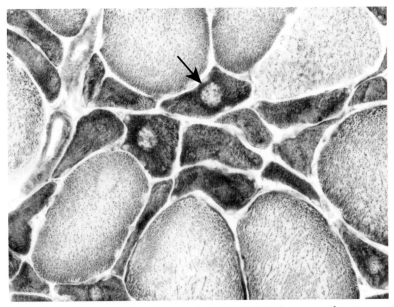

FIG. 4.35 *Target fibres (arrow) stained with NADH-TR in a case of motor neurone disease showing a dark rim around the central pale area (fibre diameter range 15–135 μm).*

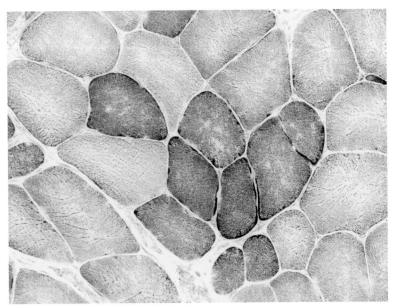

FIG. 4.36 *Moth-eaten fibres, several of which are hypertrophic, with small focal areas devoid of NADH-TR activity in a case of limb-girdle muscular dystrophy (fibre diameter range 60–115 μm).*

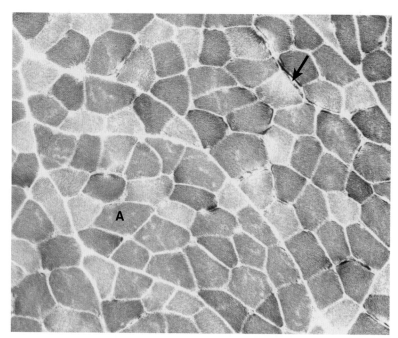

FIG. 4.37 *Poorly-defined moth-eaten effect in many fibres and some larger peripheral areas devoid of stain (arrow; NADH-TR). Fibre diameter range 30–60 μm.*

The unevenness of stain may reflect mild loss of myofibrils and a disturbance in the distribution of mitochondria (Fi g. 4.37). Minor ultrastructural disruption of the myofibrils may be seen in such cases. Staining of type 2 fibres is often uneven (Fig. 4.36) and ultrastructural studies may be needed to determine if any unevenness of stain is pathologically significant.

Ring fibres can be seen with several stains, in particular PAS and oxidative enzyme stains. In the ring fibre, the normal orientation of the myofibrils is distorted by a bundle of myofibrils, often at the periphery of the fibre, that runs at right angles to the main body of the fibre (Fig. 4.38). This gives the appearance of a striated annulet or ring around the fibre. The ring is not always peripheral, and bizarre forms may be seen in which the abnormally oriented myofibrils cross through the body of the muscle fibre. The striated annulet is often associated with an irregular mass of sarcoplasm extending outward from the ring. In frozen tissue, the ring fibres often assume a small and circular appearance and frequently stain darkly with all of the histochemical reactions. The significance of ring fibres is somewhat controversial. Although frequent in myotonic dystrophy, they are not pathognomonic of this disease.

Coil fibres, or *whorled fibres* are also characterized by disorientation of the longitudinal pattern of the myofibrils but tend to be more bizarre than the ring fibres (Fig. 4.39). They are readily identified with the oxidative enzyme reactions. At times they may form giant fibres which seem to be an aggregation of several

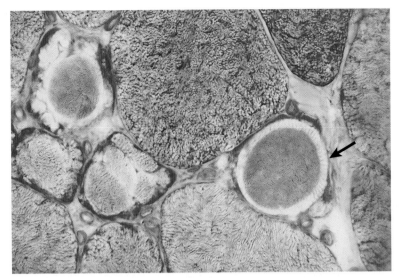

FIG. 4.38 *Ring fibres stained with PAS (arrow) in an adult case of limb girdle muscular dystrophy. Note the striations in the peripheral zone in which the myofibrils are at 90° to those in the centre of the fibre.*

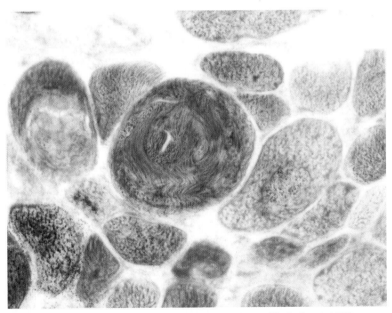

FIG. 4.39 *A whorled fibre (72 μm) with twisted myofibrils (NADH-TR).*

fibres. They commonly occur in various dystrophies and may also be found in chronic neuropathies and other disorders.

Other myofibrillar disturbances may be seen as *pale staining zones*, or a slightly different colour to surrounding areas, with routine stains such as H&E and trichrome. Electron microscopy may be needed to clarify the exact nature of such areas. Areas with an accumulation of actin filaments in some nemaline

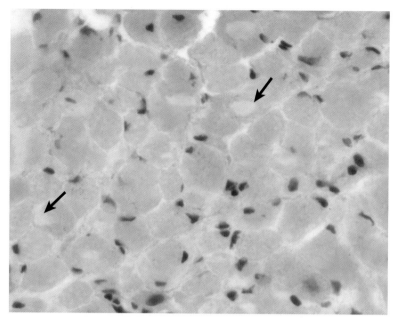

FIG. 4.40 *Pale staining zones of accumulated actin in a neonate (arrows). All fibres are less than 20 μm; H&E.*

myopathies and the granulomatous material seen in desmin-related myopathies and hyaline bodies (Barohn et al 1994a) stain in this manner (Fig. 4.40). In desmin-related myopathies, in particular those caused by mutations in the genes for desmin and αB-crystallin, these areas appear eosinophilic with H&E and may be large and devoid of oxidative enzyme stains and ATPase activity. They may extend across the whole width of the fibre and give a 'wiped out' appearance. If the section passes through such an area the whole fibre may appear devoid of enzyme activity.

Mitochondrial abnormalities

There may be abnormalities in mitochondrial structure, number, size and distribution.

Structurally *abnormal mitochondria* can be seen with various stains but electron microscopy is needed for confirmation. They are readily suspected when individual fibres show basophilic granularity (see Fig. 4.24) and an excessively intense reaction with the oxidative enzyme stain (Fig. 4.41) or peripheries are particularly intensely stained (Fig. 4.42). They occur specifically in relation to the various mitochondrial myopathies and ophthalmoplegic syndromes, but may also be an isolated and incidental feature in occasional fibres in other disorders such as dermatomyositis. In the mitochondrial myopathies the abnormal fibres are also recognized with the Gomori trichrome stain by their disruption and 'ragged-red' appearance (see Fig. 4.25).

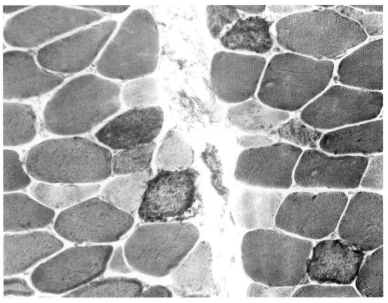

FIG. 4.41 *Fibres with abnormal mitochondria intensely stained for NADH-TR (fibre diameter range 40–100 μm).*

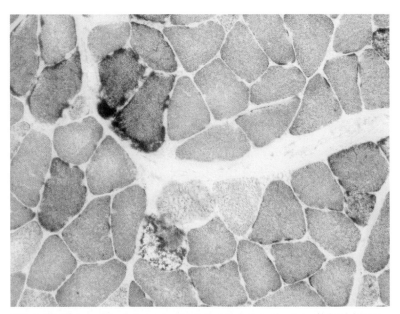

FIG. 4.42 *Fibres with abnormal mitochondria intensely stained for succinic dehydrogenase (fibre diameter range 50–80 μm).*

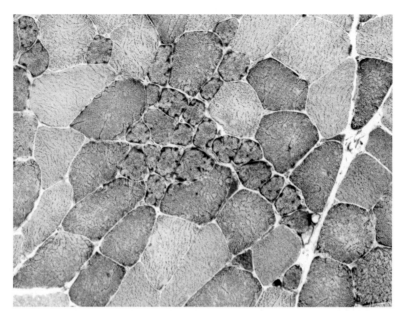

FIG. 4.43 *A group of lobulated fibres (30–50 μm) stained for NADH-TR showing peripheral aggregates of stain that are often triangular in shape.*

Lobulated fibres show a striking picture with oxidative enzyme reactions with reaction product particularly prominent at the periphery of the fibre. These areas are often triangular and are composed of many small mitochondria (Fig. 4.43). Lobulated fibres are often smaller and often type 1. They are a non-specific finding that we have observed in many conditions. They are rare in children (Guerard et al, 1985), but have been observed in some cases of the Ullrich form of congenital muscular dystrophy. They are a feature in limb-girdle dystrophy with a defect in the calpain-3 gene (LGMD2A) but can also occur in other myopathic conditions.

There is also an *aggregation of mitochondria* and oxidative enzyme activity between the central nuclei in myotubular myopathy and in some small fibres in other conditions. This is revealed as small dark centres with oxidative enzyme stains.

Tubular aggregates

This structural change has a predilection for type 2 fibres, and particularly the 2B fibres. When seen with oxidative enzymes they stain intensely. This is true with all the oxidative enzymes except succinic dehydrogenase (SDH) and menadione-linked α-glycerophosphate dehydrogenase. With these two reactions, the aggregates are unstained. With the Gomori trichrome stain, they are red, and with H&E are basophilic. In the ATPase reaction, the tubular aggregates are present in unstained areas that lack myofibrils. These structures occur in many circumstances, including periodic paralysis, exertional myalgia and the rare metabolic disorder hyperornithinaemia. In ultrastructural studies we have also observed occasional aggregates in some carriers of Duchenne dystrophy. Like so many other changes in muscle they may well be 'non-specific'. They have a distinctive appearance on electron microscopy (see Ch. 5) and are thought to be derived from the sarcoplasmic reticulum. Dysferlin and recently emerin have been shown to be associated with them (Ikezoe et al 2003; Manta et al 2004).

Cytoplasmic bodies

These are another fairly common and non-specific structural change within the muscle fibre. They may be associated with collagen vascular disease, and they are quite common in inclusion body myositis. One case has also been observed in association with habitual senna purgation. Their appearance may vary but they are usually eosinophilic and with the Gomori trichrome they have a dark-green or sometimes red appearance (Fig. 4.44). A surrounding halo can sometimes be distinguished. They have a striking appearance on electron microscopy (see Ch. 5). They usually occur in sporadic fibres but occasionally may be very extensive throughout the biopsy and may selectively involve type 2 fibres.

Rod bodies

These unusual structures are most readily seen with the Gomori trichrome stain, where they stain red, contrasting with the blue–green background stain of the muscle fibres (Fig. 4.45). They are easily missed with H&E and other routine stains and they are not demonstrated with the routine enzyme histochemical reactions. Areas where clusters of rods accumulate, such as the periphery of fibres, however, will appear negative for oxidative enzyme stains and ATPase as they lack mitochondria and myosin. On electron microscopy they appear as dense bodies with a crystalline or lattice structure and apparently arising from the Z lines (see Ch. 5).

In addition to their occurrence as a diagnostic feature in familial cases of the various forms of nemaline myopathy (see Ch. 15), rods have also been observed in a number of other situations, including central core disease (Scacheri et al 2001).

Vacuoles can occur in several conditions and they are of different types. The situations where they are most common are inclusion body myositis, glycogenoses and periodic paralysis, although absence of vacuoles in a sample does not exclude these diagnoses. Some vacuoles have detectable material within them, others appear as empty spaces. It is important to distinguish freezing artefact from this type of vacuole and also not to interpret the presence of excess lipid droplets as vacuoles (see below). Vacuoles are lined by membrane and two X-linked conditions are characterized by excessive *autophagic vacuoles*, one linked to Xq28 (Kalimo et al 1988) and the other caused by mutations in the

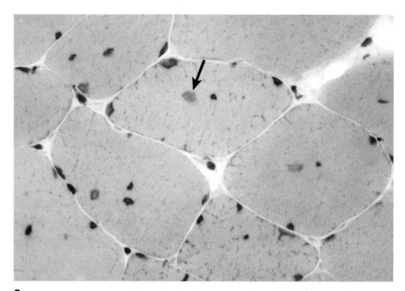

a

b

FIG. 4.44 *Cytoplasmic bodies (arrows) staining as (a) eosinophilic bodies with H&E and (b) dark-green or reddish bodies with Gomori trichrome (fibre diameter range 32–45 μm).*

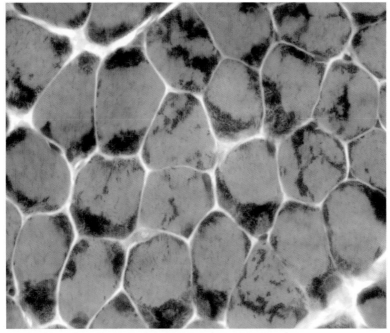

FIG. 4.45 *Clusters of red-stained nemaline rods in most fibres in a patient with nemaline myopathy caused by a mutation in the gene encoding skeletal actin (Gomori trichrome). Mean fibre diameter 26 μm.*

LAMP-2 gene, also on the X chromosome (Nishino et al 2000). Several plasmalemmal proteins, extracellular matrix proteins of the sarcolemma and the membrane attack complex localize to these vacuoles (see Ch. 6) and they have a distinctive ultrastructural appearance (see Ch. 5). Indentations of the sarcolemma also show sarcolemmal proteins and when sectioned transversely they may appear as vacuoles.

Vacuoles may have basophilic granularity associated with them, particularly at the periphery. This type of *rimmed vacuole* is typical of inclusion body myositis (Fig. 4.46). They have also been shown to be associated with a mutation in the gene for myosin heavy chain IIa on chromosome 17 (Martinsson et al 2000) in a disorder that has been grouped with other forms of hereditary inclusion body myopathy (Oldfors and Fyhr 2001).

In glycogen storage disease routine stains show a vacuolar appearance where glycogen has accumulated. In Type V (McArdle's disease) there may be a peripheral vacuolar appearance where glycogen has accumulated (see below). In severe cases of childhood cases of acid maltase deficiency (Pompe's disease) vacuoles are marked and ultrastructurally their membrane can be seen (see Ch. 5). These vacuoles do not always label with antibodies to sarcolemmal proteins and stain intensely for acid phosphatase, indicating their lysosomal origin. In milder adult cases of acid maltase deficiency the vacuoles are mainly restricted to type I fibres (Fig. 4.47).

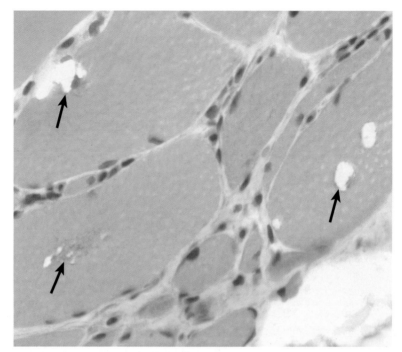

a

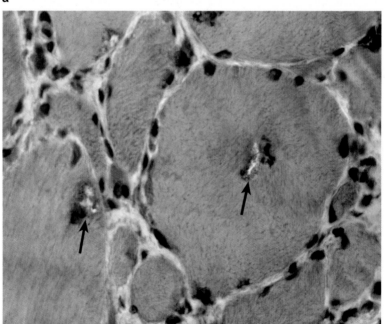

b

FIG. 4.46 *Rimmed vacuoles (arrows) in a case of inclusion body myositis stained with (a) H&E and (b) Gomori trichrome (fibre diameter range 5–75 μm).*

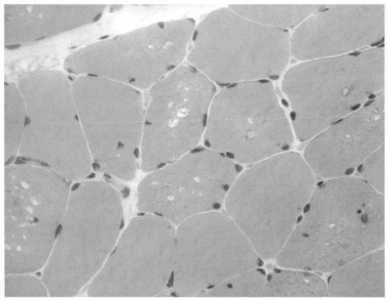

FIG. 4.47 *Multiple vacuoles in an adult case of acid maltase deficiency (fibre diameter range 45–65 μm).*

Deficiencies of enzymes

The absence of particular enzymes is of diagnostic importance. In Type V glycogenosis (McArdle's disease) there is a complete absence of phosphorylase from all fibres. This is the only disorder where this occurs and the result is unequivocal (Fig. 4.48). Immature fibres, such as those in spindles, however, express a different isoform of phosphorylase and stain with the histochemical reaction.

Staining for phosphofructokinase can also show an unequivocal absence of the protein but such cases are rare. Detection of a reduction in the enzyme may be difficult to assess histochemically and should be supported by biochemical analyses.

Myoadenylate deaminase may also show an absence of stain in the fibres but the pathological significance of this has been questioned as there is a common mutation in the normal population which leads to absence of the enzyme.

Another important situation of absence of an enzyme is cytochrome oxidase (COX). Rare cases of COX deficiency have been identified and biopsies show no or very low levels of COX by histochemistry. A more common finding is absence of stain in a few fibres (Fig. 4.49). These fibres occur in some mitochondrial disorders and in inclusion body myositis. Their number also increases with age. Type 2 fibres can show very low levels of stain with the COX technique and care is needed not to interpret these as negative fibres. The combined COX/SDH technique (see Ch. 2) is useful in such situations as fibres devoid of COX but expressing SDH are a prominent blue colour (Fig. 4.50).

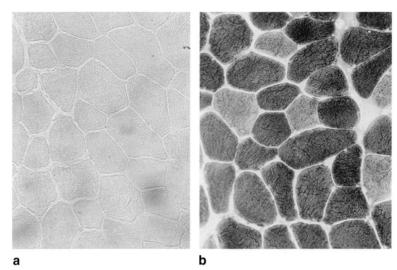

a   b

FIG. 4.48(a) *Absence of phosphorylase in a patient with McArdle's disease compared with (b) a normal fibre type pattern in control muscle stained in parallel.*

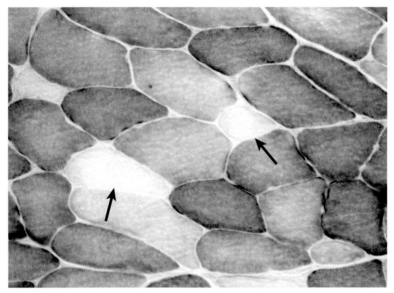

FIG. 4.49 *Fibres devoid of cytochrome oxidase activity appear white (arrows) compared with the fibre typing pattern of adjacent fibres (fibre diameter range 45–95 μm).*

Accumulation of glycogen or lipid

Glycogen accumulates in the muscle fibres in glycogenoses and is demonstrated with the PAS stain. The excess glycogen may be seen throughout the fibre, at the periphery or concentrated in the vacuolated fibres (Fig. 4.51). As glycogen is

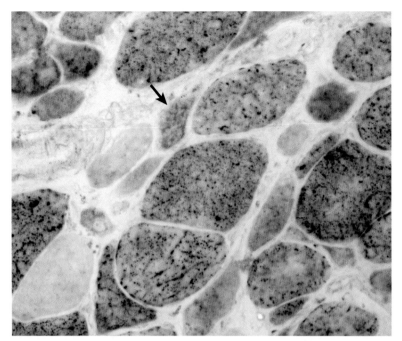

FIG. 4.50 *Three small fibres (10–20 μm) appear blue (arrow) with the combined cytochrome oxidase (COX)/succinic dehydrogenase (SDH) technique and are devoid of COX activity but retain SDH activity.*

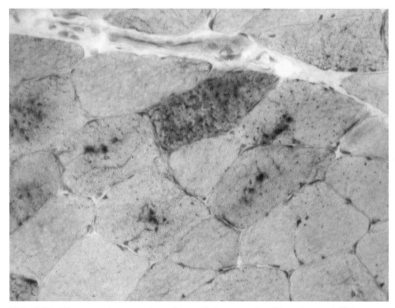

FIG. 4.51 *Glycogen in vacuoles of an adult case of acid maltase deficiency (PAS). Fibre diameter range 45–65 μm.*

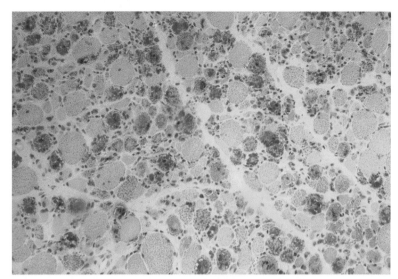

FIG. 4.52 *Accumulation of lipid stained red with oil red O in a case of carnitine deficiency.*

easily lost from fibres celloidin coating may be needed to demonstrate the excess glycogen. Lipid droplets accumulate in the fibres in carnitine deficiency (Fig. 4.52) but there is usually no detectable histochemical lipid accumulation in carnitine palmityl transferase deficiency. Both the number and the size of the droplets should be assessed but, as type 1 fibres in normal muscle show more lipid than type 2 fibres, it is not always easy to judge the amount present. For example in disorders of β-oxidation the result with oil red O or Sudan black staining may not give a clear answer. The lipid present in the fat cells in several conditions often spreads across the section and can sometimes obscure the intracellular accumulation.

Common artefacts in muscle biopsies

Artefacts in the handling of specimens and during section cutting or staining procedures can lead to difficulties in interpretation. Infiltration of the muscle with local anaesthetic or rough handling of the sample may induce rounding up and hypercontraction of the fibres. Fibres at the edge of a sample are often damaged and should be considered with caution (Fig. 4.53). If samples are kept too moist before freezing, fluid accumulates in the sample and the fibres become disrupted and vacuolated (Fig. 4.54). Mislocation of glycogen also occurs. A sample should only be kept in gauze *lightly* dampened with saline for transportation. If there is a long delay before freezing depletion of glycogen occurs. A very common artefact is the presence of ice crystals that appear as holes in the fibres (Fig. 4.55). These are induced by poor freezing of the sample and/or allowing the sample to warm up during transfer to or from the cryostat or freezer. If a

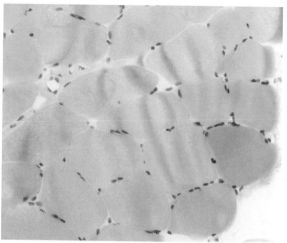

FIG. 4.53 *Artefactual hypercontraction of fibres; artefact at the edge of a section and a striped effect in some fibres caused by contraction.*

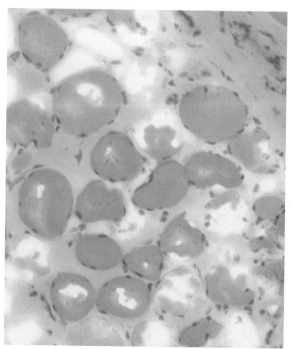

FIG. 4.54 *Disruption caused by contact with too much saline.*

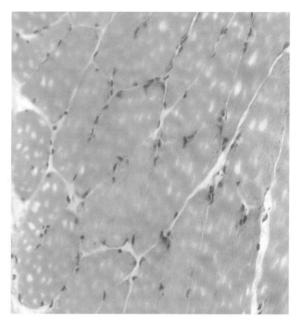

FIG. 4.55 *Holes caused by ice crystal damage.*

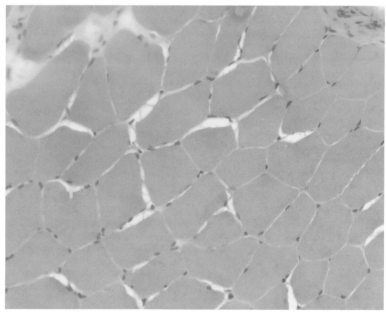

FIG. 4.56 *Shrinkage of the fibres and pulling away of the sarcolemma from the myofibrils which occurs if the sample dries out before freezing.*

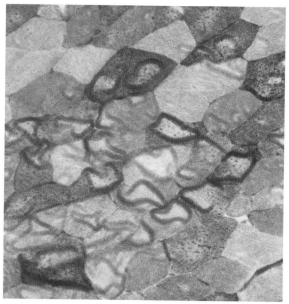

FIG. 4.57 *Artefact caused by the section lifting off the slide during staining.*

sample is particularly badly affected by freezing artefact, it can be thawed and quickly refrozen. The fibres may become round in shape but the number of holes is reduced and the overall appearance of the sample improved. It is important to distinguish freezing artefact from the pathological presence of vacuoles. Poor freezing or allowing the sample to become too dry prior to freezing causes shrinkage and the fibres pull away from the endomysium and the fibres may crack (Fig. 4.56). If the knife or guide plate is incorrectly adjusted or damaged, sections may be scratched, wrinkled or compressed. The latter may give a false impression of small fibres. Care in interpreting possible artefacts in staining, dehydration or mounting is also needed. For example, unevenness of stain may give a misleading impression, or dirt on the section may be mistaken for an inclusion. The latter, however, is always out of the plane of section and careful focusing will enable a distinction to be made. If sections lift off the slide staining intensities can vary, sometimes giving a striped or ring appearance (Fig. 4.57).

CHAPTER 5

Ultrastructural changes in diseased muscle

Skeletal muscle undergoes many changes in response to disease and trauma. With the electron microscope, the abnormalities seen at the light level can be characterized and accurately localized, and the variety of changes affecting each organelle identified. The interpretation of the pathological abnormalities observed in a muscle biopsy must take into account several factors, in particular the small sample size, possible artefacts induced by preparation and the non-specificity of the changes.

Only very small areas of tissue can be examined in the electron microscope and samples may not be representative of the muscle or of the fibre as a whole. Only part of a fibre may be pathologically affected, and frequently isolated and peculiar structures of unknown significance may be observed. Correct handling of samples is also of paramount importance to prevent artefacts. For example, fibres at the edge of blocks may be damaged and show contraction bands, or organelles may swell if the osmolarity and concentration of the buffer are not correct, or the sample is kept in contact with too much saline before fixing. Ideally muscle should be fixed at resting length for electron microscopy. This is possible for open biopsies by clamping the sample before excision or suturing each end of the muscle strip and securing this to a wooden tongue depressor or other rigid object before fixation. For needle biopsies this is not practicable but leaving the muscle to rest for 10 to 15 minutes reduces some of the contraction that occurs with fixation and does not influence the interpretation of the biopsy. Needle biopsies are therefore quite adequate for electron microscopy, particularly for qualitative pathological studies. The majority of micrographs in this chapter were obtained from needle biopsies. In general, more ultrastructural information is obtained from studies of longitudinally orientated fibres, particularly with regard to sarcomere structure. Transverse sections contain more fibres per area, however, and a good impression of fibre size and shape can be obtained from semi-thin 1 μm sections, which in general provide useful information (see Fig. 1.10; Carpenter 2001a).

The non-specificity of most ultrastructural changes makes it difficult to make a definitive diagnosis by electron microscopy alone. Muscle reacts to disease in a limited number of ways and most abnormalities can occur in a variety of disorders. Nevertheless, consistent patterns can be recognized that assist in making a diagnosis. Accurate diagnosis, however, is possible only when all clinical, histochemical, immunohistochemical, electron microscopic, biochemical and electrophysiological data are considered.

Since the previous edition of this book there has been a greater understanding of the nature of ultrastructural features and, in particular, of their molecular cause. The diagnostic role of ultrastructural studies, however, has changed very little. The main contributions of electron microscopy are:

- to help decide if a sample is normal or abnormal by looking for any subtle changes;
- to clarify the nature of a feature observed at the light level, such as nemaline rods, abnormal mitochondria or various types of inclusions or accumulated material;
- to identify structures only visible at the ultrastructural level such as nuclear inclusions, the filamentous inclusions of inclusion body myositis or tubuloreticular inclusions in capillaries.

This chapter is intended to illustrate the variety of ultrastructural changes encountered in human muscle biopsies and to serve as a practical guide to the interpretation of the changes. Table 5.1 summarizes many of the abnormalities that occur in human neuromuscular disorders and deals with the individual components of the fibres rather than the changes that occur in specific disorders. Reference to particular diseases is kept to a minimum in this section, but in subsequent chapters electron microscopic findings relevant to specific diseases will be discussed. We have retained citations of several of the early publications as a reminder of the contribution and pioneering work of morphologists to our understanding of the pathological changes in muscle, before any molecular defects were known. Further details of the occurrence of particular features can be found in reviews by Mair and Tomé (1972), Neville (1979), and Cullen and Mastaglia (1982), which have stood the test of time, and more recent texts such as Carpenter (2001a,b) and Carpenter and Karpati (2001).

Sarcolemma

A common feature is irregularity of the surface of the fibre and folding of the sarcolemma (Fig. 5.1). Such changes are often seen in situations where atrophy occurs. The basal lamina may split away from the plasma membrane and form extensive folds in the extracellular space (Fig. 5.2) or it may appear to be replicated in some areas (Fig. 5.3). Sometimes glycogen is seen between the plasma membrane and basal lamina and although this is usually only in small amounts, it can be excessive in glycogen storage diseases (Fig. 5.4).

TABLE 5.1 *Ultrastructural abnormalities in diseased muscle*

1 *Sarcolemma*

Folding

Redundant basal lamina

Thickening of basal lamina

Loss of plasma membrane

Abnormal caveolae

2 *Myofibrils and cytoskeleton*

Loss and splitting

Hypercontraction

I band loss

A band loss

Ring fibres

Cores

Filamentous bodies

Concentric laminated whorls

Z line alterations:

Streaming

Irregularities

Double Z lines

Z line loss

Rods

Cytoplasmic bodies

Granulofilamentous accumulation of desmin

3 *Nucleus*

Central location

Changes in shape

Changes in chromatin distribution

Inclusions

4 *Mitochondria*

Aggregates

Abnormal structure

Inclusions

5 *Membrane systems*

Swollen sarcoplasmic reticulum

Replication of triads

Honeycomb structures

Tubular aggregates

6 *Deposits and particles*

Excess glycogen

Excess lipid

Lipofuscin

Lipopigment

Virus-like particles

Crystalline material

7 *Other unusual structures*

Actin accumulation

Zebra bodies

Fingerprint bodies

Curvilinear bodies

Reducing bodies

Autophagic vacuoles

Membranous/myelin-like whorls

Dense tubules

Mallory body-like inclusions

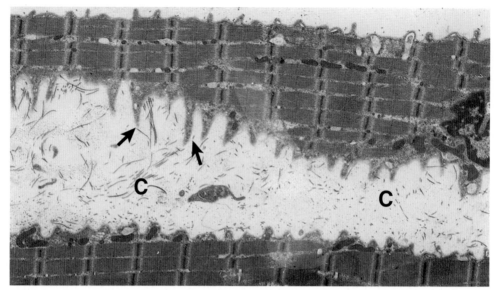

FIG. 5.1 *An atrophic fibre with sarcolemmal folds (arrows). These project into the extracellular space which contains collagen fibrils (C). Magnification in this and subsequent figures can be judged by the length of the A band which is unaltered by contraction and is 1.5–1.6 μm. (Myotonic dystrophy.)*

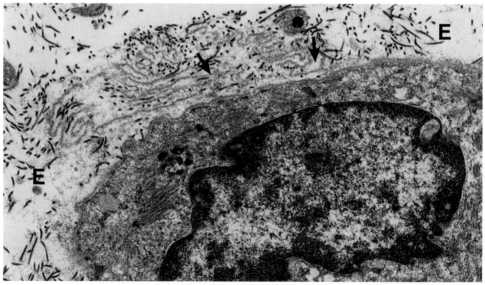

FIG. 5.2 *Peripheral region of an atrophic fibre with extensive folds of basal lamina (arrows) in the extracellular space (E). (Myotonic dystrophy.)*

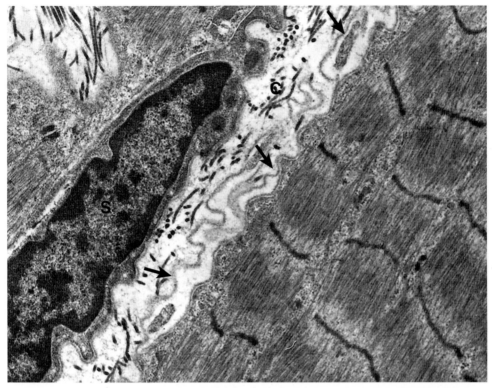

FIG. 5.3 *An additional replicated layer of basal lamina (arrows) at the periphery of an atrophic fibre. The adjacent fibre shows part of a satellite cell (S). The extracellular space between the two fibres contains longitudinally and transversely orientated collagen fibrils (C). (Spinal muscular atrophy.)*

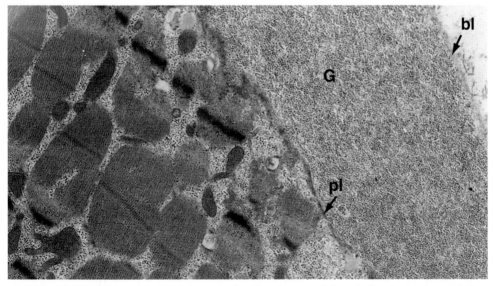

FIG. 5.4 *Glycogen accumulation (G) between the basal lamina (bl) and plasma membrane (pl). (McArdle's disease.)*

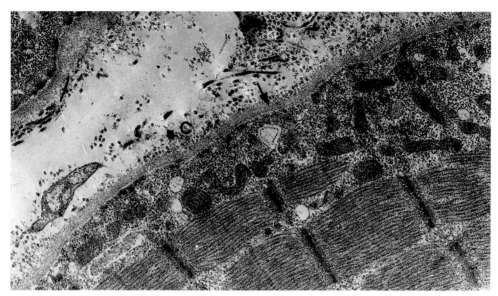

FIG. 5.5 *Thickened basal lamina of a fibre (arrow). Collagen fibrils (C) are closely applied to it on the external surface. (Limb-girdle dystrophy.)*

Redundant basal lamina is considered to be a characteristic of atrophic fibres. This is in contrast to hypotrophic fibres which have a closely adherent basal lamina. Hypotrophic fibres are believed to be small fibres in which normal growth and maturation have been arrested (Fidzianska 1976, Argov et al 1980). It is a term applied to the small type 1 fibres of congenital myopathies such as myotubular (centronuclear) myopathy, but our studies of fibres in this disorder indicate that redundant basal lamina does occur around the small fibres (see Ch. 10).

Thickening of the basal lamina also occurs and is found in a variety of neuromuscular disorders (Fig. 5.5). Thickening and duplication of capillary basal lamina is also seen in diseased muscle and is a feature of diabetes (Figs 5.6 and 5.7).

In the recessive Ullrich form of congenital muscular dystrophy caused by defects in collagen VI genes, fibrillar masses near the reticular layer may be seen which probably relate to abnormally assembled collagen VI (Ishikawa et al 2002, 2004).

The plasma membrane may also show defects. Focal breaks may be apparent (Fig. 5.8) or in necrotic fibres the plasma membrane may be lost completely (Fig. 5.9). These fibres are then only surrounded by the highly resistant basal lamina. In the search for the underlying cause of Duchenne dystrophy, now known to be dystrophin, considerable emphasis was placed on the observation of damaged plasma membranes (Mokri and Engel 1975, Carpenter and Karpati 1979, Cullen and Fulthorpe 1975), but it is a non-specific finding associated with a particular type of fibre damage and can be found in a variety of disorders (Schmalbruch 1975).

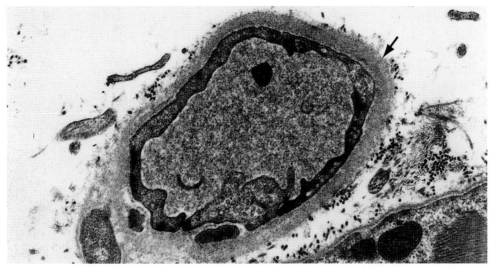

FIG. 5.6 *Capillary with thickened basal lamina (arrow). (Rheumatoid arthritis.)*

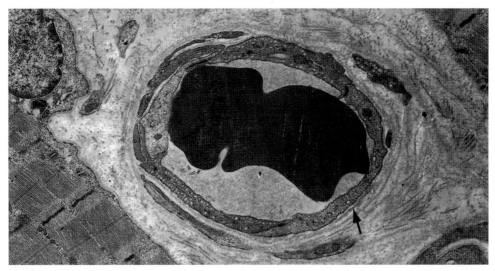

FIG. 5.7 *Capillary with replicated basal lamina (arrow). (Duchenne muscular dystrophy.)*

The plasma membrane also shows changes in disorders affecting caveolin-3 (Minetti et al 2002, Kubisch et al 2003). With transmission electron microscopy caveolae appear as small subsarcolemmal vesicles but when the gene for caveolin-3 is mutated there is impairment of caveolae formation, discontinuity of the plasma membrane, subsarcolemmal vacuoles, papillary projections and disorganization of the T system openings on the plasma membrane. Caveolin-3 and dysferlin interact (Matsuda et al 2001) and similar changes in the sarcolemma may be seen when dysferlin is deficient. In addition, deep invaginations containing basal lamina may be seen (Selcen et al 2001).

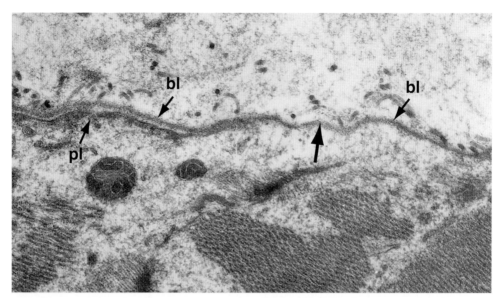

FIG. 5.8 *Focal loss of plasma membrane (large arrow). The basal lamina (bl) remains but the plasma membrane (pl) is absent from a portion of the sarcolemma (large arrow). (Possible carrier of Duchenne muscular dystrophy.)*

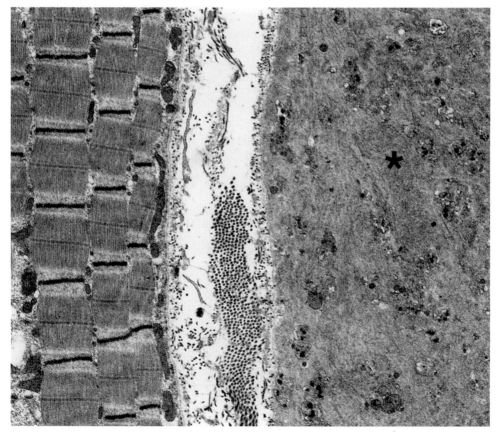

FIG. 5.9 *Necrotic fibre (*) which is only surrounded by a basal lamina. The myofibrils have been replaced by granular amorphous material. The adjacent fibre has well preserved myofibrils and the sarcolemma has both a basal lamina and a plasma membrane. (Duchenne muscular dystrophy.)*

Myofibrils and associated cytoskeleton

Loss and alterations in the myofilaments are the most common abnormalities observed in diseased muscle. Their occurrence is widespread and they have been observed in all classes of genetic and acquired neuromuscular disorders. The degree of myofilament loss and disruption is variable, depending on the nature of the disorder and the area examined. It is one of the most difficult changes to assess because even in normal muscle, departures from the classical appearance frequently occur. This is shown in Figures 5.10–5.12, which are all taken from healthy volunteers and illustrate the variety of features within normal individuals. Myofilament loss in diseased muscle may affect part or the whole of the fibre and the extent of damage varies from fibre to fibre. Therefore within a biopsy there is a spectrum of changes with fibres affected to varying degrees. Focal loss of myofilaments within a fibre may occur (Fig. 5.13) or it may be widespread and cause narrowing of the myofibrils (Figs 5.14 and 5.15). Care is needed in interpreting focal loss to ensure that changes are not just due to undulation of the myofibrils and differences in the plane of section through sarcoplasm or myofibrils. Excessive splitting of the bundles is often associated with myofibril loss (Fig. 5.15) and the space between the myofibrils is then occupied by sarcoplasmic components including glycogen, mitochondria, sarcoplasmic reticulum and T tubules.

In severely necrotic fibres, the characteristic myofilament structure is lost completely and replaced by amorphous granular material (Fig. 5.16). These fibres may contain macrophages (Fig. 5.16) and correspond to the pale disrupted fibres seen with histological and histochemical techniques. This appearance is thought to be the end stage of a series of events leading to necrosis (Cullen and Fulthorpe 1975). Earlier stages in necrosis are thought to involve the hypercontraction or overcontraction of myofibrils and probably correspond to the round, intensely stained fibres seen with light microscopy. The areas affected by hypercontraction may be focal (Fig. 5.17) or extensive (Fig. 5.18). Clumps of contracted myofibrils form and are interspersed with areas of overstretched filaments. Other organelles in these fibres also show abnormalities, and the tubular systems are often dilated and the mitochondria degenerate. Hypercontraction of myofibrils can be induced artefactually, particularly at the periphery of biopsies where handling may damage fibres. Most hypercontracted fibres seen in diseased muscle, however, are not thought to be artefactual. They are particularly common in Duchenne muscular dystrophy but also occur in a variety of other neuromuscular disorders.

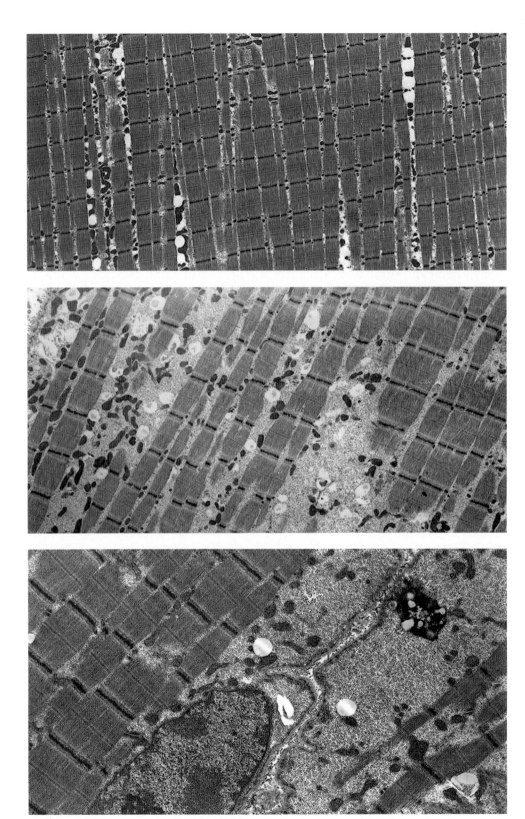

FIGS 5.10–5.12 *Sections of needle biopsies from three healthy volunteers illustrating the varying degrees of myofibrillar loss that can occur in normal muscle.*

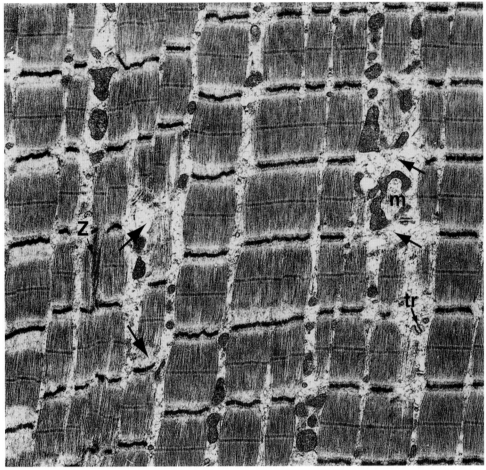

FIG. 5.13 *Focal loss of myofilaments (large arrows). The space vacated contains mitochondria (m), glycogen and displaced triads (tr). Focal Z line streaming (Z) and Z line irregularities are also present. (Unclassified congenital myopathy.)*

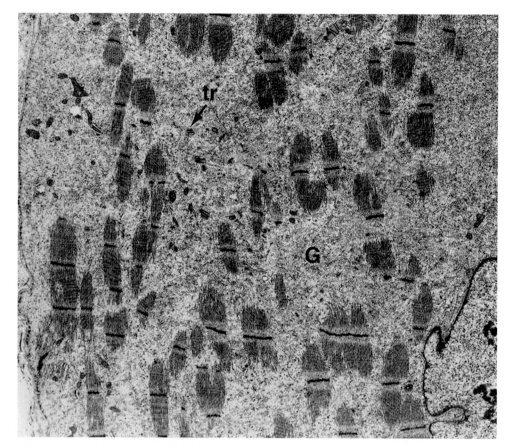

FIG. 5.14 *Extensive loss of myofibrils. The fragments that remain have retained their longitudinal orientation and glycogen (G) and triads (tr) are prominent between them. (Facioscapulohumeral dystrophy.)*

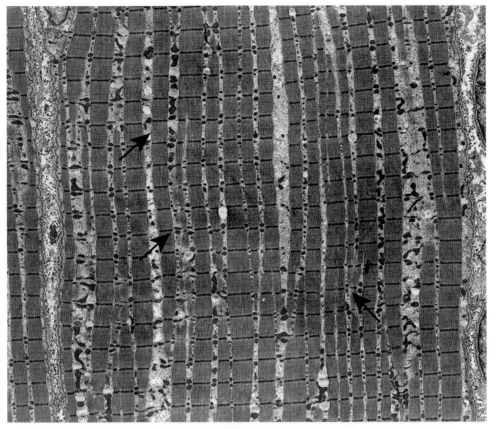

FIG. 5.15 *Narrowing and splitting of the myofibrils (arrows). Glycogen and mitochondria are prominent in the areas between the myofibrils. (Facioscapulohumeral dystrophy.)*

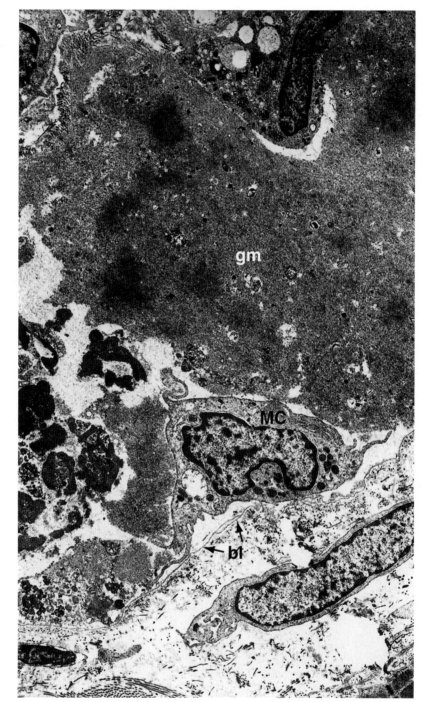

FIG. 5.16 *Necrotic granular fibre invaded by macrophages (MC). Only the basal lamina (bl) of the sarcolemma remains and the myofibrils have been replaced by granular, amorphous material (gm). (Duchenne muscular dystrophy.)*

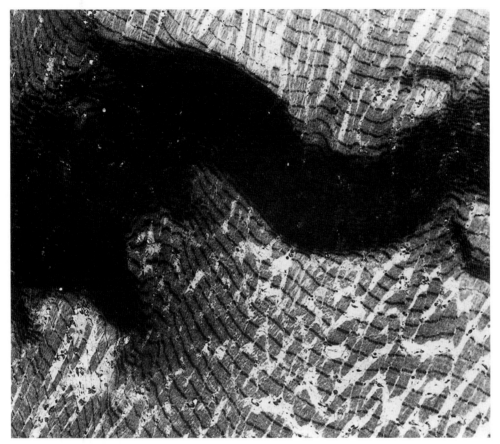

FIG. 5.17 *Focal hypercontraction of myofibrils. A dark band of very contracted myofibrils can be seen in one region of the fibre. The remaining sarcomeres are contracted but can still be distinguished. (Congenital muscular dystrophy.)*

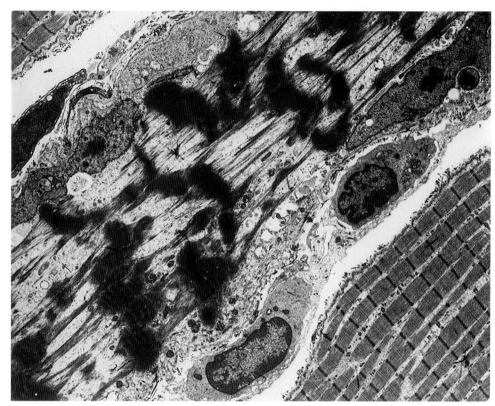

FIG. 5.18 *Extensive hypercontraction throughout one fibre. Clumps of dark myofibrillar material are interspersed with overstretched filaments. Adjacent fibres show more normal myofibrillar structure. (Infantile myositis.)*

Selective loss or abnormalities of particular regions of the sarcomere may also occur. ***Loss of I bands*** has been reported in some conditions (Cullen and Fulthorpe 1982) and is usually associated with loss of the Z line (Fig. 5.19), although remnants of the Z line may sometimes remain. As stated above, caution in interpretation is sometimes required if the plane of section has not passed completely through the whole myofibril. Sections through contracted or disorientated myofibrils may pass through filaments at one point and sarcoplasm at another, thus giving the false impression of loss. ***Loss of A bands*** (Fig. 5.20) is a rare finding in diseased human muscle, but a number of cases have been reported (Carpenter et al 1976, Yarom and Shapira 1977, Sher et al 1979, Yarom and Reches 1980) and we have observed isolated fibres with this abnormality in several conditions, including systemic lupus erythematosus, congenital muscular dystrophy, and carriers of Duchenne muscular dystrophy. It is most commonly found in patients with acute quadriplegic myopathy ('critical illness myopathy') on high doses of glucocorticoids and neuromuscular blocking agents (Danon and Carpenter 1991, Hirano et al 1992; see Ch. 23).

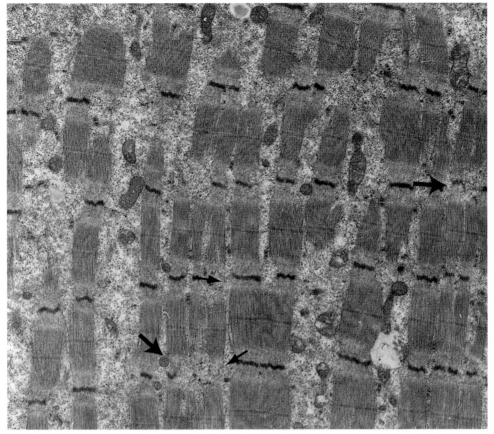

FIG. 5.19 *Loss of I bands (large arrows) from some sarcomeres. Both the Z line and I bands are absent in some areas (small arrows). The myofibrils are narrow and split. (Duchenne muscular dystrophy.)*

Myofibrils can undergo varying degrees of disorganization, disorientation and disruption. In some fibres, the normal striation pattern is lost completely but sarcomeres are still identifiable (Fig. 5.21). In others, only certain regions of the fibre are disorientated, for example in *ring fibres* (Figs 5.22 and 5.23). These unusual fibres have one or more peripheral myofibrils running at right angles to the normal axis of the fibre. The disorientated zone of myofibrils may be immediately beneath the sarcolemma (Figs 5.22 and 5.23) or be separated by an area of sarcoplasm that contains very few myofilaments. These areas are known as sarcoplasmic masses (Fig. 5.24). In some ring fibres, the disorientated myofibrils may not be peripheral throughout the fibre and bands of myofibrils at right angles to the remaining myofibrils can be seen to traverse the fibre (Fig. 5.24). Ring fibres are non-specific but are particularly common in myotonic dystrophy and some forms of limb-girdle dystrophy.

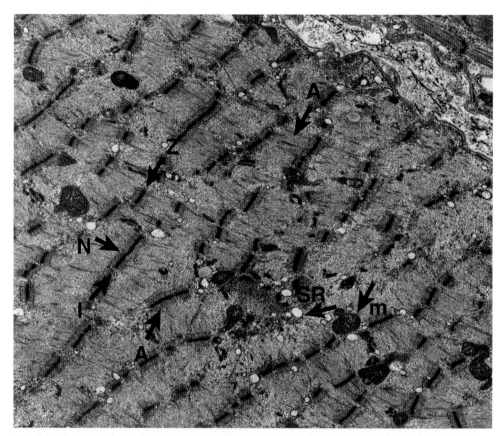

FIG. 5.20 *Extensive loss of A bands. The Z lines (Z), I bands (I) and N line (N) are retained but only fragments of A band (A) filaments span the area between them. The sarcoplasmic reticulum (SR) is slightly swollen and the mitochondria (m) present are mainly rounded and swollen. (Congenital muscular dystrophy.)*

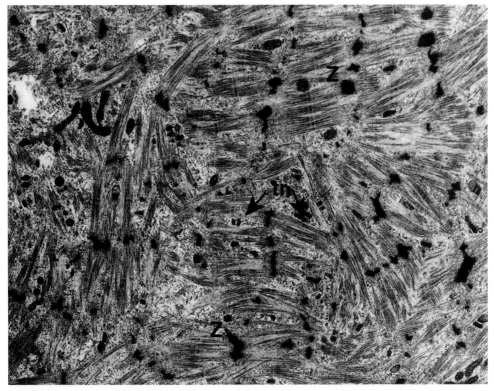

FIG. 5.21 *Disorganization of myofibrils. Sarcomeres are still identifiable but the normal striation pattern is lost. Z lines are thickened (Z) and triads displaced and replicated (tr). (Unclassified myopathy.)*

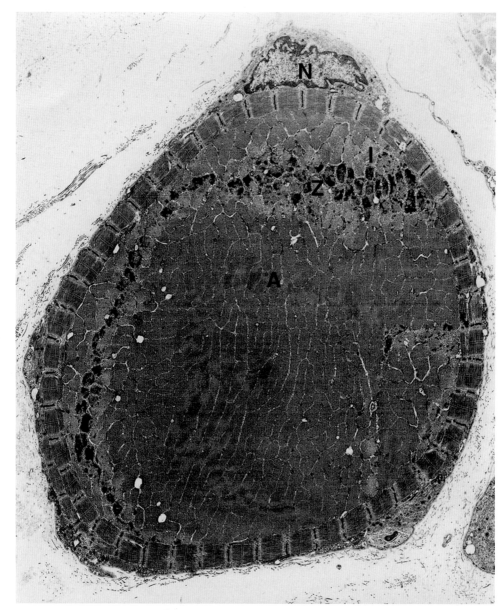

FIG. 5.22 *Transverse section of a ring fibre. The central area is transversely orientated, but a peripheral band is at 90° to this and is longitudinally orientated. The A bands (A), I bands (I) and Z lines (Z) of the transverse area are prominent and the subsarcolemmal nucleus (N) appears normal. (Myotonic dystrophy.)*

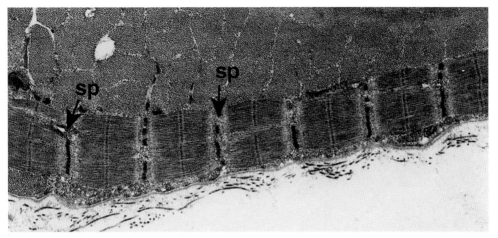

FIG. 5.23 *High power of the peripheral myofibrillar band of the same ring fibre as seen in Fig. 5.22. The normal sarcomere pattern is clear, although some splitting is present (sp).*

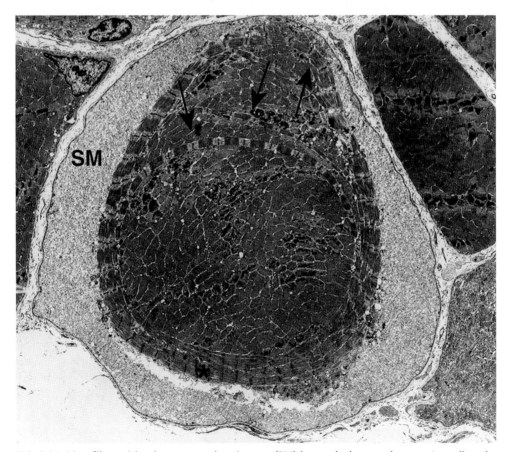

FIG. 5.24 *Ring fibre with a large sarcoplasmic mass (SM) beneath the sarcolemma. As well as the outer ring of myofibrils other bands also transect the fibre (arrows). Some sarcomeres in the peripheral ring zone are very contracted (*). (Myotonic dystrophy.)*

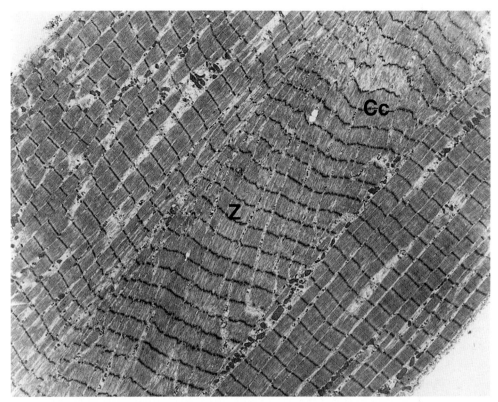

FIG. 5.25 *Structured central core (Cc). The central area is slightly disorientated and the Z line shows some irregularities (Z), but the sarcomere pattern is still distinct. Mitochondria are noticeably absent from the core but present in the relatively normal peripheral regions of the fibre. (Central core disease.)*

Restriction of myofilament disruption to focal areas is found in the formation of cores, minicores and target fibres. *Cores*, such as those found in central core disease, can be central or peripheral and may run most of the length of the fibre. They are characterized by a variable degree of myofibril disorganization and Z line streaming, and a scarcity or absence of mitochondria. Neville and Brooke (1973) recognized two pathologically distinct types of core in central core disease, the structured and the unstructured core. In the structured core, the striation pattern is preserved but the core area is slightly contracted compared with the surrounding myofibrils and shows a reduction in the number of mitochondria (Fig. 5.25). This type of core retains its myosin adenosine triphosphatase (ATPase) staining in contrast to the unstructured core in which it is lost or reduced. The banding pattern in unstructured cores is not discernible and there is usually marked myofibrillar disruption and large amounts of smeared Z line material, but mitochondria are sparse or absent (see *target fibres* below). Some authors report the occurrence of both types of cores in the same biopsy (Telerman-Toppet et al 1973, Isaacs et al 1975), but Neville (1979) considers this unusual and that it is more common to find only one type of core in a given patient with central core

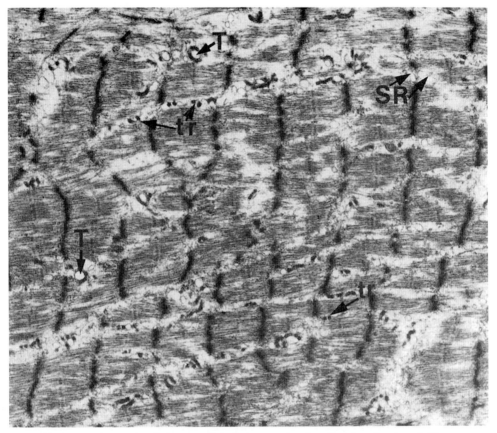

FIG. 5.26 *A central core that is intermediate between structured and unstructured. The myofibrils show disruption but the sarcomeres can still be distinguished. Triads (tr) are prominent and the T system component (T) is often dilated. The sarcoplasmic reticulum (SR) also shows some swelling. (Central core disease.)*

disease. In a case of central core disease referred to us, some cores could not easily be categorized as structured or unstructured, and were intermediate between these types (Fig. 5.26). The myofibrils of these cores showed degenerative changes but had recognizable striations. The extensive disorganization found in unstructured cores was absent. Tubular profiles were also clearly visible in these cores. These features of different types of cores probably reflect different stages of myofibrillar disruption within a spectrum.

Other clinically distinct conditions are characterized by the presence of multiple *minicores* (Engel et al 1971; see Ch. 15). These cores are small, focal areas of disruption and affect only a few sarcomeres (Fig. 5.27), or they may extend over a wider area involving several sarcomeres and myofibrils (Fig. 5.28) but they are not usually as extensive as those in central core disease. Minicores are characterized by irregularities and smearing of the Z line, and disorganization of the myofibrils. Central core disease and multiminicore disease, caused by mutations in the genes for the ryanodine receptor 1 (*RYR1*) and selenoprotein

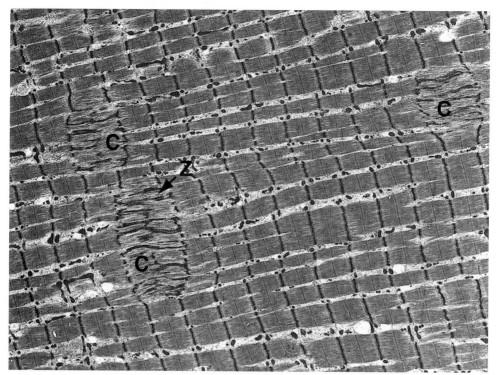

FIG. 5.27 *Minicores (c) affecting focal areas of the fibre. A few sarcomeres of some myofibrils have smeared Z line material (Z) and myofilament disruption. ('Minicore' myopathy.)*

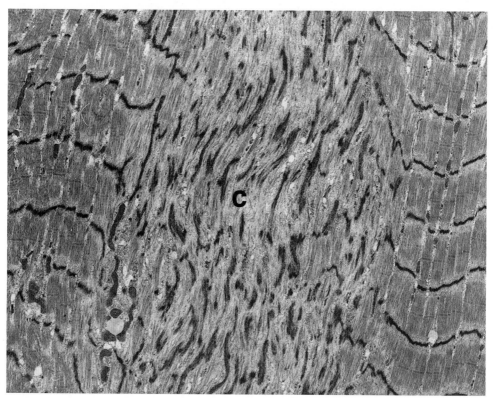

FIG. 5.28 *Large minicore (c) with excess Z line material and myofilament disruption. ('Minicore' myopathy.)*

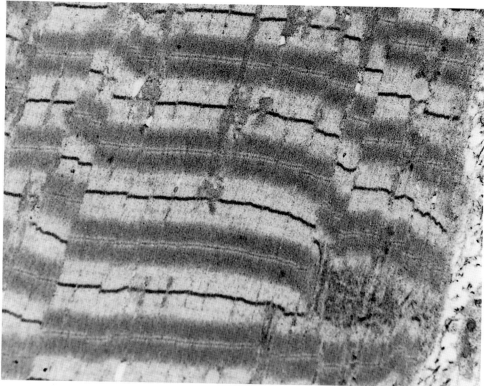

FIG. 5.29 *Misalignment of myofibrils in an area with sparse mitochondria. ('Minicore' myopathy.)*

N1 (*SEPN1*), respectively gained their names from the extent of the pathological abnormality (Jungbluth et al 2002, Ferriero et al 2002; see Ch. 15), and cores of varying dimension occur in these disorders. They are not specific for these disorders, however, and cores can be found in isolated fibres in a variety of neuromuscular disorders.

In some cores the myofibrillar disruption may be minimal and only misalignment of the striations is seen in comparison with adjacent myofibrils. These areas have a scarcity of mitochondria (Fig. 5.29) and may correspond to unevenness of oxidative enzyme stain. Caution in identifying such areas is needed, however, in samples not fixed at resting length as variable contraction of myofibrils may lead to misalignment.

Target fibres (Engel 1961) have three concentric zones that can be identified with both the light and the electron microscope and are a feature of denervated muscle. The outer zone is essentially normal except for occasional areas of Z band streaming; the intermediate zone contains myofibrils with mild Z line irregularities and swollen sarcoplasmic reticulum; and the central zone is markedly disrupted with extensive Z line material similar to unstructured cores (Fig. 5.30). If the intermediate zone is not clearly defined, the fibres are termed *targetoid*.

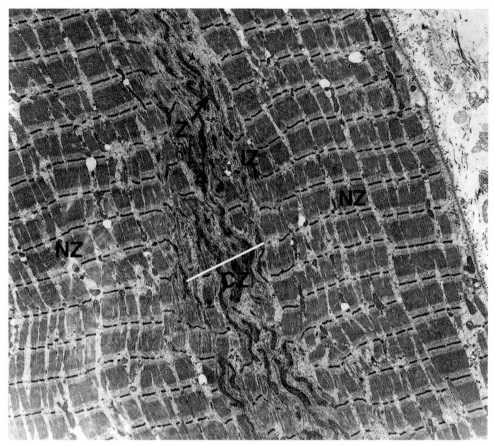

FIG. 5.30 *Target fibre with three definable areas. The outer zone shows a normal striation pattern (NZ), the intermediate zone (IZ) shows mild Z line irregularities and the central zone (CZ) has extensive areas of Z line material (Z) and no mitochondria. The central area resembles an unstructured core. (Motor neurone disease.)*

A congenital disorder has been described in which a population of *'trilaminar fibres'* with zones was found (Ringel et al 1978). In these fibres the outer zone contains mitochondria, loosely packed filaments, glycogen, ribosomes and tubular profiles; the intermediate zone consisted of a few organized myofibrils with characteristic striations; and the inner zone contained mitochondria, glycogen, osmiophilic material resembling Z line material and loosely packed filaments.

Other unusual non-specific structures which are thought to be of myofibrillar origin are filamentous bodies and concentric laminated bodies. *Filamentous bodies* are composed of tightly packed actin-like filaments (Fig. 5.31). Within a biopsy they are infrequent and when present they are often subsarcolemmal but can occur in other regions of the fibre. They have been identified in a variety of neuromuscular disorders and we have also frequently seen them in carriers of Duchenne dystrophy. They have also been recorded in normal human muscle.

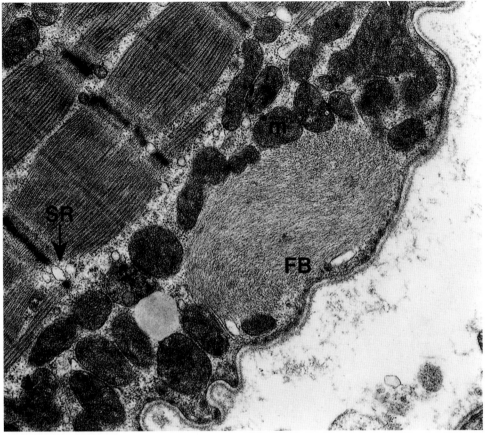

FIG. 5.31 *Filamentous body (FB) at the periphery of a fibre. It is surrounded by mitochondria (m) and the sarcoplasmic reticulum is slightly swollen (SR). (Limb-girdle muscular dystrophy.)*

Concentric laminated bodies are cylindrical structures of 3–25 concentric laminae, the centre of which may contain glycogen (Fig. 5.32). The laminae are 6–8 nm thick with a spacing of about 7.5 nm. They are considered by some workers to be of myofibrillar origin (Payne and Curless 1976), whereas others believe they are derived from mitochondria (Luft et al 1962).

Z line

Z line streaming is another very common structural alteration associated with myofibrillar damage in diseased muscle (Fig. 5.33). The number of sarcomeres involved is variable and some Z line streaming can be found in normal muscle (Meltzer et al 1976). The Z line may also show thickening (Fig. 5.34), irregularities (Fig. 5.33), duplication (Fig. 5.35) or loss (Fig. 5.33). It is also thought that the Z lines give rise to the dense rod-like structures that characterize all forms of nemaline myopathy (Shy et al 1963, Wallgren-Petterson and Laing 2000, 2001) (Fig. 5.36).

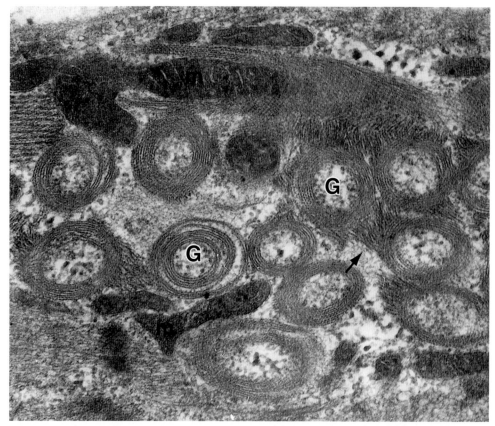

FIG. 5.32 *A cluster of concentric laminated bodies. Most of them enclose glycogen (G) and in some glycogen is present between the lamellae. Connections occur between some bodies (arrow). Mitochondria (m) are also associated with the cluster. (Polymyositis.) (Bar = 1 µm)*

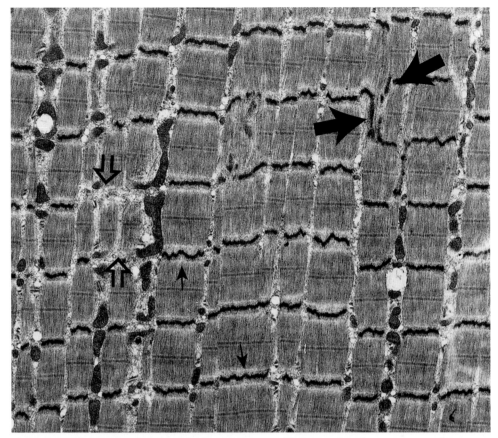

FIG. 5.33 *Z line abnormalities: focal Z line streaming affecting only a few sarcomeres (large arrows); irregular Z lines (small arrows); and loss of Z lines associated with focal loss of I band filaments (open arrows). (Spinal muscular atrophy.)*

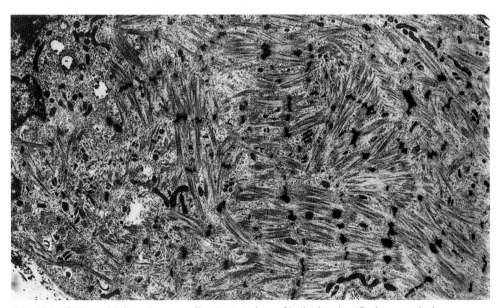

FIG. 5.34 *Thickened Z lines in some disorientated myofibrils. (Unclassified myopathy.)*

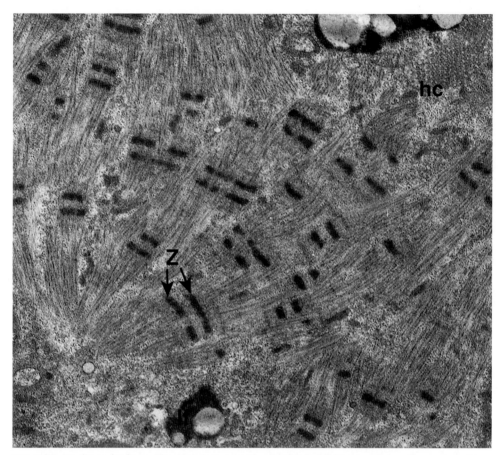

FIG. 5.35 *Duplicated Z lines. The area between the duplicated Z lines contains glycogen and is spanned by a few thin filaments. Part of a honeycomb structure is seen at the top of the micrograph (hc) adjacent to some lipofuscin (lf) which is also present near the bottom. (Carrier of Duchenne muscular dystrophy.)*

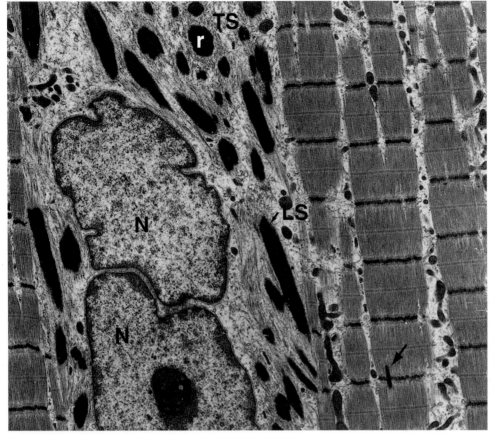

FIG. 5.36 *A group of nemaline rods (r) adjacent to two internal nuclei (N). A small rod (arrow) is also present within an I band. The rods have filaments attached and are orientated longitudinally (LS) and transversely (TS) to the long axis of the fibre. Normal Z lines are present in the myofibrils which show splitting and focal loss. (Nemaline myopathy.)*

Rods (nemaline bodies) may lie within the I band or they may extend for several sarcomeres and lie between the myofibrils (Fig. 5.37). Intranuclear rods (see below) have also been found in some severe cases with a mutation in the gene for skeletal actin (*ACTA1*; Nowak et al 1999). Continuity between rods and Z lines can sometimes be seen (Fig. 5.37). Rods frequently occur in groups which are often, but not exclusively, in the peripheral regions of the fibre. Morphological and immunocytochemical evidence strongly suggests that rods are similar to Z lines in several respects. Rods consist of closely packed filaments arranged in a lattice-like pattern (Fig. 5.38) and have a periodicity comparable to that seen in Z lines. They are composed predominantly of α-actinin; they also contain actin and have desmin at their periphery (Schollmeyer et al 1974, Yamaguchi et al 1978, 1982, Jockusch et al 1980, Goebel 1997). The occurrence of rods in occasional fibres is widespread and they have been reported in a variety of myopathies as well as in normal human extraocular muscle (Mukuno 1969) and myotendinous

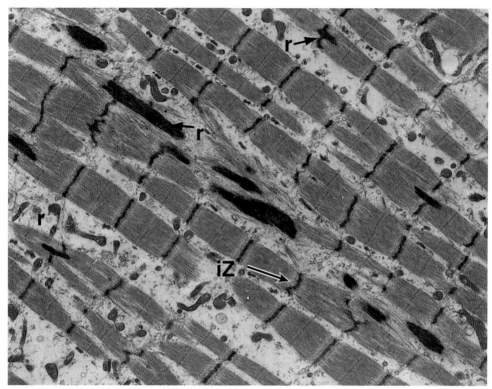

FIG. 5.37 *Rods (r), both adjacent to sarcomeres and within I bands, are continuous with Z lines. Other Z lines are irregular (iZ). (Nemaline myopathy.)*

regions (Fig. 5.39). In nemaline myopathy, they are the predominant structural abnormality and are associated with particular clinical features. A number of gene defects are now known to be responsible for the various forms of nemaline myopathy (see Ch. 15), but it is not possible at present to predict from electron microscopy which gene is mutated. The exception, however, is the presence of nuclear rods which have so far only been observed in nemaline patients with a skeletal actin mutation (*ACTA1*). Nuclear rods have, however, also been reported in epidermolysis bullosa simplex with muscular dystrophy caused by mutations in the gene for plectin (Banwell et al 1999). Studies are currently in progress to determine if the lattice structure of rods associated with each mutated gene is similar.

Cytoplasmic bodies are also thought to be an abnormality of the Z line (Macdonald and Engel 1969), and are characterized by a dense circular or oval centre and a peripheral zone of fine filaments radiating from it. Between the two zones, a pale halo of randomly orientated fine filaments is sometimes visible (Fig. 5.40). The biochemical nature of the dark core is unknown, but it is filamentous and sometimes shows structural continuity with the Z line; the radiating filaments resemble actin and continuity with adjacent myofibrils is sometimes seen (Fig. 5.41), and desmin is seen in the halo (Osborn and Goebel 1983). Occasional

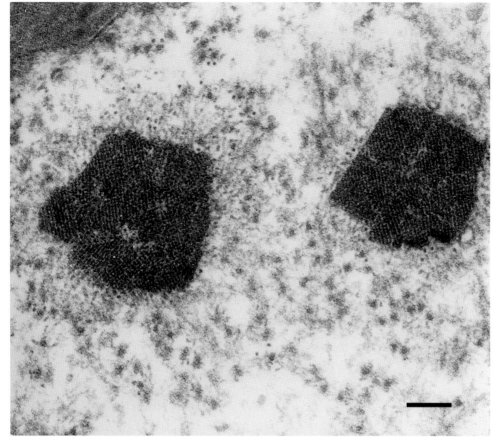

FIG. 5.38 *Transverse section through two rods showing the square lattice structure. (Nemaline myopathy.) (Bar = 0.1 μm)*

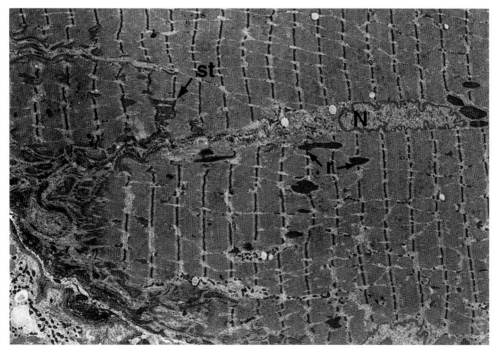

FIG. 5.39 *Rods (r) and Z line streaming (st) at a tendon region. An internal nucleus (N) is also present. (Definite carrier of Duchenne muscular dystrophy.)*

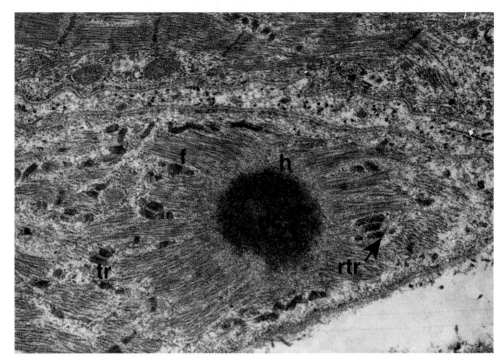

FIG. 5.40 *Cytoplasmic body with a dense core (dc) surrounded by a halo (h) and with filaments (f) radiating from it. Triads (tr) are prominent and a replicated triad (rtr) is present. (Spinal muscular atrophy.)*

cytoplasmic bodies may be found in many disorders where degeneration of myofibrils occurs and particularly where Z line abnormalities are common. They may occur singly within a fibre or in groups (Fig. 5.41) and are easily visible with routine histological stains such as Gomori trichrome (see Ch. 4). Cytoplasmic bodies are quite common in inclusion body myositis and a few cases have been reported where they are the predominant feature. This led to the distinction of 'cytoplasmic body neuromyopathy' as a disease entity (Jerusalem et al 1979). A biopsy referred to us that contained numerous cytoplasmic bodies in the muscle was from a patient who habitually took senna.

Intermediate filaments

Intermediate filaments are filaments of the cytoskeleton with a diameter of 10 nm, intermediate between that of actin and myosin. Desmin (skeletin), vimentin and syncoilin have been observed in skeletal muscle. The nuclear lamins are also intermediate filaments. Desmin is only found in muscle and is abundant in regenerating fibres and activated satellite cells (Thornell et al 1980). Rods and cytoplasmic bodies have desmin around them.

Accumulation of desmin-positive material in a group of myopathies has led to the concept of the 'desmin-related myopathies', 'surplus protein myopathies'

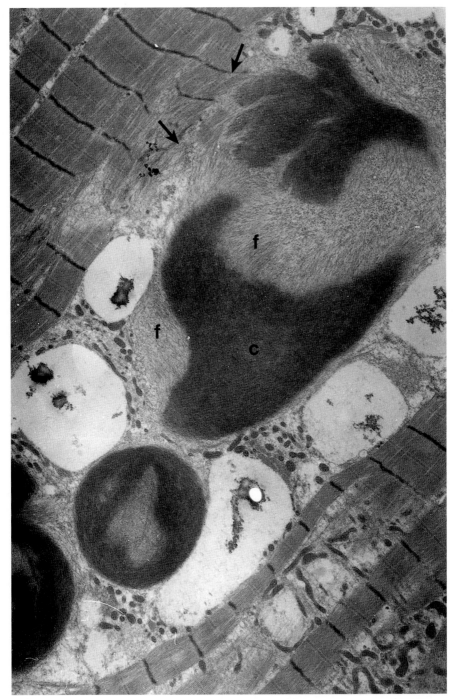

FIG. 5.41 *Group of unusual cytoplasmic bodies which show continuity with myofibrils (arrows). The core (c) is irregular in shape and not circular; no halo is present but filaments (f) radiate from the core. (Cytoplasmic body myopathy.)*

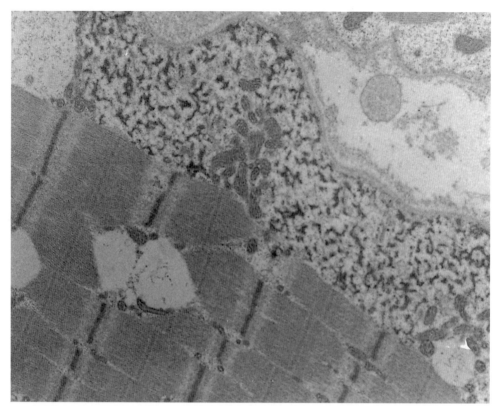

FIG. 5.42 *Accumulation of dense granulomatous material immunoreactive for desmin (Desmin myopathy.)*

and 'myofibrillar myopathies' (Goebel and Borchet 2002). In patients with a mutation in the desmin gene or the gene for the chaperone protein involved in desmin polymerization, αB-crystallin, characteristic areas of ***granulofilamentous material*** can be identified ultrastructurally (Fig. 5.42). These areas are pale with haematoxylin and eosin (H&E) and Gomori trichrome and are immunoreactive for desmin. Other proteins have also been demonstrated in these regions, including dystrophin, β-amyloid, αB-crystallin and various myofibrillar proteins (De Blecker et al 1996). Cytoplasmic bodies may also be an accompanying feature of the desmin accumulation and cases described as 'spheroid body myopathy' and sarcoplasmic bodies (Edström et al 1980) are also within this group of disorders. Many of the reported cases are familial, with a dominant pattern of inheritance. Distal weakness and cardiac involvement are common features, and cataracts are present in cases with a mutation in the αB-crystallin gene. When plectin is mutated in epidermolysis bullosa simplex with muscular dystrophy accumulations of disorganized desmin filaments occur, probably because of the impaired binding of desmin to the mutant plectin (see Schroder and Goebel 2002).

Nucleus

Changes in the myonucleus in diseased muscle include relocation, changes in shape, changes in chromatin distribution and a variety of inclusions. Within one diseased fibre, both normal and abnormal nuclei can be seen. Internal nuclei (Fig. 5.43), which occur singly or scattered through the fibres, are a common non-specific feature of neuromuscular disorders. Internal nuclei may occur in chains and can have a central position in the fibre. The sarcoplasmic areas surrounding internal nuclei may appear to be normal, or sometimes contain aggregates of mitochondria and accumulations of glycogen. Myotubular (centronuclear) myopathy is characterized by several fibres with central nuclei, and accumulations of mitochondria and glycogen (Fig. 5.44). In regenerating fibres, as in fetal fibres, nuclei are central and are often metabolically active with a prominent nucleolus.

In diseased muscle, nuclei may become irregular in shape (Fig. 5.43) and deep invaginations can occur. These sometimes give the appearance of inclusions, but they always have the typical double membrane.

Changes in chromatin condensation are associated with the activity of the fibre and the degree of damage to the fibre. Myonuclei of normal muscle often have a dense heterochromatic peripheral band with small areas of dense chromatin scattered through the nucleoplasm and a prominent nucleolus. In diseased

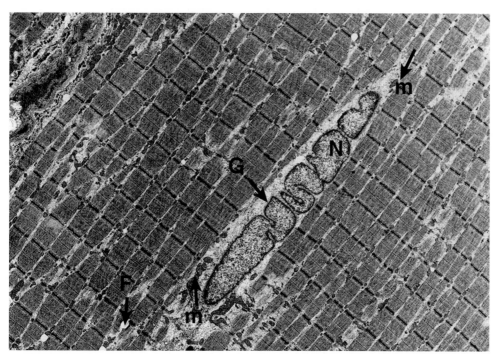

FIG. 5.43 *Irregular shaped internal nucleus (N). The area surrounding the nucleus contains glycogen (G), mitochondria (m) and a few fat droplets (F). (Facioscapulohumeral dystrophy.)*

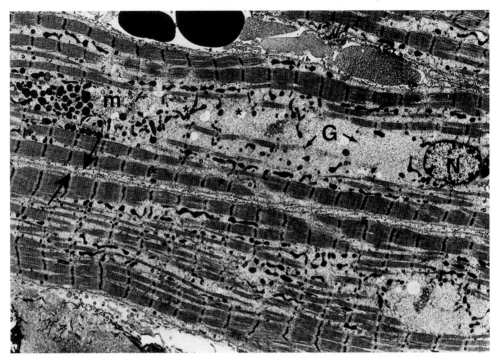

FIG. 5.44 *Two fibres in which the central zones show myofibrillar loss (*). The upper fibre has a central nucleus (N), and central accumulations of glycogen (G) and mitochondria (m). The sarcolemma of the two fibres is indicated by large arrows. (Myotubular myopathy.)*

muscle, nucleoli may be enlarged and the degree of chromatin condensation is variable. It ranges from being very dispersed (Fig. 5.45) to being highly condensed, as in pyknotic nuclei (Fig. 5.46). The chromatin can also form unusual shapes. Heterochromatin is usually attached to the nuclear membrane but in some nuclei it may be clumped and not attached to the nuclear membrane (Fig. 5.47). Such changes have been observed in apoptopic nuclei and in cases with a defect in the nuclear lamin A/C gene (Sewry et al 2001a). Changes in nuclei, including extrusion of nucleoplasm into the sarcoplasm, have also been reported in X-linked cases of Emery–Dreifuss muscular dystrophy with a defect in the emerin gene (Fidzianska et al 1998).

A variety of inclusions have also been found in nuclei of muscle fibres. Some of these resemble myofilament components, such as Z line material and rods (Jennis et al 1969, Barohn et al 1994b), or actin-like filaments; some are more tubular and a different size than myofibrillar material (Cullen and Mastaglia 1982). A feature of some severe cases of nemaline myopathy with a mutation in the actin gene is the presence of intranuclear rods (Barohn et al 1994b). The number of affected nuclei varies and cytoplasmic rods may or may not be present in addition (Fig. 5.48). Nuclear rods may also occur if the gene for plectin is mutated (Banwell et al 1999). Actin-like inclusions can occur in inflammatory myopathies such as inclusion body myositis (Fig. 5.49). Other inclusions have

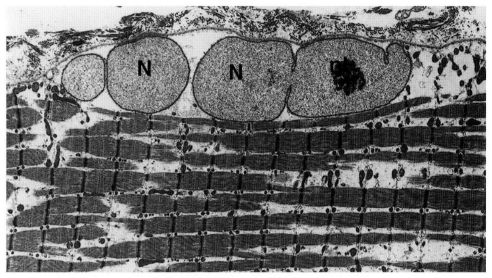

FIG. 5.45 *Peripheral nuclei (N) with dispersed chromatin. Their shape is irregular and the nucleolus (nl) of one is loosely packed. (Definite carrier of Duchenne muscular dystrophy.)*

been described as filamentous aggregates (Chou 1968, Schochet and McCormick 1973, Ionasescu et al 1975) or tubular filaments (Tomé and Fardeau 1980, Tomé et al 1981). In oculopharyngeal dystrophy, tubular filaments 8.5 nm in diameter have been observed in at least 3% of muscle fibre nuclei (Tomé and Fardeau 1980) and the authors considered them to be a characteristic morphological feature of this disorder. In oculopharyngeal dystrophy, these inclusions are restricted to nuclei, but in inclusion body myositis other larger tubular filaments (16–18 nm in diameter) are both intranuclear and sarcoplasmic (Tomé et al 1981) (Fig. 5.50). This latter type of filamentous inclusion is seen in sporadic and inherited forms of inclusion body myositis and myopathy, for example those caused by a mutation in the fast myosin *MYH2 (MyHC IIa)* gene (Martinsson et al 2000, Argov and Soffer 2002). Nuclear inclusions are generally rare but several of the reported cases and those that we have studied have been inflammatory disorders. In a study of dermatomyositis, Banker (1975) described three types of nuclear inclusions observed in sarcolemmal, interstitial cell and endothelial cell nuclei. The first is a spherical nuclear body composed of concentric fibrils, surrounded by a halo and containing a fine granular network (Fig. 5.51), the second a rod-shaped bundle of parallel filaments (Fig. 5.52) and the third type (Fig. 5.52) contains osmiophilic granules and a fibrillar cortex. Several dense osmiophilic particles of varying size may also be seen within some nuclei (Fig. 5.52).

Some intranuclear particles are thought to resemble viruses (see Fig. 5.46) (Chou 1968, Mair and Tomé 1972, Sato et al 1971, Tomé et al 1981) but no evidence has been produced to substantiate this or to suggest that they are related to a disease process. Occasionally a section may pass through the nuclear envelope itself and reveal the nuclear pores (Fig. 5.53). This may give the false impression of inclusions, whereas they are part of the normal nuclear membrane structure.

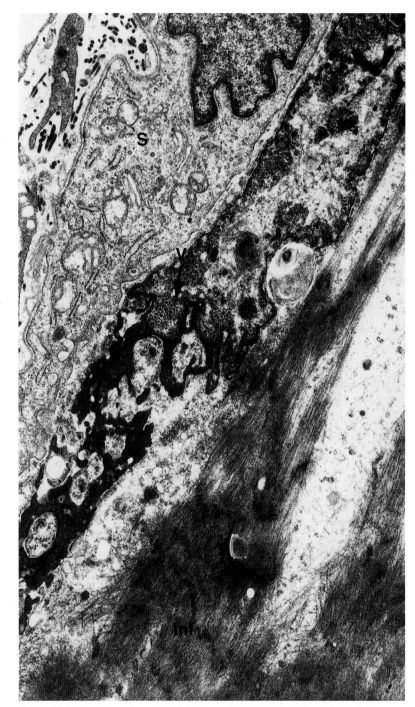

FIG. 5.46 *Pyknotic nucleus (N). The chromatin is very condensed and the nuclear envelope is disrupted. Some virus-like particles are present in one area (V). The adjacent myofibrils (mf) are hypercontracted and part of a satellite cell (S) can be seen beneath the basal lamina. (Infantile myositis.)*

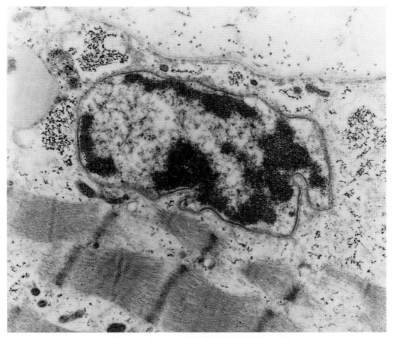

a

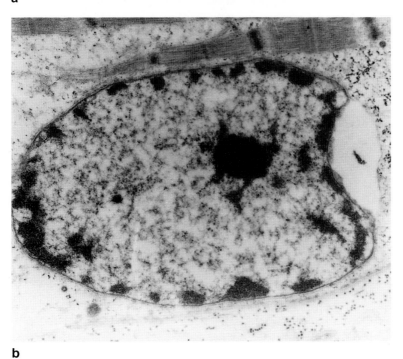

b

FIG. 5.47(a),(b) *Clumped chromatin not attached to the nuclear membrane (Autosomal dominant Emery–Dreifuss muscular dystrophy.)*

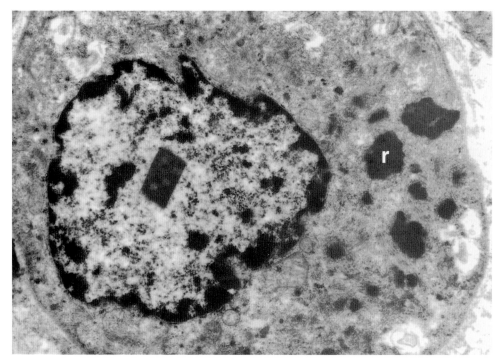

FIG. 5.48 *Nuclear rods in a case with an actin (ACTA1) mutation. Note also the cytoplasmic rods (r). (Courtesy of Professor H Goebel.)*

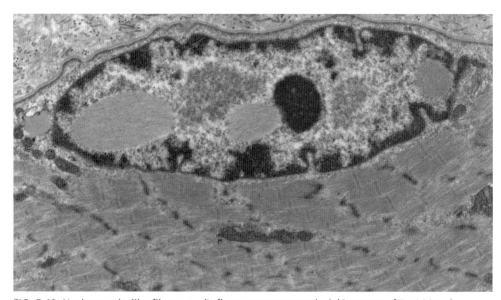

FIG. 5.49 *Nuclear actin-like filaments. (Inflammatory myopathy.) (Courtesy of Dr J Moss.)*

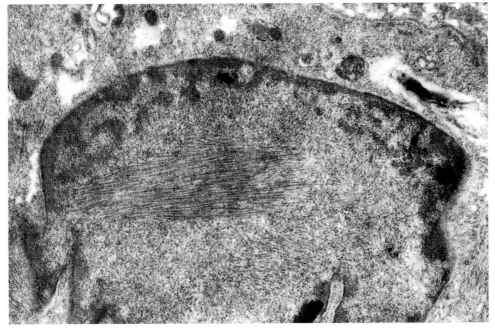

FIG. 5.50 *Typical filamentous nuclear inclusions of inclusion body myositis. (Courtesy of Dr J Moss)*

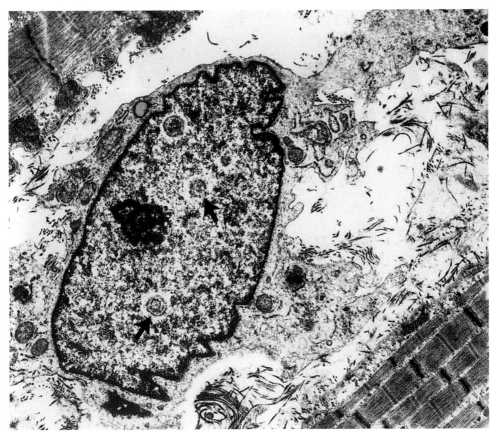

FIG. 5.51 *Spherical nuclear inclusions (arrows) surrounded by haloes in an interstitial cell. (Dermatomyositis.)*

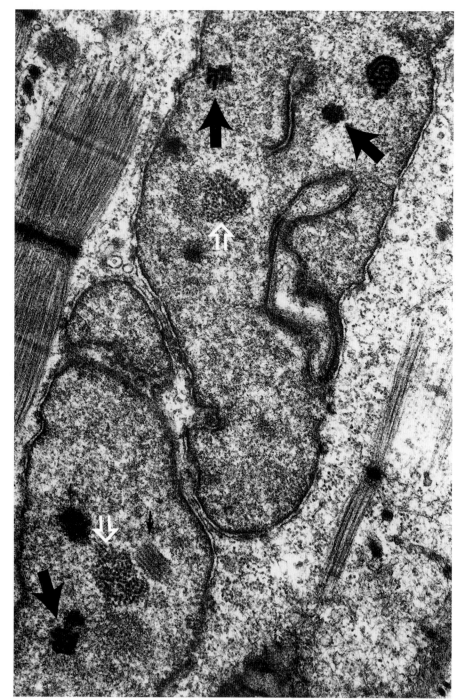

FIG. 5.52 *Irregularly-shaped nucleus with several inclusions. One is a bundle of filaments (small arrow), others are large dark osmiophilic particles (large arrows) or collections of small osmiophilic granules (open arrows). (Infantile myositis.)*

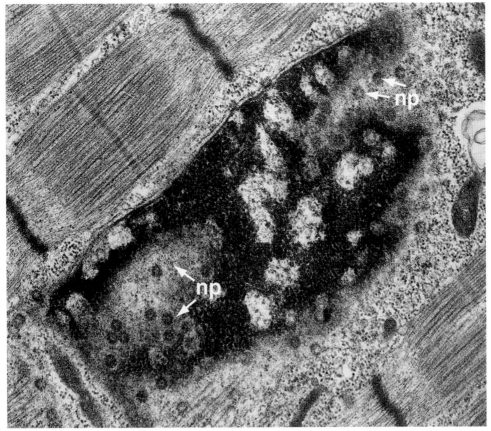

FIG. 5.53 *Internal nucleus sectioned through the nuclear envelope revealing the nuclear pores (np). (Polymyositis.)*

Mitochondria

Mitochondria in muscle, in common with many cells, can move, swell and contract. There is thus considerable variability in the number, distribution, size and shape of mitochondria in muscle. Type 1 fibres have a significantly higher volume of mitochondria than type 2 fibres, reflecting their higher oxidative metabolism (see Ch. 3). In diseased muscle, the normal position of mitochondria adjacent to the I band is often maintained, but in areas of myofilament loss they may form small groups and their shape may vary (Fig. 5.54); or there may be focal mitochondrial loss.

Subsarcolemmal aggregates may be prominent in some diseased muscle, but these are non-specific and they also occur to some extent in normal muscle. Marked aggregation of mitochondria, however, can be seen in *lobulated fibres*

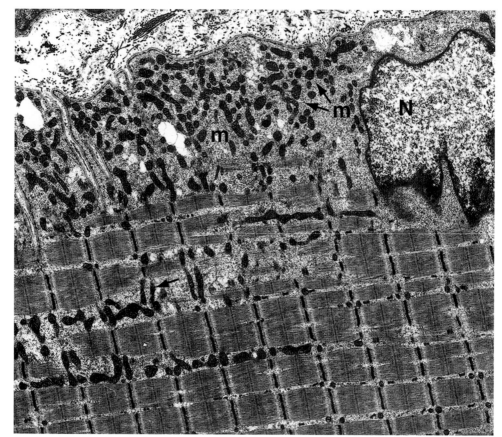

FIG. 5.54 *Subsarcolemmal accumulation of mitochondria (m) in an area with loss of myofibrils and adjacent to a nucleus (N). Focal areas of myofilament loss contain small numbers of mitochondria with varying shapes (arrow). (Definite carrier of Duchenne muscular dystrophy.)*

(Bethlem et al 1973). These fibres are characterized by large aggregates of apparently normal, often small, mitochondria towards the periphery of the fibre and in bands projecting into it. Very few mitochondria are present elsewhere (Fig. 5.55). Lobulated fibres are non-specific and have been reported in facioscapulohumeral muscular dystrophy, limb-girdle dystrophy and spinal muscular atrophy (Bethlem et al 1973). In addition, we have observed them in cases of osteomalacia, inflammatory disorders, hypothyroidism and alcoholic myopathy. They can also be a prominent feature in cases with a defect in calpain-3 (Beckmann and Fardeau 1999). They are rarely observed in children (Guerard et al 1985) but they have been observed in some cases of the Ullrich form of congenital muscular dystrophy.

Swelling of mitochondria is a phenomenon common to many injured cells, but in muscle it can occur in inadequately fixed tissue and its presence must therefore be interpreted with caution. Low amplitude swelling, however, can be recognized in diseased muscle by separation of the outer and inner membranes (Fig. 5.56). High amplitude swelling and degeneration of mitochondria can also

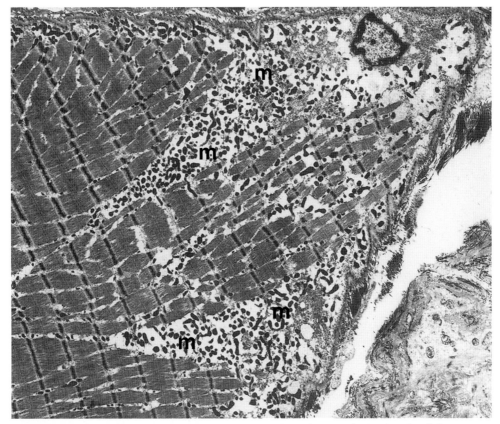

FIG. 5.55 *Lobulated fibre with prominent triangular-shaped areas of mitochondria (m) projecting into the fibre. (Unclassified myopathy.)*

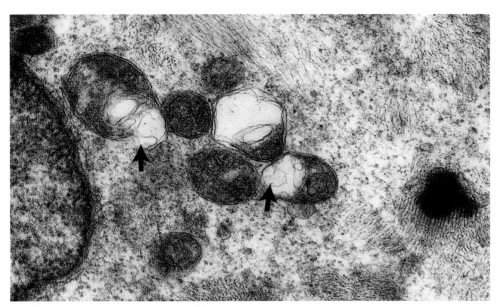

FIG. 5.56 *Low amplitude mitochondrial swelling (arrows) with separation of the inner and outer membranes. (Myopathy with abnormal mitochondria.)*

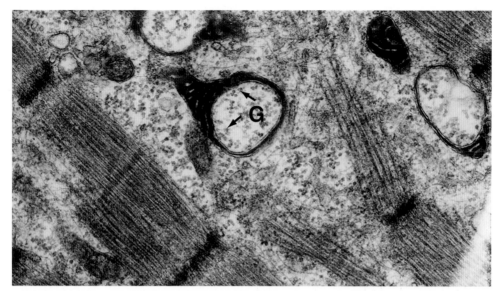

FIG. 5.57 *Swollen condensed mitochondria containing glycogen (G). (Myopathy with abnormal mitochondria.)*

be seen in a variety of situations in correctly fixed tissue, and swollen mitochondria may contain glycogen (Fig. 5.57).

Mitochondria may also show a variety of structural defects. Many neuromuscular disorders have been shown to have structurally abnormal mitochondria, but in certain cases these may be the predominant pathological feature (Morgan-Hughes 1992). A single biopsy may show several defects, which include giant mitochondria, mitochondria with branched cristae or concentric cristae, and mitochondria with inclusions (Figs 5.58–5.62). The inclusions may be of the crystalline type (Figs 5.60 and 5.61) or be osmiophilic bodies of varying size (Fig. 5.58). Enlarged and prominent mitochondrial granules, similar to those found in normal mitochondria, may also occur (Fig. 5.62). Crystalline inclusions often show connections with the inner membrane; they may appear as rectangular bodies occupying a part or the whole width of the mitochondria (Fig. 5.60) or groups of rectangular crystalline inclusions may be present within a common outer membrane (Fig. 5.61). These 'parking lot' type of inclusions are composed of four closely stacked parallel lines of equal length. One or more rectangles may be grouped within an osmiophilic border which is continuous with the inner membrane. Although several biochemical studies of muscle from cases with structurally abnormal mitochondria have been performed, no specific biochemical defect has yet been associated with any particular structural feature. This suggests that the morphological changes reflect a general alteration in the metabolic state of the fibre rather than a specific biochemical defect.

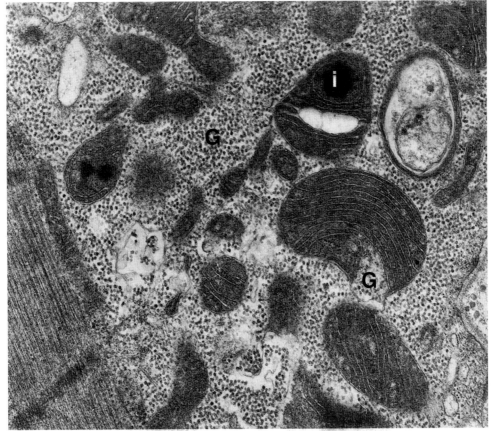

FIG. 5.58 *Enlarged mitochondria with dense inclusions (i), vacuolation and abnormal cristae. Glycogen is prominent between the mitochondria and is also present within one (G). (Duchenne muscular dystrophy.)*

Membrane systems

The sarcoplasmic reticulum (SR) and T system tubules form a complex network of membranes through the fibre which become closely associated at the triads. The abnormalities of these membrane systems in diseased muscle are mainly limited to varying degrees of dilatation or proliferation. Swelling of the SR is a common feature in pathological muscle. It is a non-specific finding, but appears to be one of the earliest changes in Duchenne muscular dystrophy (Fig. 5.63) (Cullen and Fulthorpe 1975). It can also be caused by inadequate fixation when it is usually associated with swollen or 'exploded' mitochondria. Dilatation of the T system also occurs and makes the triads prominent in some disease situations (Fig. 5.64). Triads may also be displaced from their normal position at the A/I band junction and be orientated longitudinally. Proliferation of both the T

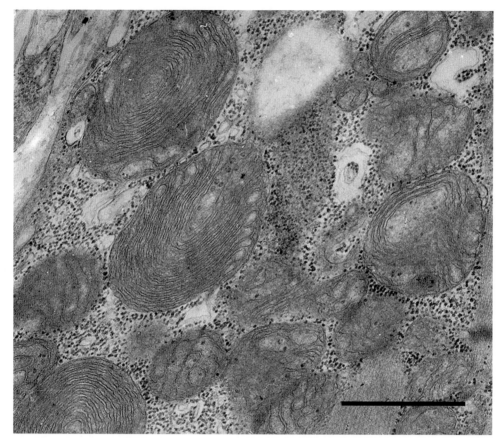

FIG. 5.59 *Abnormal mitochondria with concentric cristae. (Myopathy with abnormal mitochondria.) Bar = 1 μm*

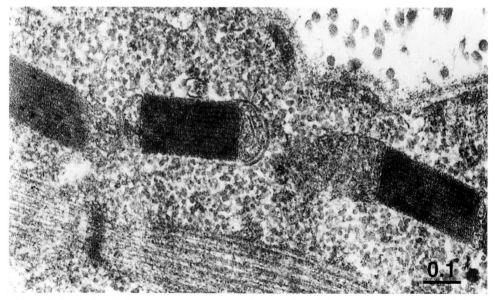

FIG. 5.60 *Crystalline inclusions occupying most of the width of the mitochondria. (Unclassified myopathy.) Bar = 0.1 μm*

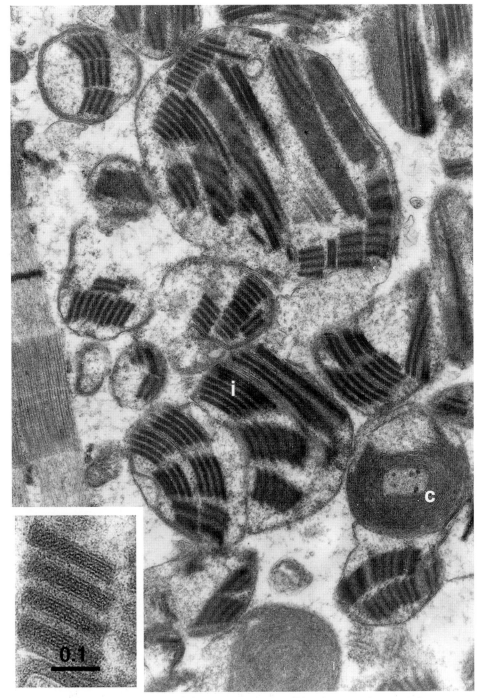

FIG. 5.61 *Enlarged mitochondria with concentric cristae (c) or groups of rectangular inclusions (i). The inset shows the rectangular inclusions are composed of four closely packed parallel lines which are bridged at intervals and surrounded by another osmiophilic membrane. (Oculocraniosomatic syndrome.) Bar = 0.1 μm*

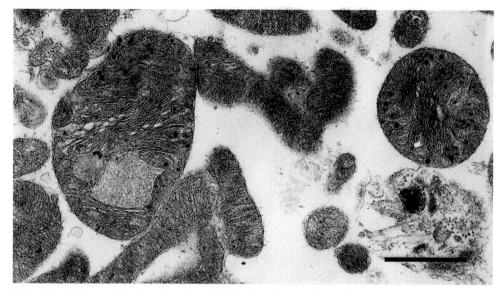

FIG. 5.62 *Enlarged mitochondria with abnormal cristae and dense granules. (Unclassified myopathy.) Bar = 1 μm*

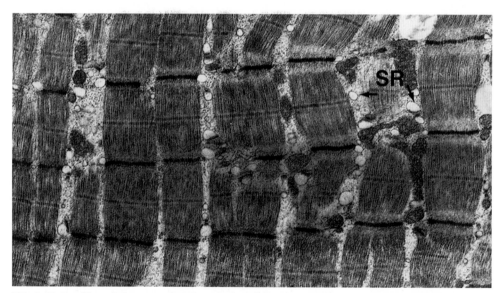

FIG. 5.63 *Swelling of the sarcoplasmic reticulum (SR). The myofibrils show focal loss. (Definite carrier of Duchenne muscular dystrophy.)*

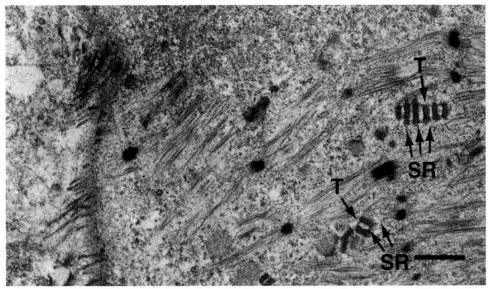

FIG. 5.64 *Replication of triads. The darker sarcoplasmic reticulum (SR) alternates with the pale T system (T) component. The T system of a single triad is also swollen. (Limb-girdle dystrophy.) Bar = 1 μm*

system and SR of the triads can give rise to tiers of closely associated membranes (Fig. 5.64). These duplicated triads have dense granular SR alternating with clear T system tubules. They are usually associated with fibre damage.

Proliferation of the T system is also thought to lead to the formation of honeycomb structures (Fig. 5.65). These are collections of closely packed tubules of different size, one large and pale with the other small and dense. In one case we have observed these in a concentric configuration (Fig. 5.66). Connections with the T system are often seen and the double tubule appearance is reminiscent of triads. Honeycomb structures occur in situations of active degeneration and regeneration.

Excessive proliferation of the SR also results in the formation of various types of tubular aggregates, which can be distinguished morphologically. One type has hexagonally packed double-walled tubules (Fig. 5.67) and it is generally accepted that they are derived from the SR. Continuity with the SR provides evidence for this (Engel et al 1970a) as does the fact that they can be immunolabelled with antibodies to the calcium activated sarcoplasmic reticulum ATPase, SERCA (Manta et al 2004), and other proteins associated with the SR, triads and calcium homeostasis (Chevessier et al 2004). Histochemical evidence by other workers, however, suggested that similar tubular aggregates also have properties of mitochondria (Pearse and Johnson 1970; Lewis et al 1971). The reason for this has never been established. Another type of tubular aggregate with similar histochemical properties has tubules haphazardly arranged and the outer membrane encompasses one or more small, discrete tubules (Fig. 5.68). In a third type of aggregate, the tubules contain a granular core and in a fourth type

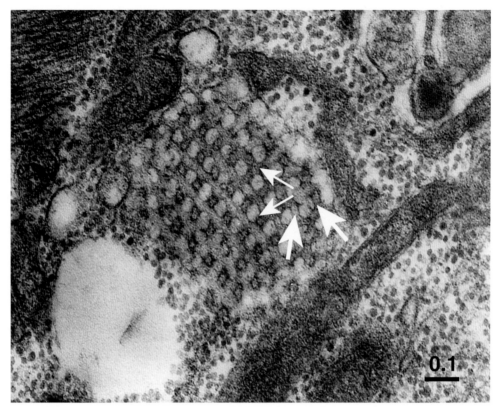

FIG. 5.65 *Honeycomb structure with two distinct tubular components (large and small arrows). (Carrier of Becker muscular dystrophy.) Bar = 0.1 μm*

filaments are regularly attached around the tubules which contain central granular material (Fig. 5.69). Tubular aggregates have been observed in several neuromuscular disorders, including in occasional fibres in carriers of Duchenne dystrophy and in biopsies from some normal individuals and ageing mouse muscle (Chevessier et al 2004). They are a common finding in cases of periodic paralysis where they are often confined to type 2 fibres. Recently, a number of antibodies have been shown to localize to tubular aggregates, including emerin, heat shock protein and dysferlin (Manta et al 2004).

Deposits and particles

Glycogen and lipid are both deposited in normal muscle in varying amounts according to the fibre type, but in disease situations excessive quantities may accumulate. In areas where filaments have degenerated, glycogen is present and in some fibres extensive subsarcolemmal accumulations occur. These are non-specific findings, but are most marked in glycogen storage diseases (see Fig. 5.4). Glycogen may also be found in membrane bound sacs which are of lysosomal origin (Engel et al 1970a). These are particularly common in adult and juvenile

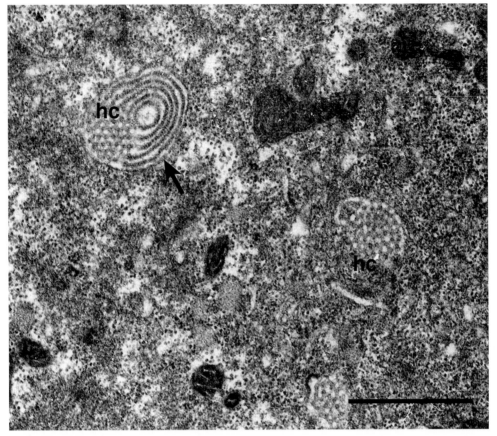

FIG. 5.66 *Several honeycomb structures (hc). One has been sectioned obliquely and shows a concentric configuration (arrow). (Limb-girdle dystrophy.) Bar = 1 μm*

forms of acid maltase deficiency (type II glycogenosis) (Fig. 5.70). Glycogen may also be found in abnormal mitochondria (see Figs 5.57 and 5.58).

Lipid droplets appear as clear or lightly stained spaces with no limiting membrane. These represent the areas where the lipid has been lost during dehydration and embedding procedures. They are found between the myofibrils and are often associated with the mitochondria. Excessive amounts of lipid may occur concurrently with other abnormalities and this is particularly striking in carnitine deficiency. In some cases, lipid storage is associated with abnormal mitochondria (Fig. 5.71).

A deposit that is common in diseased muscle and to a lesser extent in normal muscle is lipofuscin (see Fig. 5.69). It is rare in paediatric muscle but common in adults. It is considered to be the residue of lysosomal action, although lysosomes themselves are difficult to identify in muscle. Lipofuscin granules are frequently found beneath the sarcolemma and are sometimes in the perinuclear region. They appear as round or irregularly-shaped structures with vesicular inclusions in a dense osmiophilic matrix.

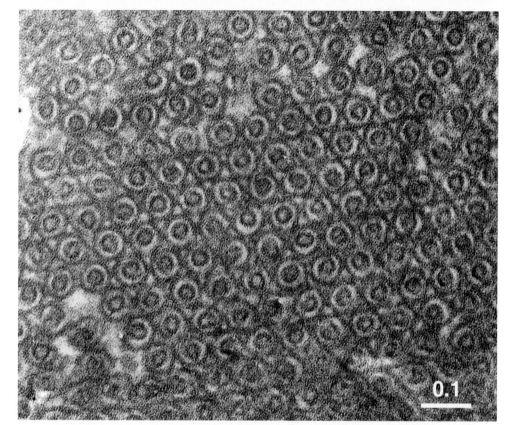

0.1

FIG. 5.67 *Tubular aggregate. Each tubule is double walled. (Periodic paralysis.) Bar = 0.1 μm*

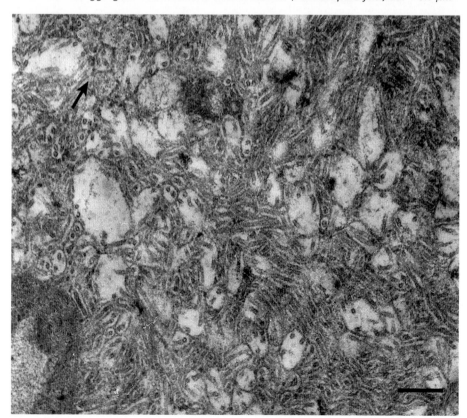

FIG. 5.68 *Aggregate of haphazardly arranged tubules. The outer membrane of the tubules often encompasses more than one smaller tubule (arrow). (Periodic paralysis.) Bar = 0.1 μm*

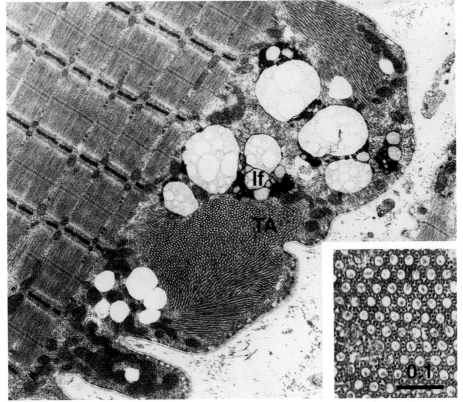

FIG. 5.69 *Subsarcolemmal tubular aggregates (TA) adjacent to lipofuscin (lf). The high power inset shows the tubules in transverse section. Each has a granular core and is surrounded by regularly attached filaments. (Definite carrier of Duchenne muscular dystrophy.) Bar = 0.1 μm*

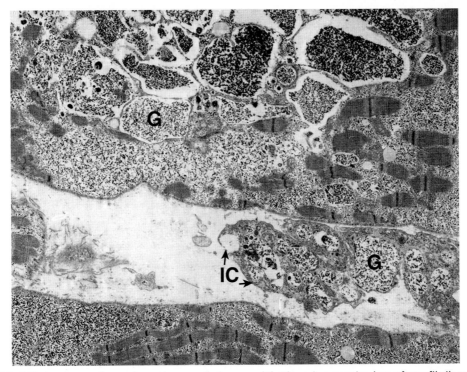

FIG. 5.70 *Large membrane bound areas of glycogen (G). There is extensive loss of myofibrils and excess glycogen is present in both the fibres and interstitial cells (IC). (Type II glycogen storage disease, Pompe's disease.)*

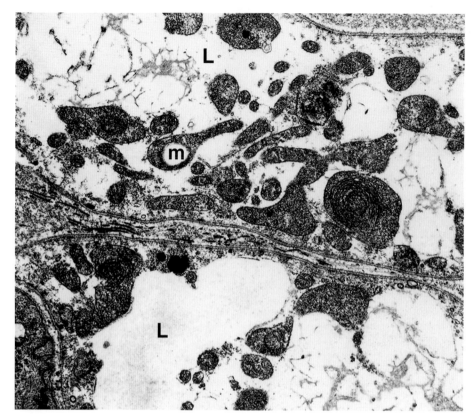

FIG. 5.71 *Excess lipid (L) associated with abnormal mitochondria (m). (Carnitine deficiency.)*

Material resembling lipopigment occurs in patients with vitamin E deficiency (Burck et al 1981; Neville et al 1983). This is in the form of dense bodies scattered in the muscle fibres (Fig. 5.72) which are positive for acid phosphatase and esterase activity, and are autofluorescent. They thus have characteristics of lysosomes and lipopigment.

Virus-like particles have occasionally been observed in skeletal muscle (see Fig. 5.46) and identifiable viruses isolated from muscle (Tang et al 1975) but this is rare. Virus-like particles may be arranged in crystalline configurations or be tubular in appearance. Although the morphological appearance of these structures resembles viruses, this has not been substantiated by tissue culture studies. A causative role for these particles has therefore not been established.

Other crystalline material has been reported in a patient with an unusual myopathy associated with xanthinuria (Chalmers et al 1969). Dense crystalline and rod-shaped structures were present in aggregates in subsarcolemmal or interfibrillar regions, and evidence suggested that the deposits may have been hypoxanthine and xanthine.

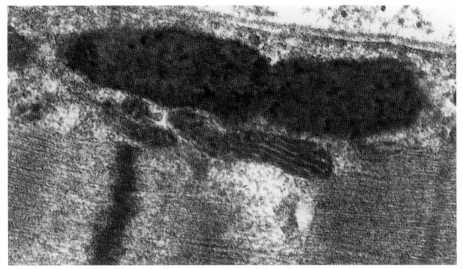

FIG. 5.72 *Dense subsarcolemmal body resembling lipopigment. (Vitamin E deficiency.)*

Other unusual structures

A variety of other ultrastructural abnormalities have been observed in skeletal muscle. Some of these are of known origin, others not, and in some instances they have led to the characterization of a disorder. In addition to the disorders and structures illustrated below, rare conditions with unusual ultrastructural features include cap disease (Fidzianska et al 1981), lamellar body myopathy, cylindrical body myopathy and sarcotubular myopathy (Jerusalem et al 1973). It is not clear whether some of these are distinct entities (see Goebel and Anderson 1999, Goebel 2002).

Actin accumulation – in the previous edition of this book (1985) we described a case of severe congenital myopathy in which several fibres had large aggregates of filamentous material resembling actin (Figs 5.73 and 5.74). In 1997 a paper describing three patients with similar features was published (Goebel et al 1997). This paved the way for the identification of mutations in the actin (*ACTA1*) gene (Nowak et al 1999). The pathological and clinical spectrum associated with actin mutations is wide (Sparrow et al 2003) and is discussed in more detail with the nemaline myopathies in Chapter 15. Nemaline rods may, or may not, occur with the actin accumulation. Actin accumulation is a feature of severe neonates and has not yet been found in any of the milder adult cases with *ACTA1* mutations (Jungbluth et al 2001). There are also neonatal cases with actin accumulation in which a mutation in the *ACTA1* gene has not been found (Wallgren-Petterson and Laing 2001, Goebel et al 2004).

    Zebra bodies are elongated filamentous structures with thin, dark bands alternating with wider dark ones (Fig. 5.75). They can be found in normal

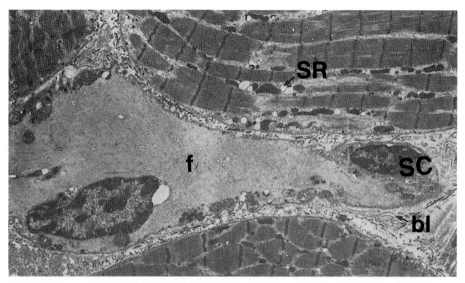

FIG. 5.73 *Accumulation of actin filaments in a severe congenital case with an ACTA1 mutation. Redundant basal lamina (bl) is present round the atrophic fibre and a satellite cell (SC) is present at one end. Adjacent fibres have moderately well preserved myofibrils and show swollen sarcoplasmic reticulum (SR).*

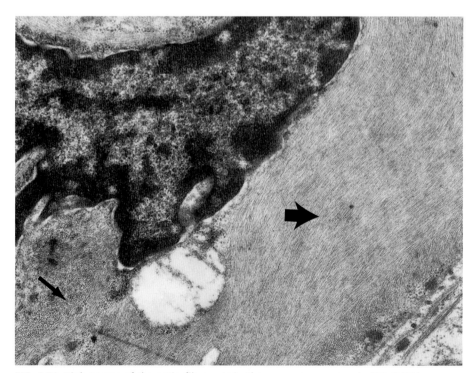

FIG. 5.74 *High power of the actin filaments in the same case as seen in FIG. 5.73 in longitudinal (large arrow) and transverse section (small arrow).*

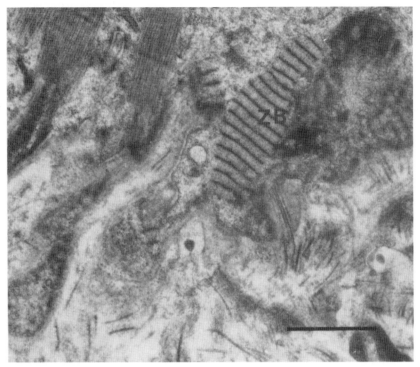

FIG. 5.75 *Zebra body (ZB) near a myotendinous junction. (Congenital muscular dystrophy.) Bar = 1 μm*

myotendinous junctions and normal extraocular muscle as well as in diseased muscle. Zebra bodies may occasionally be a prominent feature of a biopsy and this has led to the designation of 'zebra body myopathy' (Lake and Wilson 1975).

Fingerprint bodies are composed of closely packed lamellae arranged in concentric patterns resembling fingerprints (Fig. 5.76). The lamellae are spaced about 30 nm apart and each lamella has sawtooth-like projections along it. Fingerprint bodies have been found in a variety of situations, and in a case described by Engel and his colleagues (1972) they were sufficient in number for them to call the disorder 'fingerprint body myopathy'.

Curvilinear bodies are membrane-bound accumulations of short, curved membranous structures with alternating light and dark zones (Fig. 5.77). They are found in brain, skeletal muscle and other tissues in neuronal ceroid-lipofuscinosis (Batten's disease) and also in skeletal muscle in cases previously treated with chloroquine (Neville et al 1979).

Reducing bodies are oval or rounded bodies consisting of closely packed dense particles 12–16 nm in diameter. They contain clusters of glycogen granules and occasionally filamentous material (Figs 5.78 and 5.79). They do not have a limiting membrane and often lie near nuclei. Reducing bodies gain their name from the high sulphydryl content that is capable of reducing menadione-mediated tetrazolium reactions.

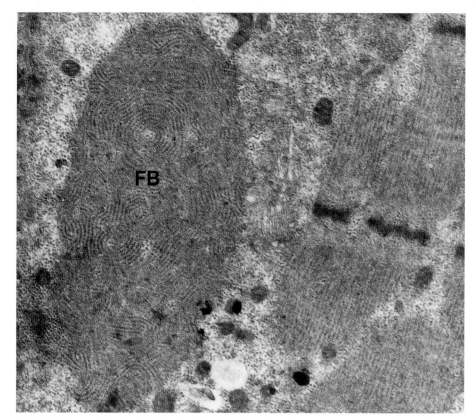

FIG. 5.76 *Fingerprint body (FB). (Definite carrier of Duchenne muscular dystrophy.)*

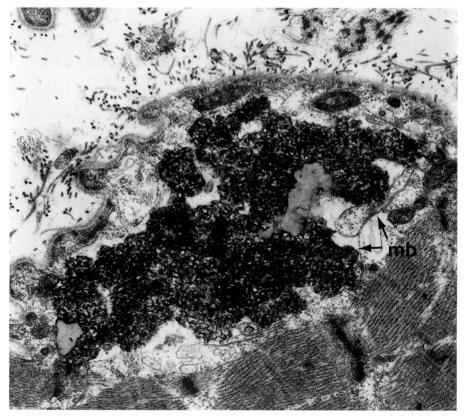

FIG. 5.77 *Curvilinear body beneath the sarcolemma. It is membrane bound (mb) and consists of short curved membranous structures. (Systemic lupus erythematosus treated with chloroquine.)*

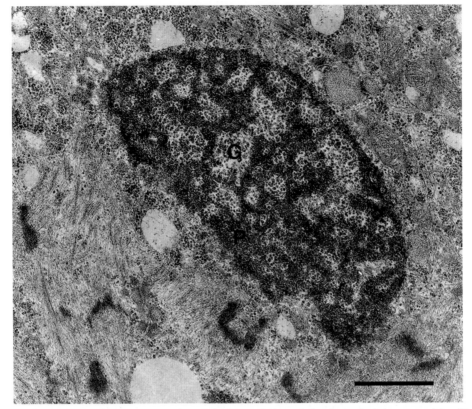

FIG. 5.78 *Transverse section of a reducing body consisting of closely packed dense particles (P) and glycogen (G). (Reducing body myopathy.) Bar = 1 μm*

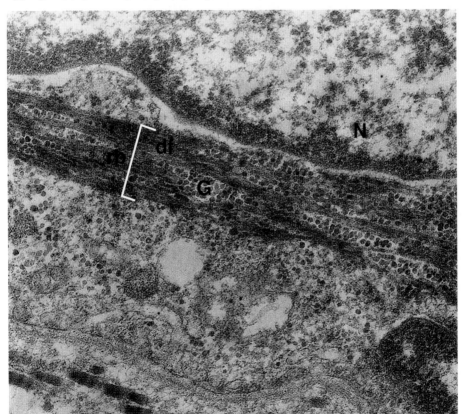

FIG. 5.79 *Longitudinal section of a reducing body (rb) near a nucleus (N). Glycogen (G) is interspersed among dense fibrillar material (df). (Reducing body myopathy.)*

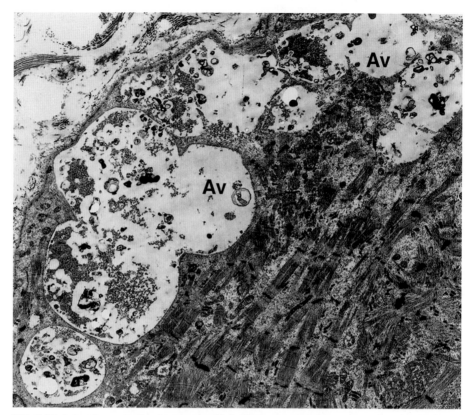

FIG. 5.80 *Extensive autophagic vacuoles (Av). These are membrane bound and contain granular and membranous cell debris. (Unclassified myopathy.)*

Autophagic vacuoles are formed when a portion of the fibre is isolated by a membrane and the contents digested by acid hydrolases. The morphology of the remaining debris or residual bodies is variable and may be dense, membranous, vesicular or granular (Figs 5.80 and 5.81), and organelles may still be identifiable. In extreme cases, the vacuolation is visible at the light level and may occupy large areas of the fibre (see Fig. 5.80). In two X-linked myopathies autophagic vacuoles have a striking and similar appearance (Fig. 5.82). One (Danon's disease) is caused by mutations in the *LAMP-2* gene (Nishino et al 2000). The other gene, linked to Xq28, is unknown (Kalimo et al 1988). The membrane of these vacuoles shows sarcolemmal proteins such as dystrophin and β-spectrin and some, but not all, may also show extracellular matrix proteins such as laminin. Vacuolated fibres also show multiple layers of basal lamina and cell debris may be present between these layers as well as in the vacuole.

Membranous whorls, or myelin-like figures, are often associated with autophagic vacuoles and are believed to be part of the lysosomal system. They are composed of collections of membranes arranged in a whorl-like manner and are of variable size (Fig. 5.83). These whorls are common in the vacuolated fibres

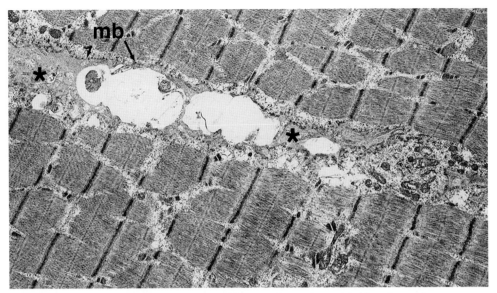

FIG. 5.81 *Vacuole in the centre of a fibre. This is membrane bound (mb) and contains PAS-positive material (*). (Hyperkalaemic periodic paralysis.)*

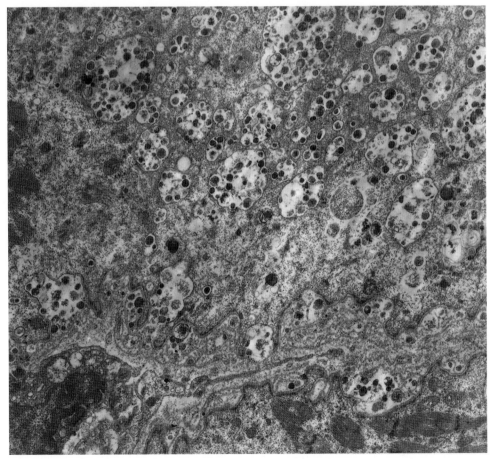

FIG. 5.82 *Vacuoles lined by plasma membrane and extracellular matrix proteins and containing dense cell debris. (Probable case of X-linked myopathy with excessive autophagy – XMEA.)*

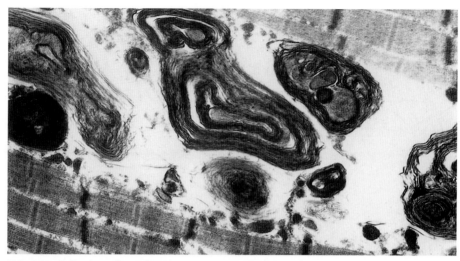

FIG. 5.83 *Collection of membranous, myelin-like figures. (Unclassified myopathy.)*

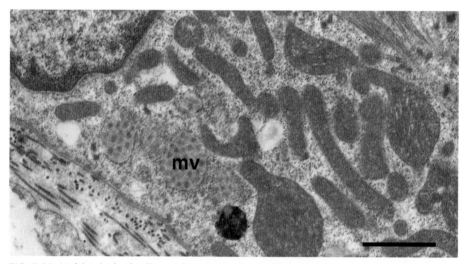

FIG. 5.84 *Multivesicular bodies at the periphery of a fibre (mv). The outer membrane encloses several small vesicles. (Unclassified myopathy.) Bar = 1 μm*

of inclusion body myositis and inclusion body myopathies and stain red with the modified Gomori trichrome technique.

Multivesicular bodies (Fig. 5.84) are a type of lysosome involved in membrane turnover and are membrane bound structures enclosing an array of small vesicles.

Dense tubules of various types may occasionally be seen, sometimes in clusters. One type has short tubules stacked in parallel array (Fig. 5.85). The individual tubules are osmiophilic and contain a granular material similar to that found in sarcoplasmic reticulum. In some instances the tubules show

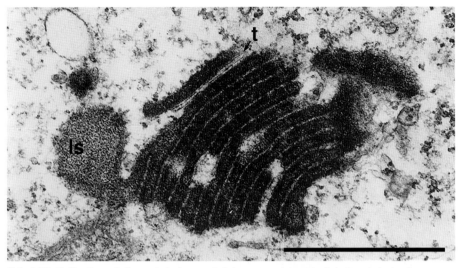

FIG. 5.85 *Collection of dense tubules containing granular material. One tubule shows a connection to a structure resembling the lateral sac of a triad (ls) and is separated from the adjacent one by a pale tubule (t). This suggests a possible origin from triads. (Myotubular myopathy.) Bar = 1 μm*

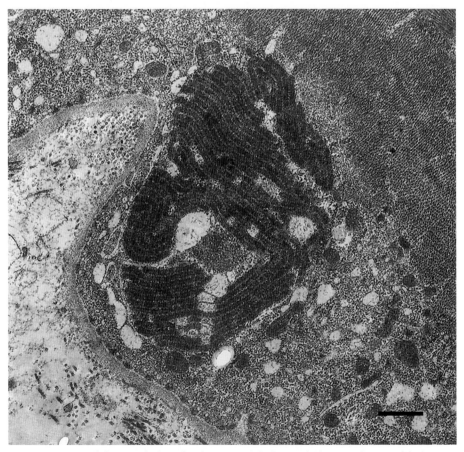

FIG. 5.86 *Array of dense tubules of unknown origin beneath the sarcolemma. (Limb-girdle dystrophy.) Bar = 1 μm*

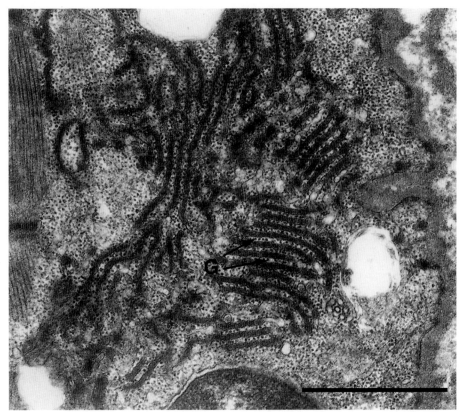

FIG. 5.87 *Collection of tubules containing filamentous material and interspersed with glycogen (G). (Duchenne muscular dystrophy.) Bar = 1 μm*

connections to structures that resemble SR. Their configuration and similar appearance to dense SR suggest that they may have developed from replicated triads that have lost the T system component. This is substantiated by the appearance of some triads in which the SR is also dense and elongated. We have only seen these collections of tubules in three cases of myotubular myopathy, but they resemble isolated structures seen in other conditions (Figs 5.86 and 5.87). Another type of dense tubule occurs round some nuclei in Marinesco-Sjögren syndrome (Fig. 5.88). These have only been observed in this syndrome but it is not yet certain if they are a consistent feature (Sewry et al 1988, Sewry 2002).

A report by Fidzianska et al (1983) described the presence of peculiar *Mallory body-like inclusions* in muscle fibres from three genetically linked children. These inclusions had a dense amorphous component, serrated filaments of 14–16.5 nm and peripherally located intermediate filaments. Retrospective examination of electron micrographs of a biopsy from a patient we studied several years ago revealed similar inclusions to those reported by Fidzianska et al (1983) (Fig. 5.89). These Mallory body-like inclusions are immunoreactive for desmin, ubiquitin and dystrophin and the disorder was categorized as a 'desmin-related

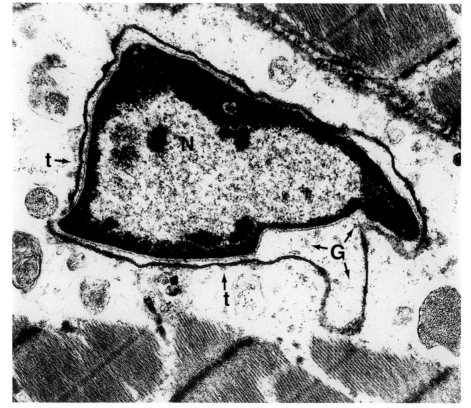

FIG. 5.88 *Nucleus (N) with condensed heterochromatin surrounded by an additional dense tubule (t). Glycogen (G) is present between the nucleus and the outer tubule and in adjacent membrane bound structures. (Marinesco-Sjögren syndrome.)*

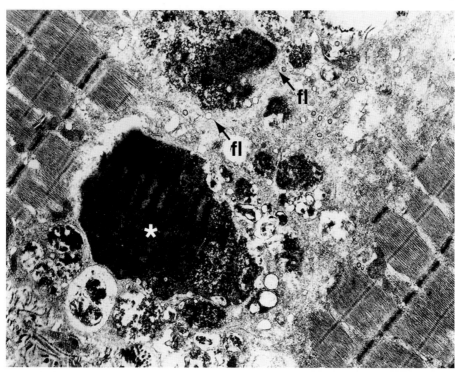

FIG. 5.89 *Mallory body-like inclusions. These have a dense amorphous component (*) and filaments (fl) associated with them. (Unclassified congenital myopathy.)*

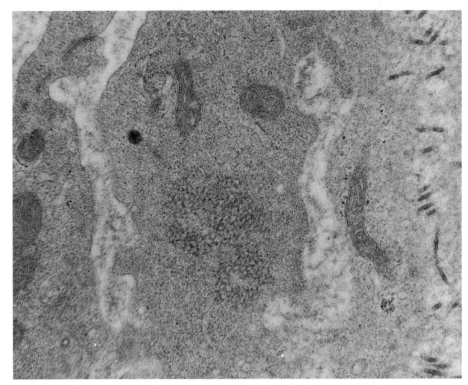

FIG. 5.90 *Tubuloreticular inclusions in an endothelial cell. (Dermatomyositis.)*

myopathy'. Recently mutations in the selenoprotein N gene (*SEPN1*) have been identified in this disorder (Ferreiro et al 2004).

Hyaline bodies – these are areas of fine rather granular material devoid of organelles but containing myosin. With routine histological stains they appear pale and stain for myosin ATPase but lack oxidative enzymes. They occur in type 1 fibres. They are a feature of a congenital myopathy but some cases are of adult onset (Cancilla et al 1971, Barohn et al 1994a). The slow myosin gene (*MYH7*) has recently been shown to be a gene responsible for these hyaline bodies (Tajsharghi et al 2003, Bohlega et al 2004, Laing et al 2005) and a recessive form has been linked to chromosome 3p, with a protein with homology to myosin heavy chain as a possible candidate (Onengut et al 2004). This disorder with myosin accumulation has been added to the group of 'surplus protein myopathies' together with desmin and actin.

Tubuloreticular structures – these undulating tubules are found in the endothelial cells of the capillaries and are a particular feature of dermatomyositis and a useful diagnostic marker (Fig. 5.90). They may also occasionally be seen in some collagen-vascular disorders (Luu et al 1989) and in patients infected with human immunodeficiency virus (HIV; Lane et al 1993). They may occur in some of the infiltrating cells in myositic conditions but they are not found in the muscle fibres themselves.

CHAPTER 6

Immunohistochemistry

Immunohistochemistry now has an essential role in the evaluation of muscle biopsies and in examining protein localization. The term 'protein expression' is often applied to describe immunohistochemical results but it should be remembered that the technique only reflects localization of a protein, not the related RNA synthesis, and the gene coding for it may not be active at the time the protein is localized. In addition, absence of labelling may sometimes be because the epitope of the antibody is masked and inaccessible. Immunohistochemistry is complementary to histology and histochemistry and the results should not be interpreted in isolation from other morphological studies and the whole clinical picture. Defects in protein localization may identify an abnormality in the gene encoding that protein (a primary defect) or they may be a secondary response to an abnormality in another gene. Immunohistochemical abnormalities related to a primary defect are of particular importance in assessing recessively inherited conditions, where both alleles are mutated. In dominant conditions expression from the normal allele may mask any alteration in the mutant allele and labelling of the normal and mutant protein may be indistinguishable; analysis of secondary defects is then particularly important. Thus, analysis of both primary and secondary abnormalities has an important role in the assessment of biopsies.

With the rapid advances in molecular medicine the number of primary defects that can be identified with immunohistochemistry is growing and there is a trend towards classifying disorders according to the protein defect (e.g. dystrophinopathy, sarcoglycanopathy, actinopathy, desminopathy). In this book, however, we have adhered to the classical clinical classification (see Ch. 8), as this still forms the basis for clinical diagnosis. This chapter aims to summarize aspects of methodology for immunohistochemistry and the analysis of proteins relevant to diagnosis, particularly using commercial antibodies that are readily available to everyone (see Table 6.1 and Sewry and Lu 2001).

Many antibodies are now available for studying diseased muscle and they have widened our understanding of pathological features, but this chapter is not intended as a comprehensive account of the myriad of features that have been identified by the application of antibodies. Emphasis will be on those currently relevant to diagnosis; aspects relating to specific disorders will be described in the appropriate chapter.

Methods for immunohistochemistry

Immunohistochemistry is used to visualize and localize specific protein components of a tissue. The principle of the technique is the specific affinity of an antibody for its antigen. Allied techniques are the labelling of glycoproteins with lectins, the labelling of receptors with a ligand such as a toxin (e.g. the specific affinity of bungarotoxin for acetylcholine receptors at neuromuscular junctions) and labelling of nucleic acids by in situ hybridization. Similar methods of detection and amplification have been developed for all these techniques but their diagnostic role is currently less than that of immunohistochemistry.

Tissue and section preparation for immunohistochemistry

As for histochemistry, all tissues should be rapidly frozen in isopentane cooled in liquid nitrogen and immunolabelling performed on cryostat sections, as described in Chapter 1. The epitope for some antibodies is destroyed or masked by fixation and unfixed frozen sections are then essential. Other antibodies may only give satisfactory results on fixed material, in which case frozen sections can be post-fixed (see below). This is rare for the antibodies currently used for the diagnosis of neuromuscular disorders. If only formalin-fixed, wax embedded material is available, various antigen retrieval techniques using pretreatment of sections with enzymes and/or microwaving can be tried. This is useful for archival material but is not the method of choice for routine studies. In our experience most antibodies for the diagnosis of neuromuscular disorders give good results on unfixed, untreated cryostat sections.

As described in chapter 1, sections collected on *Superfrost* or *Superfrost Plus* slides or uncoated coverslips can be stored until required at −20°C, or lower, if wrapped in cling-film and/or foil. This has the advantage that batches of biopsies can be labelled in parallel, which is time and cost effective, and each sample then acts as a control for the others, enabling identification of any technical problems. A batch should never consist of samples all with the same provisional diagnosis (e.g. not all potential cases of Duchenne muscular dystrophy) and a single biopsy should not be labelled in isolation. If results are needed urgently and a batch of cases cannot be assembled, or if additional or repeat studies are needed, a second sample, preferably of normal muscle, should always be included as a control. Sections should be air-dried at room temperature for about 20 minutes before use. If only a few sections from a package of stored frozen sections are required the remaining sections should not be allowed to thaw as condensation may form and freeze when the sections are returned to the freezer, resulting in artefact when the section is subsequently used.

Fixation of sections

Many antibodies when applied to muscle sections do not require fixation and this is our method of choice. Acetone or methanol, however, is frequently used for studies of muscle sections but in our experience this is unnecessary for the study of human muscle. Formaldehyde or paraformaldehyde, at various concentrations, is also sometimes used. Acetone or methanol, or permeabilization with Triton X-100 (0.05–0.2%) or saponin are often necessary for localization of inter-cellular antigens in cultured muscle cells. A fixative or permeabilization solution may affect the epitope of an antibody and if fixation is required the most suitable, and its concentration, has to be determined experimentally.

Immunolabelling and washing

Dry sections must be placed in a moist atmosphere for labelling to prevent evaporation of the small volumes of reagents as described in Chapter 1. Use of a hydrophobic pen to draw round each section is a convenient way to reduce the volume of reagents used and to prevent reagents spreading. Coverslips or slides can be placed in racks and washed collectively in a dish or they can be rinsed individually. Three rinses of buffer are required but the timing of each is variable. It can be from 3 to 5 minutes, or in the case of individual coverslips, 10 second dip washes are adequate. The staining tray shown in Figure 1.10 has a magnetic strip which holds the slides in place and is a convenient way to wash a batch of slides by gently expelling buffer from a 'squeezy' bottle over the sections for about 30 seconds. Sections must not be allowed to dry out at any stage or false results and artefact will arise. It is also important to ensure that there are no bubbles in the antibody solution when applied as no labelling will occur under the bubble.

Blocking agents

Non-specific background, which reduces the signal to noise ratio, may be a problem. Additives to the buffer, such as bovine serum albumin (BSA; 2%) or detergents (0.2% Triton X), or normal serum from the same species as the secondary antibody, can be used to block non-specific binding of secondary antibodies but as with fixatives they may affect the epitope of the antibody. Some tissue components may contain endogenous enzymes, such as peroxidase or alkaline phosphatase. For example macrophages contain endogenous peroxidase. This can be blocked with hydrogen peroxide (1%) and endogenous alkaline phosphates can be blocked with levimisole (1 mM). It can sometimes be useful to observe this peroxidase activity and to know macrophages are present without having to use specific cell markers. Endogenous biotin can be blocked by applying unconjugated avidin followed by biotin, available as a commercial kit. We find that there is rarely an advantage in using blocking agents for the study of human muscle; good washing and optimal dilution of the antibodies are more critical factors. Phosphate buffered saline (0.1 M or 0.2 M) at pH 7.2–7.4 is usually used for washing and commercially available tablets are now a convenient way to make this up.

Primary antibodies

A wide variety of primary antibodies to muscle proteins are now commercially available, in particular those that detect primary defects in muscular dystrophies (Table 6.1). Several companies sell relevant primary antibodies and most companies now have a web page. There are also various directories and hybridoma banks. Attention should be paid to the characterization of a commercial antibody as this is not always complete on data sheets, and also to the recommended storage of an antibody. If freezing is recommended an antibody should be divided into aliquots of convenient volume to avoid repeated cycles of freeze–thawing. When possible, characterization of an antibody should be checked in the original publication describing the use of an antibody, or the information obtained from the company. Dilution of a primary antibody should always be assessed by titration in each laboratory, and is dependent on such factors as supplier, poly- or monoclonal antibody, secondary antibody, time and temperature of incubation. As for washing, phosphate buffered saline at pH 7.2–7.4 is used for diluting antibodies. Incubation times can vary from 30 to 60 minutes to overnight at 4°C. The latter sometimes reduces background and lower dilutions of antibody may be possible. Both monoclonal and polyclonal antibodies are available. The former, released from hybridoma cells, recognize a single epitope and are highly specific. Polyclonal antibodies are usually purified from serum following injection of the antigen into an animal species (e.g. rabbit, goat or sheep) and recognize several epitopes on the antigen. A control not using the primary antibody is particularly important when using polyclonal antibodies (see below).

Detection systems

It is common to use an indirect detection method to visualize the primary antibody, rather than directly labelling each primary antibody with a marker. Indirect labelling gives more flexibility as it involves applying a secondary antibody against the appropriate immunoglobulin of the species in which the primary antibody was raised, and the same one can then be used to visualize several different primary antibodies. Most antibodies are immunoglobulin G (IgG) immunoglobulins but some are IgM. It is essential to use a secondary antibody to the appropriate immunoglobulin, or to use one that recognizes all classes. The secondary antibody may be directly conjugated to either an enzyme or a fluorochrome, or one conjugated to biotin can be used. The latter is then followed by streptavidin labelled with a marker of choice. This amplification technique has the advantage of enhancing the signal because of the total number of bound avidin molecules. Streptavidin directly labelled with a fluorochrome or a preformed avidin–biotin complex (ABC) may be used. Even greater enhancement is

TABLE 6.1 *Commercial antibodies and their suppliers known to work on human muscle and found to be useful for the diagnostic assessment of muscle biopsies*

Antigen	Supplier and code
β-Spectrin	Novocastra NCl-SPEC1
Dystrophin N-terminus of rod domain (amino acids 321–494)	Novocastra NCL Dys–3
Dystrophin rod domain (amino acids 1181–1388)	Novocastra NCL Dys–1
Dystrophin C-terminus last 17 amino acids	Novocastra NCL Dys–2
Dystrophin rod domain	Sigma MANDYS8
Dystrophin C-terminus	Sigma D8403 MANDRA1
α-Sarcoglycan	Novocastra NCL a-SARC
β-Sarcoglycan	Novocastra NCL b-SARC
γ-Sarcoglycan	Novocastra NCL g-SARC
δ-Sarcoglycan	Novocastra NCL d-SARC
β-Dystroglycan	Novocastra NCL b-DG
α-Dystroglycan	Upstate Biotechnology VIA4 & IIH6
Dysferlin	Novocastra NCL-hamlet 1 and 2
Utrophin	Novocastra NCL-DRP2
nNOS	Santa Cruz sc 648
Calpain-3 (immunoblots only)	Novocastra NCL- CALP-2c4
Caveolin-3	Transduction Laboratories C38320
Emerin	Novocastra NCL-emerin
Laminin α2 (80 kDa)	Chemicon MAB 1922
Laminin α2 (300 kDa)	Alexis 4H8
Laminin α2 (fragment recognized unknown)	Novocastra NCL-merosin
Laminin α5	Chemicon MAB 1924
Laminin β1	Chemicon MAB 1928 & MAB 1921
Laminin γ1	Chemicon MAB 1914 & MAB 1920

TABLE 6.1 *Continued*

Antigen	Supplier and code
Collagen IV	Southern Biotechnology 1340-01
Collagen V	Abcam ab 7406
Collagen VI	Chemicon MAB 1944 & 3303
Perlecan	Chemicon MAB 1948
Developmental myosin	Novocastra NCL MHCd
Neonatal myosin	Novocastra NCL MHCn
Fast myosin	Novocastra NCL MHCf Sigma NQ 7.5.2B
Slow myosin	Novocastra NCL MHCs Chemicon NQ 7.5.4D
Skeletal and cardiac actin	Sigma 5C5
Total actin	Sigma A4700
α-Actinin (type 1 fibres only, isoform recognized unknown)	Novocastra NCL alpha ACT
Myotilin	Novocastra NCL-myotilin
Desmin	Dako
Plectin	Santa Cruz SC 7572
SERCA 1	Novocastra SERCA-1
SERCA 2	Novocastra SERCA-2
MHC class I	Several companies W6/32 clone
Ubiquitin	Novocastra NCL UBIQ
αB-crystallin	Novocastra NCL ABCrys
N-CAM	Beckton Dickinson Leu 19
Phosphorylated tau	Sternberger Monoclonal Incorporated SM 31 & SMI 310

MHC, major histocompatibility complex; N-CAM, neural cell adhesion molecule; nNOS, neuronal nitric oxide synthase; SERCA, sarcoendoplasmic reticulum calcium ATPase

achieved with the tryamide system in which peroxidase is used to catalyse the deposition of biotin or fluorochrome-labelled tryamide close to the antigen–antibody binding site. The deposited biotin is then visualized with streptavidin conjugated to peroxidase or a fluorochrome.

The choice of label to visualize the antibody is often a matter of personal preference but it is also governed by the type of microscope available, the need for a permanent preparation, the amount and localization of the antigen and the affinity of the antibody used. Enzyme labels, such as peroxidase or alkaline phosphatase, provide permanent results and it is easier to see the overall structure of the tissue, particularly if sections are counterstained after immunolabelling. With fluorescent labels, however, it may be easier to distinguish small areas of localized antibody which appear bright against a dark background, and specificity can easily be checked by changing the excitation filter. Aqueous mountants have now improved which reduce fading, and fluorescence can be retained for several weeks or months. Good fluorescent nuclear counterstains are also now available (see below). Fluorescent methods are usually quicker to apply and avoid the use of hazardous substances such as diaminobenzamine (DAB). Double and multilabelling is easier using fluorochromes and the relationship of different antigens closely localized at the same site is more precisely determined. Illustrative examples of the use of both peroxidase and fluorochromes are given in this book.

Fluorescent labels

Several fluorochromes are now available such as fluorescein, rhodamine, Texas Red, AMCA, Cy3 and Cy5, and Alexa probes. The choice is often one of personal preference but factors such as cost, intensity, filters fitted to the microscope and fading also need to be considered. Fluorescein isothiocyanate (FITC) fades rapidly on excitation and FITC–Ig conjugates bind non-specifically to muscle components. Its use is diminishing in favour of Cy and Alexa probes (marketed by Molecular Probes) which give a particularly high signal to background ratio and are resistant to fading on storage and with excitation. Storage of the labelled sections in the dark and at 4°C helps to reduce fading. Less autoflourescence in muscle, such as that associated with blood vessels is apparent with excitations in the red region. The development of new labels encourages users to change their methods. Whilst this has obvious advantages, pathological comparisons of intensity are important and new baselines may have to be established if changes are made. Our method of choice was previously a biotin–streptavidin–Texas Red system but we now routinely use streptavidin–Alexa 594 or 488 for visualization and some reassessments of intensities have been necessary.

Enzyme labels

Secondary antibodies can be conjugated to an enzyme that can then be histochemically detected at the site of the antigen by deposition of a coloured, insoluble reaction product. Peroxidase detected with DAB has traditionally been the most used enzyme label. It produces a brown end product which is stable for long periods at room temperature, and can be enhanced with silver or nickel to produce a black end product. Other substrates that can be used include amino-ethyl carbazole (red end product) or 4-chloro-1-naphthol (blue end product). A common alternative to peroxidase is alkaline phosphatase which, with the appropriate substrate, can be visualized as a red, blue or black end product. Glucose oxidase and β-galactosidase are also useful, particularly for double labelling of two different antibodies. Amplification, as mentioned previously, can be obtained with a biotin–avidin system, either with a preformed complex, directly conjugated streptavidin alone or the tryamide system. Peroxidase antiperoxidase also provides enhancement but is now less commonly used since the wider availability of biotinylated systems. As with fluorochromes it is necessary to establish baselines and become accustomed to levels of intensity of peroxidase labelling with each antibody used.

Counterstaining and mounting

Counterstains provide an overall impression of the morphology of the tissue and can be nuclear or cytoplasmic; more commonly the former. They are not essential and their use is one of individual choice. In sections where labelling is expected to be absent, such as with dystrophin in Duchenne muscular dystrophy or mature muscle with no neonatal myosin, a nuclear counterstain can be helpful. In Emery–Dreifuss muscular dystrophy the absence of emerin from the nuclei using a peroxidase detection system is easier to assess without a counterstain. With fluorescence, however, a nuclear counterstain at a different wavelength to the one used to detect emerin can be helpful to show where the nuclei are. The choice of counterstain is dependent on the colour of the end product or fluorochrome. Haematoxylin and methyl green are common nuclear counterstains used after peroxidase. If too much haematoxylin is present it may give a pale delineation of the sarcolemma and care is then needed in assessing any very low levels of sarcolemmal proteins. For example, when assessing dystrophin in peroxidase-labelled sections from cases of Duchenne dystrophy the low levels of minor transcripts may be obscured or low levels of sarcolemmal major histocompatibility complex (MHC) class I may be difficult to identify. Fluorescence is then an advantage as the low levels are visible against the dark background. For fluorescence the nuclear counterstains most commonly used are 4′6-diamidino-2-phenylindole.2HCl (DAPI) (1 μg/mL), Hoechst dye (10 μg/mL) which are both blue under ultraviolet light, or ethidium bromide (1 μg/mL) or TOTO which are red (all available from Molecular Probes). Mountants containing a counterstain are also commercially available (e.g. with DAPI from Vector Laboratories).

The choice of mountant is also determined by the visualization marker. Sections labelled with enzymes such as peroxidase can be dehydrated in graded alcohols, cleared and mounted in synthetic resins. Fluorescent markers require aqueous mountants and several commercial ones contain antifading agents. We have found Hydromount (National Diagnostics) to be useful as this dries to hold the coverslip in place and fluorescence lasts for several weeks or months. If a glycerol-based mountant is used, which does not dry, the coverslip should be sealed and held in place by nail varnish.

Baselines for interpretation

Interpretation of results is dependent on several aspects including the visualization technique used, appropriate controls and maturity of the fibres. Results vary between different laboratories, even when using the same antibodies with the same detection conditions, and it is important that each laboratory establishes optimal conditions and baselines for each antibody, and knows how a particular antibody works in their hands. Controls are essential to check for non-specific background and to check for preservation of the tissue. An important control to check for non-specific labelling is omission of the primary antibody so that sections are only labelled with the secondary antibody and the detection reagents. Necrotic fibres often contain IgG which is detected by an anti-IgG secondary antibody and must not be confused with specific labelling.

Immunohistochemical assessment of the sarcolemma is a fundamental aspect of diagnostic muscle pathology and it is essential to know if the membrane is well preserved. Both the plasmalemma and basal lamina may be damaged or lost if the tissue is affected by freezing artefact or in pathologically damaged fibres. Sarcolemmal proteins may also be lost or reduced in postmortem material, depending on the time from death to freezing the sample. The basal lamina is more resilient than the plasma membrane and may be retained on some necrotic fibres and fibres in postmortem material, even though the plasma membrane is lost (Fig. 6.1). Plasma membrane proteins are sometimes less apparent on regenerating fibres (Fig. 6.2), and sometimes labelling within a regenerating fibre is seen with some antibodies. Studies of dystrophin and all plasma membrane proteins should always be accompanied by parallel studies of β-spectrin, as these give a good indication of the overall preservation of the sample. Similarly, any studies of basal lamina proteins should be controlled with studies of a laminin chain or a basement membrane collagen, depending on the likely nature of the disorder in question. We routinely use an antibody to laminin γ1 to assess preservation of the basal lamina as, to date, no pathological immunohistohistochemical abnormalities in its localization have been observed in skeletal muscle. For assessing components of the basement membrane, such as collagen VI, we use perlecan or collagen V.

Variation in fibre size is often more apparent in sections immunolabelled with antibodies to sarcolemmal proteins. We therefore routinely study the sarcolemma to assess this and tissue preservation, even if a defect is not suspected.

Developmental regulation of proteins

It is important to know the localization patterns of an antibody in mature, neonatal and fetal muscle, as many proteins are developmentally regulated and

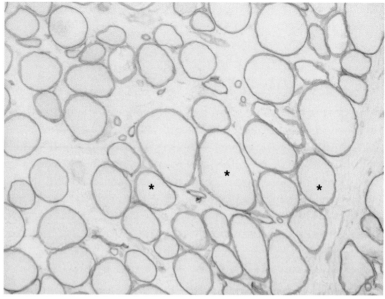

a

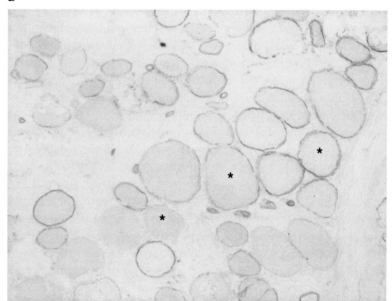

b

FIG. 6.1 *Immunoperoxidase labelling of (a) laminin α2 and (b) β-spectrin in serial sections from a case of Duchenne muscular dystrophy showing retention of the basal lamina but variable loss of β-spectrin from damaged and necrotic fibres (*). Fibre sizes range from approximately 10 to 105 μm.*

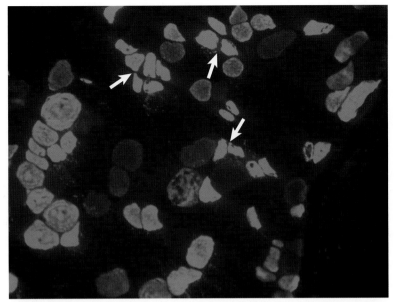

a

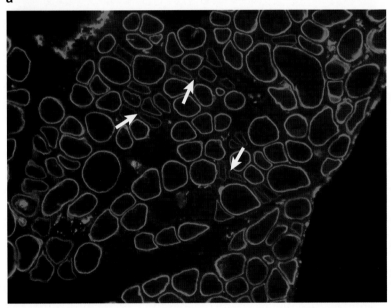

b

FIG. 6.2 *Immunofluorescent labelling of (a) neonatal myosin and (b) β-spectrin in serial sections from a case of Duchenne muscular dystrophy showing reduced β-spectrin on several regenerating fibres with neonatal myosin (arrows). Note also other fibres with neonatal myosin that have normal levels of β-spectrin.*

TABLE 6.2 *Proteins relevant to pathology whose expression changes during development*

Change of isoform
actin   cardiac → skeletal
myosin   embryonic → neonatal → fast or slow
Low expression on immature and regenerating fibres
β-Spectrin low round some small regenerating fibres
C-terminal dystrophin (sometimes)
Some dystrophin-associated proteins
Neuronal nitric oxide synthase (nNOS)
Laminin β2, extrajunctional labelling weaker in neonates
Integrin α7, extrajunctional labelling weaker in neonates
High expression on regenerating fibres*
Utrophin
Laminin α5
Neural cell adhesion molecule (N-CAM)
Vimentin
Desmin
Major histocompatibility complex (MHC) class I

*high internal labelling may also be seen

expression alters with age. In addition, a different isoform of a protein may be present at different stages of development. This is particularly important when assessing samples that may contain regenerating fibres, or samples from neonates. We summarize here our own experience with the panel of antibodies we most often use for diagnosis. This is not intended as a comprehensive account of the developmental regulation of muscle proteins but reflects developmental aspects with the antibodies used for diagnostic assessment.

Some proteins change their isoform during maturity (Table 6.2). Studies of *developmental isoforms of myosin* are useful for assessing immaturity and to help distinguish an atrophic fibre from one that is small because it is regenerating. Our studies of regenerating canine muscle showed that immature isoforms of myosin are detectable for a longer length of time than other developmentally regulated proteins such as utrophin, desmin and neural cell adhesion molecule (N-CAM) (Sewry et al 1992, Wilson et al 1994, unpublished observations). We routinely use an antibody to neonatal myosin (Novocastra MHCn) to assess maturation (Fig. 6.2) as we, and others have found this antibody detects a large number of immature fibres in dystrophic muscle; more than MHCf which probably detects a more embryonic myosin isoform and is mainly restricted to the small basophilic regenerating fibres (Goebel and Anderson 1999). In addition to regenerating fibres of variable size and number in dystrophic muscle, MHCn labels a population of fibres in neonatal muscle. This number declines with age, with a large number of positive fibres being present at birth and relatively few after 6 months of age. Some positive fibres may be seen up to 1–2 years of age but it is not yet clear whether this is within the normal spectrum of expression or if it is pathological, as all samples studied have been taken for a clinical reason and normality cannot be established beyond doubt.

The current dogma is that the presence of neonatal myosin reflects immaturity but the presence of neonatal myosin in some situations is confusing as there is evidence from work on rats that embryonic myosin can be detected immunohistochemically in denervated muscle (Jakubiec-Puka et al 1990). For example, some small fibres in motor neurone disease and the groups of small fibres in spinal muscular atrophy, both of which are thought to be non-innervated, express neonatal myosin and sometimes additional developmentally regulated proteins (Sewry 1989; see also Ch. 9). It is not known if this could reflect regeneration induced by denervation, and/or arrest in maturation and/or the re-expression of neonatal myosin induced by the pathological state. Nevertheless, studies of neonatal myosin are important for the assessment of other developmentally regulated proteins and for identifying different patterns of expression that are associated with different disorders (see below).

Another important muscle protein that changes isoform during development is *actin*. Two isoforms have been identified that differ by only four amino acids at the N-terminal region (Marston and Redwood 2003). In fetal skeletal muscle the form found in cardiac muscle is predominant and this is then replaced by the isoform of skeletal muscle. The cardiac isoform is present in the small, basophilic regenerating fibres in dystrophic muscle. It can still be detected in some fibres at birth but is rapidly lost during the neonatal period (unpublished observations). The normal time course of the switch to the skeletal isoform is currently under investigation. Accurate knowledge of the isoform recognized by a particular anti-actin antibody is essential.

It is important to assess the maturity/immaturity of muscle fibres in neonatal muscle and when regenerating fibres may be abundant. Some proteins are more highly expressed in immature muscle; others are lower (Table 6.2), as judged by antibody immunolabelling. Expression studies at the RNA level of many of these proteins are limited. *Utrophin*, the autosomal homologue of dystrophin, is high on the sarcolemma of fetal muscle fibres and on regenerating fibres (Fig. 6.3a,c). Utrophin and dystrophin are both expressed at the sarcolemma from at least 9 weeks of gestation and sarcolemmal labelling of utrophin

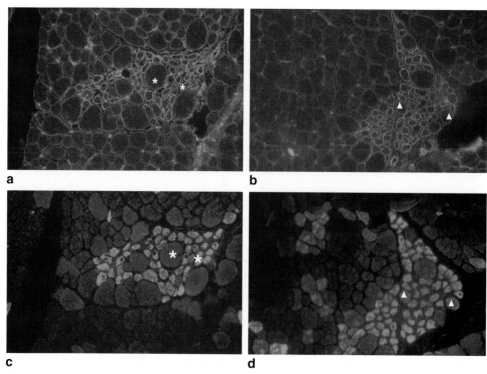

FIG. 6.3 *Labelling of (a) utrophin, (b) MHC class I antigens, and (c) and (d) neonatal myosin in a case of Becker muscular dystrophy showing utrophin and MHC class I on most fibres and particularly high levels on clusters of regenerating fibres [a and c (*), and b and d (▲) are serial areas].*

peaks at about 20 weeks of gestation (Clerk et al 1992b, 1993). After about 26 weeks of gestation and in mature muscle utrophin is no longer seen on the sarcolemma and it is confined to blood vessels and neuromuscular junctions. Utrophin has also been reported at myotendinous junctions but this is not apparent with all antibodies. In the absence of dystrophin, or reduced dystrophin, as in Duchenne and Becker muscular dystrophy, and in inflammatory myopathies, sarcolemmal utrophin is prominent (Fig. 6.3a; Helliwell et al 1992b). This assessment must take account of immaturity of the fibres by reference to the presence of neonatal myosin so that only the abnormal over-expression in mature fibres is considered. Low levels of sarcolemmal utrophin may occur in neonatal muscle that is not dystrophic and is not related to the presence of neonatal myosin (Sewry et al 1994a). The reason for this is unknown.

Laminin α 5 and MHC class I are also proteins that are high on regenerating fibres and assessment of their pathological presence again must be related to neonatal myosin (Fig. 6.3b,d). Laminin α 5 is present on fetal fibres and its presence declines during fetal development (Sewry et al 1995; see Fig. 6.9). MHC class I, however, is not present on the sarcolemma of fetal muscle fibres. All basal lamina proteins may appear to be high on regenerating fibres because of duplication of the basal lamina.

Vimentin and desmin are also high in fetal and regenerating fibres. Both are down-regulated during development; vimentin is only detected on vascular tissue in mature muscle and desmin is seen at the sarcolemma and internally in the fibres at the level of the Z line.

The *neural cell adhesion molecule* (N-CAM) is present on the sarcolemma of regenerating and non-innervated fetal fibres. Once a fibre becomes innervated during development N-CAM becomes localized to the neuromuscular junction. Non-innervated regenerating fibres with extrajunctional N-CAM also express neonatal myosin but, as pointed out previously, some small fibres in neurogenic disorders express neonatal myosin. N-CAM becomes extrajunctional following denervation (Cashman et al 1987, Figarella-Branger et al 1990), so, with the presence of both these proteins, and others associated with immaturity, it can be difficult to distinguish a denervated fibre from a regenerating one. Extrajunctional N-CAM is a common feature in Duchenne muscular dystrophy but the origin of this in relation to regeneration and innervation is not clear. Neuronal nitric oxide synthase (nNOS) is absent from the sarcolemma of denervated fibres (Gosztonyi et al 2001, Tews 2001), and the combination of comparisons of neonatal myosin, nNOS and N-CAM can be informative in distinguishing immature fibres from denervated fibres. Fibres without neonatal myosin and nNOS are likely to be denervated (see Ch. 9).

Other proteins are only weakly labelled in immature muscle. As accompanying RNA studies have not been done, the possibility that any apparent weak or reduced immunohistochemical labelling relates to masking of an epitope of a particular antibody rather than to low expression cannot be excluded. Low immunolabelling may also relate to the affinity of a particular antibody. Several sarcolemmal proteins such as β-spectrin, sarcoglycans, C-terminal dystrophin, α7 integrin and nNOS, may appear weak on some small regenerating fibres that have neonatal myosin, possibly because of immaturity and a plasma membrane that is not fully developed (Fig. 6.4). Internal labelling of small, basophilic fibres may be seen with some antibodies.

Labelling of neonatal muscle with some antibodies is also weak and may make pathological assessment difficult at this stage. For example sarcolemmal labelling of α7 integrin is low in immature muscle, and nNOS with the antibody that we use from Santa Cruz is often very weak or absent in cases under a year of age (Torelli et al 2004). Labelling of nNOS at the neuromuscular junction in immature muscle, however, is prominent. We have also noticed this weak sarcolemmal labelling in neonatal muscle with antibodies to laminin β2 which, in addition to the high expression at the neuromuscular junction (Sanes 2003), is also very prominent extrajunctionally and increases in intensity with age (Wewer et al 1997; unpublished observations). At birth blood vessels are more intensely labelled with laminin β2 than the sarcolemma but by about 3 years of age the intensities are usually comparable (see Fig. 6.9).

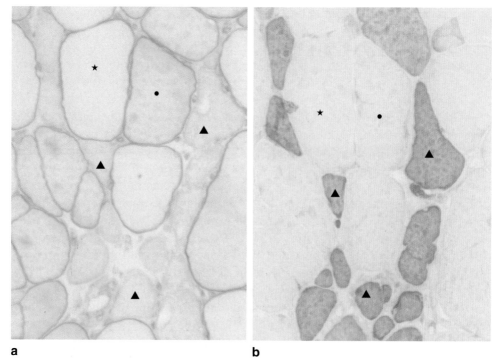

a   **b**

FIG. 6.4 *Labelling of (a) nNOS and (b) neonatal myosin in a case of limb-girdle dystrophy showing absence of detectable nNOS from regenerating fibres with neonatal myosin (▲). Note the normal sarcolemmal labelling on mature fibres (*) which range in size from about 45 to 85 μm, and the internal labelling of some of these (•) which is sometimes seen in a population of fibres.*

Use of tissues other than muscle

Although muscle is the tissue of choice, useful diagnostic information on some proteins can be obtained from other tissues. For example, skin expresses many of the extracellular matrix proteins found in muscle, and skin biopsies are a useful alternative to muscle for studying laminin α2 and collagen VI, particularly when muscle wasting is extensive (Sewry et al 1996, 1997a; see Ch. 12). Skin biopsies are also useful for studying the expression of plectin and the basal keratinocytes at the epidermal–dermal junction show a reduction or absence in epidermolysis bullosa with muscular dystrophy (Shimizu et al 1999). Similarly, emerin, which is expressed in the nuclei of many tissues, can be easily assessed in skin and oral foliate cells (Manilal et al 1997, Sabatelli et al 1998; see Ch. 13). Caution is needed using the latter, however, to ensure that the sample does not contain dead buccal cells in which the nucleus does not label. Prenatal diagnosis can be aided by studies of the immunolabelling of proteins in chorionic villi, for example in congenital muscular dystrophy caused by a primary deficiency of the laminin α2 chain ('merosin' deficient congenital muscular dystrophy; Muntoni et al 1995a; see Ch. 12) or the Ullrich form of congenital muscular dystrophy caused by mutations in collagen VI (Brockington et al 2004). Cultured fibroblasts from skin biopsies are of limited use for immunohistochemical studies but they can be useful for mitochondrial and metabolic studies and research suggests they may be useful for studying collagen synthesis (Sabateilli et al 2001). Fibroblasts can also be transfected with MyoD to convert them to muscle cells for the analysis of muscle specific proteins but this is not widely used for diagnosis. It is likely that the use of tissues other than muscle will increase in the future.

Pathological features of diseased muscle

In this section we give an overview of the immunohistochemical patterns in diseased muscle in relation to primary and secondary defects. Many of the primary defects relate to recessively inherited conditions. In dominant conditions immunohistochemical abnormalities of a protein are more difficult to detect, as the normal allele produces a normal protein product whose localization is often normal. Secondary abnormalities then have an important role. Secondary changes are also important in recessive conditions when studies of the primary protein may show equivocal results. Details in relation to specific neuromuscular disorders can be found in the appropriate chapter.

Primary defects

The number of abnormal primary protein defects that can be detected in neuromuscular disorders by immunohistochemistry is rapidly growing and is summarized in Table 6.3.

Membrane associated proteins

The gene encoding *dystrophin* was cloned in 1987 and was the first gene defect to be identified in a neuromuscular disorder (Burghes et al 1987, Koenig et al 1987). Mutations in the dystrophin gene on chromosome Xp21 cause Duchenne or Becker muscular dystrophy (see Brown and Lucy 1997). Dystrophin is a cytoskeletal protein and immunolabelling of normal muscle shows it is localized to the sarcolemma of every fibre (Fig. 6.5a). Abnormal labelling is seen in Xp21 conditions. A secondary reduction, however, can occur in some limb-girdle dystrophies (see below). The majority of cases of Duchenne dystrophy show an absence of dystrophin from most fibres, or a very marked reduction (Fig. 6.5b). This is thought to be due to disruption of the reading frame by the mutation. Isolated fibres, or small clusters, may show a normal intensity and are known as revertant fibres (Fig. 6.5c). These are fibres in which the reading frame has been maintained, skipping the mutation. In Becker muscular dystrophy the reading frame is also maintained and labelling is usually of reduced intensity on all fibres, or uneven on many fibres (Fig. 6.5d; see Ch. 10). In some Becker cases dystrophin immunolabelling may be indistinguishable from normal and then

TABLE 6.3 *Primary protein defects in neuromuscular disorders where immunohistochemistry can be informative*

Absence of a protein:	
Dystrophin	Xp21 muscular dystrophies
Sarcoglycans	Limb-girdle muscular dystrophies 2C–F
Dysferlin	Limb-girdle muscular dystrophy 2B
Caveolin-3	Limb-girdle muscular dystrophy 1A, rippling muscle disease, hyperCKaemia
Laminin α2	MDC1A ('merosin' deficient congenital muscular dystrophy)
Collagen VI	Ullrich congenital muscular dystrophy (no detectable change in Bethlem myopathy)
Intregrin α7	mild congenital dystrophy/myopathy
Emerin	X-linked Emery–Dreifuss muscular dystrophy
SERCA 1	Brody's disease
Plectin	Epidermolysis bullosa with muscular dystrophy
(Calpain-3 can only be assessed on immunoblots with the antibody from Novocastra)	
Accumulation of a protein:	
Actin	Congenital actinopathy/nemaline myopathy
Myosin	Hyaline body myopathy
Desmin	Desmin myopathy

SERCA, sarcoendoplasmic reticulum calcium ATPase

assessment of secondary changes is important. Abnormalities related to a defect in the dystrophin gene can also be seen in female carriers of Duchenne dystrophy (Fig. 6.6) and occasionally in Becker carriers (Glass et al 1992), because of random X-inactivation patterns (see Ch. 10).

Dystrophin is a large protein and it is important to use more than one antibody for assessment to avoid false results. If the epitope of an antibody lies within a region of the protein encoded by a deleted region of the gene, dystrophin will not be detected, giving the impression of Duchenne muscular dystrophy. If the reading frame is maintained, however, other domains including the C-terminal region will be present, consistent with Becker muscular dystrophy.

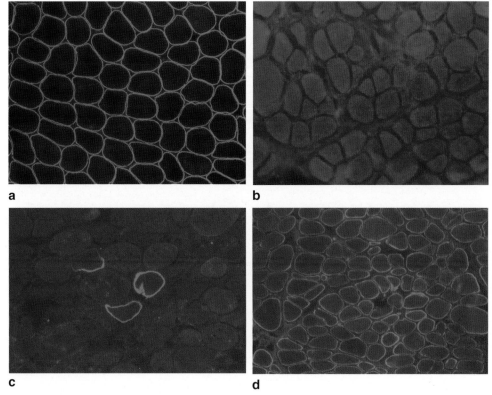

a   b

c   d

FIG. 6.5 *Labelling of dystrophin showing (a) normal sarcolemmal labelling of all fibres, (b) absent dystrophin in a case of Duchenne muscular dystrophy, (c) a few revertant fibres with dystrophin amongst fibres with an absence in a case of Duchenne dystrophy and (d) reduced labelling of most fibres in a case of Becker muscular dystrophy.*

It is therefore important when assessing a case of muscular dystrophy to use antibodies that recognize N- and C-terminal regions of dystrophin and it is usual to also include one to the rod domain of the protein. Although the majority of cases of Duchenne and Becker dystrophy conform to the frame shift hypothesis there are exceptions, and clinical severity should not be judged from dystrophin immunolabelling (Muntoni et al 1994a).

Dystrophin is associated with complexes of proteins that collectively have been called the ***dystrophin-associated proteins*** (DAPs; Straub and Campbell 1997, Lim and Campbell 1998, Ozawa et al 1998, Blake et al 2002, Michelle and Campbell 2003). All of these localize to the sarcolemma in immunohistochemical analysis. Some of these proteins are glycosylated, some are transmembrane or extracellular; others are intracellular. The DAPs are thought to provide a structural link between the subsarcolemmal actin cytoskeleton and the extracellular matrix, stabilizing the membrane during repeated contraction and relaxation. The complex may also stabilize various receptors and ion channels. The DAPs are grouped into sub-complexes (Fig. 6.7): α- and β-dystroglycan, which are post-

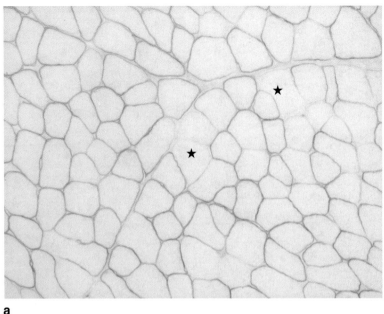

a

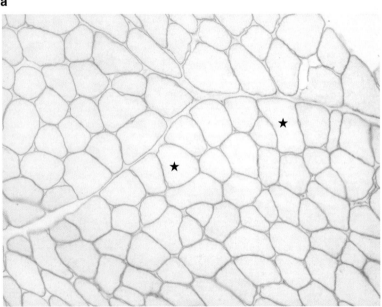

b

FIG. 6.6 *Labelling of (a) dystrophin and (b) β-spectrin in serial sections from a manifesting carrier of Duchenne muscular dystrophy showing absence of dystrophin but retention of β-spectrin from several fibres (*). Fibre sizes range from approximately 30 to 75 μm.*

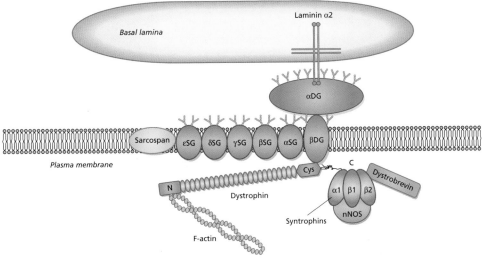

FIG. 6.7 *Diagrammatic representation of dystrophin and its associated protein complex showing how the complex links the extracellular matrix with the actin cytoskeleton. Laminin α2 in the basal lamina binds to α-dystroglycan (αDG) which binds to β-dystroglycan (βDG); β-dystroglycan binds to the cysteine rich domain of dystrophin, which in turn binds to the actin cytoskeleton. There are actin binding sites in the N- and C-terminal domains. The sarcoglycans (α, β, γ, δ, ε SG) interact with β-dystroglycan, and sarcospan is associated with the sarcoglycans although the precise interactions of all these are not yet clear. The syntrophins bind to the C-terminal domain of dystrophin and nNOS and dystrobrevin bind to the syntrophins. There is also evidence of a direct interaction of β-dystroglycan with F-actin (not shown; Chen et al 2003).*

translational products of the same gene, the sarcoglycans (α, β, γ, δ and ε) and sarcospan, the syntrophins, dystrobrevin and nNOS (Michelle and Campbell 2003, Blake and Martin-Randon 2002). A gene for another protein with homology to γ-sarcoglycan, ζ-sarcoglycan, has also been identified and it may have a role in smooth muscle and the pathogenesis of muscular dystrophy, although no mutations in humans have yet been found (Wheeler et al 2002). Defects in the genes for α, β, γ, δ sarcoglycan have been identified in forms of limb-girdle muscular dystrophies (see Ch. 11). Mutations in the gene for ε-sarcoglycan cause some cases of myoclonus-dystonia syndrome (Zimprich et al 2001, Asmus et al 2002; Han et al 2003) and it has an important role in smooth muscle where it is closely associated with β- and δ-sarcoglycan (Straub et al 2003). No defects have been identified in the gene for dystroglycan, the product of which undergoes post-translational modification to produce α- and β-dystroglycan. Secondary alterations in the glycosylation of α-dystroglycan, however, are now recognized as an important pathogenic mechanism in several forms of congenital muscular dystrophy (see below). The syntrophins are believed to be important in anchoring ion channels (Blake and Martin-Randon 2002) but no mutations in the syntrophins, dystrobrevin or nNOS have yet been found, only secondary alterations in their expression (see below).

The *sarcoglycans* (α, β, γ, δ) function as a group, so that a defect in one results in reduced expression of all four. Complete absence of one sarcoglycan, or the most severe reduction, is usually an indicator of the defective gene and helps to direct molecular analysis (Fig. 6.8). The other three sarcoglycans then show variable degrees of abnormal immunolabelling ranging from pronounced to minimal. An absence of the whole sarcoglycan complex may occur and is usually associated with a defect in the β-sarcoglycan gene (Bönnemann et al 1995). A secondary reduction of sarcoglycans occurs in Duchenne dystrophy (see below).

Other forms of limb-girdle muscular dystrophy are caused by mutations in other genes coding for proteins localized to the sarcolemma and a reduction can be detected with immunohistochemistry. An absence or marked reduction of the plasma membrane protein, *dysferlin,* can be seen in some cases of limb-girdle 2B dystrophy and Miyoshi myopathy. Dysferlin is believed to be involved in membrane fusion and repair (Bansal and Campbell 2004). Currently available commercial antibodies do not always give a clear result with immunohistochem-istry and secondary changes in dysferlin expression can also occur in other muscular dystrophies (see below). Abnormalities in dysferlin expression are often clearer on immunoblots and several proteins should be examined simul-taneously to ensure the reduction is not secondary to a primary defect in another protein such as calpain-3 or caveolin-3 (Anderson et al 1999, Anderson et al 2000, Walter et al 2003).

Caveolin-3 is the muscle specific form of caveolin and defects in its gene occur in a dominant form of limb-girdle dystrophy (LGMD1C), in rippling muscle disease and some rare cases with elevated creatine kinase (McNally et al 1998, Minetti et al 1998, Carbone et al 2000, Betz et al 2001). Caveolin-3 is a plasma membrane protein and in normal muscle it is again seen localized to the sarcolemma. An absence or reduction of the protein can be detected by immunohistochemistry.

Defects in the *LAMA2* gene encoding the *laminin α2* chain of merosin occur in the severe MDC1A form of congenital muscular dystrophy ('merosin-deficient' congenital muscular dystrophy; Helbling-Leclerc et al 1995). In normal muscle the laminin α2 chain is localized to the basal lamina of every muscle fibre. It is not present round blood vessels, in contrast to the laminin α5, β1, β2 and γ1 chains (Fig. 6.9a–e). Laminins are heterotrimers, the three chains of which are arranged in a cruciform shape and encoded by separate genes. To date, five α, three β and three γ chains have been identified, which are assembled into 14 different forms with a variable tissue distribution (Gullberg et al 1999, Libby et al 2000). Previous nomenclature referred to the chains as A, B1, B2 but this was revised to accommodate the growing number of different chains. The main variants localized to the sarcolemma are laminin-2 (often referred to as merosin; α2-β1-γ1 chains) and laminin-4 (S-merosin; α2-β2-γ1 chains). The laminin β2 chain has an organizational role at the neuromuscular junction, where it is con-centrated (Sanes 2003). Contrary to common belief, however, appreciable amounts of laminin β2 are detected on the extrajunctional sarcolemma, particularly in

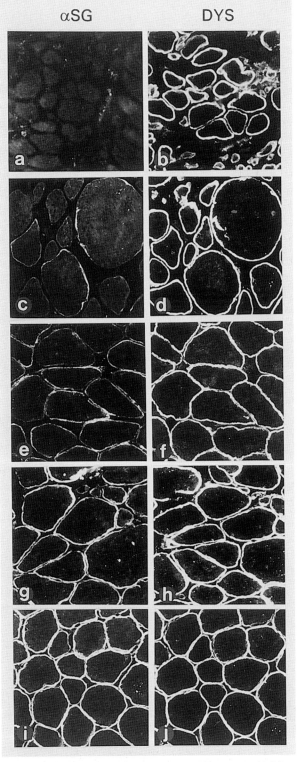

FIG. 6.8 *Labelling of α-sarcoglycan (αSG) compared with dystrophin (DYS) in cases of limb-girdle muscular dystrophy showing the variation of labelling that may be seen, ranging from absent to traces and various degrees of reduction (a–h). The bottom panel shows normal labelling in a control sample (i,j).*

mature muscle (Fig. 6.9e; Wewer et al 1997). The laminin α5 chain is detected on blood vessels and is highly expressed on immature fibres. It is down-regulated during development and only traces are detected on the sarcolemma of mature human muscle fibres (Fig. 6.9b). The clinical severity of cases with a defect in the *LAMA2* gene varies from severe to mild and this is usually reflected in the amount of protein that can be detected. Severe cases usually show an absence, or only very slight traces, of laminin α2 on the sarcolemma (Fig. 6.10a–c; Philpot et al 1995). Milder cases show only a reduction of the protein and it is then necessary to assess both N- and C-terminal epitopes of this large protein (Sewry et al 1997b; see Ch. 12). Secondary changes in laminin α2, α5 and β1 chains are discussed below. No defects in laminin γ1 have been identified and it is therefore useful for assessing the integrity of the basal lamina.

Defects in the genes that encode all three chains of *collagen VI* are responsible for dominantly inherited Bethlem myopathy and the recessive Ullrich form of congenital muscular dystrophy (Jobis et al 1996, Speer et al 1996, Bertini et al 1998, Camacho Vanegas et al 2001, Demir et al 2002). Distinct labelling of collagen VI associated with the sarcolemma is seen in normal muscle (Fig. 6.12a) and it is also seen in the perimysium and endomysium when there is excess fibrosis. As Bethlem myopathy is dominantly inherited no alteration in collagen VI immunolabelling is usually seen (Fig. 6.11). In recessive cases of Ullrich congenital dystrophy, however, collagen VI may be absent or severely reduced (Fig. 6.12b,c). In some cases this may only be a subtle change that is only apparent at the sarcolemmal (Fig. 6.12c). It is important that the good preservation of the basal lamina is controlled with parallel studies of another basal lamina protein, such as collagen IV, collagen V and/or perlecan. Collagen V has a similar localization to collagen VI, and perlecan interacts with collagen VI (see below).

Missense mutations and in-frame insertions in the gene for *perlecan* have been reported in Schwartz-Jampel syndrome (Nicole et al 2000, Arikawa-Hirasawa et al 2002). Mutations probably affect normal functioning of perlecan and immunolabelling shows that the protein is still present (see Hoffman and Pegaro 2002). Complete absence of the protein is lethal and occurs in dysegmental dysplasia with severe lack of bone growth. Perlecan has a major role in clustering of acetylcholine esterase to the neuromuscular junction and connects the basal lamina to the plasma membrane via integrins. No defects in collagen IV or V in a neuromuscular disorder have yet been found. Mutations in collagen IX are associated with epiphysial dysplasia and a myopathy (Bönnemann et al 2000).

Another primary defect in a membrane associated protein is *integrin α7* which interacts with laminin α2 (Hayashi et al 1998). Defects in the gene cause a mild disorder classified as a congenital muscular dystrophy and absence of integrin α7 is seen with a concomitant decrease in its partner, integrin β1D. This disorder is very rare and the original studies were not performed with a commercial antibody. Integrin α7β1D forms a transmembrane complex that interacts with several proteins, including laminin α2, and secondary alterations in integrins occur (see below).

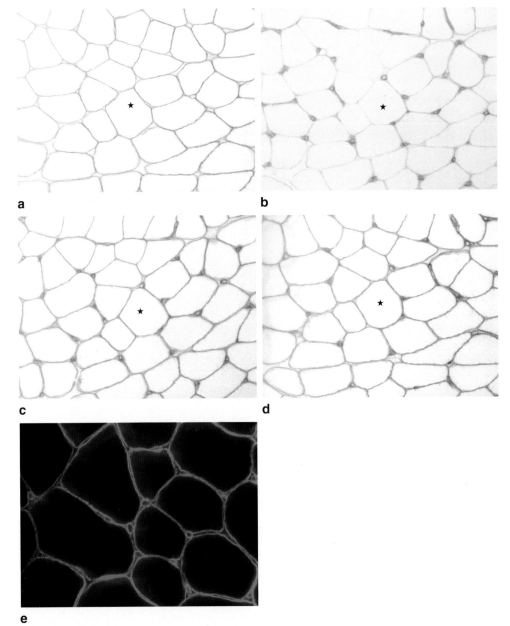

FIG. 6.9 *Immunoperoxidase labelling of (a) laminin α2, (b) laminin α5, (c) laminin β1, (d) laminin γ1 and (e) fluorescent labelling of laminin β2. Note the strong sarcolemmal labelling of α2, β1, γ1 and β2 but only traces of α5 and absence of α2 from the capillaries (a). The same fibre in a–d is marked (*).*

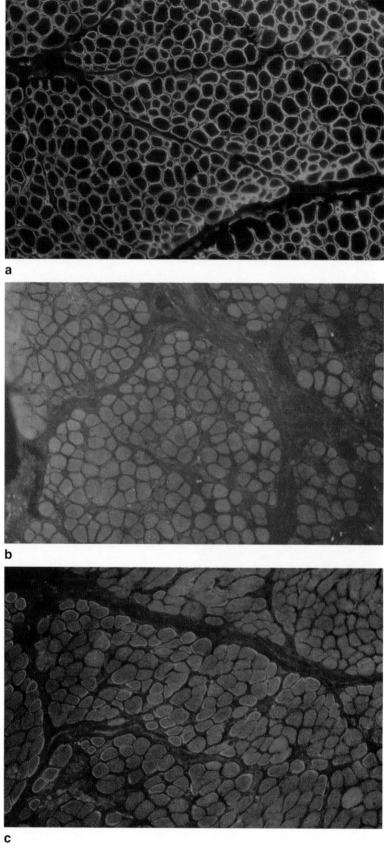

a

b

c

FIG. 6.10 *Labelling of laminin α2 showing (a) normal labelling, (b) an absence, and (c) a marked reduction in two cases with a mutation in the LAMA2 gene.*

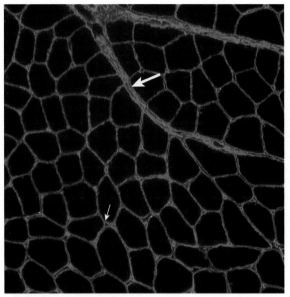

FIG. 6.11 *Normal labelling of collagen VI. Note the peripheral labelling round each fibre, labelling of the perimysium (large arrow), and labelling round capillaries (small arrow). Fibre sizes range from approximately 30 to 60 μm.*

Primary defects in nuclear proteins

Proteins of the nuclear envelope, which are responsible for the X-linked and autosomal dominant forms of Emery–Dreifuss muscular dystrophy, are those most studied in diagnostic muscle pathology. The nuclear envelope is composed of an outer and inner membrane, nuclear pore complexes and a lamina. The outer membrane is continuous with the endoplasmic reticulum and a number of proteins are integral components of the inner membrane. These proteins interact with the nuclear lamina and chromatin. *Emerin* is anchored to the inner nuclear membrane (Fig. 6.13) and mutations in the gene are responsible for the X-linked form of Emery–Dreifuss muscular dystrophy (see Ch. 13). The majority of mutations in the *STA* gene encoding emerin result in truncation of the protein which lack the C-terminal domain and result in a total absence of the protein from all nuclear membranes. This absence is easily detected by immunohistochemistry of muscle, skin or buccal cells (Manilal et al 1996, 1997, 1998, Sabatelli et al 1998). Very rare exceptions to this have been reported and emerin was seen to be reduced (Cartagni et al 1997) or mislocalized in the muscle cytoplasm (Di Blasi et al 2000).

Lamins are a principal component of the nuclear lamina and mutations in the gene for *lamin A/C* are associated with several phenotypes, including the autosomal dominant form of Emery–Dreifuss muscular dystrophy (see Ch. 13), dilated cardiomyopathy, limb-girdle muscular dystrophy 1B, familial partial

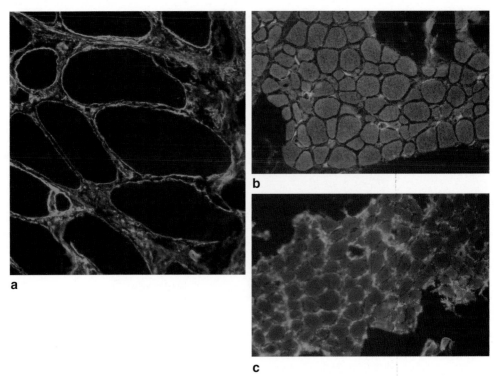

FIG. 6.12 *Labelling of collagen VI in (a) a case of Bethlem myopathy and (b) and (c) two cases of Ullrich congenital muscular dystrophy all with mutations in a collagen VI gene. Note labelling is distinguishable from normal in Bethlem myopathy (a) with strong labelling of the basement membrane and endomysium, but in one Ullrich case (b) only scant positive areas near blood vessels and absent collagen VI from the basement membrane, and a subtle reduction round some fibres in the other Ullrich case (c).*

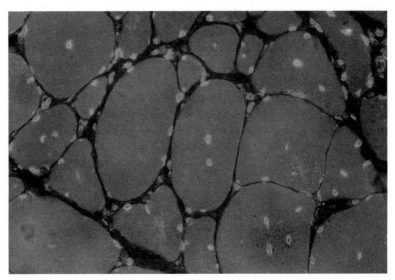

FIG. 6.13 *Immunolabelling of both peripheral and internal nuclei with emerin.*

lipodystrophy, an axonal neuropathy (Charcot–Marie–Tooth type 2B1), mandibuloacral disease, premature ageing disorders (Mounkes and Stewart 2004) and restrictive dermopathy (Navarro et al 2004). Immunolabelling of lamin A/C in dominant Emery–Dreifuss muscular dystrophy shows no detectable difference from controls. Secondary changes in laminin β1, however, may be seen (see below).

Other disorders are also caused by defects in nuclear proteins but immunohistochemistry currently has a limited role in studies of the primary protein defect. These include the survival motor neurone (SMN) protein in spinal muscular atrophy, the expansion of the genes responsible for both forms of myotonic dystrophy, and the expansion of the poly A binding protein nuclear 1 gene (*PABPN1*) in oculopharyngeal muscular dystrophy. Antibodies to PABPN1, however, have been shown to localize to the nuclear inclusions in patients with oculopharyngeal muscular dystrophy (Calado et al 2000).

Primary defects in myofibrillar and cytoskeletal proteins

Gene defects have been identified in a number of myofibrillar proteins and they are receiving increasing interest as likely candidates for several myopathies. They result in myofibrillar disorganization and collectively the term 'myofibrillar myopathy' has been used for this group of disorders. The myofibrillar myopathies highlight the importance of proteins that interact with Z line proteins and maintain sarcomeric structure (Bönnemann and Laing 2004). Mutations in myofibrillar proteins that have been identified include myosin heavy chain isoforms, actin, telethonin, myotilin, troponin isoforms, tropomyosin, titin, nebulin and the cytoskeletal proteins, desmin and plectin. The gene for the intermediate filament protein, syncoilin has also been screened as a possible candidate for myofibrillar myopathy but no mutations have been found (Selcen et al 2004). These defective proteins can all be detected by immunohistochemistry but as some relate to a dominant condition, and/or the mutations are often missense, a total absence of the protein is rarely seen. Sometimes, however, an accumulation of the protein occurs and additional secondary changes can be detected.

Myosin heavy chains are encoded by a multigene family and exist in several isoforms which are regulated in a tissue and developmental specific manner (Nguyen et al 1982, Buckingham 1985, lzumo et al 1986). The physiological fast or slow characteristics of the different fibre types relate to the respective isoforms. The major myosin heavy chain isoform in slow, type 1 fibres is encoded by the *MYH7* gene on chromosome 14. This is also the major isoform in cardiac ventricles (beta-cardiac myosin heavy chain) and mutations in the globular head are associated with familial cardiomyopathy (Seidman and Seidman 2001). Recently a mutation in the rod region has been identified in patients with no overt cardiomyopathy but a skeletal muscle myopathy with hyaline bodies (Tajsharghi et al 2003, Bohlega et al 2004, Laing et al 2005). Immunohistochemistry shows these inclusions are in type 1 fibres and contain slow myosin. This disorder has been classified as a protein surplus myosin storage myopathy

(Goebel and Borchet 2002). Mutations in the 3' domain of *MYH7* have recently been shown to cause a distal myopathy (Meredith et al 2004). Thus mutations in different domains of this gene lead to dominant disorders with varying phenotype.

Mutations in the fast myosin heavy chain IIa gene (*MYH2A*) on chromosome 17 have been found in a rare dominant disorder that was previously regarded as a variant of hereditary inclusion body myopathy because of the presence of rimmed vacuoles and the presence of 15–20 nm tubulofilamentous inclusions (Martinsson et al 2000). Immunohistochemistry of biopsies from young patients with a mutation have shown that myosin IIa is undetectable (Tajsharghi et al 2002). Older cases in this study, however, showed the presence of IIa myosin and many hybrid fibres with more than one myosin isoform. Fibres with rimmed vacuoles expressed myosin IIa. Myofibrillar disorganization and focal loss of mitochondria, particularly in 2A fibres, were also a prominent feature (Martinsson et al 2000). This suggested that there may be a relationship between abnormalities in myofibrillar proteins and the formation of rimmed vacuoles.

Although mutations in only two myosin genes have so far been identified in myopathic conditions, other members of the myosin gene family are clearly candidates for other disorders.

Mutations in the *ACTA 1* gene encoding sarcomeric skeletal muscle *actin* are now known to be associated with a broad spectrum of clinical phenotypes in forms of nemaline myopathy, ranging from severe to mild (Sanoudou and Beggs 2001, Sparrow et al 2003; see Ch. 15). Mutations can give rise to actin accumulation, with or without the typical nemaline rods, which may be nuclear and/or cytoplasmic. Accumulation of actin in association with a cardiomyopathy can occur when the gene for the cardiac actin isoform is mutated (Olsen et al 1998, Mogensen et al 1999). Mutations in the *ACTA1* gene also result in congenital fibre type disproportion (Laing et al 2005) and in a dominant congenital myopathy characterized by cores devoid of mitochondria and disrupted myofibrils and type 1 predominance, as in central core disease, but no nemaline rods (Kaindl et al 2004).

Immunohistochemical studies of *tropomyosin* isoforms in human muscle as a primary defect are limited, but mutations in the genes for α-tropomyosin and β-tropomyosin are responsible for rare dominant forms of nemaline myopathy (Laing et al 1995, Donner et al 2002). Mutations in the gene for β-tropomyosin can also cause distal arthrogryposis without the presence of rods (Sung et al 2003). The primary role of tropomyosin in relation to cardiomyopathies has also been established (Towbin 1998).

Isoforms of *α-actinin* have been characterized and mainly studied in relation to fibre typing and the rods in nemaline myopathy, rather than as a primary cause of a muscle disorder. Antibodies to α-actinin-2 label all muscle fibre types, while antibodies to α-actinin-3 only label a subset of fast fibres. A common, non-pathogenic polymorphism has been found in the gene for the α-actinin-3 (*ACTN3*; North et al 1999), which results in an absence of α-actinin-3 from all fibres. Before identification of this polymorphism, it had been suggested that the absence of α-actinin-3 might be of pathological significance in some congenital muscular dystrophies (North and Beggs 1996) but it soon became apparent that this is a non-specific finding (Vainzof et al 1997).

Titin and nebulin are two of the largest proteins described, both of which exist as multiple isoforms resulting from differential splicing (Millevoi et al 1998, Gregorio et al 1999). They are believed to have a role in maintaining myofibrillar alignment and contribute to the elasticity of the myofibrils. The genes for both proteins are located on chromosome 2q and mutations in the nebulin gene are responsible for one of the more common forms of nemaline myopathy (Wallgren-Petterson et al 1995, Pelin et al 1999). Commercial antibodies to nebulin show retention of the protein but research studies with an antibody corresponding to the SH3 region of nebulin have shown an absence in a few severe cases of nemaline myopathy, which can help direct molecular analysis (Sewry et al 2001b, Wallgren-Petterson et al 2002). Titin is the defective protein in limb-girdle dystrophy 2J which is characterized by tibial involvement (Hackmann et al 2002, 2003). As with nebulin, absence of the whole titin protein does not occur but a non-commercial antibody raised against the defective exon, the last exon of this giant gene, has shown an absence (Hackmann et al 2002). Secondary abnormalities in nebulin expression occur in Duchenne dystrophy and prior to the identification of the dystrophin gene, nebulin was thought to be the primary defective gene product (Wood et al 1987), but was subsequently found to be an artefact.

Mutations affecting other myofibrillar proteins in which immunohistochemistry has been used to study the primary protein include *telethonin*, responsible for limb-girdle muscular dystrophy 2G, *myotilin* responsible for limb-girdle muscular dystrophy 1A and a myofibrillar myopathy, and slow *troponin T*, responsible for a rare form of nemaline myopathy (Speer et al 1992, Hauser et al 2000, Moreira et al 2000, Johnston et al 2000, Selcen and Engel 2004). The prevalence of these defects is not known, as only a few affected cases have been reported. Recent studies, however, suggest that mutations in the gene for myotilin may be a more common cause of myofibrillar myopathy than previously thought (Selcen and Engel 2004). The mutations were all missense and myotilin was still detected. The mutations were found in the same serine-rich exon 2 as in limb-girdle muscular dystrophy 2A, but these disorders have a different phenotype and pathology. As in other myofibrillar myopathies, cardiac involvement was found to be common and also peripheral neuropathy. Mutations in the gene for a fast isoform of *troponin I* on chromosome 11 cause a form of distal arthrogryposis (Sung et al 2003) but there is currently no immunohistochemical data on the expression of the protein.

The cytoskeletal protein *desmin* is involved both primarily and secondarily in a group of myofibrillar myopathies often collectively referred to as 'desminopathies' or 'desmin-related myopathies'. Both missense mutations and deletions in the gene for desmin have been identified (Goldfarb et al 1998, Dakalas et al 2000). Inheritance is often dominant but recessive cases are also known. Age of onset is variable and cardiomyopathy is a frequent complication. Antibodies to desmin show accumulation in fibres that do not express neonatal myosin, distinguishing them from regenerating fibres with high desmin. A characteristic accumulation of electron dense granulomatous material is seen at the ultrastructural level (see Ch. 5) and additional features include cytoplasmic and spheroid bodies. Histochemical staining for oxidative enzymes and adenosine triphosphatase (ATPase) show extensive areas that lack activity and have a 'rubbed out' appearance. Vacuoles may also be seen. Similar features are seen when the gene for the chaperone protein **αB-crystallin** is mutated (Vicart et al 1998). This small heat shock protein is involved in desmin polymerization and is thought to be involved in the protection of the intermediate filament network from stress-induced damage. It is not possible to identify the primary gene defect by looking at the pathology; accumulations of desmin and αβ-crystallin, and the granulomatous material are seen in both conditions. Cardiomyopathy also occurs in both, but a distinguishing clinical feature is the presence of cataracts in cases with a mutation in the gene αB-crystallin.

The gene for *plectin* is mutated in the rare skin blistering recessive disorder, epidermolysis bullosa simplex with muscular dystrophy (Gache et al 1996, Smith et al 1996). Plectin is believed to have a role in anchoring desmin to the periphery of the Z lines. Immunolabelling of skin and muscle with antibodies to plectin shows an absence or reduction and a secondary accumulation of desmin can occur (Shimizu et 1999, Schröder and Goebel 2002).

Primary defects in enzymes

Several primary enzyme defects are known to cause a neuromuscular disorder but it is often more important to examine the activity of the enzyme biochemically rather than its localization by immunohistochemistry. Immunoblots, however, are useful for studying enzymes such as *calpain-3,* which is defective in limb-girdle muscular dystrophy 2A (Richard et al 1995). This disorder is unusual amongst the limb-girdle muscular dystrophies in not being caused by a membrane-associated protein. Calpain-3 is an enzyme located in the cytosol of the fibre and in the nucleus, and it binds to the C-terminus of titin. Absence or reduction of calpain-3 using a commercial antibody from Novocastra can be detected on immunoblots in limb-girdle muscular dystrophy 2A but it cannot be localized by immunohistochemistry with this antibody (Anderson et al 1998). It is important to distinguish primary from secondary changes in calpain-3 (see below).

Primary defects of ion channels

The two ion channels that have been studied by immunohistochemistry are the ryanodine receptor 1 (RYR1) and the sarco(endo)plasmic reticulum calcium ATPase (SERCA). Mutations in the *RYR1* gene on chromosome 19q occur in central core disease and malignant hyperthermia (Quane et al 1993, McCarthy et al 2000, see Ch. 15). Malignant hyperthermia is also linked to several other loci (Loke and MacLennan 1998). Not all cases of central core disease appear to be susceptible to malignant hyperthermia but patients are always advised of the potential risk. The ryanodine receptor is a large ligand-gated calcium-release channel with an essential role in excitation–contraction coupling. It has several C-terminal transmembrane loops in the membrane of the sarcoplasmic reticulum and cytoplasmic regions that interact with the voltage-gated dihydropyridine receptor of the T tubule. Genotype–phenotype correlations suggest that mutations in the transmembrane C-terminal region of *RYR1* are more commonly, but not exclusively, associated with central core disease, whereas malignant hyperthermia is more often associated with N-terminal hot-spots (Monnier et al 2001; Tilgen et al 2001; Davis et al 2003). Most mutations in the *RYR1* gene are missense and dominantly inherited so total absence of the protein is not seen. Limited immunohistochemical studies of the RyR1 protein have been reported and they are not currently used for diagnosis. A secondary accumulation of several proteins, however, can be useful for visualizing the cores (Sewry et al 2002).

Brody's disease, characterized by stiffness and exercise-induced pain (Brody 1969), is caused by mutations in the ATP2A1 gene encoding the sarcoplasmic reticulum calcium ATPase, SERCA1 (Odermatt et al 1996). SERCA1 is confined to fast fibres and SERCA2 to slow fibres. Thus, antibodies to these show a checkerboard pattern in normal muscle (Fig. 6.14). In Brody's disease an absence of SERCA1 from the fast fibres can be detected. Proteins, such as sarcolipin, that are associated with SERCA are candidates for Brody's syndrome, which clinically resembles Brody's disease, but no mutations have yet been found (Odermatt et al 1997).

Secondary defects

A large number of publications describe the wide variety of secondary alterations in protein localization and expression that occur in diseased muscle as a consequence of a primary defect in another gene, such as those described above. In this section we concentrate on those that we have found to be of diagnostic value and situations where antibodies can clarify the nature of a structure (Table 6.4).

Membrane associated proteins

The use of *β-spectrin* as a control has already been discussed. It is used to assess the preservation of the plasmalemma and its closely associated cytoskeleton, so that the presence of other membrane proteins can be judged. β-Spectrin is lost from necrotic fibres (see Fig. 6.1) and if there is artefactual damage to the membrane, such as freezing artefact or freeze–thawing, labelling of the sarcolemma may be weak, uneven or disrupted. Weak labelling of some regenerating fibres has been discussed in the section on development. The internal membranes of split fibres and branched fibres and myotendinous junctions label with antibodies to many plasmalemmal and basal lamina proteins (Fig. 6.15). Invaginations of the sarcolemma when sectioned transversely, for example at myotendinous

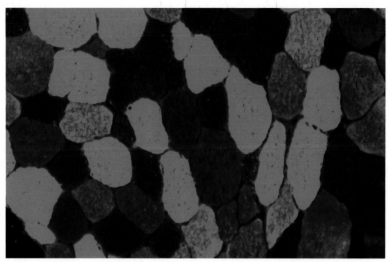

FIG. 6.14 *Labelling of SERCA 1 which is higher in type 2 (fast) fibres. Note the three grades of intensity with this antibody.*

TABLE 6.4 *Proteins that show a secondary change that is useful for diagnosis and can be studied with commercial antibodies*

Dystrophin
Sarcoglycans
Utrophin
Neuronal nitric oxide synthase (nNOS)
Laminin α2
Laminin β1
Laminin α5
α-Dystroglycan
Neonatal myosin
Desmin accumulation
Major histocompatibility complex (MHC) class I
Tau accumulation

junctions, may sometimes be confused with vacuoles. The labelling of true vacuoles, however, is dependent on their origin. Those of lysosomal origin, such as in acid maltase deficiency or those derived from the sarcoplasmic reticulum, do not usually label with β-spectrin and other sarcolemmal proteins, whilst the autophagic vacuoles in Danon's disease (*LAMP-2* mutation) and the other X-linked disorder with similar pathology, X-linked myopathy with excessive autophagy (see section on vacuoles in Ch. 4 and the ultrastructural features in Ch. 5), show the presence of plasma membrane proteins on most vacuoles and of basal lamina proteins on some (Fig. 6.16).

Dystrophin rarely shows a secondary reduction in well preserved muscle. An exception is in recessive limb-girdle dystrophy 2E with a defect in β-sarcoglycan (Bönnemann et al 1995). It may occasionally occur when other sarcoglycans are defective (Vainzof et al 1996) but usually immunolabelling of dystrophin is indistinguishable from normal in limb-girdle muscular dystrophies. If dystrophin is reduced in a female patient careful distinction from a Duchenne carrier is needed. Utrophin may then be useful (see below). Reduced labelling of dystrophin has also been reported in Fukuyama congenital muscular dystrophy (Arikawa et al 1991) and in early immunohistochemical studies we observed it in inflammatory myopathies (Sewry et al 1991). Weak labelling with antibodies to the C-terminus of dystrophin (such as the monoclonal antibody DYS2 from Novocastra raised against the last 17 amino acids) may be apparent in some neonatal samples, possibly because of differential splicing at the C-terminus of the gene. Dystrophin labelling of internal membranes mirrors that of β-spectrin. Labelling of dystrophin and most proteins of the dystrophin-associated glycoprotein complex is enhanced at neuromuscular junctions (Fig. 6.17) and structures such as cytoplasmic bodies may label (Helliwell et al 1994).

Utrophin is an autosomal protein encoded by a gene on chromosome 6. It has considerable sequence and structural homology to dystrophin, and is ubiquitously expressed in a variety of tissues (see Brown and Lucy 1997). In normal skeletal muscle it is localized to blood vessels, including capillaries, peripheral nerves and neuromuscular junctions, and myotendinous junctions with some antibodies. As discussed previously, it is highly expressed on the sarcolemma of regenerating fibres in a variety of disorders (see Fig. 6.3). Over-expression of utrophin on mature fibres occurs in Duchenne and Becker muscular dystrophy, symptomatic carriers of Duchenne dystrophy and inflammatory myopathies (Fig. 6.3; Helliwell et al 1992b; Sewry et al 1994b). Asymptomatic carriers may also show some utrophin. Young cases of Duchenne and Becker dystrophy tend to show less sarcolemmal utrophin and careful assessment of fibre maturity may then be needed (Taylor et al 1997a). Although the presence of utrophin is a useful marker for assessment of Xp21 disorders, it is not specific and sarcolemmal labelling can be detected in a variety of other conditions, including other muscular dystrophies, some neonates and in muscle adjacent to tumours (Sewry et al 1994a, 2005b). The reasons for this are not known but current research on utrophin is aimed at elucidating the factors that up-regulate utrophin and its possible therapeutic potential in Duchenne dystrophy. Two full length isoforms of

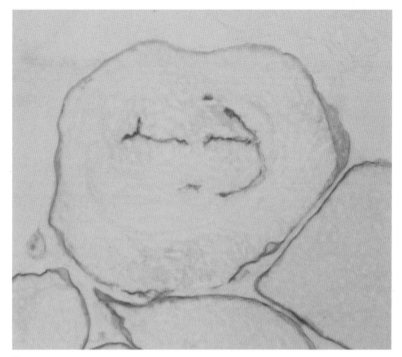

a

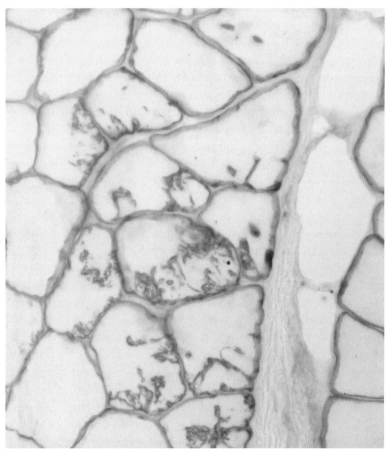

b

FIG. 6.15 *Labelling of internal membranes with (a) β-spectrin in a whorled hypertrophic fibre (150 μm) and (b) laminin α2 at a myotendinous junction. Fibres approximately 30–55 μm.*

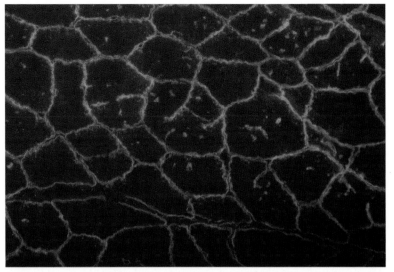

a

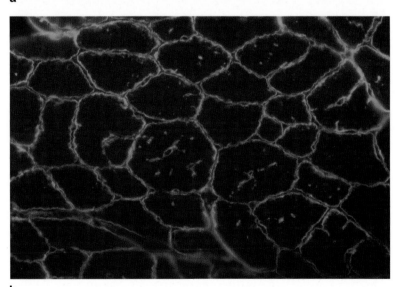

b

FIG. 6.16 *Labelling of (a) dystrophin and (b) laminin α2 in serial sections from a case resembling X-linked myopathy with excessive autophagy. Note the internal labelling with invaginations and vacuoles many of which have both proteins.*

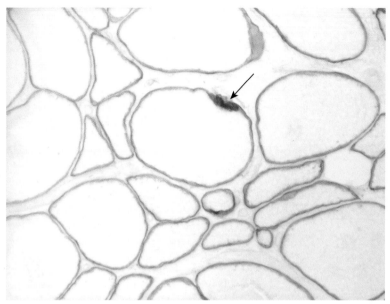

FIG. 6.17 *Enhanced labelling of dystrophin at a neuromuscular junction (arrow) on a fibre approximately 80 µm in diameter.*

utrophin, A and B, have been identified (Burton et al 1999) and the up-regulated isoform in human dystrophic muscle and the isoform at the sarcolemmal of fetal and regenerating fibres is the A form (Sewry et al 2005b).

Most proteins of the ***dystrophin-associated complex*** show a secondary reduction in Xp21 disorders. We have recently found immunolabelling of nNOS to be useful in the assessment of Becker muscle dystrophy as sarcolemmal labelling is absent when there is a mutation in the rod domain 'hot-spot' (Torelli et al 2004). Sarcolemmal nNOS is also absent in cases of Duchenne dystrophy. Labelling on larger blood vessels, however, is retained. Whether this relates specifically to nNOS or the use of a particular polyclonal antibody is not clear. Other DAPs show a variable reduction on the sarcolemma in Xp21 disorders. When there is a primary defect in one sarcoglycan gene all components of this complex show a reduction.

Labelling of nNOS is also useful in the assessment of neurogenic disorders as evidence suggests denervated fibres lose sarcolemmal nNOS but it gradually reappears following reinnervation (Gosztonyi et al 2001, Tews 2001).

In limb-girdle muscular dystrophies secondary reductions have suggested a relationship between some proteins and care in identifying the primary defect is then necessary. For example, dysferlin and calpain-3 can both show a secondary reduction when the gene for either is mutated (Anderson et al 2000, Vainzof et al 2001). Similarly, a reduction in caveolin-3 can occur when the primary defect is in the gene for dysferlin, suggesting an interaction (Matsuda et al 2001, Walter et al 2003). Calpain-3 is very susceptible to degradation and this must also be taken into consideration in interpreting results. Commercial antibodies from Novocastra to calpain-3 are only suitable for assessment of immunoblots.

A secondary modification in the *O*-glycosylation of **α-dystroglycan**, a dystrophin-associated protein (DAP), is now recognized as an important pathogenic mechanism in various forms of congenital muscular dystrophies (see Ch. 12; Muntoni et al 2002a, Michelle and Campbell 2003, Muntoni et al 2004c). Mutations in several genes encoding proven or putative glycosyltransferases result in abnormal glycosylation of α-dystroglycan. These include POMGnT, POMT1, Fukutin, Fukutin-related protein and LARGE (Michelle and Campbell 2003, Muntoni and Voit 2004). Commercial antibodies to glycoslyated epitopes of α-dystroglycan are available but none are currently available to the core protein and studies on the latter are research-based at present (Brown et al 2004). In normal muscle both are localized to the sarcolemma. Caution and carefully controlled studies are needed for the interpretation of results with current commercial antibodies to α-dystroglycan, as different batches can give variable results. Despite this, different disease-associated patterns of dystroglycan expression are emerging. In Xp21 disorders, antibodies to the core protein and glycosylated epitope of α-dystroglycan both show a reduction, as both α- and β-dystroglycan are reduced, in common with other proteins of the DAP complex. In the various forms of congenital muscular dystrophy β-dystroglycan shows normal sarcolemmal localization when the plasmalemma is well preserved, but α-dystroglycan is altered. The core protein is usually retained, except in Walker-Warburg syndrome caused by mutations in the *POMT1* gene, where little, if any, is detected (Jimenez-Mallebrera et al 2003a). Variable degrees of reduced glycosylation are seen in muscle-eye-brain disease (mutations in the *POMGnT1* gene), Fukuyama congenital muscular dystrophy (mutations in the gene for fukutin), limb-girdle muscular dystrophy 2I and congenital muscular dystrophy 1C (MDC1C, mutations in the fukutin-related protein) and congenital muscular dystrophy 1D (MDC1D, mutations in the *LARGE* gene) (see Muntoni and Voit 2004). In MDC1C and limb-girdle dystrophy 2I there appears to be a correlation between the residual α-dystroglycan and clinical severity (Brown et al 2004). Epitope masking of α-dystroglycan also occurs and can give the appearance of reduced immunolabelling. Many of the extracellular matrix proteins are highly glycosylated and the epitopes for the antibodies used to localize them are not known. It is possible that alterations in the glycosylation of these proteins also occurs and may also result in abnormal immunolabelling.

Several *extracellular matrix proteins* show secondary alterations and with the primary defects discussed above they highlight the pathological importance of the extracellular matrix (Muntoni and Sewry 1998, Sewry and Muntoni 1999). Various types of collagen, such as types III, V and VI are detected in the perimysium and endomysium, and are prominent when connective tissue is excessive (Fig. 6.18). Collagen type I is mainly restricted to the perimysium, although a little may be seen in the endomysium in Duchenne dystrophy (Duance et al 1980, Stephens et al 1982). The distribution of fibronectin is similar to that of collagen type III. In normal muscle several collagen types are constituents of the

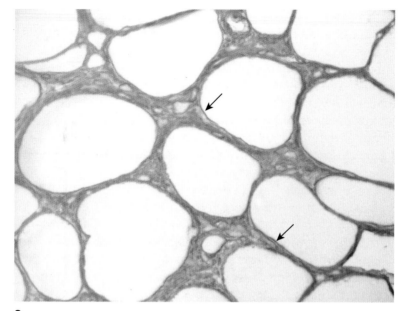

a

b

FIG. 6.18 *Labelling of (a) collagen V and (b) collagen VI in serial sections showing a distinction of the basement membrane (arrows) and excess labelling of the endomysium with both antibodies.*

basement membrane and appear round each fibre at the sarcolemma. In normal muscle the periphery of each fibre is clearly delineated by antibodies to proteins such as collagen types IV, V, VI, laminins, perlecan and nidogen (Fig. 6.19). They are also seen in the extracellular matrix round blood vessels. When connective tissue is excessive the sarcolemmal labelling of collagen types V and VI is usually more prominent than that of the adjacent endomysium (Fig. 6.18). Architectural features involving the sarcolemma, such as splits and whorls and indentations, show extracellular matrix proteins associated with them. Some vacuoles also do, depending on their origin (see Fig. 6.15 and section on β-spectrin). Other collagens are also expressed in skeletal muscle, such as types XV and XVIII, but their distribution in pathological states is not known.

Secondary changes in some laminin chains are seen in various muscular dystrophies, in particular various forms of congenital muscular dystrophy (Muntoni and Voit 2004). Laminin α2, a receptor for α-dystroglycan, shows a secondary reduction in Fukuyama congenital muscular, muscle-eye-brain disease, congenital muscular dystrophy type 1B, linked to chromosome 1q, and MDC1C caused by mutations in the gene for the fukutin-related protein. Interestingly, the allelic limb-girdle dystrophy 2I caused by defects in the same gene often shows normal sarcolemmal labelling of laminin α2 on sections but a marked reduction on immunoblots (Bushby et al 1998). The reason for this is not yet apparent.

Laminin β1 is reduced on the sarcolemma, but not the blood vessels, in some dominant conditions, in particular Bethlem myopathy and autosomal dominant Emery–Dreifuss muscular dystrophy (Fig. 6.20; Merlini et al 1999, Sewry et al 2001a). It has also been reported in other dominant myopathies originally thought to be genetically distinct (Taylor et al 1997b, Li et al 1997) but recent molecular studies have shown that several of these cases are part of the phenotypic spectra of Bethlem myopathy and Emery–Dreifuss muscular dystrophy. Reduced laminin β1 has also been observed in facioscapulohumeral muscular dystrophy and some recessive cases of limb-girdle muscular dystrophy 2I. Reduction of laminin β1 is age dependent and has only been seen in affected adults and adolescents, not young children. A more subtle reduction in laminin β1, with normal localization of laminin α2 and γ1, may only be seen on fibres at the periphery of fascicles, on the sarcolemma adjacent to the perimysium (Fig. 6.21). This is not a consistent feature in all biopsies, and it is not yet clear if it is pathological or if it might relate to the presence of different interacting proteins at this site, such as different integrins or different laminin variants.

The laminin β2 chain shows a secondary reduction in MDC1A when the laminin α2 chain is defective (Cohn et al 1997). This is also apparent in chorionic villus samples from affected fetuses and raises the possibility that the laminin-4 heterotrimer as well as laminin-2 could be abnormal, as both heterotrimers contain the α2 chain (Muntoni et al 2003).

Laminin α5 on the sarcolemma is higher in cases with a primary defect in laminin α2 (MDC1A) and is often higher than normal muscle in Xp21 dystrophies and inflammatory myopathies. As expression of laminin α5 is

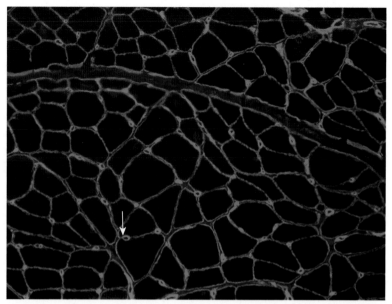

a

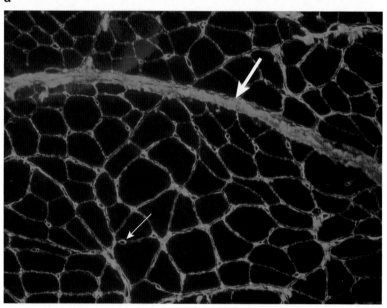

b

FIG. 6.19 *Double labelling of (a) perlecan (red) and (b) collagen VI (green) in the same section. Note perlecan and collagen VI at the sarcolemma and round capillaries (small arrows) but only collagen VI in the perimysium (large arrow).*

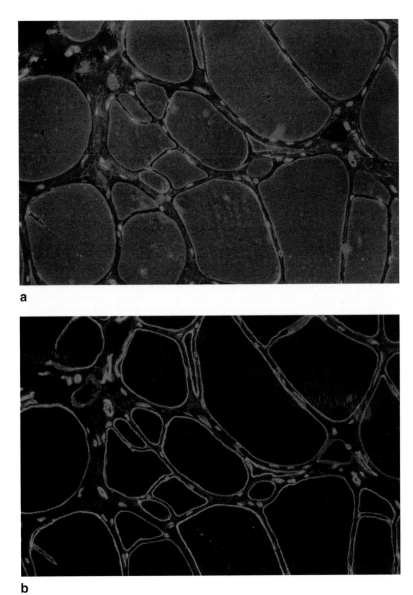

a

b

FIG. 6.20 *Serial areas showing (a) reduced laminin β1 on the sarcolemma but normal labelling of capillaries and (b) normal labelling of laminin γ1.*

developmentally regulated, some of this may relate to regeneration and immaturity and careful correlation with neonatal myosin is needed.

Integrins are a family of transmembrane glycoprotein receptors each with an α and β chain. To date 18 α and 8 β chains have been identified which associate into at least 24 different dimers. Diversity is increased still further by alternative splicing which gives rise to more chains. *Integrin α7β1D* is the major integrin receptor of skeletal muscle and is enriched at myotendinous and neuromuscular junctions (Mayer 2003). It interacts with laminin α2 and α-dystroglycan, and as

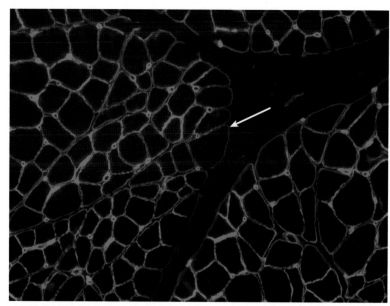

FIG. 6.21 *Reduced labelling of laminin β1 at edge of fascicles only (arrow).*

well as the primary defect in integrin α7 described above, secondary alterations occur when these are affected. Thus a primary or secondary reduction of laminin α2 is accompanied by a reduction in labelling of integrin α7β1D (Hodges et al 1997, Vachon et al 1997, Cohn et al 1999). In contrast, in Duchenne muscular dystrophy labelling of integrin α7β1D is reported to be higher than normal and its up-regulation, like utrophin, has been proposed as a possible therapy (Burkin et al 2001). As the availability of chain specific antibodies increases it is likely that studies of integrin expression will expand.

Major histocompatibility proteins (MHC) are also of diagnostic importance. Normal mature muscle fibres express minimal or no detectable MHC class I or class II or β_2-microglobulin but all are detectable on endothelial cells of blood vessels, and the capillary network is clearly visible (Appleyard et al 1985, McDouall et al 1989). MHC class I and β_2-microglobulin are expressed by regenerating fibres in all disorders, but not fetal fibres (see Fig. 6.3). Careful correlation with the expression of neonatal myosin, to take account of regeneration, is therefore needed when MHC class I is assessed. Over-expression of MHC class I is an important tool for assessing inflammatory myopathies as it is overexpressed on the sarcolemma, and sometimes internally in the fibres, in all forms of inflammatory myopathy (Appleyard et al 1985, McDouall et al 1989, Karpati et al 1988). This is apparent even when pathological features are minimal and there is no inflammatory cellular reaction (Fig. 6.22; Topaloglu et al 1996). Over-expression of MHC class I, however, is not specific to inflammatory myopathies and it is also sometimes seen in Xp21 muscular dystrophies (Appleyard et al 1985) and in limb-girdle muscular dystrophy 2B with a defect in dysferlin (Fanin and Angelini 2002, Confalonieri et al 2003), in which inflammatory cells may be

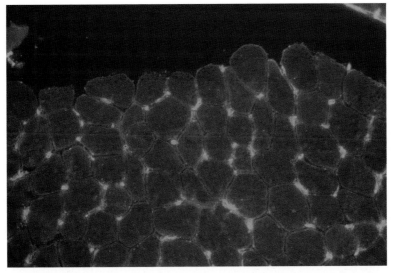

a

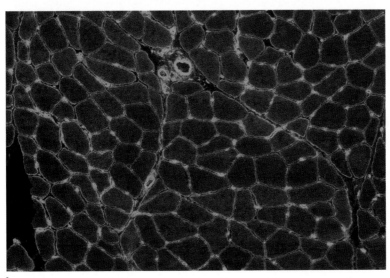

b

FIG. 6.22 *Major histocompatibility complex class I in (a) normal muscle where it only labels blood vessels and (b) a child with dermatomyositis showing sarcolemmal and internal labelling in the absence of marked pathology.*

present. We have also observed low levels of sarcolemmal expression in some neonates and occasionally in a variety of undefined conditions. As cytokines can up-regulate MHC class I these may have a role in this non-specific expression. MHC class II antigens are not usually expressed on fibres in diseased muscle (Appleyard et al 1985, McDouall et al 1989) but they too can be induced by cytokines and it does occur but to a lesser extent than class I expression (Zuk and Fletcher 1988, Bartoccioni et al 1994).

Deposition of ***immunoglobulins and complement*** occurs in necrotic fibres and in inflammatory myopathies, the muscular dystrophies and myasthenia gravis (Engel & Biesecker 1982, Isenberg 1983, Morgan et al 1984). The membrane attack complex complement C5b-9 (MAC) is deposited on fibres in X-linked vacuolar myopathy (Villanova et al 1995) and in endothelial cells it is an early feature of dermatomyositis (Emslie-Smith and Engel 1990). Isenberg (1983) suggested that immunoglobulin deposition can be used to distinguish myopathic from neuropathic disorders. Studies of myasthenia gravis have shown immunoglobulin and complement (C3 and C9) at motor endplates (Engel et al 1977), providing evidence for antibody-dependent complement-mediated injury at the postsynaptic membrane.

A variable number of ***inflammatory cells*** are a feature of myositic conditions and they may also occur in several muscular dystrophies. They are common in Xp21 dystrophies, limb-girdle dystrophy 2B with a defect in dysferlin and facioscapulohumeral muscular dystrophy. Immunohistochemistry can be used to define the cell types using antibodies to specific cell differentiation markers (CD markers). The most useful are those that recognize all T cells, CD8 and CD4 T cells, B cells and macrophages (Arahata and Engel 1984, 1988a, b, Engel and Arahata 1984). The distribution and proportion of T and B cells has been found to differ between perivascular and endomysial areas with T cells, in particular CD8 cytotoxic T cells, being more prevalent than B cells in endomysial areas. The reverse occurs with B cells. In polymyositis and inclusion body myositis, but not dermatomyositis, CD8 T cells and macrophages invade apparently non-necrotic fibres (Arahata and Engel 1988a). In practice, the type of myositis is rarely diagnosed by this type of assessment but it can be useful to study the types of cells present.

Secondary changes in the expression of ***myosin heavy chain isoforms*** are also useful for assessment of biopsies and reflect the plasticity of muscle. Myosin heavy chains are encoded by a multigene family and exist in several isoforms which are regulated in a tissue and developmental specific manner (Nguyen et al 1982, Buckingham 1985, Izumo et al 1986). In addition, hormones such as thyroxine, activity and innervation can influence and induce isoform transitions (see Pette and Vrbova 1992). During development, embryonic and neonatal (fetal) isoforms are replaced by the adult fast and slow forms (Whalen et al 1981, Butler-Browne et al 1990). In normal human muscle the majority of fibres express either a slow or fast myosin heavy chain isoform, corresponding to the histochemical type 1 and 2 fibre types, respectively (Fig. 6.23). The slow isoform is the same as the beta cardiac isoform and in human muscle the fast 2A and 2X heavy chains are expressed. The 2B myosin isoform has not been detected in the human muscles studied. In diseased muscle hybrid fibres expressing more than one isoform are common, and an excessive number can be used as a marker of abnormality (Fig. 6.24). This co-expression accounts for the poor differentiation of fibre types that is sometimes seen in the muscular dystrophies with the myosin ATPase technique at pH 9.4, as the method cannot distinguish between the enzymes associated with each myosin isoform.

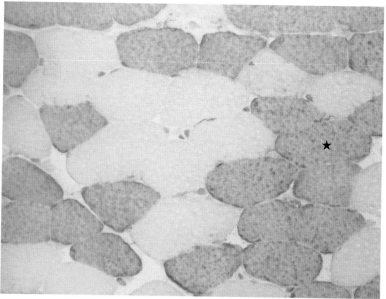

a

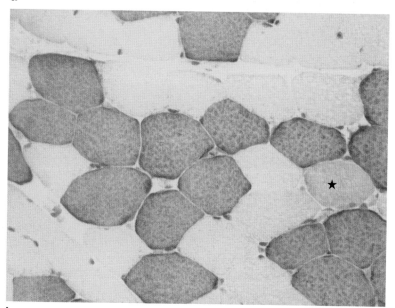

b

FIG. 6.23 *Labelling of (a) fast myosin and (b) slow myosin, showing a normal reciprocal two-fibre pattern. Most fibres show either fast or slow myosin but one fibre with intermediate labelling of slow myosin (*) co-expresses some fast myosin.*

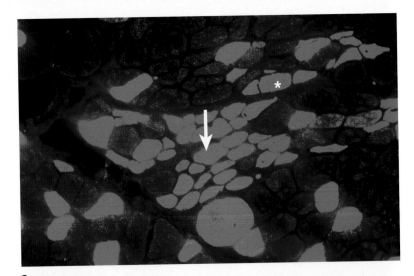

a

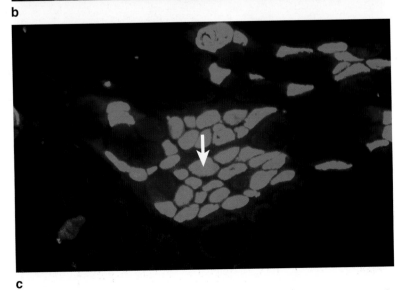

b

c

FIG. 6.24 *Labelling of (a) fast, (b) slow and (c) neonatal myosin in a case of Becker muscular dystrophy showing a group of regenerating fibres that co-express all three isoforms (arrows). Note also the occasional fibre that co-expresses fast and slow myosin (*).*

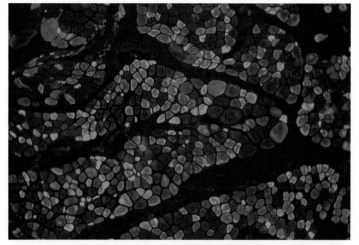

a

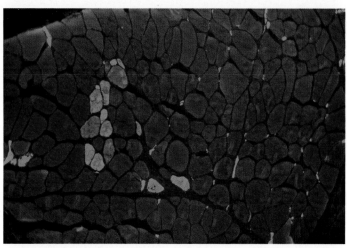

b

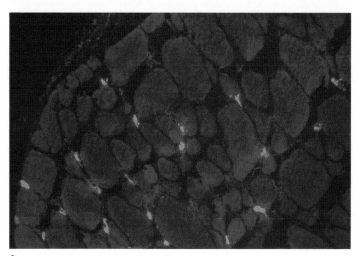

c

FIG. 6.25 *Differing numbers and distribution of fibres with neonatal myosin. Note in (a) the large population of diffusely distributed positive fibres of varying size in a case of Duchenne muscular dystrophy, in (b) a cluster of positive fibres and scattered very small fibres in a case of Becker muscular dystrophy, and in (c) only scattered very small fibres in a case of nemaline myopathy.*

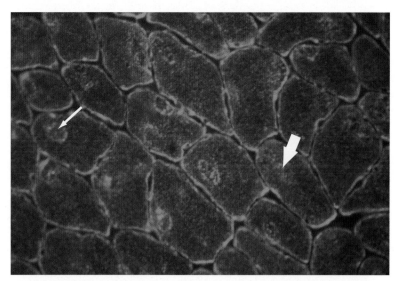

FIG. 6.26 *Labelling of desmin in a case of central core disease. Note the desmin around some cores (small arrow) and accumulation of desmin in others (large arrow).*

Embryonic and neonatal myosin is rarely expressed in adult skeletal muscle and is useful as an indicator of immaturity. Neonatal myosin is present in a large population of fibres at birth and the number declines over the first few months after birth. A few may still be detected up to 1 year of age in samples that show no detectable abnormality. It is not clear if this is part of the normal spectrum of development, or if it might reflect an abnormality, as all the samples studied have been taken because of a suspected neuromuscular problem.

Embryonic and neonatal myosin heavy chains are abundant in regenerating fibres. Neonatal myosin is also expressed in an appreciable proportion of non-basophilic fibres in the muscular dystrophies and is frequently co-expressed with fast and/or slow isoforms in a variety of disorders, particular the muscular dystrophies (Fig. 6.24). Small fibres in several disorders including spinal muscular atrophy, congenital muscular dystrophy and many of the perifascicular fibres in dermatomyositis also express neonatal myosin. Some of these fibres, therefore, may not be atrophic, as is commonly thought, but may be immature fibres. The presence of neonatal myosin in denervated muscle has been discussed previously (see section on developmental regulation). The size and number of fibres with neonatal myosin in pathological muscle varies and, as they often relate to regeneration, they can be a useful reflection of muscle damage. In severe muscular dystrophies, such as the Duchenne form, a large diffuse population of fibres of variable size and showing variable intensity of labelling, is seen (Fig. 6.25a). In Becker muscular dystrophy clusters of positive fibres may occur in some areas with very small positive fibres diffusely distributed elsewhere (Fig. 6.25b). These very small fibres with neonatal myosin are a common feature in congenital myopathies (Fig. 6.25c). They are easily detected using fluorescent

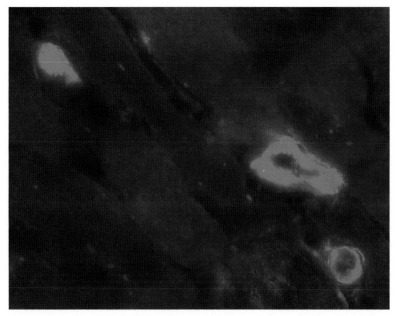

FIG. 6.27 *Accumulation of phosphorylated tau in a case of inclusion body myositis.*

markers but may be less easily seen if peroxidase with haematoxylin is used as the nucleus may nearly fill the whole diameter of these very small fibres.

An *accumulation of a protein* may also be useful to assess. For example high levels of desmin are not only seen in regenerating fibres but also in myofibrillar myopathies or when there are structural defects such as cores or hyaline bodies. Cores with disruption of myofibrils show accumulation of several additional proteins such as γ-filamin, myotilin and ubiquitin (Fig. 6.26; Schröder et al 2003, Sewry et al 2002). In disorders characterized by rimmed vacuoles, such as inclusion body myositis and the various forms of hereditary inclusion body myopathies, several proteins found in the brain of patients with Alzheimer's disease accumulate (Askanas and Engel 2001, Oldfors and Fyhr 2001). These include phosphorylated neurofilaments (tau), ubiquitin, β-amyloid precursor protein, prion protein and presilin (Fig. 6.27).

CHAPTER 7

How to read a biopsy

When the pathologist is asked to evaluate a muscle biopsy, much of the interpretation is based on his or her previous experience and the recognition of similarities between the biopsy and muscle from known diseases. In some instances, such as an advanced dystrophy or a spinal muscular atrophy, the changes may be striking and unequivocal. In others the changes may be more subtle and a systematic approach is required in the evaluation and interpretation. Once the pathology is defined, correlation with clinical features is essential and the pathology must be interpreted in the light of this. A muscle biopsy is only one piece of the jigsaw and has to be considered together with the family history, the clinical history and presentation, and the results of any other investigations. Knowledge of serum creatine kinase levels (CK), for example, is a useful indicator; no case of Duchenne muscular dystrophy has a normal CK, whereas levels are usually normal in congenital myopathies and neurogenic disorders. Knowledge of the distribution of muscle weakness, cardiac involvement, respiratory difficulties, abnormalities in brain magnetic resonance imaging (MRI), contractures and joint laxity are also valuable. Clinical spectra are widening with advancing molecular diagnoses and this has led to a wider appreciation of pathological features seen in muscle biopsies. There is frequently a lack of concordance between the severity of the pathological change and the degree of clinical disability, which places a constraint on the pathologist in giving a prognostication for a particular disease process. It is safer to define the type of pathological change and leave the assessment of clinical severity and prognosis to the clinician. Relating the pathology to the clinical picture is paramount to diagnosis. For example, an overtly dystrophic picture in a 6-month-old infant with hypotonia from birth may confirm the diagnosis of congenital muscular dystrophy, whereas a similar picture in a 14-year-old boy who was ambulant until the age of 10 would be characteristic of Duchenne muscular dystrophy. Similarly, an identical pathological picture is seen in a severely affected infant with Werdnig–Hoffmann disease (spinal muscular atrophy; SMA I) as in a milder case with later onset and better motor function and prognosis (SMA II).

There are considerable advantages if the clinician assessing the patient can also review the biopsy with the pathologist, and then provide a comprehensive diagnosis of the patient. This has always been our policy and gives continuity between the clinical diagnosis and other investigations.

During the preparation of the first edition of this book, a chapter was added, almost as an afterthought, which reflected many discussions and arguments on various aspects of interpretation of muscle pathology. It represented a synthesis of the approach to the interpretation of changes in a biopsy which we thought might be helpful, particularly to the novice in muscle pathology.

While retaining the same basic format as before, we have revised and extended the content of this chapter and added a new section on immunohisto-chemistry. Our aim is to summarize the main pathological features and to give a synopsis of their relevance. Subsequent chapters will give more detail on individual disorders. Part I attempts to place the biopsy into a normal or abnormal category and, if abnormal, to try and characterize the abnormality as myopathic/dystrophic or neurogenic, or some other pathological change. Part II attempts to provide a more specific diagnosis, based on comparison with the classical changes found in individual disorders. The sequence of features is expressed in the form of a flow sheet and is based primarily on the routine histological stains, haema-toxylin and eosin (H&E), and Gomori trichrome, and the histochemical reactions for oxidative enzymes and adenosine triphosphatase (ATPase) and the additional techniques mentioned in Chapter 2. Parts III and IV provide a similar approach to immunohistochemistry and electron microscopy, respectively.

Part I

1 *Histological stains:* With careful overall inspection of the stained sections it should be possible to answer the following:

(a) Is the biopsy normal or abnormal?

Pay particular attention to:
> Overall pattern of the muscle bundles
> Shape and size of fibres
> Position of nuclei
>> peripheral, number that are internal, central
> Presence of focal changes in individual fibres
>> necrosis/overstained hypercontracted fibres
> Distribution of connective and adipose tissue
> Presence/absence of inflammatory cells

(b) Is the abnormality gross and obvious, or minimal?

(c) Is the abnormality diffuse or focal?

2 *Histochemical reactions:* The following additional information should be obtained from the histochemical preparations:

(a) Reduced nicotinamide adenine dinucleotide-tetrazolium reductase (NADH-TR):
Differentiation into fibre types
Selective fibre involvement
Architectural changes within the fibres:
intermyofibrillar network pattern
cores
moth-eaten fibres
coiled or whorled fibres
ring fibres
Aggregation of stain peripherally or internally
Excessive granularity or intensity of reaction product

(b) Cytochrome oxidase (COX); in addition to above:
Absence of stain in some fibres

(c) Succinic dehydrogenase:
Presence of reaction product in fibres devoid of COX
Excess reaction product

(d) ATPase:
Fibre typing
Size, shape, proportion and distribution of respective fibre types
Selective fibre type involvement

(e) Periodic acid-Schiff (PAS):
Distribution of glycogen
Presence of ring or coil fibres
Absence of stain in some fibres ('white' fibres)

(f) Oil red O (ORO):
Distribution of lipid droplets
Excess lipid within fibres
Size of lipid droplets
Excess lipid outside the fibres
Artefact due to surface spreading of lipid droplets

(g) Enzymatic activity (all-or-none reaction)
Deficiency of:
Phosphorylase
Phosphofructokinase
Adenylate deaminase

(h) Enzyme activity:
Acid phosphatase associated with vacuoles
Alkaline phosphatase in perimysium

Borderline changes: One common difficulty is assessing the significance of pathological changes in borderline cases. Thus one may attach different significance to the presence of one or two internal nuclei in occasional fibres, one or two internal nuclei in many fibres, many internal nuclei in occasional fibres and many internal nuclei in many fibres.

The following 'flow sheet' is an attempt to provide a systematic interpretation of individual changes in the course of analysing a muscle biopsy.

H&E, Gomori trichrome

Feature	Implication
Fibre size	
Changes in fibre size	Biopsy is abnormal
Changes random and diffuse	Myopathy/dystrophy
Two distinct populations of small and large fibres	More characteristic of denervation or of type specific atrophy or a congenital myopathy
Presence of small angulated fibres	Suggests denervation
Presence of small group atrophy	Denervation
Presence of large group atrophy	Denervation
Presence of perifascicular atrophy	Dermatomyositis
Nuclei	
Internal nuclei in more than:	
3% of the fibres	Mild non-specific abnormality in adults, may be significant in children
10% of the fibres	Suggests myopathy but is seen occasionally in chronic neuropathy
30% of the fibres	Suggests a chronic dystrophy
60% of the fibres	Think of myotonic dystrophy
Centrally-placed	Think of myotubular myopathy or congenital myotonic dystrophy or central core disease
Pyknotic nuclear clumps	Indicates fibre atrophy, more common in denervation but also consider myotonic dystrophy and other chronic dystrophies
Fibres	
Presence of necrotic fibres	More common in dystrophies and some myopathies, rare in congenital myopathies, occasionally seen in denervation such as SMA III

H&E, Gomori trichrome (Continued)

Feature	Implication
Clusters of necrotic fibres	Dystrophy
Isolated necrotic fibres	Metabolic myopathy
Fibre splitting	Common in dystrophies, particularly limb-girdle forms
Basophilic fibres	If present to any degree suggests a myopathy. If in small groups think of a dystrophy
Phagocytosis	Suggests a dystrophy, but may be seen in chronic neuropathies
Cellular reactions	
Presence of inflammatory cells	Suggests a myopathy; when profuse think of inflammatory myopathies, facioscapulohumeral dystrophy and dysferlinopathy. Can occur in Duchenne dystrophy. Distinguish normal neurovascular bundle and regeneration from inflammatory response
Fibrosis	
Confined to perimysium	Abnormal if abundant in an adult
Increased in endomysium	Abnormal
Mild	Non-specific but more common in myopathies; can occur in SMA III
Moderate	Suggests a dystrophy; can also occur in some congenital myopathies
Severe	Think of a dystrophy
Other structures	
Are the vessels abnormal in size and number?	Significance is the same as in routine pathology (i.e. periarteritis etc.); also think of inflammatory myopathies
Are the nerves abnormal?	Lack of trichrome staining may indicate a myelination problem; changes of fibrosis
Are muscle spindles abnormal?	Requires specialist knowledge
Presence of rods	Suggests nemaline myopathy; may also occur in core myopathies
Presence of vacuoles	Excessive in some glycogenoses; May have associated basophilia or red material with the trichrome stain in inclusion body myositis/myopathies; Lined by sarcolemmal proteins in some vacuolar myopathies; Invaginations of sarcolemma may appear as vacuoles; Amyloid may be helpful

NADH-TR reaction

Feature	Implication
Presence of target fibres	Suggests reinnervation and thus indirectly, denervation
Presence of targetoid fibres	A less specific abnormality seen in both myopathies and denervation
Presence of central cores or peripheral cores	When numerous, suggests central core disease. Isolated cores difficult to distinguish from targetoid fibres
Presence of minicores	Consider core myopathies; may occur in different clinical syndromes (see Chs 12 and 15)
Large 'wiped out' areas devoid of stain	Think of desmin-related myopathy
Uneven distribution of stain	May relate to uneven distribution of mitochondria and/or myofibrillar disruption
Presence of moth-eaten and whorled fibres	Non-specific abnormality if a minor change. When numerous suggests a myopathy. When profuse consider a chronic dystrophy
Lobulated fibres	Non-specific but common in limb-girdle 2A (calpainopathy); rare in children
Presence of dark-centred fibres	Indicates clusters of mitochondria; seen in myotubular myopathy
Presence of tubular aggregates	Seen in a variety of disorders but when profuse consider the periodic paralyses
Presence of small **dark** angulated fibres	Suggests denervation but are also seen in polymyositis, facioscapulohumeral dystrophy and oculopharyngeal dystrophy and they may contain neonatal myosin

ATPase reaction, pH 9.4

Feature	Implication
Fibre type pattern indistinct	Frequent in Duchenne dystrophy; also seen in central core disease
Fibre type predominance	Type 1 fibre predominance is common in most myopathies
Atrophy	Both types small suggests denervation
Type 1 atrophy	Seen in myotonic dystrophy, and several congenital myopathies, may be smaller in laminopathies
Type 2 atrophy	Non-specific and may reflect disuse of the muscle. May be induced by corticosteroid therapy
Largest fibres of one type	In motor neurone disease (amyotrophic lateral sclerosis) largest fibres are usually type 2; in chronic neuropathy type 1; in SMA type 1
Fibre type grouping	Pathognomonic of reinnervation and thus denervation. Must be distinguished from type predominance
Ring fibres present in any of the stains (including PAS)	When numerous, suggests a chronic myopathy such as limb girdle dystrophy or myotonic dystrophy

Other stains

Acid phosphatase present in vacuoles	Acid maltase deficiency
Absence of **phosphorylase**	Type V glycogenosis (McArdle's disease)

Part II

In completing Part I, some idea will have been obtained as to whether an abnormal biopsy is due to a myopathic process or secondary to denervation. A few biopsies will not fit clearly into either category. Part II is concerned with placing the biopsy into a more specific diagnostic category. The biopsies will be considered under the headings: neurogenic, myopathic and others, and those *additional* changes that seem characteristic of the particular disease will be listed.

1 *Neurogenic biopsies*

    (a) Spinal muscular atrophy:
        Severe infantile spinal muscular atrophy
        (Werdnig–Hoffmann disease/SMA I)
        Intermediate severity spinal muscular atrophy

(late infantile/juvenile/SMA II)
　　large group atrophy
　　rounded atrophic fibres of both types
　　hypertrophied fibres mostly type 1 (ATPase)
Mild spinal muscular atrophy (Kugelberg-Welander disease/SMA III)
　　hypertrophic fibres often type 2
　　type grouping
　　structural changes and internal nuclei in large fibres
　　mild 'myopathic' changes, including fibrosis

(b) Motor neurone disease:
　　Type 2 fibre hypertrophy
　　Type 2 fibre predominance
　　(Type 2 fibre atrophy if upper motor neurone involvement severe)

(c) Chronic neuropathy:
　　Type 1 fibre hypertrophy
　　Type 1 fibre predominance
　　'Myopathic' changes

(d) Simple neuropathy:
　　No specific changes apart from the general ones of denervation

2 Myopathic biopsies

(a) Duchenne dystrophy:
　　Wide variation in fibre size
　　Most fibres rounded
　　Necrotic fibres
　　Phagocytosis
　　Endomysial fibrosis
　　Basophilic fibres, often in clusters
　　Hypercontracted fibres
　　Internal nuclei increased but not a marked feature
　　Mild aggregation of oxidative enzyme stains
　　Fibre typing indistinct
　　Split fibres
　　Whorled fibres

(b) Becker dystrophy:
　　Increased variability in fibre size
　　Split fibres
　　Whorled fibres
　　Hypercontracted fibres
　　Endomysial fibrosis
　　Groups of small fibres
　　Necrosis and phagocytosis sometimes less than Duchenne
　　Basophilic fibres

(c) Limb-girdle dystrophy:
　　Good fibre type differentiation

Extensive fibre splitting
Excessive internal nuclei
Variable amount of fibrosis
Sometimes less basophilia and phagocytosis than Duchenne
Moth-eaten fibres common
Ring and coil fibres common
Lobulated fibres in adult cases

(d) Facioscapulohumeral dystrophy:
Large fibres often type 2
Groups of small fibres
Endomysial fibrosis variable
Inflammatory response common
Small angulated fibres (may be the only abnormality)
Moth-eaten and whorled fibres
Changes often focal and inconspicuous
Occasionally extensive pathological change

(e) Congenital muscular dystrophy:
Forms with severe disability:
  variation in fibre size
  extensive endomysial fibrosis
  extensive adipose tissue
  necrosis but may not be apparent
  type 1 predominance
Forms with mild disability:
  variation in fibre size, may be mild
  endomysial fibrosis and adipose tissue, may be mild
  necrosis may be present
Immunohistochemistry essential (see below)

(f) Myotonic dystrophy:
Type 1 fibre atrophy
Excessive internal nuclei, central in congenital cases
Ring fibres; sarcoplasmic masses
Moth-eaten fibres

(g) Oculopharyngeal dystrophy:
Many rimmed vacuoles
Excessive internal nuclei

(h) Inflammatory myopathies:
Hypertrophied fibres rare
Perifascicular atrophy in dermatomyositis
Necrosis
Phagocytosis
Moth-eaten whorled fibres
'Ghost fibres'
Inflammatory cells (not universal)
Reduced number of capillaries (dermatomyositis)

Rimmed vacuoles in inclusion body myositis
Alkaline phosphatase in perimysium
Fibres devoid of cytochrome oxidase in inclusion body myositis (but
may relate to ageing)
Immunohistochemistry essential (see below)

3 Other biopsies

(a) Myasthenia gravis:
Focal type 2 fibre atrophy
Lymphorrhages

(b) Periodic paralyses:
Tubular aggregates
Vacuoles

(c) Mitochondrial myopathy:
'Ragged-red' or granular fibres in Kearns–Sayre syndrome
Fibres devoid of cytochrome oxidase activity

(d) Central core disease, nemaline myopathy, reducing body myopathy:
Distinctive pathological change implied in the name of the disease
Selective type 1 fibre involvement
Type 1 fibre atrophy
Type 1 fibre predominance or uniformity
Internal nuclei, may be central
Fibrosis may be present
Extensive adinose tissue may be present

(e) Myotubular myopathy:
Diagnose only if:
Prominent single central nuclei in transverse section (may only affect
10–20% of fibres owing to spacing of nuclei). Exclude congenital
myotonic dystrophy
Dark central aggregation of stain with NADH-TR
Central 'hole' with ATPase

(f) Congenital fibre type disproportion:
Childhood biopsy in which type 1 fibres are smaller than type 2 (which
may be hypertrophic; also consider other congenital myopathies)

(g) Type V glycogenosis (McArdle's disease)
Negative histochemical reaction for phosphorylase

Part III

Immunohistochemistry

Assessment of a biopsy using immunohistochemical techniques is now essential.
Several gene defects result in a change in the respective protein, particularly in
the recessive muscular dystrophies. Secondary alterations can also be useful

indicators. This section summarizes the localization in normal muscle of proteins relevant to diagnosis and the significance of their immunolabelling in neuromuscular disorders using a panel of commercially available antibodies.

Key

DMD = Duchenne muscular dystrophy
BMD = Becker muscular dystrophy
LGMD = limb-girdle muscular dystrophy
CMD = congenital muscular dystrophy

Protein	Interpretation
β-Spectrin	
Uniform sarcolemmal labelling on all fibres	Normal, indicates good preservation of plasma membrane
Reduced on small fibres	If fibres also express fetal myosin indicates regenerating fibres
Reduced on many fibres in neonates	May reflect immaturity
Absence from whole or part of fibre	Necrotic fibre
Internal labelling	May occur on vacuoles, invaginations of sarcolemma and splits
Dystrophin	
Uniform on sarcolemma of all fibres with all antibodies	Normal
Absent from fibres without β-spectrin	Necrotic fibres
Absent from most fibres with all antibodies	DMD
Present only on small clusters or a few isolated fibres	DMD with revertant fibres
Very weak labelling on most fibres	DMD expressing minor transcripts of dystrophin
Uneven/patchy labelling on most fibres	BMD
Reduced intensity on most fibres	BMD
Intensity on all fibres similar to controls	BMD not excluded
Labelling with antibodies to C-terminal domain but other domains absent	Possibly BMD with a deletion affecting the exons not detected (clinical severity cannot be predicted)

Protein	Interpretation
Dystrophin (cont'd)	
Mosaic pattern of positive/negative fibres and areas with reduced labelling in a female	Manifesting DMD carrier
Reduced labelling with an absence of all sarcoglycans	Consider β-sarcoglycan gene defect
Internal labelling	May occur on vacuoles, invaginations of sarcolemma, splits and cytoplasmic bodies
Sarcoglycans (α, β, γ, δ)	
Uniform on sarcolemma with all antibodies	Normal
All reduced	DMD/BMD or LGMD
Absence of only one with reduction of the others	LGMD with a mutation in the gene for the absent protein
Absence of all	Possibly β-sarcoglycan gene mutation
Internal labelling	May occur on vacuoles, invaginations of sarcolemma and splits
β-Dystroglycan	
Uniform on sarcolemma of all fibres	Normal
Reduced on most fibres	DMD/BMD
α-Dystroglycan glycosylated epitope (controls essential)	
Uniform on sarcolemma of all fibres	Normal
Reduction on most fibres	DMD, feature of several forms of CMD (equivocal results in some cases)
Utrophin	
Only blood vessels, nerves and neuromuscular junctions labelled	Normal
Sarcolemma of small fibres with fetal myosin	Regenerating fibres
Sarcolemmal labelling of many mature fibres	DMD, BMD or myositis; May occur in some LGMDs

Protein	Interpretation
Laminin	
Laminin α2 (merosin)	
Uniform on sarcolemma of all fibres. Blood vessels not labelled. Nerves labelled	Normal
Uniform on fibres with no dystrophin	Necrotic fibre
Absence from sarcolemma and nerves	Primary 'merosin' deficient CMD
Traces on a few fibres	Usually primary 'merosin' deficient CMD
Reduced expression on several fibres	Primary or secondary defect of 'merosin'
Internal labelling	May occur on vacuoles, invaginations of sarcolemma and splits
Laminin α5	
Traces on sarcolemma High expression on blood vessels	Normal
High expression on fibres with fetal myosin	Regenerating fibres
High expression on mature fibres	Over-expression (seen in 'merosin' deficient CMD and DMD)
Laminin β1	
Uniform on sarcolemma and same intensity as blood vessels	Normal
Reduced sarcolemma labelling compared with blood vessels	Seen in some LGMD2I cases and some dominant conditions (e.g. Bethlem myopathy and dominant Emery–Dreifuss muscular dystrophy)
Internal labelling	May occur on vacuoles, invaginations of sarcolemma and splits
Laminin γ1	
Uniform on sarcolemma and same intensity as blood vessels	Normal
Internal labelling	May occur on vacuoles, invaginations of sarcolemma and splits

Protein	Interpretation
Myosin heavy chains	
Fetal/neonatal myosin	
All fibres unlabelled	Normal mature muscle
Several positive fibres in a patient under 1 year (whole fibre labelled)	Immaturity in a neonate
Many positive fibres of varying size and intensity	Dystrophic muscle
Clusters of positive fibres in some areas with very small ones elsewhere	Consider BMD
Only very small positive fibres	Mild damage in congenital myopathies
Fast and slow myosin heavy chains	
Diffuse 2-fibre checkerboard pattern	Normal; most fibres with fast or slow myosin only
Fibre type grouping	Reinnervation following denervation
Predominance of slow myosin	Common myopathic feature
Uniformity of slow myosin	Congenital myopathy e.g. central core disease also common in Duchenne muscular dystrophy
Co-expression of more than one isoform in same fibre	Fibre type conversion or regeneration or a time point during maturation
Calpain-3	
	*Antibodies only suitable for immunoblotting; absent or reduced when calpain gene mutated, secondary reduction may occur when dysferlin gene mutated, reduced if muscle degraded
Dysferlin	
Uniform sarcolemmal labelling	Normal
Absence on sections	May indicate mutation. Reduction better assessed on immunoblots. Secondary changes in amount can occur

*this refers to the antibody marketed by Novocastra, other commercial antibodies may be suitable for sections but have not been assessed

Protein	Interpretation
nNOS	
Uniform sarcolemmal labelling Internal labelling may be present	Normal
Absent from sarcolemma	DMD or BMD with mutation in rod domain 'hot-spot'
Blood vessels labelled	
Caveolin-3	
Uniform sarcolemmal labelling of all fibres and blood vessels	Normal
Absence or reduction	LGMD1C Rippling muscle disease HyperCKaemia
Collagen VI	
Uniform sarcolemmal labelling, labelling of endomysial and perimysial tissue and blood vessels	Normal (most cases of Bethlem myopathy look normal; Ullrich CMD not excluded)
Absent	Ullrich CMD
Reduced, particularly at sarcolemma	Possibly Ullrich CMD
MHC class I	
Sarcolemma negative, blood vessels labelled	Normal
Sarcolemma of all/most fibres labelled (some labelling may also be internal)	Myositis or DMD or dysferlinopathy (distinguish by clinical history)
Fibres with fetal myosin	Regenerating fibres
Membrane attack complex (C5–9)	
No labelling of fibres or blood vessels	Normal
Labelling of necrotic fibres	Non-specific abnormality
Labelling of capillaries	Dermatomyositis
Emerin	
All nuclei labelled	Normal
All nuclei negative	X-linked Emery–Dreifuss

Protein	Interpretation
Nuclear lamins	
All nuclei labelled	Normal; mutation in gene for lamin A/C not excluded
Desmin	
Accumulation in small fibres with neonatal myosin	Regenerating fibres
Accumulation in fibres without neonatal myosin	Abnormality seen in desmin-related disorders and rare cases of laminopathies; may accumulate in or line cores
The following proteins can be assessed in skin biopsies and can be useful	
Laminin α2	
Present at dermal/epidermal junction, on sebaceous glands, and nerves; blood vessels not labelled	Normal
Absent from dermal/epidermal junction and nerves	Primary 'merosin' deficient CMD
Reduced at dermal/epidermal junction; nerves labelled	May be secondary 'merosin' deficiency
Laminin α5 and γ1	
At dermal/epidermal junction, on sebaceous glands, and nerves; blood vessels labelled	Normal
Laminin β1	
At dermal/epidermal junction, on sebaceous glands, and nerves; blood vessels labelled	Normal
Reduced at dermal/epidermal junction; nerves and blood vessels labelled	Primary or secondary 'merosin' deficiency
Collagen VI	
Present in dermis and round blood vessels and nerves	Normal, defect in collagen VI genes not excluded
Absent	Consider Ullrich CMD
Emerin	
All nuclei labelled	Normal
Absence from all nuclei	X-linked Emery–Dreifuss muscular dystrophy
Areas of positive and negative nuclei	Carrier of X-linked Emery–Dreifuss if patient female

Analysis of laminin α2, collagen VI and emerin in chorionic villus samples can also be useful in prenatal diagnosis

Part IV

Electron microscopy

The ultrastructural changes encountered in neuromuscular disorders are often non-specific, as has been emphasized in Chapter 5. This, however, does not detract from the potential role that electron microscopy has to play. As a sole diagnostic technique, its use is limited to situations where a disease is characterized by an ultrastructural feature, such as rods in nemaline myopathy, or where a feature can only be seen at the ultrastructural level, such as the filamentous inclusions in inclusion body myositis. It is also of value in helping to decide whether a biopsy is normal or abnormal and in clarifying features seen at the light microscopical level.

As with light microscopy, the evaluation of a muscle biopsy by the electron microscopist is largely based on experience but this section is designed to help the newcomer to the field. It aims to provide a guide to the examination of a biopsy that will contribute more than an aesthetic collection of electron micrographs.

Selection of biopsy for electron microscopy

Electron microscopy is a time-consuming technique in both the preparation of sections and their examination, and it is usually necessary to select the biopsies for ultrastructural examination. A sample from all biopsies, however, should be fixed and embedded for electron microscopy in case they are required. The selection of biopsies should be based on the light microscopical features and an affirmative answer to the following questions:

Light microscopy	Additional information from electron microscopy
Does the biopsy appear normal?	Ultrastructural features may be abnormal
Are ragged red fibres present?	Mitochondrial abnormalities may be present
Does Gomori trichrome stain show red inclusions?	Rods, cytoplasmic bodies, sarcoplasmic bodies or tubular aggregates may be present
Does Gomori trichrome stain show rimmed vacuoles?	Suggests presence of membranous whorls; filamentous inclusions of inclusion body myositis may be present
Do NADH-TR preparations show loss of stain in some fibres?	Cores or disruption of myofibrils may be present
Do NADH-TR preparations show fibres with excess stain?	Mitochondria may be abnormal

Light microscopy	Additional information from electron microscopy
Is PAS stain excessive?	Excess glycogen may be present
Do fibres show excess ORO stain?	Lipid storage; mitochondria may be abnormal
Are there pale or dark staining areas in some fibres with H&E or Gomori trichrome?	Accumulation of myofibrillar material may be present (e.g. actin or desmin)
Are there any unusual inclusions or features that cannot be interpreted?	Electron microscopy may reveal their nature

Semi-thin sections

The area examined in an ultrathin section is small and often contains only a few fibres. A bigger sampling area can be examined in a semi-thin, 0.5–1 μm section. These are stained with toluidine blue and observed with a ×60 or ×100 oil immersion lens. The detail seen in these sections is very good and it is possible to identify many features, including individual myofibrillar bundles, the position of mitochondria and fat, chromatin distribution and the presence of unusual structures. These sections give a good overall impression of the biopsy, particularly with regard to the myofibrils, and they enable selection of an interesting area to be made (see Fig. 1.11). Ultrastructural studies should therefore always be preceded by examination of semi-thin sections. These may even produce the required answer to a problem without the need for detailed electron microscopy studies.

Sampling area

The number of blocks chosen for examination depends on the nature of the disorder. In a situation where a population of fibres contains an unusual structure, one block may provide the answer required. In another situation where the pathological changes are minimal, it may be necessary to look at several blocks; in these biopsies it is particularly important to remember the limitations of sampling.

Ultrastructural changes

Although the abnormalities observed in a biopsy are usually non-specific, certain patterns of change and the presence of particular structures may limit the number of possible conditions and contribute to the final diagnosis. The following flow sheet lists the main features to be assessed when examining a biopsy, and their possible implications.

Feature observed	Implications
Sarcolemma	
Is it folded?	Atrophic fibres; contraction artefact
Redundant basal lamina	Atrophic fibre
Loss of plasma membrane	Necrotic fibre
Myofibrils	
Focal loss in isolated fibre	May occur in normal muscle
Extensive loss in several fibres	Abnormal biopsy
Mild loss in some fibres	Difficult to assess, look for other abnormalities
Hypercontraction	Common in dystrophies, sometimes seen in chronic neurogenic disorders; can be artefactual
Z and I band loss	Common in myopathies
Misalignment of striations	May be artefact but may relate to a core; look for presence of mitochondria
Accumulation of actin filaments	Nemaline myopathy with mutation in *ACTA1* gene
Cores	Look for structured and unstructured forms
Filamentous bodies	Occasionally seen in normal muscle. If frequent, abnormal
Concentric laminated whorls	Rare; not seen in normal muscle
Z line streaming and irregularities	Non-specific abnormality, assess number of fibres affected and number of affected areas per fibre; common abnormality in core myopathies and nemaline myopathy
Rods	Numerous in nemaline myopathies. Can occur in central core disease. Found in normal myotendinous junctions; occasional cores may occur in other disorders
Cytoplasmic bodies	Rare; usually isolated; numerous in cytoplasmic body myopathy and common in inclusion body myositis
Nuclei	
Irregular shape	Shape can be affected by contraction

Feature observed	Implications
Nuclei (cont'd)	
Chromatin distribution	Diseased muscle often shows active nuclei with prominent nucleoli. Pyknotic nuclei common in denervation and chronic degenerative disorders
Clumped chromatin not attached to nuclear membrane	Apoptotic nuclei; can occur in Emery–Dreifuss muscular dystrophies
Dense encircling membrane	Only seen in Marinesco–Sjögren syndrome
Intranuclear rods	Seen in nemaline myopathy with a mutation in *ACTA1* gene
Filamentous inclusions	Actin-like filaments found in some myositic conditions; 8.5 nm filaments in oculopharyngeal dystrophy exclusively in nuclei; 16–18 nm filaments in inclusion body myositis in nuclei and cytoplasm
Mitochondria	
Small, peripheral aggregates of normal mitochondria	May occur in normal muscle
Large, peripheral aggregates of normal mitochondria	Found in lobulated fibres; occasional fibres in several disorders
Swollen and disrupted	If universal and sarcoplasmic reticulum (SR) also affected, fixation artefact
Abnormal structure	Isolated fibres with abnormal mitochondria sometimes seen in several disorders. If many fibres affected, suggests metabolic myopathy
Membrane systems	
Swollen SR	Common in dystrophies. If mitochondria also very swollen, may be due to fixation artefact
Duplicated triads	Damaged fibre
Honeycomb structures	Found in active areas of degeneration and regeneration
Tubular aggregates	Occasionally seen in isolated fibres, also in normal muscle. A feature of periodic paralysis

Feature observed	Implications
Deposits and particles	
Glycogen	Excessive in glycogen storage disease; may be membrane bound. Accumulates in areas with myofibrillar loss
Lipid	Droplets usually appear as white areas. Droplets near mitochondria in normal muscle; excessive in carnitine deficiency myopathy
Lipofuscin	Common in perinuclear regions; found in normal muscle; more abundant in adults; increased in diseased muscle
Lipopigment	Small, granular bodies in vitamin E deficiency
Other unusual features	
Zebra bodies	May occur in normal myotendinous junctions; characteristic of zebra body myopathy
Fingerprint bodies	Isolated ones found in several disorders; common in fingerprint myopathy
Curvilinear bodies	Found in muscle in Batten's disease and patients treated with chloroquine
Reducing bodies	Can be seen at the light level with menadione α-glycerophosphate; so far restricted to a specific congenital myopathy
Concentric laminated whorls	Occasional, non-specific feature
Myeloid/membranous whorls	Stain red with Gomori trichrome; non-specific abnormality; feature of rimmed vacuoles in inclusion body myositis/myopathy
Autophagic vacuoles	Common in several disorders where myofibre breakdown occurs
Vacuoles lined with sarcolemmal proteins and containing dense granular material	X-linked vacuolar myopathies
Dense tubules	A stacked variety has been seen in myotubular myopathy; other types occasionally seen in several disorders
Granular material with ATPase activity but lacking oxidative enzymes and visible with Gomori trichrome	Hyaline body myopathy (mutation in slow myosin *MYH7* gene)

Feature observed	Implications
Other unusual features (cont'd)	
Dense granulofilamentous material and desmin accumulation	Desmin-related myopathy (possible mutation in desmin or αB-crystallin gene)
Focal peripheral areas with fragments of myofibrillar material that are devoid of ATPase activity but contain desmin	Cap disease
Capillaries	
Tubular reticular inclusions in endothelial cells	Dermatomyositis, occasionally seen in systemic lupus erythematosus
Thick basal lamina	Diabetes mellitus

SECTION 2

Pathological muscle: individual diseases

CHAPTER 8

Classification of neuromuscular disorders

The first section of this book covered techniques and general aspects of interpretation of pathological changes. We now turn our attention to specific disorders and the variable role muscle biopsy has in them. In some conditions, such as spinal muscular atrophy, myotonic dystrophy and facioscapulohumeral muscular dystrophy molecular analysis is very reliable and a muscle biopsy has very little to contribute from a diagnostic point of view. In other disorders, such as myasthenia gravis, diagnosis is based on clinical and electrodiagnostic evaluation. In others, however, such as the various muscular dystrophies and the congenital myopathies, there are clinical similarities and a biopsy makes an important contribution to providing a definitive diagnosis.

In addition to the well-defined pathological changes that occur in various neuromuscular disorders, skeletal muscle may also be directly or indirectly involved in many acute or chronic diseases. Biopsy may reveal striking and unexpected changes in situations where involvement of muscle is not clinically apparent. It is also possible that even such common symptoms as the aches and pains which accompany so many illnesses, or the weakness following periods of bedrest, may be associated with marked biochemical, histochemical or structural changes within the muscle.

In this section we shall try to cover systematically the pathological changes in the known inherited and acquired neuromuscular disorders. We also include in this edition a chapter on the pathological effects of drugs and various toxins as there is a growing awareness of this, and the pathologist needs to bear in mind possible effects of both prescribed drugs and abuse of various substances.

The molecular revolution has led to the identification of many gene defects and the protein products responsible for neuromuscular disorders (Dalkilic and Kunkel 2003). Proteins located in every part of a muscle fibre have been found, the extracellular matrix, the plasma membrane, the cytoskeleton, the Golgi, the internal membrane systems, nuclei, myofibrils, neuromuscular junction and the cytosol (summarized in Figs 8.1–8.3). The discovery, over 15 years ago, that mutations in the gene encoding dystrophin are responsible for Duchenne and Becker

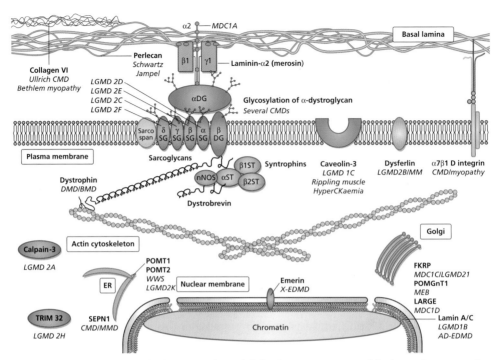

FIG. 8.1 *Diagram showing the large number of defective genes responsible for various muscular dystrophies and the localization of their proteins. (See p. xi for abbreviations.)*

muscular dystrophy paved the way for recognizing the role of plasma membrane proteins and led to the identification of defective interacting proteins, such as the sarcoglycans and laminin α2, that cause other muscular dystrophies. Several muscular dystrophies encompassing some limb-girdle muscular dystrophies and congenital muscular dystrophies could be explained on the basis of this complex of interacting sarcolemmal proteins linking the extracellular matrix to the cytoskeleton, the dystrophin-associated protein complex (Fig. 8.1). This concept has had to be broadened with the discovery that proteins not in this complex cause other muscular dystrophies. For example various forms of limb-girdle dystrophies are caused by defects in other membrane proteins such as dysferlin and caveolin-3, in the myofibrillar protein telethonin, and in the enzyme calpain-3, and mutations in the nuclear membrane proteins emerin and lamin A/C are responsible for Emery–Dreifuss forms of muscular dystrophy. It is also now recognized that abnormal post-translational modification of proteins, in particular glycosylation, can result in various forms of congenital muscular dystrophy, many of which also have brain involvement because of the essential role of this process in the brain as well as muscle. The number of genes and their protein products involved in glycosylation pathways that are responsible for a neuromuscular disorder is rapidly growing (Fig. 8.1).

Defects in various myofibrillar proteins have been identified in a number of early and late onset disorders with a wide spectrum of phenotypes (Fig. 8.2).

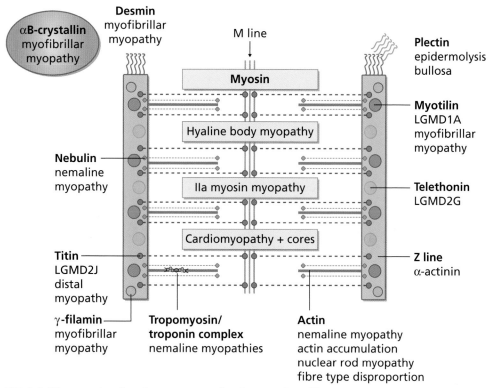

FIG. 8.2 *Diagram showing the genes encoding intermediate filaments and sarcomeric proteins that are defective in myofibrillar myopathies (interactions not shown).*

Other components of the sarcomere and their interacting proteins are good candidates for further investigations. With the clinical similarities in these disorders, pathological assessment of muscle with a variety of techniques has an important role.

Diagnosis of many of the ion channel disorders, and neuromuscular junction and axonal defects (Fig. 8.3) relies on clinical evaluation and electrophysiology, and pathological studies of muscle rarely contribute additional diagnostic information. A notable exception to this is defects associated with the calcium-release channel, the ryanodine receptor of the sarcoplasmic reticulum, which is defective in central core disease. Pathology has a major role in studies of this and other congenital myopathies and a wide spectrum of pathological changes are now known to be associated with them. A biopsy, however, will often be taken before a final diagnosis has been arrived at. Some metabolic disorders are also not easily identified by pathological studies but as some can be, such as those with structurally abnormal mitochondria or lipid or glycogen storage, pathological examination may be pursued.

The wide spectrum of defective proteins that have been identified and the interactions between them has challenged the traditional classification of neuromuscular disorders based on clinical features. Diseases are often now referred

MUSCLE BIOPSY

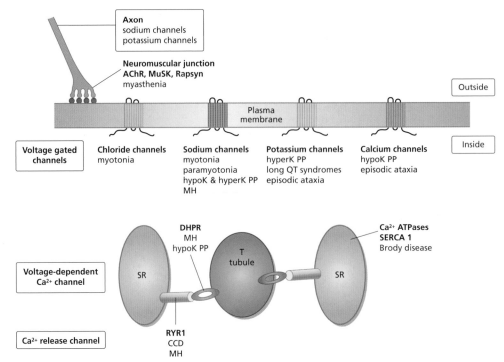

FIG. 8.3 *Diagram showing the defective genes responsible for ion channel disorders. (See p. xi for abbreviations.)*

to on the basis of the protein defect, such as dystrophinopathy, sarcoglycanopathy and actinopathy, and according to the pathogenic mechanisms. The traditional boundaries of a muscular dystrophy, myopathy and neuropathy have become ill-defined by the molecular developments in the field. In this book, however, we have still adhered to the traditional clinical classification. Clinical symptoms lead to the referral of a patient and these are assessed before a gene or protein defect has been identified. We therefore feel it is still relevant to the pathologist to adhere to a classification based on clinical features. Undoubtedly, a combination of a detailed clinical and family history, together with the pathological features, can lead to identification of the causative gene defect but molecular analysis is not usually the starting point.

CHAPTER 9

Neurogenic disorders

There are a large number of inherited and acquired clinical disorders caused by a defect in upper or lower motor neurones or the peripheral nerve. These include amyotrophic lateral sclerosis (ALS; upper and lower motor neurones), hereditary motor and sensory neuropathies (HMSN; motor and sensory neurones and peripheral nerves), the spinal muscular atrophies (SMA; lower motor neurones) and inflammatory peripheral neuropathies. Several causative genes have been identified and inheritance may be dominant or recessive. About 10% of cases of ALS (motor neurone disease) are familial with autosomal dominant inheritance. In a proportion of these (approximately 15–20%) there is a mutation in the Cu/Zn superoxide dismutase (*SOD-1*) gene.

The hereditary peripheral neuropathies are a heterogeneous group of disorders encompassing several clinical syndromes with dominant or recessive inheritance. Many of these still carry the eponymous titles of the clinician who described them (e.g. Charcot–Marie–Tooth) but the advent of molecular genetics has led to reclassification and the identification of several different inherited types. A useful website for these advances is *http://molgen-www.uia.ac.be/cmtmutations/*. Detailed clinical and electrophysiological studies and studies of sural nerve biopsies are required to direct molecular analysis and muscle biopsies usually contribute very little to this. The study of sural nerves is a specialized field beyond the scope of this book and details can be found in a variety of text books (e.g. Midroni and Bilbao 1995, King 1999, Dawson et al 2003, Dyck et al 2005).

Changes in the muscle as a result of a denervating process are similar, irrespective of the site of the lesion, be it in the neurone or the peripheral nerve, and it is rarely possible to precisely define the disorder from a muscle biopsy, although certain patterns are suggestive. Careful clinical and electrophysiological investigations often give a clue to the defective gene and muscle biopsies are now performed less often in neurogenic disorders. For example, molecular analysis of the survival motor neurone (*SMN*) gene identifies the majority of cases with spinal muscular atrophy and severity and prognosis is based on clinical features not muscle pathology.

Some neurogenic atrophies, however, may mimic some muscular dystrophies or myopathies, such as distal myopathies. Muscle pathology can then be useful in differential diagnosis and particular patterns of change may be revealed with histological and histochemical techniques. Immunohistochemistry may contribute to the interpretation of secondary changes in the muscle but the primary gene product is not usually studied in the muscle. As mentioned above, changes in relation to the nerve may be informative; for example, abnormalities in the sensory sural nerve in the diagnosis of peripheral neuropathies. We describe here the general characteristics of denervated muscle. These are the changes seen in chronic disorders such as ALS and can be distinguished from the early onset childhood disorders such as SMA. As the pathology in the different forms of SMA is variable this is described in detail and a muscle biopsy may well be performed in advance of a molecular diagnosis or in cases where a neurogenic problem is not initially suspected.

General pathological features of denervated muscle

Diseases which involve the motor neurones are associated with a characteristic set of pathological changes in human muscle. Denervated muscle fibres shrink in size but there may be little change in the internal architecture of the fibres. Even the cross-striations of individual atrophic muscle fibres are preserved until late in the atrophic process. The basal lamina round individual fibres often remains as the fibre shrinks and becomes folded (see Ch. 5 on electron microscopy). In chronic conditions such as ALS the atrophic fibres have an angular shape (Fig. 9.1), in contrast to the rounded shape of the atrophic fibres in SMA. All that may be visible of some atrophic fibres in chronic denervation is a clump of nuclei which may be pyknotic (see Fig. 4.21). Pyknotic sarcolemmal nuclei may also be seen along the course of a pre-existing fibre.

Since one motor nerve supplies many muscle fibres, denervation will result in atrophic fibres scattered at random in a biopsy. These atrophic fibres are often clustered into groups, and the number of fibres within these groups increases with increasing severity of denervation, until whole fascicles may be rendered atrophic. The presence of this 'small group' or 'large group' atrophy is pathognomonic of denervation (see Figs 9.1 and 9.3 and see section on SMA).

Two populations of muscle fibres are seen in denervated muscle: atrophic ones that are denervated and those that are relatively normal in size or hypertrophied. Histographic representation of this frequently shows a bimodal or twin-peaked configuration (see Ch. 4). This occurs because not all motor neurones are involved simultaneously. Fibres supplied by an intact motor nerve will obviously not atrophy and compensatory hypertrophy may occur as they take over the function of the atrophic muscle fibres which have lost their motor

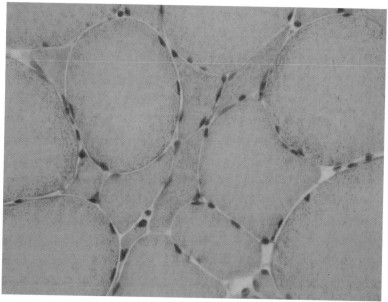

FIG. 9.1 *A small group of angulated atrophic fibres (diameter range 10–35 µm) and more rounded hypertrophied fibres (diameter size range 90–120 µm) in a case of amyotrophic lateral sclerosis. Note also the absence of endomysial connective tissue (H&E).*

supply. In addition, surviving nerves may sprout and reinnervate clusters of denervated fibres, causing them to enlarge again.

All the changes described above can be seen with routine stains such as the Gomori trichrome and haematoxylin and eosin (H&E). In addition histological examination of nerves present in a sample may reveal changes such as loss of myelin or fibrosis (Fig. 9.2). In chronic denervation histochemical reactions are particularly useful in demonstrating the angular atrophic fibres (Fig. 9.3). Atrophic angulated fibres stain intensely with techniques for oxidative enzymes, suggesting they are type 1 fibres (Fig. 9.3) but with adenosine triphosphatase (ATPase) staining or immunolabelling of myosin isoforms they may be of either type (Fig. 9.4). This is an important distinction, and a diagnosis of a denervating disease should not be made unless the atrophy involves both fibre types. In addition, these denervated fibres tend to have a positive esterase but negative acid phosphatase reaction, in contrast to regenerating or necrotic fibres which are strongly positive for both enzyme reactions. Denervated fibres may also lose their glycogen content and appear unstained and white with periodic acid-Schiff (PAS). With immunohistochemistry some, but not all, angulated fibres may show neonatal myosin and some may co-express fast myosin (Fig. 9.4). As discussed in Chapter 6, it is possible this reflects re-expression of neonatal myosin rather than immaturity resulting from regeneration, but the possibility of regeneration stimulated by denervation cannot be excluded. Immature and non-innervated fibres, such as regenerating fibres, show neural cell adhesion molecule (N-CAM) on all the sarcolemma, whereas on normal mature fibres it is confined to the

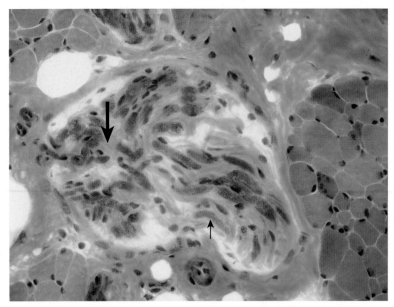

FIG. 9.2 *An abnormal nerve (diameter 170 μm) stained with Gomori trichrome in a case with peripheral neuropathy. Note the excess connective tissue (large arrow) and loss of red stained myelin from some axons (small arrow).*

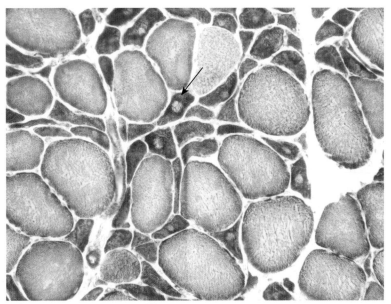

FIG. 9.3 *Darkly stained angulated atrophic fibres (diameter range 20–45 μm) in a case of amyotrophic lateral sclerosis. The paler fibres show two intensities of staining and are hypertrophic (diameter range 80–135 μm). Note several atrophic fibres show cores (arrow). These are not clearly identifiable as target fibres but the rim of some cores is a little more intensely stained (NADH-TR).*

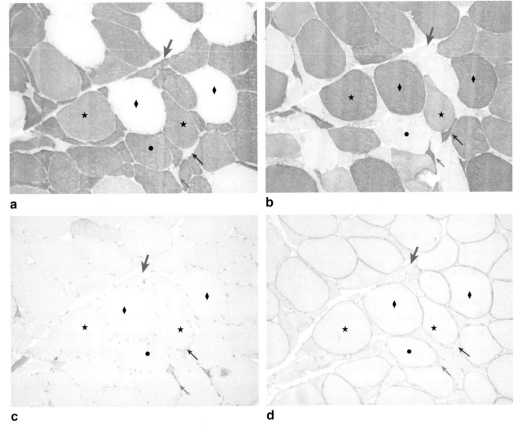

FIG. 9.4 *Serial areas from a case of amyotrophic lateral sclerosis immunolabelled with antibodies to (a) slow myosin, (b) fast myosin, (c) neonatal myosin and (d) nNOS. Note the absence of nNOS from all the atrophic fibres (size range 5–35 μm) which are of both types (arrows). Atrophic fibres with fast myosin show variable amounts of neonatal myosin (slow only = green arrows; fast and neonatal = light and dark blue arrows). Some larger fibres show slow (•) or fast (♦) myosin only, whilst others (diameter range 65–135 μm) show co-expression of slow and fast myosin (★) None of the larger fibres shows neonatal myosin. The same fibre in each section is marked with the same symbol.*

neuromuscular junction (Cashman et al 1987, Walsh and Moore 1985). Denervated fibres also show extrajunctional N-CAM but, in contrast, neuronal nitric oxide synthase (nNOS) is not detected and reappears after reinnervation (Gosztonyi et al 2001; Fig. 9.4). Assessment of nNOS must always take account of immaturity as nNOS is absent from immature fibres (see Ch. 6) but the combination of nNOS, N-CAM and neonatal myosin can help to distinguish denervated fibres from those that may be immature.

As has been pointed out earlier (see Ch. 3), the motor nerve has an important role in determining the particular type of muscle fibre. Thus, motor neurones may be thought of as supplying either type 1 or type 2 (slow or fast) motor units. Although it should be possible to have a denervating disease selectively involving a single type of motor neurone, this is not found in human disorders and

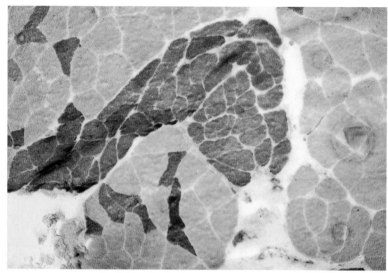

FIG. 9.5 *A group of darkly stained type 2 fibres surrounded by pale type 1 fibres in a case of amyotrophic lateral sclerosis (ATPase 9.4).*

both fibre types undergo denervation. If this criterion is used in making the diagnosis of denervation, it safeguards against diagnosing denervation in a patient showing, for example, selective fibre type atrophy from other causes.

Grouping of fibres of the same type is pathognomonic of denervated muscle and results from collateral sprouting of the surviving nerves which reinnervate the denervated fibres. Some idea of prognosis may be obtained from the presence of type grouping, since extensive fibre type grouping, in association with very little fibre atrophy, should imply good compensation of the denervating process and thus a milder or more chronic process. It is important to distinguish fibre type predominance from fibre type grouping, especially in a small sample, and groups of both types should be present to make a diagnosis of denervation (Fig. 9.5). Grouping may sometimes be difficult to assess and it may not be very obvious in all biopsies from neurogenic conditions (Fig. 9.6). Co-expression of myosin isoforms may also make fibre type grouping difficult to define in sections stained for ATPase (see Figs 9.4 and 9.12).

Another change seen in denervating diseases is the presence of target fibres (Engel 1961). In some biopsies the dark rim round the pale zone devoid of oxidative enzyme activity may not be prominent and the fibres then have an appearance similar to a fibre with a central core (Fig. 9.3; see also Fig. 9.11). These core-like areas can occur in fibres of varying size (see section on SMA) and are usually focal lesions, rarely extending down the whole length of a fibre. The possibility has been raised, based on experimental studies in animals, that target fibres may represent reinnervation rather than denervation of the fibre (Dubowitz 1967). Perhaps the fact that they are seen in profusion in diseases such as acute recovering neuropathies or chronic peripheral neuropathies, in which reinnervation is a prominent part of the picture, supports this view.

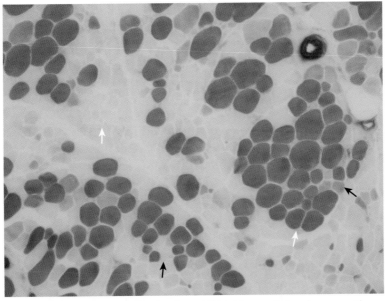

FIG. 9.6 *Mild fibre type grouping in a child with a peripheral neuropathy. Atrophic fibres are of both types (black arrows) and there is a group of type 1 and type 2 fibres (white arrows; ATPase 4.3). Fibre diameter range 10–50 μm.*

Other architectural changes such as moth-eaten fibres and whorled fibres may occasionally be seen with oxidative enzyme stains. Excess endomysial connective tissue is not usually a feature of denervated muscle but can occur, particularly in chronic conditions. Internal nuclei may also be seen in some hypertrophic fibres. These features, in the absence of fibre type grouping, may make it difficult to distinguish from a 'myopathic' appearance (see section on SMA).

Spinal muscular atrophy

One of the most common forms of neurogenic atrophy is spinal muscular atrophy with an incidence of about 1:10 000 births. It is an autosomal recessive condition in which the degenerative process affects the anterior horn cells of the spinal cord. The genetic defect is in the survival motor neurone (*SMN*) gene on chromosome 5q and over 95% of SMA patients have a deletion affecting exon 7 and 8 of the telomeric copy of the SMN gene (*SMN1*). The sequence of the centromeric gene (*SMN2*) is almost identical and severity of the disorder correlates with the amount of protein produced by the variable number of copies of *SMN2*. Current therapeutic strategies are aimed at the up-regulation of centromeric *SMN2*. The SMN gene product has an important role in assembly of a spliceosomal complex and in pre-RNA splicing, and may also have a neuron-specific function (Gubitz et al 2004). The affected region of chromosome 5 is complex and other genes, which are also duplicated and have telomeric and centromeric copies, may also be deleted, in particular, the neuronal apoptosis inhibitory protein gene (NAIP) and p44. The high proportion of patients with a deletion involving exon 7 and 8 of *SMN1* provides a reliable molecular screen that identifies the majority of SMA cases and also heterozygous carriers. The presence of exon 7 and 8, however, does not totally exclude a diagnosis of SMA, as a few atypical cases with mutations outside this region have been documented (Skordis et al 2001, Cusco et al 2004). The reliability of molecular analysis has revolutionized diagnosis of SMA and the role of muscle biopsy has diminished. Muscle biopsies, however, may be taken in cases where the diagnosis is less obvious clinically. No deletions of *SMN1* have been found in patients with lower motor neurone disease but it has been suggested that there is a significantly higher incidence of deletions of exon 7 of centromeric *SMN2* in these patients than in the normal population (Echaniz-Laguna et al 2002).

Other genes are responsible for clinical syndromes related to SMA. Some have more distal rather than proximal muscle involvement, and some are asymmetrical or more focal in presentation. Some of the adult forms have a dominant inheritance and there is also a separate X-linked bulbospinal form with a benign course and associated facial fasciculation, severe muscle cramps and gynaecomastia (Kennedy's disease, Kennedy et al 1968), caused by a CAG nucleotide expansion of the first exon of the androgen receptor on chromosome Xq13 (La Spada et al 1991). A severe X-linked form with associated arthrogryposis maps to Xp11 (Kobayashi et al 1995) and a distinct autosomal recessive form, with severe diaphragmatic and respiratory involvement (diaphragmatic spinal muscular atrophy with respiratory distress; SMARD), is caused by mutations in the gene encoding immunoglobulin microbinding protein 2 (*IGHMBP2*) on chromosome 11q13-q21 (Grohmann et al 2001). The severe diaphragmatic involvement is a useful distinguishing clinical feature from classical chromosome 5 SMA, in which the diaphragm is selectively spared, in spite of severe involvement of the intercostal muscles. Cases with ponto-cerebellar hypoplasia may also resemble SMA clinically and pathologically (Muntoni et al 1999), but have associated features of central nervous system involvement, and were shown not to be associated with the *SMN1* gene (Dubowitz et al 1995).

In this section we shall cover the muscle pathology associated with the three main clinical groups of autosomal chromosome 5 SMA, both the cases manifesting the classical features and those where these may be less obvious.

Three main clinical groups, types I, II and III, have been arbitrarily defined on relative severity and whether the ability to sit or stand unaided and walk is achieved (see below). There is clinical variability within each group, and some cases are not easily categorized into these rigid groups (Dubowitz 1991, 1995b, Munsat 1991, Munsat and Davies 1992). Some clinicians distinguish cases with a mild adult onset as a fourth group whilst others include these within the spectrum of SMA III. Type I SMA (Werdnig–Hoffmann disease) is the severest form with onset in utero or early infancy and patients are never able to sit and usually die in the first year and rarely survive beyond 2 years. In type II (intermediate SMA) onset is usually between 6 and 12 months and the ability to sit unsupported is achieved but they fail to stand. The clinical spectrum of SMA III (Kugelberg–Welander), who achieve ambulation, is broad ranging from onset in the second year of life, with little or occasionally with marked progression, to adult onset with mild progression. Differential diagnosis from a myopathic condition is important in these cases. The typical features of each group are summarized in Tables 9.1, 9.2 and 9.3.

Although there is marked variation in severity, the basic clinical pattern is similar in all types, with symmetrical weakness, affecting lower limbs more than upper, and proximal muscles more than distal. The cranial nerves are relatively spared except in the more severe forms, and there is usually no facial weakness. Fasciculation of the tongue, however, is common, especially in type II. There is no associated sensory or long tract involvement.

Type I (Werdnig–Hoffmann disease)

This is the severest form with early onset, often in utero or early infancy, in which paralysis of the trunk and limbs is very marked. The infant is hypotonic and does not achieve the ability to lift the head or to sit. Active movements of the limbs are usually confined to the feet and toes and the forearms and hands. The legs are more severely paralysed than the arms. Tendon reflexes are absent. The face is relatively spared and may appear normal, but there is often associated bulbar weakness, with difficulty in swallowing and a weak cry. The intercostal muscles are also affected whereas the diaphragm is spared, so that breathing is mainly diaphragmatic with associated costal recession. These children usually die of respiratory infection before the age of 1 year, though some may survive into their second year or rarely even longer. Cardiac muscle is not affected.

Type II (intermediate spinal muscular atrophy)

This is a milder juvenile form, of intermediate severity, where the child passes the early motor milestones normally and is able to maintain a head posture and to sit unaided, but is unable to take weight on the legs and never achieves the ability to stand or walk unaided. Clinical onset is usually later, often between 6 and 12 months of age, but in some, weakness may already be noted earlier and even in the neonatal period. The legs are again more severely affected than the arms, which may at times be practically normal or have only slight weakness confined to the shoulder muscles. There is variable weakness of the intercostal muscles and the cranial nerves tend to be spared. However, fasciculation and atrophy of the tongue is common, without associated symptoms. A coarse tremor of the hands is also noted in many cases. The weakness tends to be non-progressive and in most cases the prognosis is good. Some children with a similar distribution and degree of limb weakness may also have marked

TABLE 9.1 *Features of severe type I spinal muscular atrophy (Werdnig–Hoffmann disease)*

Onset

In utero or within the first few months of life

Clinical features

Severe hypotonia

Severe limb and axial weakness

Poor head control

Bell-shaped chest and diaphragmatic breathing

Respiratory problems which often lead to pneumonia and early death

Sucking difficulties

Weak cry

Motor ability

Sitting and weight-bearing never achieved

Investigations

Creatine kinase normal

Electromyogram features of denervation with large amplitude polyphasic potentials

Motor nerve conduction velocity normal or reduced (electrophysiological studies are now rarely necessary with the advent of molecular diagnosis)

Muscle pathology

Large groups of atrophic fibres

Fibre type grouping

Large fibres type 1

Uniform atrophy

Some samples from early cases may show minimal change (pre-pathological)

TABLE 9.2 *Features of intermediate type II spinal muscle atrophy*

Onset

Usually between 6 and 12 months

Clinical features

Hypotonia

Symmetrical weakness of legs, predominantly proximal

Fasciculation of tongue

Tremor of hands

Diminished or absent tendon jerks

Joint laxity, particularly of hands and feet

Scoliosis

Respiratory problems

Motor ability

Able to sit

Unable to stand unaided or walk

Investigations

Creatine kinase normal or occasionally mild elevation

Electromyogram features of denervation and reinnervation with large amplitude polyphasic potentials and fasciculation

Normal nerve conduction velocity (electrophysiological studies are now rarely necessary with the advent of molecular diagnosis)

Muscle pathology

Similar to type I spinal muscular atrophy

Large group atrophy

Fibre type grouping

Hypertrophic fibres type 1

TABLE 9.3 *Features of spinal muscle atrophy type III (Kugelberg–Welander disease)*

Onset

From second year of life

In childhood, adolescence or adulthood

Clinical features

Weakness static or may be progressive

Difficulty running, jumping and climbing stairs

Waddling gait

Flat footed

Difficulty rising from floor (Gowers' manoeuvre)

Hand tremor (variable)

Tongue fasciculation (variable)

Joint laxity, particularly of hands and feet

Motor ability variable

Able to walk but may be limited

Investigations

Creatine kinase normal or moderately elevated

Electromyogram features of denervation and reinnervation with large amplitude polyphasic potentials

Normal nerve conduction velocity

Muscle pathology

Variable

Minimal change, or small or large group atrophy with grouping of normal size or hypertrophied type 1 fibres

Architectural changes – whorls, cores, splits

May be difficult to distinguish from limb-girdle dystrophy

intercostal weakness and are then likely to have respiratory infections and accordingly a poor prognosis. Scoliosis is a common complication.

Type III (Kugelberg–Welander disease)

This is the mildest form in which onset is later and ambulation is achieved. Weakness is mainly confined to the proximal muscles of the lower limbs and clinically the picture is very similar to a limb-girdle muscular dystrophy. Fasciculation may be seen in the tongue but rarely in peripheral muscles. The tendon reflexes may be normal or diminished. The course is usually benign, with little tendency for deterioration in most cases. Some do show progressive increase in weakness over a long period and this may lead to loss of ambulation. On the other hand, some cases seem to improve with time, probably as a result of compensating reinnervation of muscle and supportive management. Although bulbar symptoms are not a usual feature of the Kugelberg–Welander syndrome, some cases have been reported with associated bulbar involvement of long duration.

Clinically it is difficult to draw clear-cut dividing lines between the above three forms of disease. The very severe Werdnig–Hoffmann and the very mild Kugelberg–Welander varieties are clearly identifiable but the borderline cases are more difficult to categorize. This led to the suggestion of subdividing each type on a scale of 1 to 10 based on clinical severity (Dubowitz 1995b).

Histology and histochemistry

Severe and intermediate spinal muscular atrophy types I and II

The pathological changes seen in muscle biopsies in the severe infantile and intermediate forms are so similar that they will be discussed together. It is not possible to distinguish between types I and II on muscle pathology; the distinction is a clinical one.

Atrophic fibres occur in all biopsies, often in large groups, and these are interspersed with fascicles of hypertrophic fibres (Fig. 9.7). The shape of the atrophic fibres is usually round, in contrast to the angulated shape in other forms of neurogenic atrophy such as ALS (see Figs 9.1 and 9.3).

With histochemical reactions, the atrophic fibres are type 1 and 2 and the large fibres usually show uniformity of reaction and are invariably type 1 fibres (Fig. 9.7). Many of the grouped atrophic fibres may appear as type 2 with ATPase at 9.4 because of co-expression of more than one isoform of myosin (see Fig. 9.12). The fibre uniformity suggests that they are not unaffected normal fibres, but fibres reinnervated by sprouting of the surviving nerves. The hypertrophy may be a compensatory effect resulting from these fibres taking over the function of the atrophic fibres.

The overall histological and histochemical pattern in infantile SMA is remarkably consistent but the extent of atrophy may vary in different parts of the muscle. Some bundles may be composed entirely of normal-sized fibres,

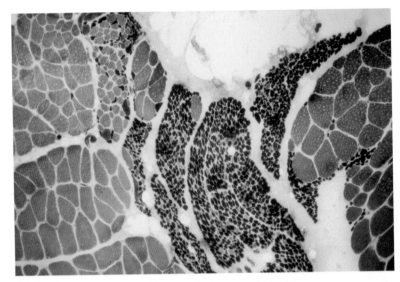

a

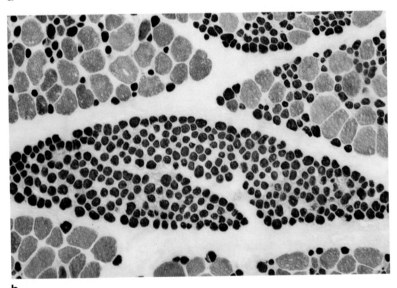

b

FIG. 9.7(a),(b) *Atrophy of both fibre types in two cases of SMA I stained with ATPase 9.4. Most of the larger fibres are type 1 and many of the atrophic fibres appear as type 2 fibres because of co-expression of neonatal myosin. Note also the rounded shape of the atrophic fibres compared with the atrophic fibres in ALS (compare Figs 9.1 and 9.3).*

others entirely of atrophic fibres. If a sample is small it might consist entirely of small or of normal fibres, or of fibres of one type. In occasional early cases of severe SMA I cases the classical features of group atrophy and fibre type grouping may not be present in that particular sample (Fig. 9.8). This has been referred to as pre-pathological SMA, in view of the unequivocal clinical picture, now supported by deletions in the *SMN1* gene.

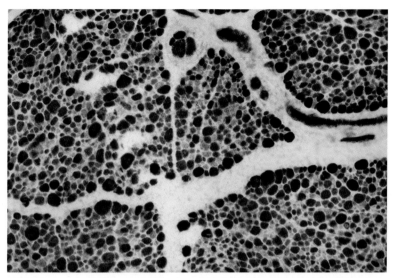

FIG. 9.8 *A neonatal case of SMA1 aged 11 days showing a pre-pathological state without classical fibre type grouping. The small fibres are of both types and many of the hypertrophied fibres are type 1 (ATPase 4.3).*

Muscle spindles may be numerous in infantile SMA. Nuclear changes, such as pyknotic or internal nuclei, however, are rare in severe or intermediate SMA. Evidence of degeneration and necrosis is also not a feature. The perimysium is often wide and there may be foci of adipose tissue, but excess endomysial connective tissue is not a feature of SMA. Similarly, architectural changes within the fibres such as targets or whorls are rare in the severe forms.

Mild spinal muscular atrophy type III (Kugelberg–Welander)

The clinical spectrum of the mild cases with Kugelberg–Welander syndrome is wide, ranging from childhood to adult onset. Similarly, the pathological changes are also variable, with or without the classical features of denervation.

Group atrophy may occur but the number of atrophic fibres per cluster tends to be less than in the severe forms but can at times also be extensive (Fig. 9.9). Fibre type grouping also occurs (Fig. 9.10), and type 2 predominance may be a feature. Architectural changes such as cores, target fibres, whorled fibres and split fibres and internal nuclei may also be seen (Fig. 9.11).

Some biopsies from mild cases show unequivocal denervation changes, whilst others may show very little pathology or be difficult to distinguish from a myopathy or muscular dystrophy. Some of these milder cases may also have a mildly elevated serum creatine kinase level. Focal groups of atrophic fibres are common in Becker and facioscapulohumeral muscular dystrophy and it is important to assess the overall pattern of change in the biopsy as a whole with regard to fibrosis, degeneration and the distribution of fibre types. It is important to distinguish type 1 fibre predominance, which is common in the dystrophies,

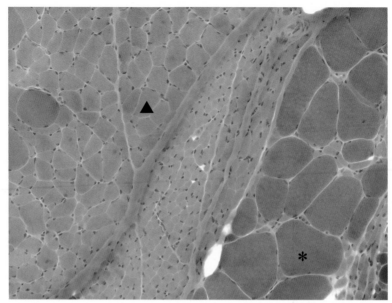

FIG. 9.9 *Case of SMA III (Kugelberg–Welander disease) aged 2.5 years showing large group atrophy (many fibres less than 10 μm). Note also the group of hypertrophic fibres (*; up to 100 μm in diameter) and the area with many fibres of normal size (▲; Gomori trichrome).*

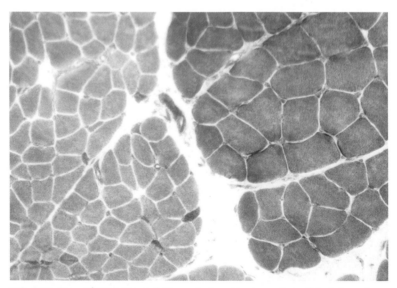

FIG. 9.10 *Case of SMA III aged 16 years showing grouping of dark type 1 and paler type 2 fibres and some isolated atrophic fibres (NADH-TR). Fibre diameter range 15–140 μm.*

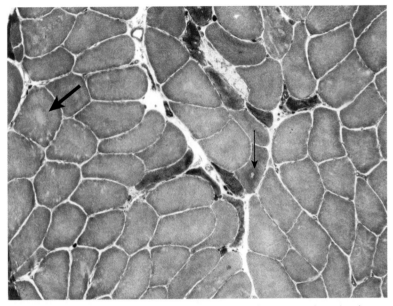

FIG. 9.11 *Case of SMA III aged 5 years showing a few intensely stained angulated atrophic fibres, and cores (large arrow) and targets (small arrow) in some paler type 2 fibres (NADH-TR). Fibre diameter range 10–60 μm.*

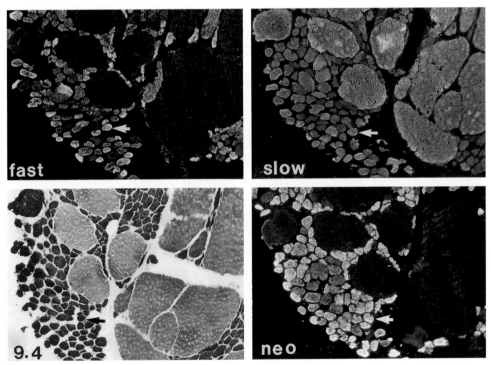

FIG. 9.12 *Serial sections from a case of SMA III aged 7 years showing co-expression of fast, slow and neonatal myosin in several of the atrophic fibres which stain as type 2 with ATPase at pH 9.4 (arrow). Note also the larger fibres only express slow myosin.*

from fibre type grouping. Note should also be taken of the results from ancillary investigations such as creatine kinase and electromyography.

Immunohistochemistry

Immunohistochemistry in relation to fibre types reflects the histochemical properties and shows that the hypertrophic fibres have a slow phenotype. Atrophic fibres co-express fast, slow and neonatal myosin in various combinations (Fig. 9.12). In the early onset cases this neonatal myosin might reflect an arrest in maturation but this is less likely in older cases and is probably the result of denervation. This is supported by the fact that other developmentally regulated proteins such as desmin and vimentin are only detected in some, but not all, the atrophic fibres (Sewry 1989, Soussi-Yanicostas et al 1992). N-CAM, which is confined to neuromuscular junctions on innervated fibres, becomes extrajunctional on denervated fibres (Cashman et al 1987, Walsh and Moore 1985, Sewry 1989). As pointed out previously, nNOS is lost from the sarcolemma of denervated fibres and reappears following reinnervation (Goszytonyi et al 2001, Tews 2001; see Fig. 9.5) and can be a useful marker of denervation. The full spectrum of nNOS changes in all forms of SMA is not yet clear.

The SMN protein is localized in nuclei, to structures known as gems, but their number has not been correlated with severity, although severity is related to the total amount of SMN protein.

CHAPTER 10

Muscular dystrophies and allied disorders I: Duchenne and Becker muscular dystrophy

Background

Although the advent of molecular genetics has totally transformed the diagnostic confirmation of Duchenne and Becker muscular dystrophy, we thought it worth retaining some historical background and clinical description of these classical muscular disorders.

Duchenne muscular dystrophy (DMD) has been recognized as a clinical entity since the nineteenth century. In 1868 Duchenne gave a detailed account of 13 male patients with progressive muscle weakness. Onset was in childhood, weakness was initially worse in the lower limbs and lumbar region, and was accompanied by hypertrophy of some muscles. He also took muscle samples from these cases using a biopsy needle that was the forerunner of the type we use today (see Ch. 1), and noted the marked proliferation of connective tissue and adipose tissue. Although the disease is attributed to Duchenne, earlier descriptions had in fact been made by the London physician, Meryon and by Conte and Gioja in Italy (Meryon 1852, Conte and Gioja 1836). Meryon's life and work has been researched and published (Emery and Emery 1995), and Conte's contribution has been celebrated by Nigro with the establishment of a Conte Foundation (1986). Meryon described the pathological features of autopsy samples from his cases and pointed out the necrotic nature of the muscle but apparent normality of the nervous system. He also suggested that the sarcolemma was principally at fault, and that genetic transmission was through females and only affected males.

In 1879 Gowers presented clinical observations on 21 personal cases and reviewed the descriptions of over 100 cases of others. He observed and illustrated the unusual way affected boys get up off the floor by climbing up their legs – the Gowers' manoeuvre. Despite the advances in clinical management over the years Gowers' masterly description of the devastating effects of the disease is still very apt (see Dubowitz 1995a).

In 1955 Becker and Kiener described cases with similar features to Duchenne dystrophy but milder in severity. There have been several subsequent reports on similar cases of Becker muscular dystrophy (BMD) and in 1984 it was shown by linkage analysis to be allelic to DMD on the short arm of the X chromosome (Kingston et al 1984).

DMD is one of the most common neuromuscular disorders with a prevalence of approximately 1 in 3500 live male births. The gene is highly prone to mutations and likely to be the childhood disorder most often seen by a muscle pathologist. The Becker form is less common with a predicted prevalence of 1 in 17 500 live male births (Emery 1991), although within the general population as a whole their prevalence is similar, as BMD patients live longer.

The previous edition of this book, published in 1985, was written before the explosion in molecular science and the underlying cause of the disease was not known. At that time all that was known was that the locus for DMD was on the short arm of the X chromosome at Xp21 and that the Becker form was probably allelic. Since that time the gene responsible for both has been cloned and its protein product named dystrophin (Koenig et al 1987, Hoffman et al 1987). Considerable knowledge on the consequences and types of mutations in the gene, and the relationship of dystrophin to other proteins, has been acquired, but the precise function of dystrophin is still unknown. Clinical management has greatly improved over the years and various therapeutic strategies are being investigated, but there is still no cure and the relentless progression of the disease in Duchenne patients inevitably leads to premature death. The gene for dystrophin was the first to be identified in a neuromuscular disorder and there are several texts documenting its cloning (see Emery 1993, Karpati et al 2001, Brown and Lucy 1997, Bushby and Anderson 2001). Muscle biopsies are an important component of the assessment of a patient with a muscular dystrophy and immunohistochemistry is now an essential component of differential diagnosis.

Clinical features

The clinical manifestations of DMD and BMD are now well known and documented (see Dubowitz 1995a). The aim of this summary (see Table 10.1) is to draw attention to features that should alert pathologists and they may find helpful in arriving at a diagnosis. Neonatal screening of serum creatine kinase activity (CK) can detect affected cases at birth but clinical abnormalities are not usually apparent until the child starts to walk. Motor milestones such as sitting, standing and walking are often delayed and about 50% of cases of DMD are late walking (beyond 18 months of age). Contractures of the Achilles tendons and hip flexors are early features of DMD, and result in toe-walking. They have a charac-

TABLE 10.1 *Main features of Duchenne (DMD) and Becker muscular dystrophy (BMD)*

Clinical features

Manifests within the first 5 years

Delayed motor milestones

Progressive proximal weakness

Contracture of Achilles tendon resulting in toe-walking

Waddling gait, lumbar lordosis

Difficulty running, hopping, jumping

Difficulty rising from floor (Gowers' manoeuvre)

Difficulty going up stairs

Calf hypertrophy

Cramps – BMD rather than DMD

Ambulation

Lost by 12 years – DMD

Ambulant beyond 16 years – BMD

Creatine kinase

Usually grossly elevated (10–50 times normal)

Elevated at birth

Associated features

Cardiomyopathy (invariable in DMD by late teens; variable in BMD)

Intellectual impairment (30% of DMD; rare in BMD)

Nocturnal hypoventilation

Scoliosis

Respiratory failure by late teens in DMD

Pathology

Clinical severity cannot be assessed from pathology

Necrosis, regeneration, fibrosis, wide variation in fibre size

Split fibres

Dystrophin usually absent in DMD

Dystrophin usually present but abnormal in BMD, some exceptions to this

Reduction of all dystrophin-associated proteins

teristic waddling gait and lumbar lordosis. Scoliosis occurs after loss of ambulation and may require surgical intervention. Duchenne and Becker boys are prone to falls and get up with the typical Gowers' manoeuvre. Duchenne boys are usually unable to jump or hop but these may be achieved in a Becker patient. Muscle weakness is proximal more than distal and greater in the legs than the arms and is steadily progressive. Hypertrophy of calf muscles is an early feature, but not specific to DMD and BMD. This is a pseudohypertrophy (a term coined by Duchenne), resulting from an increase in fibrotic and adipose tissue. Cramps on exercise may also be a feature and in some mild cases of BMD this may be the presenting feature. Rhabdomyolysis may also occur and, although a particular feature of some metabolic problems, should not mislead the pathologist. There may be a delay in learning to speak and a variable degree of non-progressive intellectual impairment in about 30% of DMD patients, but is rare in cases of BMD.

In the past, most Duchenne boys died before the age of 20 years, but better management, in particular non-invasive respiratory support at the onset of respiratory failure, has considerably improved life expectancy with survival into the mid 20s. Cardiac involvement is present in most cases of DMD by the late teens and is common in BMD.

Several serum enzymes are elevated in DMD and estimation of CK is the most sensitive and reliable and is grossly elevated. In both DMD and BMD levels are usually very high, 50–100 times the normal level, and they are particularly elevated early in the disease and may drop during its course. Levels of less than 10 times the normal are more likely to be associated with other forms of muscular dystrophy. Rare cases of BMD presenting with cramps and myalgia have been reported with normal CK but it is not clear if all these were molecularly proven (Samaha and Quinlan 1996). Most cases presenting with cramps have a raised CK but some cases that are relatively asymptomatic with a mutation can have a normal CK. There is no reported case of DMD with normal CK. The level of CK does not correlate with clinical severity and equally high levels occur in both DMD and BMD.

Clinical severity is variable in both DMD and BMD, and may even vary in members of the same family who carry the same mutation. The distinction between DMD and BMD is a clinical one and is based on the degree of weakness and the age at which ambulation is lost. Classical Duchenne patients are almost invariably off their feet by the age of 12 years, whereas Becker patients are ambulant to 16 years or beyond. The severity of BMD is very wide and several cases have been documented that have minimal muscle weakness and lead near normal lives for decades. At the severe end of the Becker spectrum there are patients approaching the Duchenne type in severity but who remain ambulant after 12 years of age and go off their feet before 16 years of age, or later. These so-called 'intermediate' cases often have atypical mutations, particularly in the 5′ region of the dystrophin gene, and they highlight the value of muscle biopsy and of examining protein expression (see below).

Histology and histochemistry

The classical histological changes in DMD and BMD are: rounding of the fibres; diffuse variation in fibre size, with hypertrophy and atrophy of fibres; necrosis and subsequent loss of fibres; basophilic regenerating fibres; densely stained hypercontracted fibres; increased internal nuclei; proliferation of endomysial and perimysial connective tissue; increased adipose tissue; and sometimes an increased cellular response (Fig. 10.1a–d). These features collectively are often referred to as 'dystrophic' and they reflect the progressive loss of muscle and

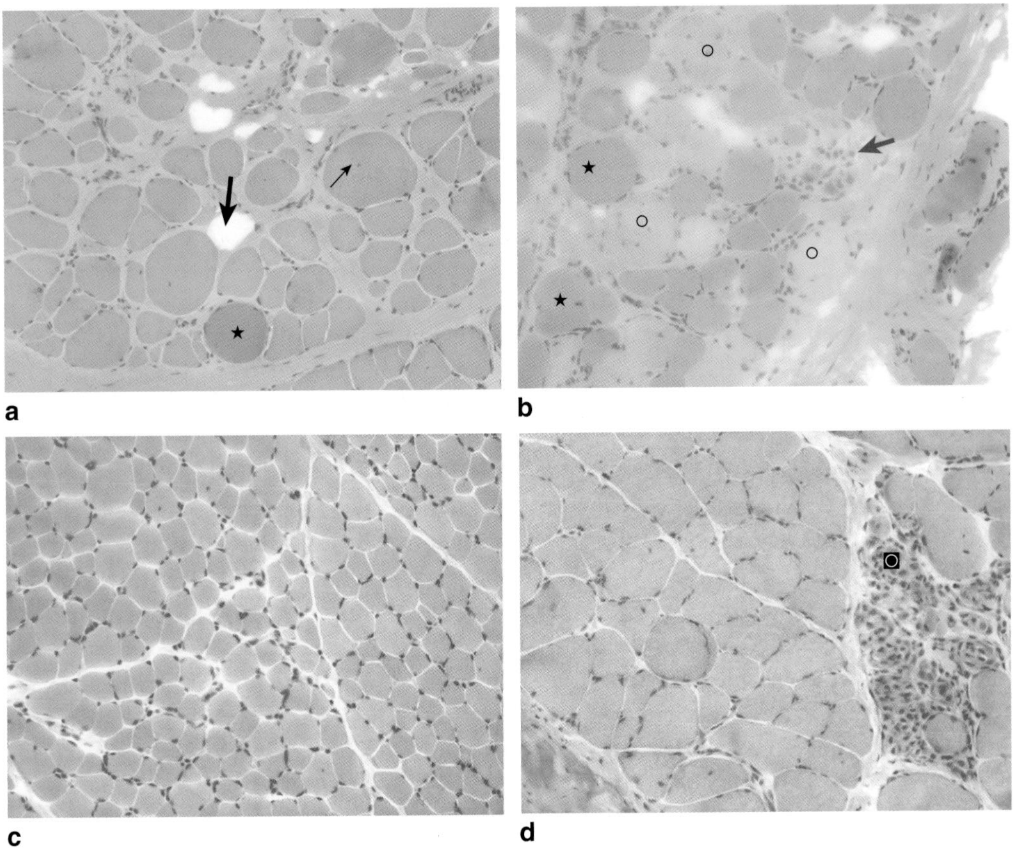

a b c d

FIG. 10.1 *Sections stained with H&E from (a), (b) two cases of Duchenne muscular dystrophy aged 9 and 6 years respectively and (c), (d) two cases of Becker muscular dystrophy aged 4 and 6 years respectively showing typical dystrophic features. In (a) there is a wide variation in fibre size (range 10–90 μm); the fibres are round in shape and have excess connective tissue round most of them. A few internal nuclei (small arrow), a darkly stained hypercontracted fibre (*), and a little adipose tissue (large arrow) are also shown; in (b) there are several pale necrotic fibres (o), a few basophilic fibres (green arrow) and several hypercontracted fibres (*; up to 80 μm in diameter); in (c) from the 4-year-old Becker patient the same features are present but are less pronounced (fibre size range 15–60 μm); in (d) the necrotic fibres are invaded by macrophages (◙) (fibre size range 30–95 μm).*

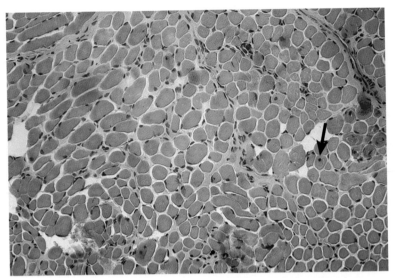

FIG. 10.2 *Muscle biopsy from a 6-month-old preclinical case of Duchenne muscular dystrophy. Note the abnormal features even at this stage, in particular variation in fibre size, increased endomysial connective tissue, adipose tissue and internal nuclei (arrow; H&E).*

necrotic nature of the tissue. Care should be exercised in describing muscle as 'dystrophic' when only excess connective tissue is present as this can occur in the absence of necrosis. Clinical severity cannot be judged from the degree of pathology; it is not possible to distinguish Duchenne and Becker dystrophy on the basis of histology alone (see Fig. 10.1a,d).

Pathological changes can be seen in DMD even at a few months of age when there are no clinical manifestations of the disease, other than elevated CK (Fig. 10.2). The changes can, however, be pronounced at a few months of age. As the disease progresses regeneration fails to keep pace with necrosis and the muscle is gradually replaced by connective and adipose tissue (Fig. 10.3). Abnormalities in BMD as young as a year can also be seen.

Attempts have been made to identify pathological changes in the muscle of potentially dystrophic male fetuses but these are equivocal and difficult to assess (Toop and Emery 1974, Emery 1977). Immunolabelling of dystrophin in at risk fetuses, however, can be useful (see below; Clerk et al 1992a,b).

Changes in fibre size

All cases show variation in fibre size, which is often marked. Fibre morphometry is rarely necessary when assessing cases of DMD as the size variation is usually obvious. In some mild BMD cases, however, variation may be less apparent but is usually present. The smallest fibres (less than 5 μm) may be barely visible with routine histological stains but may be more apparent with immunolabelling (see below). Some hypertrophic fibres (Fig. 10.4) can be extremely large (>200 μm)

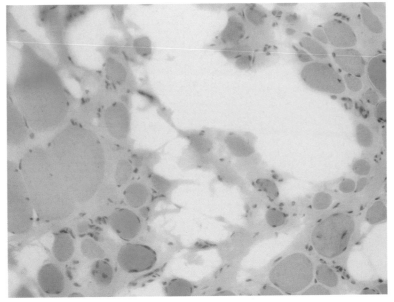

a

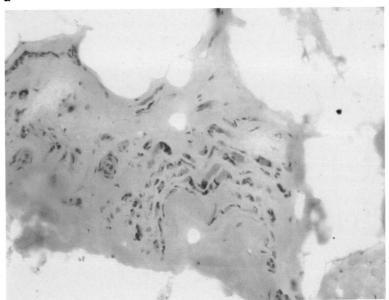

b

FIG. 10.3 *Two sections of advanced muscular dystrophy from (a) an 18-year-old case of Duchenne muscular dystrophy and (b) a 28-year-old case of Becker muscular dystrophy who were both re-biopsied to assess their dystrophin status. (a) Extensive adipose tissue is shown with some residual muscle fibres; (b) shows extensive fibrotic material containing fragments of fibres (H&E).*

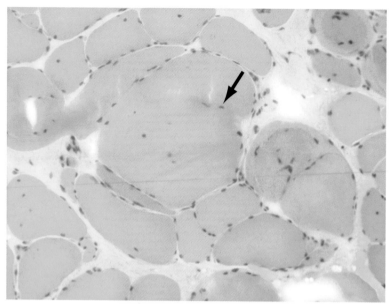

FIG. 10.4 *A very hypertrophic fibre 250 μm in diameter that shows splits and multiple internal nuclei some of which are associated with the splits (arrow). Note also the adjacent split and whorled fibre (H&E).*

and almost give the impression of several fibres joined together. Branching of fibres occurs and contributes to the variation in fibre size (see Fig. 10.1a).

Abnormalities in distribution

The size variation is diffuse with no groups of large fibres. Occasionally clusters of small fibres may be seen and this has sometimes been put forward as evidence of denervation (Fig. 10.5). Many of these fibres express neonatal myosin so may be regenerating, but this alone does not distinguish them from non-innervated or denervated fibres (see Ch. 6). The overall picture, however, is myopathic and there are never any signs of reinnervation or fibre type grouping.

Fibre typing

Fibre type differentiation is usually impaired. With oxidative enzymes it is often indistinct (particularly in DMD, and less so in milder/BMD cases) and most fibres show an intensity intermediate between normal type 1 and type 2 fibres. Fibres devoid of cytochrome oxidase are rare but can occur. Fibre typing with ATPase is also not always clear, particularly at pH 9.4, although it may be visible with acid preincubation. This poor differentiation is probably due to the presence of more than one myosin isoform in several fibres (see below). When fibre typing is visible type 1 fibres (slow fibres) often predominate, a common myopathic feature (Fig. 10.6). 2C fibres are also common and the basophilic regenerating

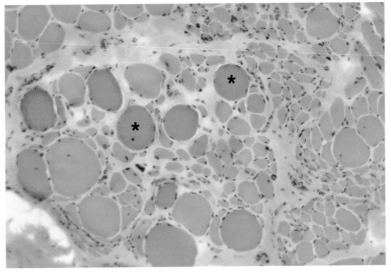

FIG. 10.5 *Clusters of small fibres in a case of Becker muscular dystrophy which are sometimes mistaken for denervation. Note also the darkly stained hypercontracted fibres (*) and the excess fibrous tissue (H&E).*

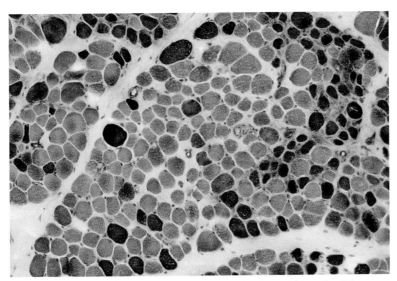

FIG. 10.6 *Biopsy of a case of Duchenne muscular dystrophy stained for ATPase at pH 9.4 showing variation in size of both fibre types and a marked predominance of the pale type 1 fibres. Several of the dark type fibres are 2C fibres in this section and were also dark when stained for ATPase with acid preincubation at pH 4.6 and 4.3.*

fibres stain as 2C fibres. The variation in fibre size affects both main fibre types (Fig. 10.6), although the largest fibres in young patients may more frequently be type 2.

Changes in sarcolemmal nuclei

Internal nuclei displaced from their normal sarcolemmal position are common but the number of affected fibres is not as great as in some other muscular dystrophies (see Fig. 10.1a). Multiple internal nuclei within one fibre in cross-section are rare in children with DMD but may occur in BMD and are common in other forms of muscular dystrophy. An exception is the large fibres with splits in which there may be multiple internal nuclei, many of which are associated with the splits (see Fig. 10.4). Regenerating, basophilic fibres may have large internal vesicular nuclei with a prominent nucleolus and pale nucleoplasm (Fig. 10.7).

Degeneration and regeneration

Necrotic fibres may be isolated or clustered and phagocytes are often seen within them. The necrosis is often segmental and only affects a portion of the fibre. Necrotic fibres appear pale with haematoxylin and eosin (H&E) staining and with the trichrome technique (see Fig. 10.1b,d), but may retain their differential myosin content. The large, round hypercontracted fibres that are intensely stained with histological techniques are damaged fibres (see Figs 10.1a and 10.8). There is still controversy as to their significance but they are a particular feature of DMD and BMD and sometimes more easily seen with the Gomori trichrome stain. Fibres that lack glycogen are also common in DMD but they are not a specific feature and probably represent a stage in muscle damage, prior to necrosis. Regenerating, basophilic fibres may also occur in clusters or be diffuse through the sample (Fig. 10.7). A variable number of fibres that are not basophilic show neonatal myosin and may be at various stages of regeneration (see below).

Fibrosis

Both perimysial and endomysial fibrosis is variable in extent and is a consistent feature of DMD and BMD. In early cases it may only be slight but it is often pronounced, and it is not uncommon to see all fibres surrounded by endomysial connective tissue (Fig. 10.8). Excess adipose tissue is often perimysial but it can also occur in the endomysium.

Cellular reactions

A variable number of cells of different type may be apparent in a Duchenne or Becker sample. Areas of necrosis frequently appear cellular with a mixture of macrophages, T cells and myoblasts, and mast cells are also common.

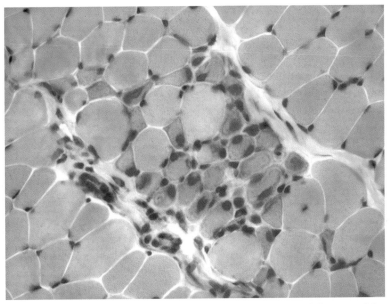

FIG. 10.7 *A cluster of blue basophilic regenerating fibres with large nuclei (size range 15–20 μm) in a case of Becker muscular dystrophy (H&E).*

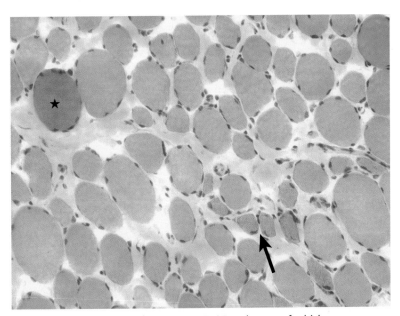

FIG. 10.8 *Rounded fibres (size range 25–85 μm) most of which are surrounded by excess connective tissue and fat in a case of Duchenne muscular dystrophy. Note also the dark hypercontracted fibre (*) and a few slightly basophilic fibres (arrow; H&E; compare with Fig. 10.1b).*

Architectural changes

Whorling of the myofibrils is common, particularly in the hypertrophic fibres (Fig. 10.9a). These are seen well with oxidative enzyme stains such as reduced nicotinamide adenine dinucleotide-tetrazolium reductase (NADH-TR). Moth-eaten fibres (Fig. 10.9b) and varying degrees of disruption of the myofibrils may also be apparent, although less so than in other dystrophies, and some aggregation of oxidative enzyme stains may be seen (Fig. 10.9a). Core-like areas devoid of mitochondria are infrequent in DMD and BMD but do occur.

Immunohistochemistry

Dystrophin

Cloning of the gene responsible for DMD and BMD and localization of its protein product, dystrophin, to the sarcolemma led the way to the revolution in muscle pathology that has occurred during recent decades (see Brown and Lucy 1997, Karpati 2002). The gene for dystrophin is one of the largest known with 2.5 Mb of DNA and 79 exons. It has some very large introns and the transcribed mRNA is 14 kb. Transcription of the gene is thought to take about 16 hours. The full length protein has a predicted molecular mass of 427 kDa and has four main domains (Fig. 10.10); the commercial antibodies commonly used recognize epitopes in these different domains (see Table 6.1; Fig. 10.10). The N-terminus is an actin binding domain; the large rod domain has 24 spectrin-like repeats and four hinge regions; the cysteine rich domain binds β-dystroglycan; and the C-terminal domain binds syntrophin, dystrobrevin and probably also F-actin and α-actinin. The dystrophin gene has at least eight promotors which give rise to different isoforms of different molecular mass (Fig. 10.11), and there is considerable splicing at the 3′ end. The various isoforms of dystrophin are differentially expressed in skeletal, cardiac and smooth muscle, fetal muscle and neural tissue. It has been suggested that the mental retardation that occurs in about 30% of cases may relate to involvement of the brain isoforms. In skeletal and cardiac muscle the full length transcripts from 5′ promotors are the most important and antibodies corresponding to the different domains of the protein show uniform labelling of the sarcolemma of all fibres in normal muscle, and in non-Xp21 disorders. The various isoforms of dystrophin share a common C-terminus (Fig. 10.11) and antibodies with epitopes in this region (e.g. DYS2 from Novocastra) recognize all isoforms. On immunoblots using antibodies to the N-terminus or rod domain (e.g. DYS1) dystrophin appears as a doublet, probably representing the 427 and 400 kDa muscle isoforms. With antibodies to the C-terminus (e.g. DYS2) dystrophin is seen as a single band on immunoblots (DYS3 does not recognize denatured dystrophin on immunoblots).

Dystrophin is a cytoskeletal protein that lies on the cytoplasmic face of the plasma membrane. It interacts with the actin cytoskeleton and a complex of other proteins, the dystrophin-associated proteins (Fig. 10.12). It is believed to act as a

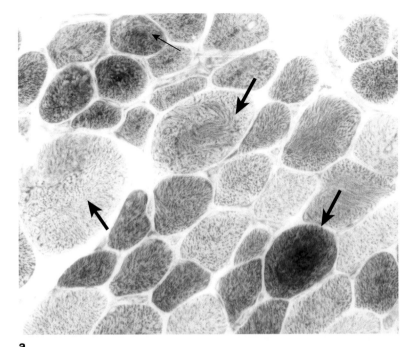

a

b

FIG. 10.9 *Various architectural changes revealed with staining for NADH-TR. Note in (a) variable degrees of whorling of myofibrils (large arrows) and aggregation of stain (small arrow; fibre size range 10–60 μm), and in (b) some moth-eaten fibres (28–32 μm) with areas that lack stain (arrow). Fibre typing is clear in (a) but less distinct in (b).*

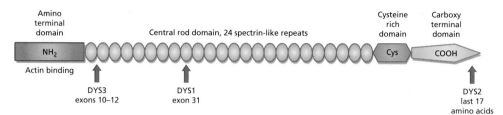

FIG. 10.10 *Diagrammatic representation of the dystrophin gene showing the four main domains and the position of the epitopes of the Novocastra DYS1, DYS2 and DYS3 antibodies.*

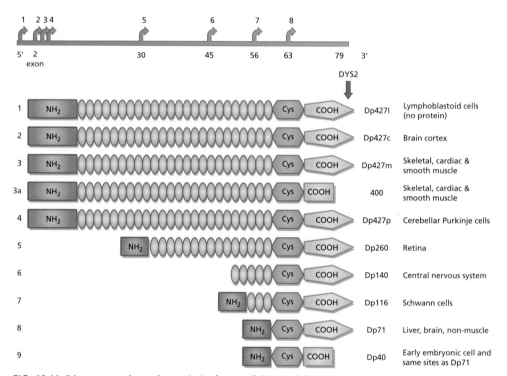

FIG. 10.11 *Diagram to show the main isoforms of dystrophin produced from different promoters and expressed in different tissues. Note the presence of a common C-terminus in many of them which will be detected by antibodies recognizing a C-terminal epitope such as DYS2. No protein has been identified from the transcript in lymphoblastoid cells and evidence suggests it is an artefact of PCR.*

link between the extracellular matrix and the cytoskeleton, stabilizing the membrane during contraction. The complex probably also has a role in signalling, anchoring of ion channels and organization of the acetylcholine receptors at the neuromuscular junction. These interactions probably account for a number of the secondary changes in protein expression that are seen in DMD when dystrophin is abnormal (see below).

About two-thirds of identified mutations in the dystrophin gene are deletions, about one-third are point mutations, and a small proportion are duplications (see Brown and Lucy 1997). Point mutations are difficult to identify with

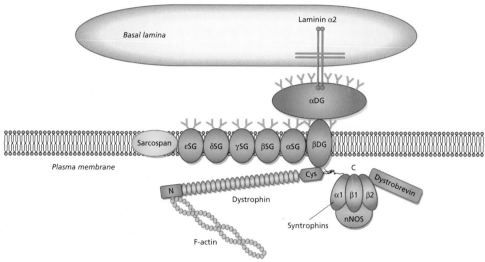

FIG. 10.12 *Diagrammatic representation of dystrophin and its associated protein complex showing how the complex links the extracellular matrix with the actin cytoskeleton. Laminin α2 in the basal lamina binds to α-dystroglycan (αDG) which binds to β-dystroglycan (βDG); β-dystroglycan binds to the cysteine rich domain of dystrophin, which in turn binds to the actin cytoskeleton. There are actin binding sites in the N- and C-terminal domains. The sarcoglycans (α, β, γ, δ, ε SG) interact with β-dystroglycan, and sarcospan is associated with the sarcoglycans although the precise interactions of all these are not yet clear. The syntrophins bind to the C-terminal domain of dystrophin and nNOS and dystrobrevin bind to the syntrophins. There is also evidence of a direct interaction of β-dystroglycan with F-actin (not shown; Chen et al 2003).*

standard polymerase chain reactions (PCR) but immunohistochemistry easily identifies all mutations that lead to a stop codon and result in an absence of protein (see below). There is no correlation between the size or type of mutation and severity; some extensive deletions have been identified in BMD patients (England et al 1990), whereas point mutations can cause DMD. A mutation may occur in any part of the gene but two 'hot-spots' where mutations are clustered have been identified. One involves exon 44 (the common mutation causing BMD is a deletion of exons 45–47), the other involves exons 2–7.

Mutations affect the amount of protein formed. In most cases of DMD dystrophin is not detected on the majority of fibres. In contrast, most cases of BMD show reduced and/or uneven labelling of muscle fibres (Fig. 10.13). This difference is explained by the effect the mutation has on the reading frame and whether it halts or maintains transcription. In the majority of DMD cases the reading frame is disrupted, while in BMD it is maintained, allowing RNA to be transcribed and translated into protein (Fig. 10.14). About 95% of cases conform to this dogma but there are several exceptions. Thus, it is unreliable to make a diagnosis of DMD or BMD based only on molecular analysis, emphasizing the importance of examining protein expression in muscle biopsies. Notable exceptions to the reading frame hypothesis are cases with deletions of exons 3–7, which is a frame-shift deletion and should result in no expression of dystrophin

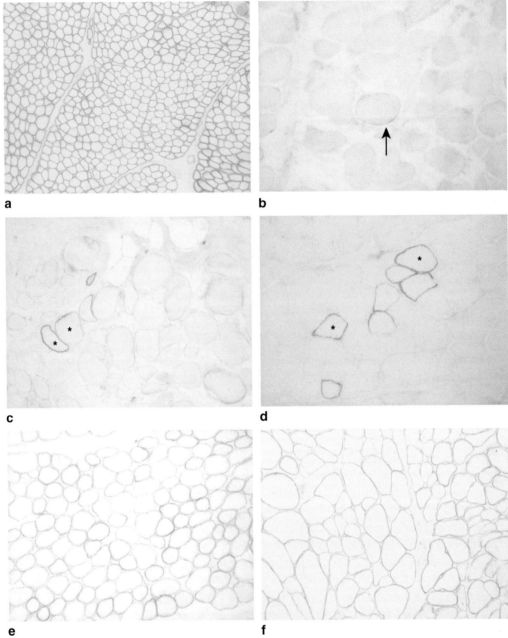

FIG. 10.13 *Immunolabelling of dystrophin using a peroxidase label in (a) control muscle, (b)–(d) three cases of Duchenne muscular dystrophy and (e), (f) two cases of Becker muscular dystrophy. Note the normal sarcolemmal labelling in (a) which was labelled at the same time as (b) which shows virtually no dystrophin except very slight traces on an occasional fibre (arrow); (c) shows revertant fibres (*) some of which are not completely labelled and traces of dystrophin on several fibres; in (d) there is only labelling of revertant fibres (*); (e) and (f) show reduced and uneven labelling of several fibres. Fibre size ranges: (a) 10–30 μm, (b) 20–45 μm, (c) 15–90 μm; (d) revertants 20–35 μm; (e) 15–30 μm; (f) 25–105 μm. A counterstain has intentionally not been used on these sections to make the low levels of dystrophin easier to see.*

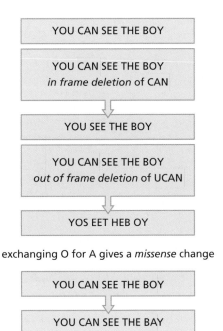

FIG. 10.14 *Diagram to explain the reading frame hypothesis. Each amino acid is coded by a triplet of nucleotides, represented here by words of three letters. If some letters (nucleotides) are deleted but the 'message' is still intelligible when the letters regroup into threes the deletion is said to be 'in-frame'. If rearrangement of the letters following a deletion results in nonsense the message comes to a stop and is said to 'out-of-frame'. Some mutations result in the replacement of a single letter (nucleotide) which can change a word (amino acid). This is a missense mutation the effect of which depends on the importance of the word (amino acid) within the 'message' as a whole.*

and a severe phenotype. These cases, however, show some expression of protein because splicing restores the reading frame (Fig. 10.15; Gangopadhyay et al 1992). These patients often have a phenotype intermediate between Duchenne and Becker dystrophy. Other exceptions also involve 5′ exons, around exon 3, and cases with very large deletions (Muntoni et al 1994a). In general, most cases of DMD show an absence of the C-terminus, whilst in most cases of BMD it is preserved. Exceptions, however, have been reported (Gangopadhyay et al 1992, Clemens et al 1992, Helliwell et al 1992a, Goldberg et al 1998).

Very low levels of dystrophin expression can be detected in some DMD cases, probably from minor transcripts of the gene (see Fig. 10.13b,c), and dystrophin is particularly prominent on fibres known as 'revertant' fibres (Fig. 10.13c,d). The expression on these fibres is of normal intensity and arises from restoration of the reading frame. It is still a matter of debate whether the restoration is a genomic event, or if it results from exon skipping. The size of the dystrophin protein varies between revertant fibres, suggesting different splicing events in the gene, but fibres in a single cluster tend to be similar (Lu et al 2000). Thus not all revertant fibres are labelled with all antibodies to dystrophin. They all lack the region corresponding to the deletion. The number of revertant fibres in a biopsy is variable; some have none, others a few isolated ones, and others have

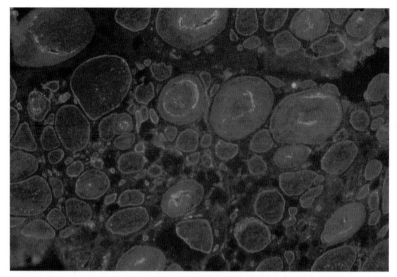

FIG. 10.15 *Immunofluorescent labelling of dystrophin in a case with a deletion of exons 3–7. This is an out-of-frame deletion but the reading frame has been restored by splicing resulting in some expression of dystrophin. The phenotype of this patient was intermediate between Duchenne and Becker muscular dystrophy and he was still ambulant at 16 years of age.*

several in clusters. The number has been reported to show no correlation with severity (Fanin et al 1992), but in limited biopsy samples this is difficult to assess accurately. In some fibres only a focal portion of the sarcolemma may appear to be 'revertant' and it may not be seen down the entire length of a fibre.

Immunohistochemistry of dystrophin in BMD patients may show uneven sarcolemmal labelling, an overall reduction on most fibres, with or without occasional fibres with intense labelling, or very little detectable difference from normal (Fig. 10.16a–d). Assessment of secondary changes (see below) and immunoblots can then be informative. Immunoblots are used to examine the quantity of a protein and its molecular mass. In BMD a deletion will reduce both, and a multiplex system enables simultaneous comparison of several proteins (Anderson and Davison 1999). Immunoblotting is rarely sensitive enough to detect a change in molecular mass in cases with a small deletion. Although immunoblotting is a powerful tool, as with all techniques, it must be correctly controlled. In practice it is rarely of diagnostic value to assess dystrophin by immunoblotting in cases of DMD as the absence of protein can easily be shown on sections by immunohistochemistry. Some cases of DMD show a faint band of dystrophin on blots and it has been suggested the quantity may explain some of the variation in severity in DMD (Nicholson et al 1993a,b). Many BMD patients have a deletion in the rod domain 'hot-spot' (exons 45–47) and secondary changes detected on sections will identify these (see below). In cases of BMD with a point mutation, which are not easily identified by standard molecular techniques, and with little change in dystrophin detectable on blots, secondary changes may be helpful in differential diagnosis (see below and Ch. 11).

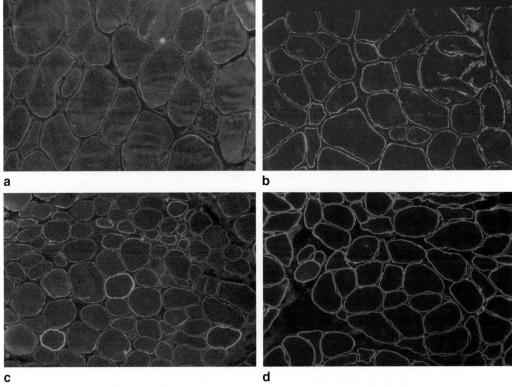

FIG. 10.16 *Immunofluorescent labelling of dystrophin to show the variable amount that can be seen in Becker muscular dystrophy patients. In (a) labelling is weak and uneven on several fibres; (b) shows a little more but labelling is still weak; in (c) most fibres are moderately labelled and a few show an almost normal intensity and might have different exons present in a similar way to revertant fibres; in (d) it is difficult to distinguish labelling from normal.*

As the position and size of the mutations in the dystrophin gene vary it is essential to use antibodies that correspond to more than one domain, to avoid false-negative results. If a deletion encompasses the epitope of an antibody, labelling cannot occur and might give the impression of DMD. A mutation that maintains the reading frame, however, will preserve the C-terminal region, in keeping with BMD (Fig. 10.17). Exon specific antibodies can be useful in identifying the region of a small deletion (Thanh et al 1995). In practice, it is common to use antibodies to an N-terminal, rod and C-terminal domain (see Ch. 6). As mentioned previously, an important role of immunocytochemistry is shown in DMD cases where the deletion cannot easily be detected by standard molecular techniques. In these cases the absence of protein is easy to detect by immunohistochemistry.

It is important to always assess the integrity of the plasma membrane when assessing dystrophin, as this may be damaged for a variety of reasons and proteins associated with it are then undetectable. Parallel studies with an antibody to β-spectrin have become the standard for assessing the preservation of the plasmalemma and the periphery of each fibre is intensely labelled (Fig. 10.18). Exceptions, however, are necrotic fibres, which often lose their plasma membrane, and small regenerating fibres that may show weak labelling of β-spectrin (Fig. 10.18).

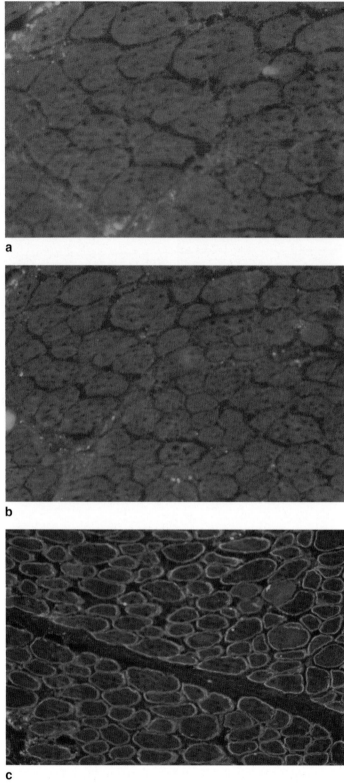

a

b

c

FIG. 10.17 *This patient had a large deletion that removed the epitopes for the DYS3 and DYS1 antibodies from Novocastra so there is no labelling of dystrophin in (a) or (b). The C-terminal domain shown labelled with DYS2 in (c) was still present. This case shows the importance of using antibodies to N- and C-terminal domains. This patient was an exception to the reading frame hypothesis and had a severe phenotype despite the presence of C-terminal dystrophin.*

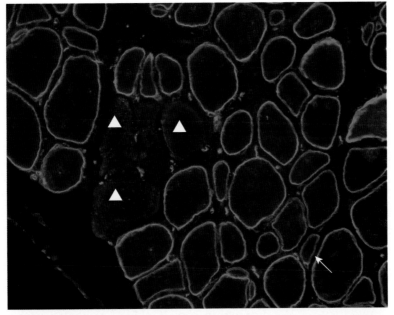

a

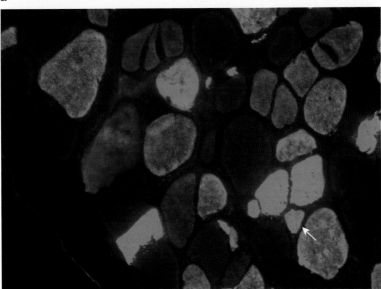

b

FIG. 10.18 *Serial areas labelled with antibodies to (a) β-spectrin and (b) neonatal myosin. Spectrin is absent from necrotic fibres (▲) and low on some small fibres regenerating fibres that show neonatal myosin (arrow). Normal sarcolemmal labelling is apparent on most fibres indicating that the cytoskeleton is preserved on the majority of fibres. Fibre size range 15–85 μm.*

X-linked cardiomyopathy

Some cases of cardiomyopathy with minimal skeletal muscle weakness are caused by mutations in the dystrophin gene (Ferlini et al 1999). Skeletal muscle biopsies show near normal immunolabelling of dystrophin but it is abnormal in cardiac muscle. Products from C-terminal promotors may be detected in the heart and also utrophin (Muntoni et al 1995b). In cardiac muscle, in contrast to skeletal muscle, sarcolemmal proteins are also detectable on T tubules. The difference in dystrophin expression in these rare X-linked cases has been explained by differential splicing in skeletal and cardiac tissue. Muntoni et al (1995b) showed that a mutation in the promotor in exon 2 gave rise to different events in skeletal and cardiac muscle. In skeletal muscle a splicing event occurred that allowed the downstream Purkinje cell promotor to be used, resulting in good expression of this form of dystrophin. In cardiac muscle this did not occur resulting in an absence of dystrophin.

These cases of X-linked cardiomyopathy are rare, and the mutations seem to be of Italian origin. In a screen of 80 cases of cardiomyopathy by immunohistochemical studies of cardiac samples, we did not find any that appeared to be caused by mutations in the dystrophin gene (Gobbi et al 1998).

Secondary immunohistochemical changes in Duchenne and Becker muscular dystrophy

The abnormal expression of dystrophin in DMD and BMD is associated with secondary abnormalities in the expression of other proteins and these can be helpful in differential diagnosis and in distinguishing the secondary reductions that occur in some limb-girdle dystrophies (see Ch. 11). The proteins most useful for diagnosis are those of the dystrophin-associated complex, utrophin and myosin isoforms.

Dystrophin-associated protein complex

In DMD and BMD all proteins of the sarcolemmal complex associated with dystrophin show reduced sarcolemmal labelling compared with normal, although the degree of this reduction is variable. We have observed that there appears to be more retention of the sarcoglycans and β-dystroglycan in some cases of DMD than in others, but this has not been quantified and any clinical significance is not known. Antibodies to both the core protein and glycosylated epitopes of α-dystroglycan show a reduction, in keeping with an overall reduction of dystroglycan. Dystroglycan is encoded by a single gene on chromosome 3 and post-translation modification gives rise to α- and β-dystroglycan. β-Dystroglycan binds to dystrophin via its C-terminus and the transmembrane part binds to the heavily glycosylated α-dystroglycan which in turn binds to the laminin α2 chain (see Figs 10.12 and 8.1). In other forms of muscular dystrophy it is the glycosylation of α-dystroglycan that is particularly affected (see Chs 11 and 12). The

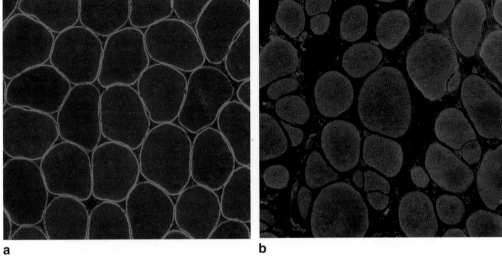

a b

FIG. 10.19 *Labelling of nNOS in (a) control muscle and (b) a case of Duchenne muscular dystrophy. Note there is virtually no sarcolemmal nNOS in the Duchenne case. Fibre size range 20–95 µm.*

syntrophins and dystrobrevin bind to the C-terminal domain of dystrophin and form a sub-complex with neuronal nitric oxide synthase (nNOS). Labelling of the syntrophins and dystrobrevins is reduced in DMD but sarcolemmal nNOS is usually absent with the antibody we use (see Ch. 6). Labelling on large blood vessels is retained, and traces may be detectable on a few fibres but generally there is very little sarcolemmal labelling of nNOS (Fig. 10.19). This is particularly useful in the diagnosis of BMD as we have found that patients with a deletion in the rod domain hot-spot (exons 45–47) also show this clear absence (Torelli et al 2004). Cases of BMD with a duplication in the hot-spot domain retain nNOS.

Utrophin

Utrophin, in contrast to the dystrophin-associated proteins, is overexpressed on the sarcolemma in DMD and BMD (Helliwell et al 1992b, Taylor et al 1997a) and it may be a useful diagnostic aid in cases of Becker dystrophy where dystrophin shows minimal reduction. The abnormal sarcolemmal utrophin expression is related to age, and cases of Xp21 dystrophies less than about 2 years of age may show very little sarcolemmal expression on mature fibres, in contrast to older cases where it is usually abundant (Fig. 10.20; Taylor et al 1997a). Although many cases of Becker dystrophy show over-expression of utrophin it is now apparent that this is not a universal feature and not specific to Xp21 dystrophies. We have also observed it in limb-girdle muscular dystrophy 2I (Sewry et al 2005a; see Ch. 11). As utrophin is also expressed on regenerating fibres, careful correlation with the expression of neonatal myosin is needed so that only the abnormal expression on mature fibres is considered. Two full length transcripts of utrophin

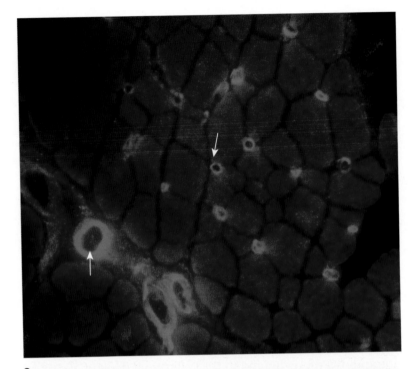

a

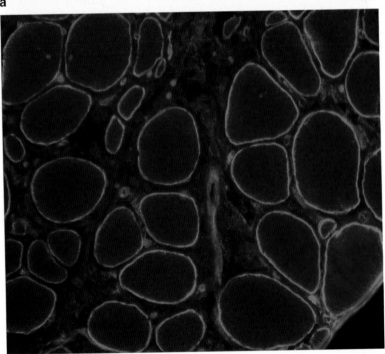

b

FIG. 10.20 *Utrophin labelling in (a) control muscle where it is confined to blood vessels including capillaries (arrows) and (b) a case of Duchenne muscular dystrophy in which most fibres show utrophin on the sarcolemma. Fibre size ranges (a) 10–20 μm; (b) 20–85 μm.*

have been identified from alternative promotors, A and B (Burton et al 1999). The isoform on the sarcolemma of fibres in DMD, on fetal muscle fibres and neuro-muscular junctions is A-utrophin. B-utrophin is confined to blood vessels (Weir et al 2002; Sewry et al 2005b).

Myosin isoforms

Embryonic and neonatal myosin isoforms are abundant in regenerating fibres. Neonatal myosin (detected by the Novocastra MHCn antibody) is expressed in an appreciable proportion of non-basophilic fibres, particularly in DMD (Fig. 10.21). Very small regenerating fibres also label with the antibody MHCd (Novocastra) and probably detect an embryonic myosin isoform. Caution in interpreting the presence of small fibres is needed as they may not be atrophic fibres if they express neonatal myosin and may be regenerating fibres. The size and number of fibres with neonatal myosin, and intensity of labelling, are vari-able in DMD and the distribution may differ from BMD. In DMD there is often a large population of labelled fibres, diffusely distributed throughout the sample. In BMD clusters of labelled fibres can be seen with very small positive fibres scattered amongst unlabelled fibres (Figs 10.21 and 10.22). Neonatal myosin is frequently co-expressed with fast and/or slow isoforms and this co-expression accounts for the poor differentiation of fibre types with the myosin ATPase tech-nique at pH 9.4 (Fig. 10.22).

Carriers of Duchenne and Becker muscular dystrophy

In the previous edition of this book details of the many changes that can be seen in carriers of DMD and BMD were given. Following identification of the dystro-phin gene, molecular analysis is now used whenever possible, particularly in cases where the mutation in the proband is known, and muscle biopsies are performed less frequently. We have retained here a summary of the histological and histochemical pathological changes in carriers and highlight the importance of dystrophin immunohistochemical analysis for distinguishing a female carrier from a female with limb-girdle muscular dystrophy.

Female carriers of DMD usually show no symptoms of the disease, but may on occasion show minor features such as enlargement of a calf muscle (often unilateral), or muscle cramps; or some may have overt muscle weakness and be as severe as a boy with DMD. The variability in the clinical and subclinical manifestations can be explained by the Lyon hypothesis of random inactivation of one X chromosome in every cell, which could be the mutated or the normal X chromosome.

CK levels are an important indicator of carrier status. Only about 70% of carriers, however, have elevated serum CK so a normal level does not exclude the possibility of a carrier. On the basis of the actual level of the normal CK,

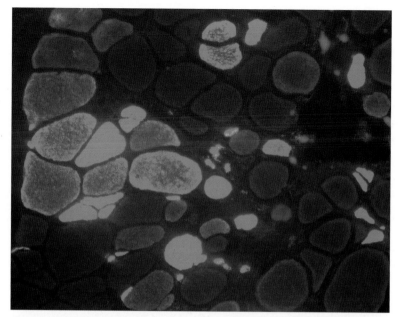

a

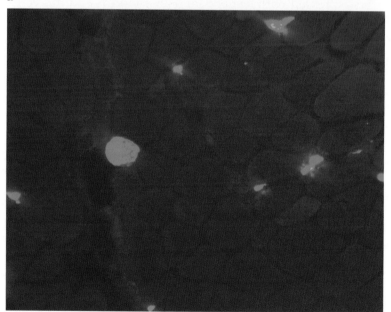

b

FIG. 10.21 *Labelling of neonatal myosin in a case of (a) Duchenne muscular dystrophy and (b) Becker muscular dystrophy. Note the many positive fibres of varying size and intensity in the Duchenne but only a few small positive fibres in the Becker.*

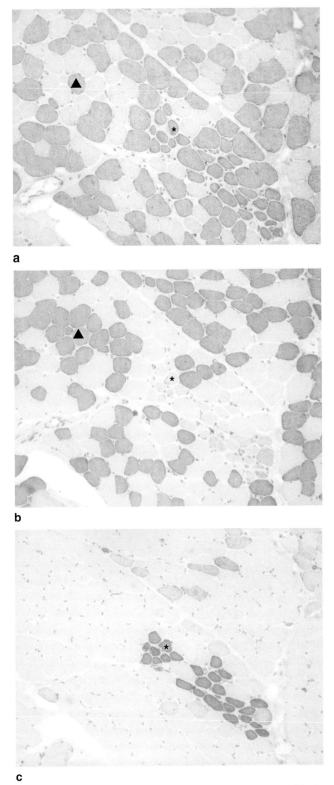

FIG. 10.22 *Labelling of serial sections with antibodies to (a) fast myosin, (b) slow myosin and (c) neonatal myosin in a case of Becker muscular dystrophy. Note the cluster of regenerating fibres (*) with neonatal myosin that also contain fast myosin and slight traces of slow myosin. Some fibres without neonatal myosin show both fast and slow myosin (▲). In this patient the hybrid fibres are of intermediate intensity with slow myosin but this is not always the case. Fibre size range of mature fibres 10–45-μm.*

taken on separate occasions, in comparison with the control range, and the application of Bayesian theory taking account of the status of relatives in the previous generations, a risk factor can be calculated for a possible carrier (Emery 1980).

Histological and histochemical abnormalities can be detected in muscle biopsies in some definite carriers but not in others. Moreover, unequivocal changes may be present even when CK levels are normal. The pathological changes include abnormal variation in fibre size, splitting of fibres, occasional basophilic fibres, internal nuclei, phagocytosis and proliferation of endomysial connective tissue, unevenness of the staining pattern with staining for NADH-TR (Fig. 10.23). Commonly, however, the features are equivocal and trying to determine their significance can be difficult. Quantitative evaluation of the changes in needle muscle biopsies from a series of potential carriers in comparison with normal female controls suggested that this approach was useful, particularly when combined with electron microscopy and CK levels (Maunder-Sewry and Dubowitz 1981).

The application of antibodies to dystrophin has had a major impact on the identification of manifesting carriers. Manifesting carriers invariably show fibres or parts of fibres that lack dystrophin (Fig. 10.24), often described as a mosaic pattern, because of the random inactivation of one X chromosome in each nucleus. It is important to establish that these fibres have a well preserved plasma membrane with parallel studies of β-spectrin (Fig. 10.24). Nuclei with the active normal X chromosome will express dystrophin in contrast to those in which the X carries a mutation in the gene for dystrophin. If there is abnormal skewing of X inactivation such that many of the abnormal X chromosomes are active then a female will manifest the disease. In asymptomatic carriers this skewing does not occur and only subtle changes in dystrophin are detectable or only occasional isolated negative fibres seen (Clerk et al 1991). These changes may be accompanied by the presence of occasional fibres with utrophin (Sewry et al 1994a). In manifesting carriers with a mosaic pattern of dystrophin utrophin is present on fibres both with and without dystrophin but expression of the dystrophin-associated glycoproteins is reduced on the dystrophin-negative fibres (Sewry et al 1994a). In our experience, if the histological abnormalities in a biopsy from a female are pronounced but dystrophin immunolabelling appears normal, the patient is unlikely to be a DMD carrier.

Morphological changes can be detected in BMD carriers but manifesting BMD carriers are rare. All daughters of affected BMD patients will be carriers and identification of the precise mutation is then important. Dystrophin expression has been studied in BMD carriers, but not extensively, and the diagnostic value of dystrophin studies in them is not clear (Glass et al 1992).

Carriers of DMD and BMD are susceptible to cardiomyopathy. Regeneration of fibres from satellite cells with a normal X in skeletal muscle will reduce the number of dystrophin-negative fibres with time. Cardiac muscle, however, cannot regenerate and X inactivation patterns probably have a greater effect with retention of the mosaic pattern. Skeletal muscle fibres are syncytial and dystrophin

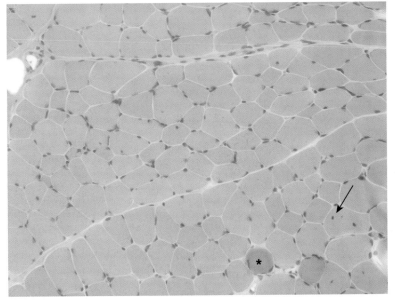

a

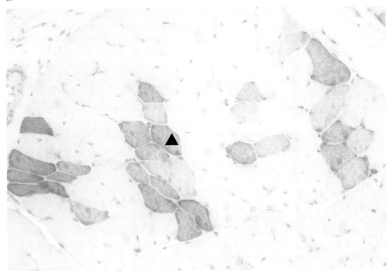

b

FIG. 10.23 *Muscle biopsy from a manifesting carrier stained with (a) H&E and (b) labelled with an antibody to neonatal myosin. Note the pathological features of variation in fibre size, internal nuclei (arrow), hypercontracted fibres (*) (fibre size range 20–65-μm) and the clusters of fibres with neonatal myosin (▲). (Fibre size range 15– 40 μm.)*

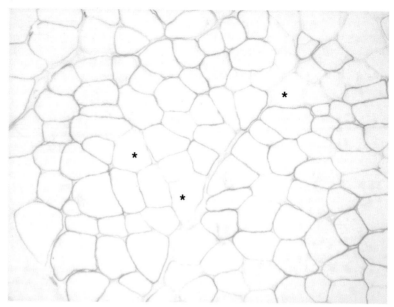

a

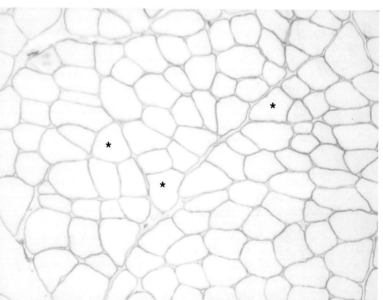

b

FIG. 10.24 *Serial sections labelled with antibodies to (a) dystrophin and (b) β-spectrin in the manifesting carrier of Duchenne muscular dystrophy shown in Fig. 10.23. Note the reduced or absent dystrophin but presence of β-spectrin on several fibres (*). Fibre size range 30–70 µm.*

produced from normal nuclei can, to some extent, spread down a fibre to compensate for the abnormal nuclei.

Females with Duchenne muscular dystrophy

Although DMD is a recessive X-linked disorder, females with a chromosomal translocation affecting the dystrophin locus will manifest the disease and be as severely affected as an affected boy. Such females were crucial to the identification of the gene locus (see Emery 1993). Muscle biopsies from these females show the typical morphological features of DMD. As the X chromosome carrying the translocation is usually the active chromosome, dystrophin is absent in muscle biopsies from these females, but it is not certain if this is a feature of all cases with a translocation.

CHAPTER 11

Muscular dystrophies and allied disorders II: Limb-girdle muscular dystrophies

Background

Heterogeneity in the muscular dystrophies has long been recognized (Erb 1884). The wide application of molecular techniques and the Human Genome Project has identified a growing number of clinical entities and their gene and protein defects. The limb-girdle muscular dystrophies (LGMD) are a diverse group of disorders with either autosomal dominant or autosomal recessive inheritance (Table 11.1). Dominant forms have been classified as LGMD1 and recessive forms as LGMD2. An alphabetical suffix has been assigned for each locus and allows for addition of new discoveries. Currently 7 dominant and 11 recessive forms caused by mutations in different genes have been identified. The common clinical feature of all LGMDs is progressive weakness of the pelvic and shoulder muscles, although distal wasting in the lower limbs is also a feature of some (e.g. LGMD2A, calpainopathy and LGMD2B, Miyoshi myopathy, dysferlinopathy). The facial muscles are not usually involved. Other features are variable and we have attempted to summarize those that can alert the pathologist to a particular type of LGMD (Table 11.2). Detailed clinical details of each type of LGMD is beyond the scope of this book and can be found in various textbooks and reviews (e.g. Bushby 1999, Karpati et al 2001, Piccolo et al 2002). Difficulties in classification of LGMDs arise because of allelic variations with clinical extremes or clearly different phenotypes resulting from defects in the same gene. For example mutations in the gene encoding the fukutin-related protein (FKRP) cause LGMD2I and a severe form of congenital muscular dystrophy (MDC1A; see Ch. 12); the gene for dysferlin is responsible for LGMD2B presenting with limb-girdle weakness and for Miyoshi myopathy, which presents with selective distal weakness. Genotype–phenotype correlations and a broadening of our understanding of pathogenesis are beginning to clarify aspects of this but the mechanisms of gene modification are still far from understood. In this book we have adhered to a clinical classification, rather than one based on the protein defect, as the clinical features are fundamental to diagnosis, and direct molecular analysis and patient management (see Ch. 8).

TABLE 11.1 *Distinct limb-girdle muscular dystrophies (LGMD) and their gene and protein defects*

LGMD	Gene locus	Defective protein
Dominant forms		
LGMD1A	5q31	Myotilin
LGMD1B	1q11-q21	Lamin A/C
LGMD1C	3p25	Caveolin-3
LGMD1D	6q23	?
LGMD1E	7q	?
LGMD1F	7q 32.1-q32.2	?
LGMD1G	4q21	?
Recessive forms		
LGMD2A	15q15.1	Calpain-3
LGMD2B/Miyoshi	2p13	Dysferlin
LGMD2C	13q12	γ-Sarcoglycan
LGMD2D	17q 12-q21.33	α-Sarcoglycan
LGMD2E	4q12	β-Sarcoglycan
LGMD2F	5q33-q34	δ-Sarcoglycan
LGMD2G (very rare)	17q11-q12	Telethonin
LGMD2H (very rare)	9q31-q34	TRIM 32
LGMD2I	19q13.3	Fukutin-related protein
LGMD2J (very rare)	2q31	Titin
LGMD2K	9q34	POMT1

Histology and histochemistry

The overall pattern of pathology is usually dystrophic with variation in fibre size, necrosis and regeneration, splitting and branching of fibres, internal nuclei, and often an increase in connective tissue and architectural change. As with all muscle disorders, the degree of pathology does not correlate with clinical severity. It is not possible to classify a case of LGMD, or distinguish LGMD from

TABLE 11.2 *Main features of limb-girdle muscular dystrophies*

Onset

Childhood or adult

Clinical features

Difficulty with gait, running, climbing steps

Lordosis

Variable progressive weakness, may be as severe as Duchenne

Tightening of Achilles tendons (toe-walking)

Inability to walk on toes (LGMD2B/Miyoshi only)

Scapular winging (prominent in LGMD2A and LGMD2C–2F)

Muscle hypertrophy in some

Calf wasting (LGMD1A, LGMD2A)

Cramp on exercise (especially LGMD2C–2F and 2I)

Ambulation

Often retained but may be lost

Creatine kinase

Mild to gross elevation; moderate in dominant forms; very high in LGMD2B and 2I

Associated features

Cardiomyopathy common in dominant forms, and LGMD2E, 2F, and 2I

Pathology

Necrosis, regeneration, fibrosis, wide variation in fibre size

Lobulated fibres (common in LGMD2A)

Abnormalities in expression of primary defective protein immunohistochemically; immunoblot analysis very important; secondary alterations in protein expression of diagnostic value

Duchenne muscular dystrophy (DMD) or Becker muscular dystrophy (BMD) or a carrier of DMD, based on histology and histochemistry alone and immunohistochemistry is essential.

Changes in fibre size

Fibres may be round in shape and all forms show an abnormal variation in fibre size that is usually obvious (Fig. 11.1). Hypertrophied fibres are common and this may be marked, especially in some adults. The hypertrophied fibres often show splits or appear branched in longitudinal sections. Some of the size variation seen in transverse sections is due to this branching. In contrast to DMD, the hypertrophied fibres are rarely hypercontracted and heavily stained in LGMD. Groups of small fibres, as in BMD, are not usually seen, but can occur. Multiple splitting may sometimes give the impression of a group of small fibres (Fig. 11.2). In cases of LGMD1B we have noted a tendency for the type 1 fibres to be generally smaller in diameter than type 2 (Sewry et al 2001a) but this is not a specific feature.

Changes in fibre typing

As with many muscular dystrophies, type 1 fibres (with slow myosin) are often predominant and fibre typing may be more distinct than in DMD (see Fig. 11.5b). With adenosine triphosphatase (ATPase) type 2B fibres may be deficient but it is not clear how this observation relates to myosin content as many fibres co-express more than one form of myosin isoform (see below).

Nuclear changes

Internal nuclei can be profuse is some cases and multiple within the cross-section of one fibre (Fig. 11.3a). As with DMD, nuclei are often associated with the internal splits in a fibre (Fig. 11.3b). Nuclear clumps may be seen in chronic cases. The nuclei of regenerating, basophilic fibres may be large (Fig. 11.1b) and vesicular with a prominent nucleolus and pale nucleoplasm.

Degeneration and regeneration

Necrotic fibres and basophilic regenerating fibres are frequently seen which may be in clusters or isolated (Fig. 11.1). Necrotic fibres are not a universal feature, which may reflect sampling problems, but a high prevalence of fibres with neonatal myosin suggests muscle damage (see below). Basophilic fibres may be less frequent than in DMD.

Cellular response

Phagocytosis is associated with necrosis. Inflammatory cells are a particular feature of LGMD2B (dysferlinopathy) and cases have sometimes been misdiag-

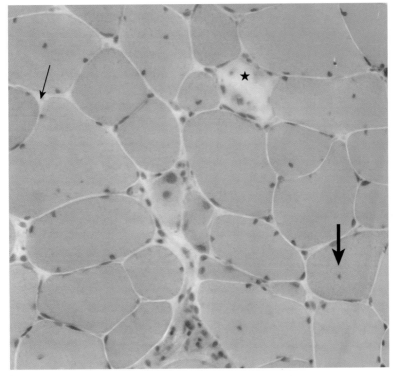

a

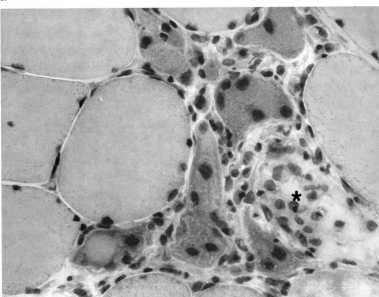

b

FIG. 11.1 *A case of limb girdle dystrophy aged 39 years showing (a) a wide range variation in fibre size (10–100 μm) with necrosis (*), excess internal nuclei (large arrow) and a little endomysial connective tissue (small arrow); and in (b) a necrotic fibre invaded by macrophages (*) and a cluster of regenerating basophilic fibres (mean diameter 30 μm) with large nuclei and surrounded by mononuclear cells of various types (H&E).*

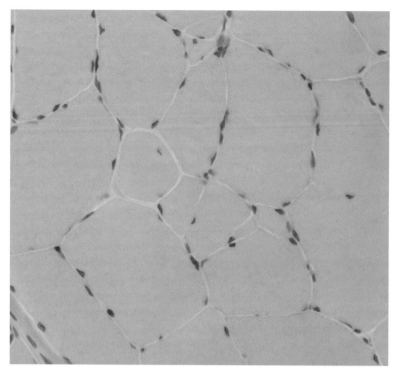

FIG. 11.2 *An area with several splits giving the impression of a group of small fibres (limb girdle dystrophy 2I; H&E). Fibre diameter range of non-split fibres 50–80 µm.*

nosed as a myositis (Fanin and Angelini 2002). Inflammatory cells are rare in other forms of LGMD but areas of necrosis may appear cellular because of regeneration and the presence of myoblasts/myotubes. Excess endomysial connective tissue is usually present but the extent is variable (Fig. 11.4).

Architectural changes

Moth-eaten and whorled fibres are common in LGMD and ring fibres may be seen. The latter, however, are not specific for LGMD. Lobulated fibres can also occur, especially in LGMD2A, but they can also occur in other disorders (Fig. 11.5a). Various degrees of aggregation of tetrazolium stain may be seen, sometimes with some resemblance to lobulation (Fig. 11.5b). Vacuoles can be observed in some cases and in LGMD1A rimmed vacuoles have been reported with basophilia around them (Hauser et al 2000).

Immunohistochemistry

Alterations in the expression of the primary protein defect of several LGMDs can be demonstrated by immunohistochemistry and immunoblotting, in particular in the recessive forms. With the large number of genes and exons involved in

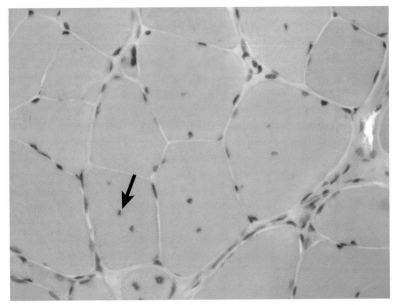

a

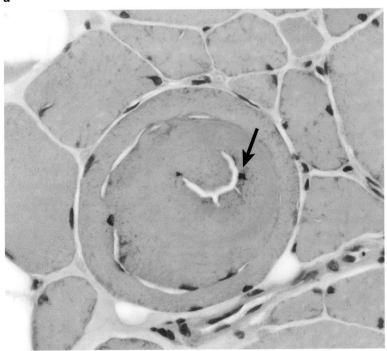

b

FIG. 11.3 *(a) Fibres with multiple internal nuclei (arrow); limb-girdle dystrophy 2I aged 13 years (H&E); fibre diameter 15–95 µm. (b) A round hypertrophied fibre with internal nuclei associated with splits (arrow); limb-girdle dystrophy 2I aged 10 years (H&E).*

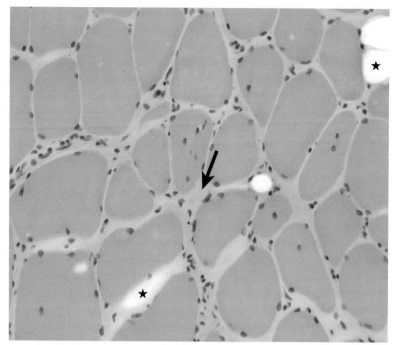

a

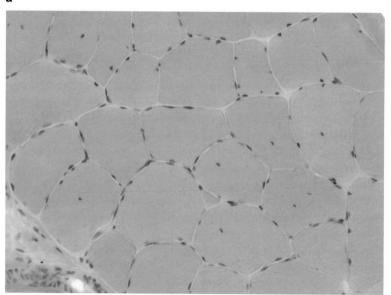

b

FIG. 11.4(a),(b) *Two cases of limb-girdle dystrophy showing different degrees of fibrosis. In (a) most fibres are surrounded by endomysial connective tissue (arrow); fibre diameter range 15–110 μm, note also a little adipose tissue (*) but in (b) there is very little endomysial connective tissue. Fibre diameter range 20–100 μm.*

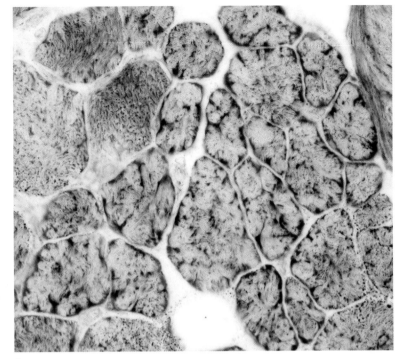

a

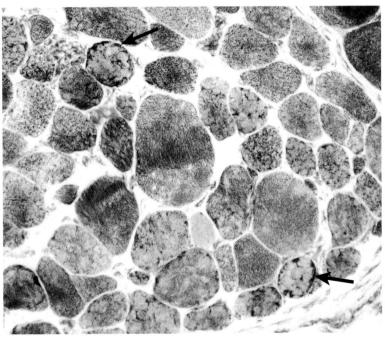

b

FIG. 11.5 *(a) Lobulated fibres (20–50 μm in diameter) in a case of limb-girdle dystrophy 2A; (b) fibres with aggregation of stain in a slightly similar manner to lobulated fibres (arrows); limb-girdle dystrophy 2C (NADH-TR). Fibre diameter range 10–90 μm.*

LGMDs, analysis of protein expression is an important way to direct molecular analysis and to identify the most likely defective gene. In this section we discuss the primary and secondary abnormalities in relation to each form of LGMD.

Dominant limb-girdle muscular dystrophies

As in many other dominant conditions, the primary defect may not lead to a detectable alteration in protein localization or quantity, as the normal allele produces a normal product. Many of the mutations are missense and protein is still formed from the mutated allele.

In **LGMD1A**, caused by mutations in the gene for myotilin, an immunohistochemical alteration can only be seen in rare cases when both alleles are affected (Hauser et al 2000). Myotilin is associated with the Z line and nemaline rods occur. There is clinical overlap with some molecularly undefined cases of adult onset nemaline myopathy which raises the possibility that myotilin might be responsible. Myotilin is also responsible for a form of myofibrillar myopathy which is clinically and morphologically distinct from LDMD1A (Selcen and Engel 2004; see Ch. 16).

In **LGMD1B** there is no detectable alteration in the expression of the nuclear protein lamin A/C or in emerin in muscle biopsies. Mutations in the lamin A/C gene are now known to be associated with a wide spectrum of clinical phenotypes in addition to LGMD1B, including autosomal dominant Emery–Dreifuss muscular dystrophy, familial partial lipodystrophy, an axonal neuropathy (Charcot–Marie–Tooth type 2B1), mandibuloacral disease and premature ageing disorders (Mounkes and Stewart 2004). There is clearly clinical overlap between LGMD1B and autosomal dominant Emery–Dreifuss muscular dystrophy, including cardiac conduction defects, and the two conditions are considered allelic.

Mutations in the gene encoding caveolin-3 are responsible for three phenotypes, **LGMD1C, rippling muscle disease and cases with persistent high creatine kinase (hyperCKaemia)**. LGMD1C is characterized by mild to moderate proximal muscle weakness and exercise-induced cramps. Cramps following exercise are also a feature of rippling muscle disease, the particular feature of which is percussion-induced muscle contraction in a rippling fashion. Patients with hyperCKaemia have minimal muscle weakness or symptoms. Reported cases of all three conditions to date are heterozygous, consistent with dominant transmission, but, in contrast to many dominant conditions, a reduction in the primary protein product, caveolin-3 can be observed with immunohistochemistry and immunoblotting (Minetti et al 1998, Hauser et al 2000, Herrmann et al 2000). The reduction is particularly pronounced in cases of LGMD1C (Ho and Brown 2002). In normal muscle, caveolin-3 is localized to the sarcolemma and labelling is normal in other forms of muscular dystrophy (Fig. 11.6; Crosbie et al 1998), and is not affected by polymorphic changes in the caveolin-3 gene (McNally et al 1998, de Paula et al 2001).

Caveolin-3 is the muscle specific member of the caveolin family, which are principal components of caveolae. Caveolae are small invaginations of the plasma

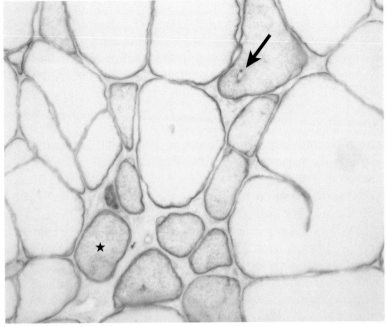

FIG. 11.6 *Normal labelling of caveolin-3 on all fibres (diameter range 20–60 µm). Note the indentation of the sarcolemma and the vacuole-like area which is probably also an indentation (arrow). The small fibres have slight internal labelling (*) and may be regenerating fibres with neonatal myosin (limb-girdle dystrophy 2I).*

membrane found in many cell types and they are believed to be involved in membrane trafficking and signal transduction (see Ch. 5). Evidence suggests caveolin-3 interacts with dysferlin and secondary changes in dysferlin occur in patients with a mutation in the caveolin-3 gene (Matsuda et al 2001, Capanni et al 2003). This interaction raises the possibility that caveolin-3 could, like dysferlin, be involved in membrane repair. The plasma membrane shows ultrastructural abnormalities when caveolin-3 is mutated (Minetti et al 2002; see Ch. 5).

The proteins responsible for **LGMD1D–1G** have, to date, not been identified and there are no immunohistochemical data in these conditions.

Recessive limb-girdle muscular dystrophies

The recessive forms of LGMD are more frequent than the dominant forms, in particular LGMD2A and LGMD2I in our patient population. LGMD2G, LGMD2H and LGMD2J are rare and have only been described in a few families. The gene defects affect a variety of proteins including an enzyme (calpain-3), myofibrillar proteins (telethonin, titin), and components of the dystrophin-associated glycoprotein complex. It remains to be seen if there is a common factor that links them.

LGMD2A is caused by defects in the gene encoding the enzyme calpain-3, which is present in the sarcoplasm of the fibre. The disorder usually has a slow progression and distal muscle involvement is common. Calpain-3 has a nuclear translocation sequence, suggesting nuclear localization, and it also binds to a C-terminal region of titin (Baghdiguian et al 1999, Sorimachi et al 1995). Commercial antibodies to calpain-3 are only suitable for studies by immunoblotting and not for immunohistochemistry, and interpretation must take account of secondary changes that can occur when the primary defect is in dysferlin, and those resulting from degradation (Anderson et al 1998, 2000, Vainzof et al 2001). A normal quantity of calpain-3 on an immunoblot does not exclude a defect in the gene (Anderson et al 1998).

LGMD2B and Miyoshi myopathy are clinically distinct but both are caused by defects in the gene for dysferlin. The differences in phenotype are not understood and can even occur within one family with the same mutation. Both are characterized by a very high CK, 10–150 times the normal level. Distal weakness and inability to walk on tip-toe are features of Miyoshi myopathy, and proximal upper and lower limb weakness develop as the disease progresses. In LDMD2B, however, proximal weakness is present at onset. Onset is usually in adolescence or early adulthood and some patients lose ambulation.

In normal muscle dysferlin is localized to the sarcolemma and a reduction in intensity of labelling can be seen in LGMD2B and Miyoshi myopathy. Some internal labelling of fibres may also occur. The commercial antibodies, however, give a clearer indication of quantity on immunoblots. As pointed out previously, immunoblots are also important for distinguishing secondary alterations in dysferlin, as these can occur when either the gene for calpain-3 or caveolin-3 is defective (Anderson et al 2000, Matsuda et al 2001, Vainzof et al 2001, Capanni et al 2003), and also in other muscular dystrophies (Piccolo et al 2000).

A secondary feature associated with defects in dysferlin is the occurrence of inflammatory cells and the sarcolemmal expression of major histocompatibility complex (MHC) class I antigens. The distinction from a myositis is then based on clinical history.

LGMD2C–LGMD2F are often referred to as the sarcoglycanopathies as the mutations affect members of the sarcoglycan complex, which is associated with dystrophin (α-, β-, γ- and δ-sarcoglycan) (Fig. 11.7). All the sarcoglycans are transmembrane glycoproteins with a small intracellular domain, a single transmembrane domain, and a large extracellular domain. The nomenclature of the sarcoglycans has been confusing and has changed and developed over the years, as additional genes have been identified. The Greek lettering (α, β, γ, δ), however, has now been uniformly adopted. Campbell and co-workers originally introduced a terminology that reflected the molecular mass of these proteins and their membership of the dystrophin-associated glycoprotein (DAG) complex (e.g. 50DAG, 35DAG; Ervasti and Campbell 1991), whereas Ozawa and the Japanese group, who had also identified the same proteins, used a numerical terminology with subdivisions with 'A' as prefix (A0–A5; e.g. A3a, A3b; Yoshida and Ozawa 1990). The first member of the complex to be identified was the 50-DAG protein

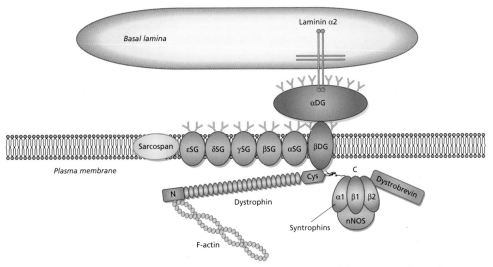

FIG. 11.7 *Diagrammatic representation of the sarcolemmal dystrophin-associated protein complex that links the basal lamina with the actin cytoskeleton. Laminin α2 in the basal lamina binds to heavily glycosylated α-dystroglycan (αDG) which binds to β-dystroglycan (βDG); β-dystroglycan binds to the cysteine rich domain of dystrophin, which in turn binds to the actin cytoskeleton. The sarcoglycans (α, β, γ, δ, ε SG) are transmembrane proteins that interact with β-dystroglycan, and sarcospan is associated with the sarcoglycans, but the precise interactions of all these are not yet clear. The syntrophins bind to the C-terminal domain of dystrophin and nNOS and dystrobrevin bind to the syntrophins. There is also evidence of a direct interaction of β-dystroglycan with F-actin (not shown; Chen et al 2003). Defects in the genes for α-, β-, γ-, δ-sarcoglycan result in limb-girdle dystrophy 2C–2F (see Table 11.2) and secondary defects in other components are involved in other forms (see text).*

(now known as α-sarcoglycan), and absence of the protein was identified before the gene was cloned. It was originally named adhalin after the Arabic name for muscle (Fardeau et al 1993). The second member of the complex to be identified was named 35-DAG, reflecting its molecular mass (now known as γ-sarcoglycan). This was followed by identification of a protein with a molecular mass of 43 kDa that was associated with 50- and 35-DAG. Confusion then arose as a different protein with a molecular mass of 43 kDa, and also associated with dystrophin, had already been named 43-DAG (now known as β-*dys*troglycan). Similarly, another protein with molecular mass of 35 kDa was identified (δ-sarcoglycan). It should be remembered that early papers on '43-DAG' are in fact referring to the protein now known as β-dystroglycan. It was soon appreciated that the proteins responsible for LGMDs act as a complex and were given the name 'sarcoglycan' with a Greek prefix (α, β, γ, δ). The dominant LGMDs were designated LGMD1 and the recessive forms LGMD2. The four sarcoglycanopathies, LGMD2C–2F, were assigned letters in the order in which the genes were identified (Table 11.3).

In smooth muscle ε-sarcoglycan replaces α-sarcoglycan and forms a different complex with β- and δ-sarcoglycan (Straub et al 1999). This raises the possibility of smooth muscle involvement in the sarcoglycanopathies and perhaps

TABLE 11.3 *The genes and proteins of the sarcoglycan complex*

Name	Gene locus	Protein	Molecular mass (kDa)
LGMD2C	13q12	γ-Sarcoglycan	35
LGMD2D	17q12-q21.33	α-Sarcoglycan	50
LGMD2E	4q12	β-Sarcoglycan	43
LGMD2F	5q33-q34	δ-Sarcoglycan	35
Myoclonus dystonia	7q21	ε-Sarcoglycan	50

explains some of the phenotypic differences between them. For example cardiac function is impaired in patients with defects in the β- and δ-sarcoglycan genes which might relate to effects on smooth muscle in the aorta (Gnecchi-Ruscone et al 1999). The cardiomyopathic hamster has a mutation in the first exon of the δ-sarcoglycan gene and is used as an animal model for this form of muscular dystrophy (Nigro et al 1997). ε-Sarcoglycan, in common with the other sarcoglycans, is present on the sarcolemma of skeletal muscle fibres but, in contrast to the others, it is also detected on blood vessels. Mutations in the gene for ε-sarcoglycan cause myoclonus-dystonia syndrome (Zimprich et al 2001, Asmus et al 2002, Han et al 2003) but there are no commercial antibodies to this protein and studies of it are limited. No pathogenic mutations have been identified in the gene encoding ζ-sarcoglycan. Similarly, sarcospan (25 kDa) is another protein thought to be associated with the sarcoglycans and is a component of the dystrophin-associated glycoprotein complex, but no pathogenic defects in its gene have been identified yet (Crosbie et al 1997).

LGMD2C is often the most severe of this group of LGMDs and has been described as 'Duchenne-like' or 'severe childhood autosomal recessive muscular dystrophy' (SCARMD), with loss of ambulation in some cases. It was first described in North Africa and a defect in the γ-sarcoglycan gene should be suspected in any LGMD patient with this ethnic origin. Mutations in the α-sarcoglycan gene can also lead to a severe phenotype. The latter are the most common and mutations in the δ-sarcoglycan gene the rarest. In the UK Caucasian population, defects in sarcoglycans are rare, but are more common in our other ethnic groups.

Immunohistochemistry has shown that the sarcoglycans act as a complex, such that a defect in one gene causes a secondary reduction in protein expression of all of them. The reduction may be minimal or pronounced as illustrated in Figure 11.8. A total absence of one sarcoglycan, or the one with most reduction, is usually indicative of a gene defect in the one that is absent (Fig. 11.9). A total absence of all sarcoglycans is more likely to indicate a primary defect in the β-sarcoglycan gene (Bönnemann et al 1995). Careful correlation with normal labelling of sarcoglycans is needed and variable affinity of each antibody must be

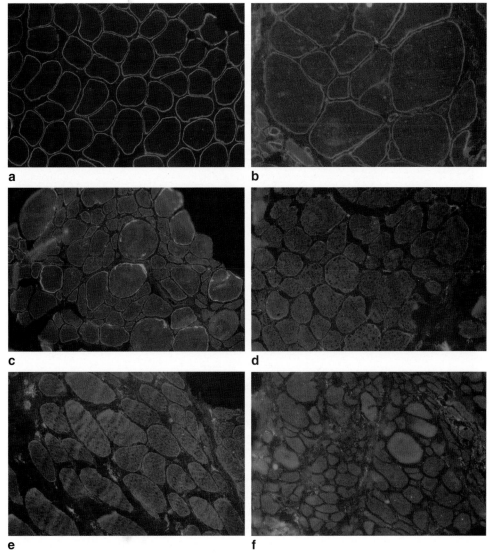

FIG. 11.8 *Immunolabelling of α-sarcoglycan showing the varying degrees that can be seen in patients with defects in the sarcoglycan genes compared with a control (a). In (b) most fibres show reduced labelling; in (c) some fibres have retained moderate labelling whilst others have very little; (d) and (e) show only very slight traces but this suggests the primary defect is less likely to be in the α-sarcoglycan gene; (f) shows a complete absence of α-sarcoglycan from all fibres in a case with a confirmed mutation in the α-sarcoglycan gene (LGMD2D). The other cases had mutations in other sarcoglycan genes and the reduction of α-sarcoglycan a secondary phenomenon.*

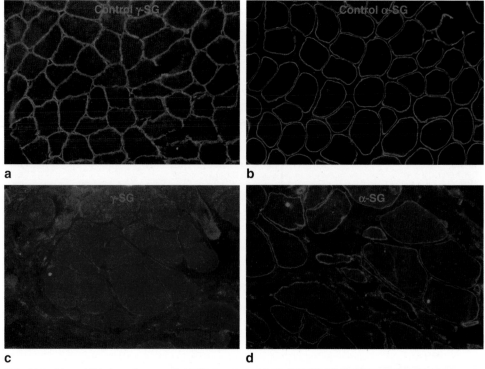

FIG. 11.9 *(a) and (b) show immunolabelling or γ- and α-sarcoglycan (γ-SG, α-SG) in control muscles with normal labelling; (c) shows absence of γ-sarcoglycan in a case with a proven mutation (LGMD2C) and (d) shows a secondary reduction of α-sarcoglycan in the same case. Labelling of β- and δ-sarcoglycan also showed a secondary reduction in this case.*

taken into account. Dystrophin immunolabelling is usually normal in sarcoglycanopathies but a secondary reduction can occur when the β-sarcoglycan gene is the primary defect. It is important to examine sarcoglycans in conjunction with dystrophin as a secondary reduction of sarcoglycans occurs in DMD and BMD. As the sarcoglycans act as a complex it is questionable whether all four need to be examined on a routine basis. It is our practice to routinely label two of them (α and β or γ-sarcoglycan) and to examine the others if results and the phenotype warrant it.

Immunohistochemistry has revealed other secondary changes. Overexpression of utrophin is rare in sarcoglycanopathies but can occur (Fig. 11.10; Sewry et al 1994c). Labelling with antibodies to myosin isoforms shows a predominance of fibres with slow myosin, several fibres of varying size with neonatal myosin (probably reflecting muscle damage and regeneration; Fig. 11.11), and co-expression of more than one isoform in several fibres.

LGMD2G is extremely rare and so far only identified in the Brazilian population. Telethonin was absent in the patients studied and no secondary defects have been reported so far. Rimmed vacuoles are a feature in this form of LGMD (Moreira et al 1997, 2000).

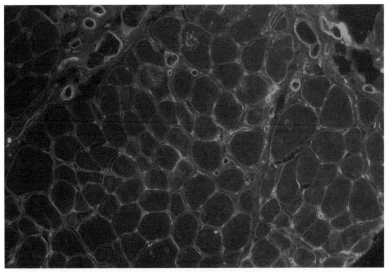

FIG. 11.10 *Immunolabelling of utrophin in a case of LGMD2C showing labelling of the sarcolemma of most fibres.*

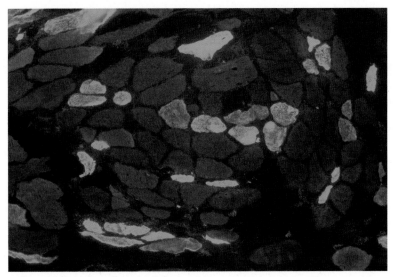

FIG. 11.11 *Several fibres positively immunolabelled for neonatal myosin in the same case of LGMD2C as in Fig. 11.10.*

LGMD2H is also very rare and so far has only been described in the Hutterite Canadian population (Weiler et al 1998). There are no reported studies on the expression of the defective protein, TRIM 32. The protein is a putative E3 ubiquitin ligase, possibly involved in the tagging of target proteins with ubiquitin ready for degradation.

In the UK Caucasian population **LGMD2I** is probably the most common form of LGMD (Poppe et al 2003). The clinical spectrum of LGMD2I is wide, even within one family, and patients can present in childhood, adolescence or adulthood (Mercuri et al 2003). Some are Duchenne-like and lose ambulation in their teens; others remain ambulant and can resemble BMD, which can be misleading. Dilated cardiomyopathy is common and respiratory failure is also a complication. The defective gene on chromosome 19 encodes a protein that has been named the fukutin-related protein (FKRP) because of its sequence homology to fukutin, the defective protein in Fukuyama congenital muscular dystrophy (see Ch. 12). Mutations in the FKRP gene are also responsible for a severe form of congenital muscular dystrophy (MDC1C; Brockington et al 2001a,b; see Ch. 12). LGMD2I patients are often homozygous or heterozygous for a common mutation (C826A, leading to Leu276Ile change; Poppe et al 2003) and the presence of this mutation seems to determine severity. It has not been found in the severe MDC1C cases. It has been suggested that this common mutation may be a founder mutation that has dispersed among populations of European origin (Frosk et al 2005). FKRP is present in many tissues with high levels in skeletal and cardiac muscle, and is targeted to the Golgi apparatus. Sequence homology suggests it is a member of the glycosyltransferase family and that it has a role in glycosylation.

Muscle biopsies show dystrophic features with variation in fibre size (see Fig. 11.3a), several fibres with neonatal myosin and fibres co-expressing more than one isoform of myosin (Fig. 11.12). Dystrophin immunolabelling is usually normal. Some cases show a secondary reduction of laminin α2 (Fig. 11.13) but this may only be apparent on immunoblots, and not on sections (Bushby et al 1998). Laminin β1 labelling on the sarcolemma may also be reduced but normal on blood vessels (Fig. 11.13). This reduction may be subtle and may only be apparent in adolescents and adults, not young children. Sometimes a reduction in laminin β1 is only seen on the sarcolemma adjacent to the perimysium on fibres at the periphery of fascicles, but it is not yet clear if this is pathologically significant (see Fig. 6.21). It is not, however, a universal feature of pathological specimens and laminin γ1 labelling on these fibres is of normal intensity. Reduction of laminin β1 is not specific to LGMD2I and has been observed in other conditions, in particular Bethlem myopathy and autosomal dominant Emery–Dreifuss muscular dystrophy. Over-expression of utrophin is often a useful secondary marker of BMD but this now appears to be less specific than originally thought, and we have noted that cases of LGMD2I can also show utrophin on the sarcolemma of mature fibres (Fig. 11.14; Sewry et al 2005a). Distinguishing BMD and LGMD2I can then be difficult but as many cases of BMD have a mutation in the rod domain hot-spot, they lack sarcolemmal neuronal nitric oxide synthase (nNOS), in contrast to LGMD2I in which nNOS is present (Fig. 11.14).

An important secondary alteration in LGMD2I is a reduction in labelling of the glycosylated epitope of α-dystroglycan. Hypoglycosylation of α-dystroglycan is now known to be a pathological mechanism in several neuromuscular disorders and several causative genes have been identified in congenital muscular dystrophies (Muntoni et al 2002, Michele and Campbell 2003; see Ch. 12). This has led to the introduction of the term 'dystroglycanopathy' but it should be

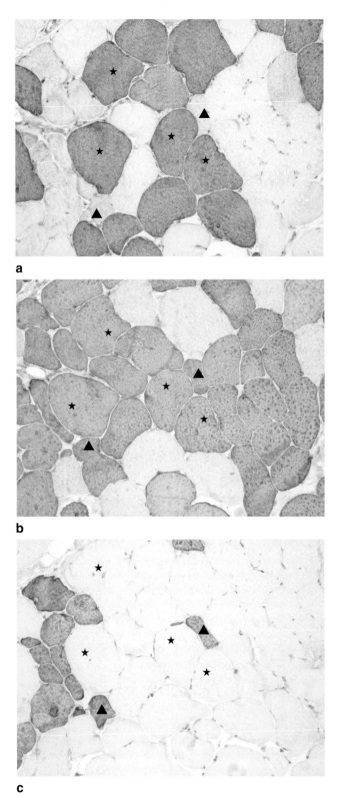

FIG. 11.12 *Immunolabelling of (a) slow myosin, (b) fast myosin and (c) neonatal myosin in a case of LGMD2I (fibre diameter range 30–140 μm). Note the fibres that co-express slow and fast myosin (*) and those that co-express fast and neonatal myosin (▲). There are no fibres in this field that co-express all three isoforms but this can occur in basophilic regenerating fibres (see Fig. 6.24).*

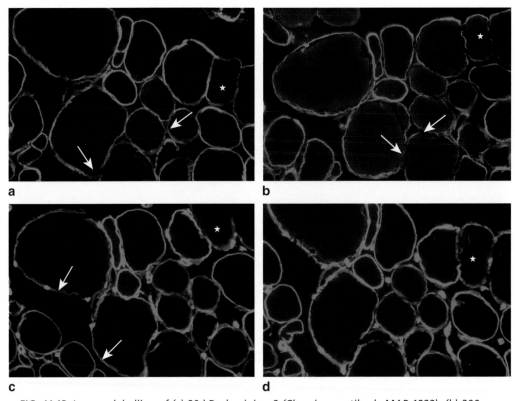

FIG. 11.13 *Immunolabelling of (a) 80 kDa laminin α2 (Chemicon antibody MAB 1922), (b) 300 kDa laminin α2 (Alexis antibody 4H8), (c) laminin β1 and (d) laminin γ1 in serial section in a 10-year-old case of LGMD2I. Note the slight reduction of laminin α2 which is more apparent with 4H8 and the reduction of laminin β1 on some fibres (arrows). Reduced laminin β1 is often not seen in children. Some fibres show a reduction of all three chains (*) and may have a damaged basal lamina or it may be pathological. Careful comparison with other antibodies that label the sarcolemma is then needed. Fibre diameter range 20–160 μm.*

remembered that the alterations in dystroglycan in all conditions is a secondary phenomenon, whereas in 'dystrophinopathies', 'sarcoglycanopathies' and 'actinopathies' the term refers to the primary defect. It remains to be established if the hypoglycosylation of α-dystroglycan is of similar importance in all phenotypes. Dystroglycan is a sub-complex of the dystrophin-associated complex and α-dystroglycan is a ligand for laminin α2. Post-translational cleavage of the gene transcript for dystroglycan gives rise to two subunits, the transmembrane β-dystroglycan subunit and α-dystroglycan, to which it binds (see Fig. 11.7). α-Dystroglycan undergoes *N*-linked and extensive *O*-linked glycosylation but to a variable extent in different tissues. The predicted molecular mass is 75 kDa but because of variable glycosylation it appears as a wide band on immunoblots and it has a molecular mass of 156 kDa in muscle but 120 kDa in brain.

Two commercial monoclonal antibodies to α-dystroglycan are available (Upstate Biotechnology, IIH6 and VIA4), which both recognize glycosylated

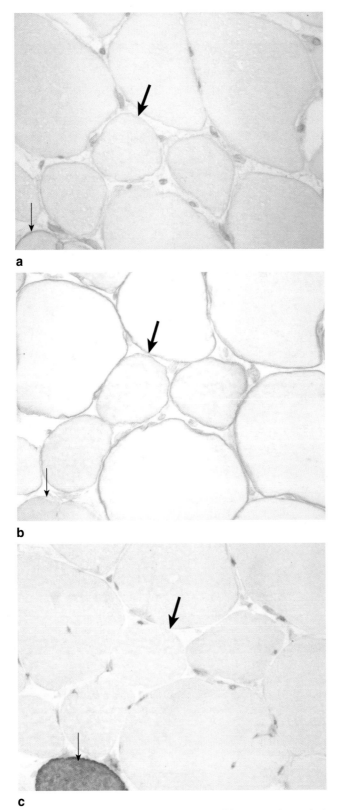

FIG. 11.14 *Immunolabelling of (a) utrophin, (b) nNOS and (c) neonatal myosin in a case of LGMD2I. Note low levels of utrophin on all mature fibres with no neonatal myosin which also show normal labelling of nNOS (large arrows). The small arrow indicates part of an immature fibre with neonatal myosin, no nNOS and slightly more utrophin. Fibre diameter range 55–90 µm.*

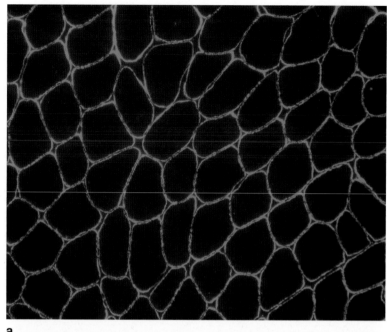

a

b

FIG. 11.15 *Immunolabelling of α-dystroglycan using antibody IIH6 (Upstate Biotechnology) showing (a) normal labelling and (b) reduced labelling on several fibres in a case of LGMD2I with a mutation in the FKRP gene (same case as Fig. 11.13).*

epitopes. Control sections labelled in parallel are essential when assessing α-dystroglycan and batches of the antibodies have been found to vary and give different results. Optimal conditions for each batch should therefore be determined. Labelling of β-dystroglycan on the majority of fibres is normal in LGMD2I and is also an important control. If the sarcolemma is damaged for any reason immunolabelling of several sarcolemmal proteins may appear reduced or absent. Dystrophin binds to β-dystroglycan and secondary changes in the latter usually only occur when dystrophin is reduced. A reduction in α-dystroglycan is apparent in most LGMD2I cases, either on immunoblots or sections. In some cases the reduction is unequivocal but in others it may be subtle (Fig. 11.15). There seems to be a correlation between clinical severity and the degree of hypoglycosylation which is less marked in cases of LGMD2I than in MDC1C, a severe form of congenital muscular dystrophy (Brown et al 2004; see Ch. 12). There are currently no commercial antibodies to the core protein of α-dystroglycan but research studies have shown that it is retained in LGMD2I (Brown et al 2004). In DMD the whole dystroglycan complex is reduced because dystrophin is absent. Thus labelling of α-dystroglycan with IIH6 and VIA4, the core protein and β-dystroglycan is all reduced in DMD.

Tibial involvement is the hallmark of **LGMD2J**, caused by mutations in the gene for titin (Hackman et al 2002, Udd et al 2005). It has been classified with other distal myopathies, including Welander myopathy and the Nonaka type, which is allelic to hereditary inclusion body myositis (Barohn and Griggs 2001). Mutations in the titin gene give rise to a late onset dominant distal myopathy, as well as this earlier onset limb-girdle form with a homozygous mutation, and cause a cardiomyopathy (Gerull et al 2002, Itoh-Sato et al 2002). Recessive LGMD2J is very rare and has been described in the Finnish population. Vacuoles may be present in the dominant form but are not a universal feature, and muscle biopsies show no accumulation of tau or β-amyloid, which are associated with rimmed vacuoles in other conditions. Titin is still detectable with commercial antibodies but an antibody raised specifically against the mutated last exon of this giant gene shows an absence (Udd et al 2005). Titin has binding sites for calpain-3 and telethonin and a secondary reduction in calpain-3 occurs in both LGMD2J and the dominant disorder caused by mutations in the titin gene.

LGMD2K. This is another rare variant, characterised by proximal muscle weakness, microcephaly, mental retardation, a hypertrophic phenotype, and marked elevation of serum CK. The defective gene is POMT1 (Balci et al 2005), which is also responsible for the Walker Warburg syndrome (see Ch. 12).

CHAPTER 12

Muscular dystrophies and allied disorders III: Congenital muscular dystrophies

History and background

The term congenital muscular dystrophy (CMD) has been widely used to describe a group of infants with weakness and hypotonia from birth or within the first few months of life. Severe, early contractures are common and most cases have delayed motor milestones. Detailed clinical studies combined with pathological and molecular studies have revolutionized this field and led to the characterization of several conditions and identified a novel pathogenic mechanism in muscle that involves the modification of proteins by glycosylation. An international consortium and workshops sponsored by the European Neuromuscular Centre (ENMC) have made a major contribution to the advances in the field (see Dubowitz 1994, Dubowitz and Fardeau 1995, Dubowitz 1996, 1997, 1999, Muntoni and Guicheney 2002, Muntoni et al 2003b). All currently identified forms have an autosomal, recessive mode of inheritance (with the exception of rare de novo dominant cases with the Ullrich form of CMD, see below). The clinical features, severity and progression are variable in the different entities (Tables 12.1–3), in particular with regard to the degree of involvement of the central nervous system.

Despite the name, and the sometimes striking pathological picture, some cases remain relatively static or progress only very slightly, and indeed some cases may actually improve with time, passing various motor milestones and even achieving the ability to walk. The muscle biopsy may look considerably worse than the clinical picture and one may be surprised that a patient with such extensive pathological change in a limb muscle may actually be ambulant. In no circumstances, therefore, should the biopsy picture be used as an index of severity of the disease or as a basis for prognosis.

To some extent the name 'dystrophy' is a misnomer, as unequivocal necrosis is not always a feature but fibrosis and the presence of adipose tissue are often marked and suggest loss of muscle fibres. It is difficult, however, to suggest an alternative name since a non-specific term such as 'congenital myopathy' is used

TABLE 12.1 *Summary of the main clinical features of the congenital muscular dystrophies associated with defects in sarcolemmal proteins*

Features common to all forms of CMD

Onset in utero, at birth or within a few months of life

Hypotonia

Muscle weakness

'Merosin deficient' congenital muscular dystrophy (MDC1A)

Never able to walk unaided, sitting achieved

Axial weakness plus proximal > distal limb weakness

Weakness usually non-progressive

White matter changes on brain MRI in all cases by 6 months

Intelligence normal but may be reduced in cases with structural brain changes

Epilepsy common

Feeding difficulties common

Spinal rigidity and scoliosis frequently develop

Respiratory complications and respiratory failure common

Pronounced elevation of creatine kinase (CK)

Ullrich congenital muscular dystrophy

Hyperlaxity of distal joints

Contractures of proximal joints

Dislocation of hips

Delayed ambulation, achieved in some but not all

Additional features:
    round face with prominent ears
    hyperkeratosis; abnormal scar formation
    respiratory complications
    prominent calcanei
    scoliosis

CK normal or mildly elevated

Integrin α7 deficiency (very rare)

Delayed motor milestones

Mild muscle weakness

CK normal

TABLE 12.2 *Summary of the main clinical features of the congenital muscular dystrophies associated with defects in proteins that affect the glycosylation of α-dystroglycan and have a secondary reduction in laminin α2*

Fukuyama congenital muscular dystrophy
Prevalent in Japan
Severe generalized muscle weakness at birth
Standing with support achieved, rarely ambulant
Progressive contractures and scoliosis
Hypertrophy of calves, quadriceps and tongue
Severe brain involvement with type II lissencephaly
Cerebellar cysts
Severe mental retardation
Epilepsy in most cases by age of 3 years
Ocular involvement in about 50% of cases
Dilated cardiomyopathy from second decade
Respiratory failure in second decade
Pronounced elevation of CK

Muscle-eye-brain disease (MEB)
Neonatal presentation
Variable severity (mild to severe)
Sitting and ambulation achieved in milder but not severe cases
Muscle hypertrophy
Joint contractures
Severe brain involvement with type II lissencephaly
Cerebellar cysts, flat brain stem
Severe mental retardation
Severe myopia and eye involvement
Epilepsy in about 30%

Walker–Warburg syndrome (WWS)
Most severe form of congenital muscular dystrophy, short life expectancy
Very severe muscle weakness at birth
Contractures at birth or soon after
Severe structural brain changes with type II lissencephaly
Cerebellar cysts, brain stem hypoplasia and hydrocephalus
Severe eye abnormalities with microphthalmia, cataracts, glaucoma, hypoplastic optic nerve
Pronounced elevation of CK

MDC1C ('FKRP' congenital muscular dystrophy)
Severe muscle weakness at birth
No contractures at birth
Sitting delayed but usually achieved
Walking with support may be temporarily achieved
Progressive respiratory muscle weakness
Hypertrophy of leg muscles and tongue
Normal brain and intelligence in milder cases
Severe cases have structural brain changes and mental retardation
Severe cases may have eye involvement and resemble MEB or WWS
Dilated cardiomyopathy
Pronounced elevation of CK

MDC1D (LARGE gene, rare, one reported case)
Severe muscle weakness at birth
White matter changes
Subtle structural brain changes
Severe mental retardation at age 17 years
Moderately elevated CK

MDC1B is not included in this table as the gene has not been identified (see text). In common with the above disorders muscle biopsies from the few cases identified show abnormal glycosylation of α-dystroglycan and a secondary reduction of laminin α2

TABLE 12.3 *Summary of the main clinical features of the congenital muscular dystrophy (CMD) with rigid spine associated with a defect in selenoprotein N1 of the endoplasmic reticulum (RSMD1)*

Axial hypotonia in first year of life

Normal motor milestones

Ambulation usually achieved and maintained into adulthood

Rigidity of spine in most cases

Progressive scoliosis

Nasal speech

Pronounced respiratory insufficiency leading to respiratory failure

Normal or mild elevation of CK

Clinical, pathological and molecular overlap with multi-minicore disease and Mallory body myopathy

Clinical and pathological overlap with Ullrich CMD (UCMD)

for conditions defined by particular structural features (see Ch. 15). The amount of actual muscle tissue is low in CMDs so there is thus some kind of 'dystrophic' process, with a reduced number of muscle fibres, for whatever reason, even though the process may not be one of necrosis.

The incidence of CMD is difficult to estimate as the identification of cases, the clinical spectrum and number of disease entities are increasing. There is also significant geographical variation in the incidence of the various forms. For example the CMD described by Fukuyama (Fukuyama et al 1960) is one of the most common forms of muscular dystrophy in Japan after Duchenne dystrophy, because of a founder effect, but is very rare elsewhere in the world. In contrast, mutations in the gene for the fukutin-related protein responsible for congenital muscular dystrophy type 1C (MDC1C) and limb-girdle muscular dystrophy type 2I (LGMD2I) (see Ch. 15) are common in the Northern European population but rare in Asia. An epidemiological study in North East Italy estimated the incidence of CMD to be 4.65×10^{-5} with a prevalence of 8×10^{-6} (Mostacciuolo et al 1996), indicating that CMD is one of the most common neuromuscular disorders. These figures are undoubtedly an under-estimate in the light of recent developments. The clinical phenotype has provided the basis for the classification of the variants of CMD and in 1994 the first ENMC workshop on CMD was convened to define and designate individual syndromes for genetic study (Dubowitz 1994). A distinction was made between 'classical' cases without intellectual retardation and structural brain changes and those with overt central nervous involvement. This was a heterogeneous group clinically, some cases being generally hypotonic whereas others had marked contractures. A proportion of cases also had changes in the white matter of the brain on computed tomography or magnetic resonance imaging. In the group with central nervous system involvement, three syndromes were identified: Fukuyama congenital muscular dystrophy (FCMD), muscle-eye-brain disease (MEB; Santavuori et al 1989) and Walker–Warburg syndrome (WWS; Dobyns et al 1989) were distinguished on the degree of mental retardation, eye involvement and structural brain changes such as cobblestone lissencephaly. A major step forward the same year was the finding of abnormal expression of laminin α2 (also referred to as merosin) in nearly half of the cases of 'classical' CMD (Tomé et al 1994). This correlated closely with the more severe cases with inability to walk unaided, contractures of the muscles, and white matter changes on brain imaging. The cause was later found to be a primary defect in the *LAMA2* gene encoding laminin α2 on chromosome 6q (Hillaire et al 1994, Helbling-Leclerc et al 1995; see below). A secondary reduction in laminins, in particular laminin α2, had already been observed in FCMD (Hayashi et al 1993) and this is now known to also occur to other forms of CMD (see Muntoni and Voit 2004; see below). The early linkage data that emerged justified the clinical division of the different forms of CMD with brain involvement. FCMD linked to chromosome 9q (Toda et al 1994), and MEB and WWS did not link to either the 6q or 9q loci, and were later shown to link respectively to regions on chromosome 1p and a separate region on 9q from Fukuyama (Table 12.4; see Voit and Tomé 2004; Muntoni and Voit 2004).

Molecular analysis soon led to the identification of the actual genes responsible for the various forms and to date defects in 12 different genes have been shown to cause a CMD (Table 12.4). These can be grouped according to the type of protein the gene encodes (Muntoni and Voit 2004); laminin α2, collagen VI and integrin α7 have an important role at the sarcolemma; *O*-mannosyl transferase type 1, 2 (POMT1, POMT2), *O*-mannosyl β-1-2-*N*-acetylglucosaminyl transferase (POMGnT1), fukutin, fukutin-related protein (FKRP) and the product of the LARGE gene have a role in glycosylation of α-dystroglycan and may act on it; and selenoprotein N1 (SEPN1) is an enzyme in the endoplasmic reticulum of unknown function. There is still further genetic heterogeneity as some cases do not carry a defect in any of the currently identified genes. As is apparent in Tables 12.1–3 there is considerable clinical overlap between the different forms and a similar phenotype may arise from a defect in more than one gene (Muntoni 2005). For example, severe cases with defects in the gene for FKRP can result in a phenotype that resembles MEB or WWS. In addition, it is not always possible to distinguish a primary gene defect that may only have a mild effect on protein expression from a secondary one. This adds to problems for the pathologist and emphasizes the importance of combining pathological and clinical data in trying to direct molecular analysis and arrive at an accurate diagnosis.

The nomenclature of the CMDs (MDC1A–1D) has been assigned by the Online Mendelian Inheritance in Man database (OMIM). As the acronym CMD had already been assigned to cardiomyopathies, MCD has had to be used. As

TABLE 12.4 *Genetically identified forms of congenital muscular dystrophy*

Common disease name	Abbreviation	Gene symbol	Gene locus	Protein	Protein type
'Merosin deficient' CMD	MDC1A	LAMA2	6q	Laminin α2	Extracellular matrix
Ullrich syndrome	UCMD1	COL6A1	21q22	Collagen VI	Extracellular matrix
	UCMD2	COL6A2	21q22	Collagen VI	Extracellular matrix
	UCMD3	COL6A3	2q37	Collagen VI	Extracellular matrix
Integrin α7 deficiency		ITGA7	12q13	Integrin α7	Transmembrane (plasma membrane)
Fukuyama CMD	FCMD	FCMD	9q31-q33	Fukutin	Possible substrate for glycosyltransferase
Muscle-eye-brain disease	MEB	POMGnT1	1p3	O-mannose β-1,2-N-actetyl-glucosaminyl-transferase	Glycosyltransferase
Walker–Warburg syndrome	WWS	POMT1 POMT2	9q34 14q24.3	Protein-O-mannosyl-transferases	Glycosyltransferase
–	MDC1B	?	1q42	?	?
–	MDC1C	FKRP	19q1	Fukutin-related protein	Possible phosphosugar transferase
–	MDC1D	LARGE	22q12	LARGE	Possible glycosyltransferase
Rigid spine syndrome	RSMD1	SEPN1	1q36	Selenoprotein N1	Glycoprotein of reticulum endoplasmic

yet, there is no neuromuscular disorder designated MDC2. The original clinical terms for the forms with severe brain involvement are still in use and clinically appropriate (Fukuyama; MEB; WWS).

We summarize here the main pathological features of muscle biopsies in the various forms of CMD but this is an ever expanding field and there are undoubtedly more features to find. For further clinical details and citation of original articles readers are referred to some of the recent reviews (Muntoni and Voit 2004, Voit and Tomé 2004, Muntoni et al 2004, Jimenez-Mallebrera et al 2005).

General pathological features of congenital muscular dystrophies

As the various forms of CMD share common pathological features, we summarize these collectively here and then cover the individual disorders together with the application of immunohistochemistry. It is not possible to identify a particular form of CMD from the histological and histochemical features alone. Representative views of the typical features seen in CMDs are shown in Figure 12.1.

All CMDs show an abnormal variation in fibre size and the shape of the fibres is often rounded. Fibre atrophy is common and hypertrophied fibres, which may be split, occur in some cases. Internal nuclei occur but are not numerous. The amount of fibrosis and adipose is variable but both may be very extensive. The presence of endomysial connective tissue around individual atrophic fibres can help distinguish these fibres from the group atrophy seen in spinal muscular atrophy (SMA). One biopsy in our series of 'merosin deficient' MDC1A cases had a surprising similar histological appearance to a case of SMA but the grouped atrophic fibres were surrounded by endomysial connective tissue (Fig. 12.2).

Necrotic fibres and basophilic regenerating fibres may be seen, particularly in early stages of the disease, but not in all cases. Inflammation is rare but there has been a report of a case where it was sufficient to suggest an inflammatory myopathy (Pegoraro et al 1996). Fibre typing with histochemical techniques may be indistinct or show a predominance of type 1 fibres. Oxidative enzyme staining may show disruption of myofibrils and abnormalities in mitochondrial distribution, including aggregation or minicores (Fig. 12.1g,h). Both these have been noted in particular in Ullrich CMD and the form associated with rigid spine (RSMD1), caused by mutations in the genes for collagen VI and SEPN1, respectively.

In addition to focal myofibrillar disruption (minicores), electron microscopy reveals abnormalities of the basal lamina (Minetti et al 1996, Ishii et al 1997, Yamamoto et al 1997, Saito 1999) and Fardeau et al 1978a observed that there were fewer satellite cells in CMD patients compared with controls.

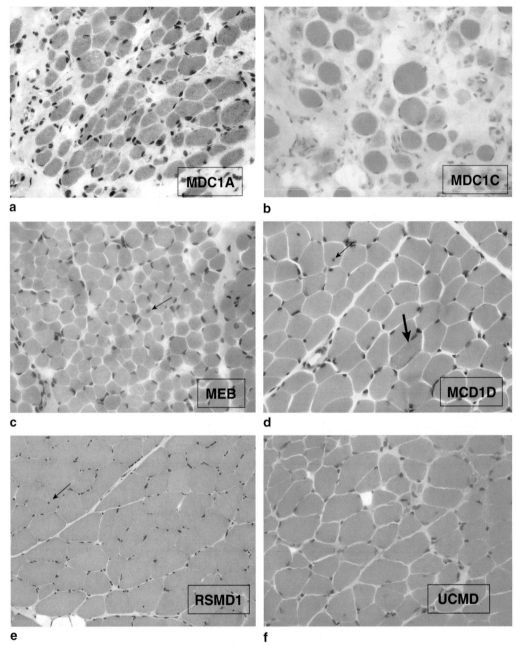

FIG. 12.1(a)–(h) *Representative views from various forms of congenital muscular dystrophy showing the general features. (a) Merosin deficient CMD (MDC1A); (b) MDC1C (fukutin-related protein); (c) muscle-eye-brain disease (MEB); (d) MDC1D (LARGE); (e) and (g) a case of rigid spine with muscular dystrophy (RSMD1); (f) and (h) two cases of Ullrich congenital muscular dystrophy (UCMD); (a)–(f) Haematoxylin and eosin (H&E); (g) and (h) NADH-TR. Variation in fibre size is present in all of them and there is a variable amount of endomysial connective tissue and occasional internal nuclei (small arrows). (d) Occasional basophilic slightly granular fibres are shown (large arrow).*

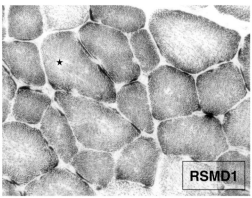
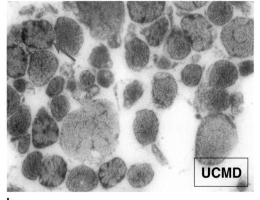

RSMD1

UCMD

g   h

FIG. 12.1 *Continued in (g) note the unevenness of stain in several fibres (*) and (h) the aggregation of stain, resembling that seen in lobulated fibres (red arrow).*

Congenital muscular dystrophies associated with sarcolemmal proteins

A primary deficiency of laminin α2 ('merosin deficiency'; MDC1A) is caused by a mutation in the *LAMA2* gene on chromosome 6q. It has been quoted as representing 30–40% of all cases and being one of the most common forms. This figure, however, was based on the original screening by various international groups, before the identification of other causative genes. From the experience of our own patient pool we have had very few new cases with a LAMA2 defect in recent years but an increasing number with other gene defects, especially collagen VI, responsible for the Ullrich form of CMD (see below).

Cases of MDC1A invariably present at birth, or soon after. The hypotonia and muscle weakness may be associated with failure to thrive and respiratory and feeding problems. Contractures may be present but severe arthrogryposis is rare. Patients with a complete absence of laminin α2 protein rarely achieve the ability to walk independently but are usually able to sit unsupported. Those with only a partial reduction of protein usually show a milder phenotype (Sewry et al 1997b). Thus, as with many disorders, some residual localization of protein produces a milder phenotype than a complete absence. Serum CK levels are always elevated and abnormal white matter changes are invariably seen with T_2-weighted MRI of the brain by the age of 6 months. To date, all patients with a total absence of laminin α2 and a mutation in the *LAMA2* gene have shown increased signal intensity in the white matter. Although the white matter changes resemble a leukodystrophy with dysmyelination, loss of myelin has not been shown, and the abnormalities most likely represent abnormal myelination rather than loss of myelin. Some cases also show structural brain changes but not of the type in other forms of CMD (Philpot et al 1999; Table 12.1).

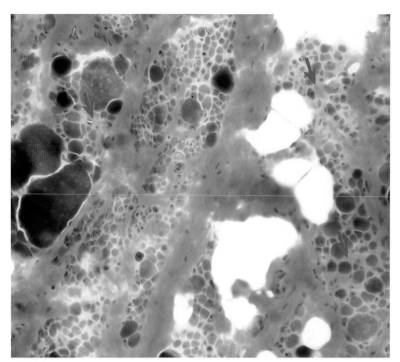

FIG. 12.2 *A case of merosin deficient CMD (MDC1A) showing large groups of atrophic fibres and hypertrophic fibres. Although the appearance is a little similar to spinal muscular atrophy there is obvious connective tissue between the atrophic fibres (arrows) and the hypertrophic fibres are hypercontracted and heavily stained which distinguish it as a CMD (Gomori trichrome).*

Laminins are components of the basal lamina and all 12 variants that have been identified are composed of a heterotrimer of an α, β and γ chain. The increasing diversity of laminin variants led to a numbering system for the nomenclature of each heterotrimer, replacing the previous names of merosin (M), laminin A, B1 and B2. The most abundant trimers in muscle are laminin-2 (merosin; composed of α2-β1-γ1 chains) and laminin-4 (S-merosin; composed of α2-β2-γ1 chains). Thus mutations in the gene for laminin α2 affect both variants. The presence of laminin α2 on the sarcolemma of cardiomyocytes probably accounts for the cardiac problems in some cases. Laminin α2 is also present on Schwann cells, in association with laminin β2 and γ1 (laminin-4), and mutations in the *LAMA2* gene affect motor nerve myelination, reducing motor nerve conduction velocities (Shorer et al 1995). Sensory nerve function, however, is unaffected. In the brain laminin α2 is present on blood vessels but it is not detected on blood vessels in muscle (see Ch. 6).

Immunohistochemical studies are essential for the analysis of all cases of CMD, to visualize and localize various proteins. Immunolabelling of laminin α2 in cases with a mutation in the *LAMA2* gene may show a complete absence, slight

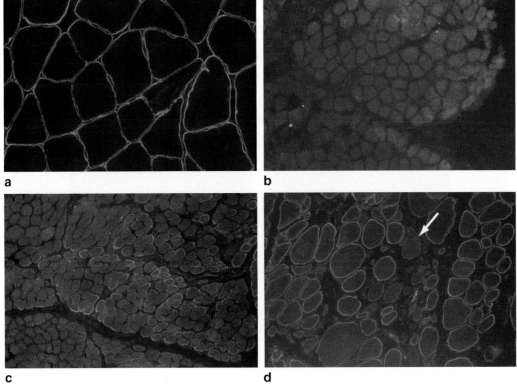

FIG. 12.3 *Immunolabelling of laminin α2 in (a) control muscle and (b), (c) and (d), three molecularly proven cases of MDC1A showing varying degrees of protein expression with a total absence in (b), traces on some fibres in (c), and partial expression in (d) (arrow).*

traces on a few fibres, or a reduction on several fibres (Fig. 12.3). The latter is often more apparent with an antibody to the N-terminal fragment of the protein (Fig. 12.4). Laminin α2 is processed into two fragments when denatured for immunoblots, one of 80 kDa and one of 300 kDa. The commercial antibody from Chemicon recognizes the 80 kDa fragment and is the only commercial antibody that works adequately on immunoblots. The antibody from Alexis (4H8) has been shown by immunoprecipitation to recognize the N-terminal 300 kDa fragment, substantiated by the studies of He et al (2001), and often shows the partial reduction of laminin α2 better than the Chemicon antibody (Sewry et al 1997b). Like the Alexis antibody to the 300 kDa fragment, the antibody from Novocastra (NCL-MER3) also shows the partial reduction better than the one from Chemicon, but this antibody does not recognize denatured laminin α2 on immunoblots and its epitope has not been mapped. Evidence from a patient with gene mutations in the *LAMA2* gene, however, indicates that the epitope is on the C-terminal LG3 or LG4 globular domain (He et al 2001). This antibody should not therefore be sited as recognizing the N-terminus, as frequently occurs in the literature.

80 kDa　　　　**300 kDa**

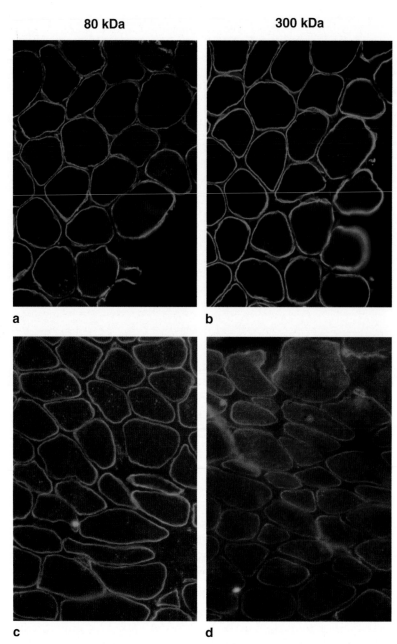

a　　　　　　　b

c　　　　　　　d

FIG. 12.4 *Immunolabelling of laminin α2 with separate antibodies to the 80 and 300 kDa fragment in: (a) and (b) a control; and (c) and (d) a case of MDC1A with a partial deficiency showing more strikingly with the antibody to the 300 fragment (from Alexis).*

It is important to examine laminin α2 on nerve axons if they are present in a sample. Normal nerves show laminin α2 round each axon and in cases of MDC1A with an absence of sarcolemmal laminin α2 it is also absent from the axons. In rare cases, however, laminin α2 may appear almost normal on the sarcolemma but be absent from the nerve (Deodata et al 2002).

In MDC1A the deficiency of laminin α2 is a primary effect caused by mutations in the *LAMA2* gene. In several other forms of CMD a secondary reduction occurs as a consequence of a mutation in another gene (see below). In milder cases it may be difficult to distinguish this secondary reduction from a primary partial reduction. An important distinguishing feature, however, is the presence of white matter changes on brain MRI, as this is a consistent feature in cases with *LAMA2* mutations, over the age of 6 months.

Secondary immunohistochemical features are of diagnostic relevance. Laminin α5 is over-expressed on mature fibres in MDC1A. This protein, however, is developmentally regulated (see Ch. 6) and is high on immature fibres (Sewry et al 1995). It is therefore important to make comparisons with an antibody to neonatal myosin so that immature and/or regenerating fibres can be excluded from the assessment. The commercial antibody that is often used (clone 4C7) was originally thought to recognize the laminin α1 chain (previously known as laminin A) but Tiger et al (1997) showed that it is probably the α5 chain that is recognized by this antibody.

No detectable difference in the labelling of laminin β1 and γ1 is usually seen in MDC1A and these can be used to control for good preservation of the basal lamina. Similarly, labelling of β-spectrin, dystrophin and its associated proteins is usually normal. In contrast, laminin β2 shows a reduction on the sarcolemma (Cohn et al 1997). Interpretation of this, however, also has to take immaturity of the fibres into consideration (see Ch. 6). The integrin complex α7β1D and α-dystroglycan are also reduced on the sarcolemma in MDC1A, which is thought to result from the deficiency of laminin α2, as both of these interact with laminin α2.

Labelling of myosin isoforms shows that fibres with neonatal myosin are abundant. As necrosis, and by inference regeneration, are not always marked features, the presence of neonatal myosin in some fibres may not always be a reflection of regeneration (see Chs 6 and 10). Biopsies from cases of CMD are often taken when they are very young and it is possible that some neonatal myosin reflects a lack of maturation. As in many muscular dystrophies, fibres with slow myosin are often predominant and some may co-express fast myosin.

Laminin α2 is also expressed in *skin* at the epidermal/dermal junction on the base of the keratinocytes, on the sensory nerves and round hair follicles (Sewry et al 1996), thus skin biopsies can be useful for diagnosis (Fig. 12.5). Skin biopsies are particularly useful in cases where muscle is not available and in cases with pronounced muscle wasting, in which a muscle biopsy is likely to yield very few muscle fibres for assessment. In some cases the reduction of laminin α2 may appear greater in skin than muscle.

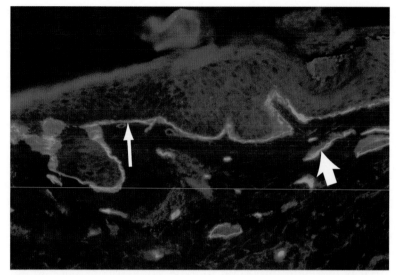

a

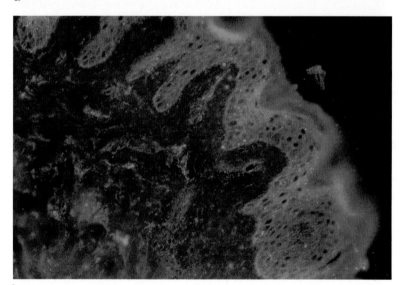

b

FIG. 12.5 *Immunolabelling of laminin α2 in skin biopsies from (a) a control and (b) a case of MDC1A. Note the positive labelling on the basal keratinocytes at the junction of the epidermis and dermis (small arrow) in the control and labelling of sensory nerves (large arrow) but a total absence of laminin α2 in the case of MDC1A at the junction.*

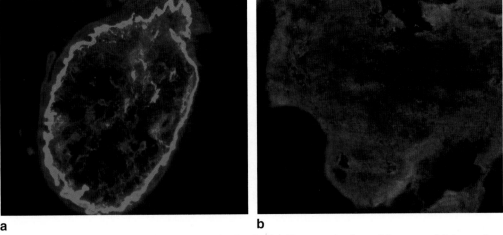

a b

FIG. 12.6 *Immunolabelling of laminin α2 in chorionic villus samples from (a) a normal fetus and (b) a fetus with MDC1A homozygous for a* LAMA2 *mutation showing a total absence of laminin α2.*

Prenatal diagnosis of cases of MDC1A is aided by studies of the expression of laminin α2 in chorionic villus samples (Naom et al 1997, Vainzof et al 2005) and affected fetuses show a complete absence of laminin α2 (Fig. 12.6). It is important, however, to establish that there is an absence, or near absence, of laminin α2 in muscle or skin in the proband, as the expression of laminin α2 in chorionic villi of fetuses with a partial deficiency is not known. Laminin β2 is also reduced in chorionic villi of affected fetuses, suggesting that as in muscle, the laminin-4 variant may have a pathogenic role as well as laminin-2 (see Muntoni et al 2003).

Ullrich congenital muscular dystrophy (UCMD) is caused by defects in the genes encoding ***collagen VI*** (*COL6A1, COL6A2, COL6A3*). These patients typically present with hypotonia and muscle weakness in the neonatal period. They often have a rounded face and prominent ears. Associated features include kyphosis of the spine, torticollis, dislocation of the hips and proximal contractures. Distal joints show striking hyperlaxity and protruding calcanei are common. Skin typically shows follicular hyperkeratosis and cheloid formation may occur. Maximum motor ability is variable with a proportion of patients never achieving ambulation. Respiratory insufficiency develops in most cases in the first or second decade. Creatine kinase levels are often normal or only slightly elevated (Table 12.1).

Early molecular characterization of UCMD cases with defects in genes for collagen VI indicated a recessive mode of inheritance (Camacho et al 2001), and it was believed that dominant mutations caused milder Bethlem myopathy (see Ch. 13). This distinction, however, is not universal and some severely affected patients with dominant mutations have been identified, as well as milder cases with recessive mutations in the *COL6A2* gene (Pan et al 2003, Baker et al 2005,

Lampe et al 2005). It is now thought that UCMD and Bethlem are part of a clinical spectrum and that the effect of a particular mutation on the production and function of collagen VI determines severity.

Collagen VI is composed of three chains, α1, α2, α3, each encoded by a different gene. Mutations in all three genes have been identified. The three chains assemble intracellularly into a monomer and prior to secretion into the extracellular space they form antiparallel dimers which then associate into lateral tetramers. In the extracellular matrix the tetramers associate end to end and form a microfibrillar network that interacts with other proteins, including fibronectin, decorin, biglycan, perlecan, collagen IV and the chondroitin sulphate proteoglycan NG2 receptor.

Immunohistochemical labelling of collagen VI can be a useful diagnostic aid as some cases show an unequivocal reduction compared to normal (Fig. 12.7). In others, however, the reduction may be subtle and may only be apparent at the sarcolemma, with normal intensity of the endomysium (Fig. 12.8). Even when endomysial collagen is increased in controls, the distinct sarcolemmal labelling can be distinguished from that in the endomysium (Fig. 12.7). Ultrastructural studies have shown that collagen VI microfibrils are absent from areas adjacent to the sarcolemma (Ishikawa et al 2002, Ishikawa et al 2004). As well as in the perimysium and endomysium, collagen VI in normal muscle is also seen round blood vessels, including capillaries, round axons and in the perineurium. In UCMD collagen VI round axons and blood vessels may be absent or reduced but this is not a universal feature. As assessment of the basal lamina is of particular importance for collagen VI, it is essential to control for good preservation. This can be done with single or double labelling with an antibody to laminin γ1, collagen IV or V, or perlecan. Although perlecan interacts with collagen VI and a secondary reduction might be expected, sarcolemmal labelling is normal when collagen VI is reduced. Damage to both the plasma membrane and basal lamina can arise from poor freezing or storage of the tissue or sections, and an absence of several basal lamina proteins in addition to collagen VI should be interpreted with caution.

Collagen VI is expressed in most connective tissues and its presence in skin can be studied immunohistochemically and a clear reduction may be seen in some affected cases (Mercuri et al 2002; Kirschner et al 2005). Normal immunolabelling of collagen VI in muscle or skin, however, does not exclude a defect in a gene for collagen VI. Research studies suggest that changes in collagen VI may be more easily observed in cultured skin fibroblasts (Jimenez-Mallebrera, personal observations) than in biopsy tissues. There is also evidence from studies of cultured fibroblasts that the interaction with fibronectin may be abnormal in some cases (Sabatelli et al 2001). Assessment of skin fibroblasts may become a useful test for directing molecular studies.

Immunolabelling of collagen VI in chorionic villus samples can also be useful for prenatal diagnosis (Brockington et al 2004; Fig. 12.9) but as with laminin α2 interpretation must be related to that in the proband and linkage data.

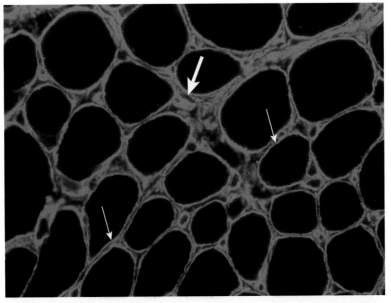

a

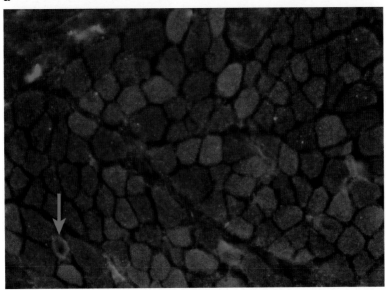

b

FIG. 12.7 *Immunolabelling of collagen VI in (a) control and (b) a case of Ullrich congenital muscular dystrophy (UCMD). Note that the labelling of the endomysial connective tissue (large arrow) can be distinguished from that of the sarcolemma (small arrows) in the control but both are absent in the cases of UCMD. The case of UCMD shows labelling of a blood vessel (green arrow) but not of the capillary network.*

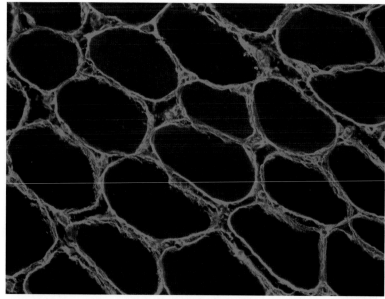

a

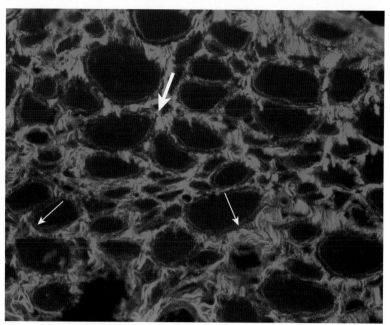

b

FIG. 12.8 *Immunolabelling of collagen VI in (a) a control and (b) a case of Ullrich congenital muscular dystrophy which shows prominent labelling of the endomysial connective tissue (large arrow) but very reduced labelling of the sarcolemma (small arrows).*

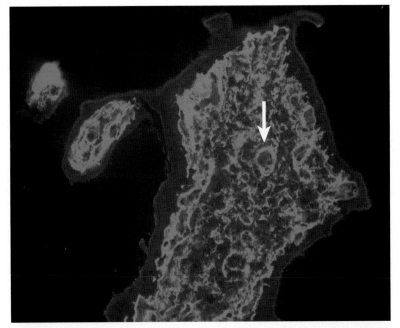

a

b

FIG. 12.9 *Immunolabelling of collagen VI in choronic villus samples from (a) a normal fetus and (b) a fetus with Ullrich congenital muscular dystrophy. Note the strong mesenchymal labelling in the control and the presence of blood vessels (arrow) but the disrupted and reduced labelling in the affected fetus.*

Integrin α7 deficiency

Integrins are transmembrane heterodimers composed of α and β chains. The complex on the sarcolemma of muscle fibres is composed of the α7 and the muscle specific β1D chains. The integrin α7 chain is a ligand for laminin α2 making it an obvious candidate for a neuromuscular disorder. Defects in the gene encoding integrin α7 result in a very rare disorder currently classified with the congenital muscular dystrophies but it is clinically and pathologically a mild myopathic condition (Hayashi et al 1998), although transgenic mice with an absence of integrin α7 show a progressive muscular dystrophy (see Mayer 2003). The patients described by Hayashi et al (1998) showed delayed motor milestones with no brain involvement, a normal CK, and only mild myopathic histological defects in the muscle, with variation in fibre size and no fibrosis or necrosis. Only three recessive cases were identified by the Japanese group. They demonstrated an absence of integrin α7 from the sarcolemma and blood vessels in an immunohistochemical screen of a large number of muscle biopsies. No additional cases have been reported since publication of the original article. Difficulties in pathological studies arise because integrin α7 appears to be developmentally regulated and is low in neonatal muscle, at a time when biopsies from CMD patients are often taken. Antibodies to integrin α7 used to date are polyclonal, limited in supply and not commercially available. Integrin β1D shows a concomitant decrease when α7 is absent, but commercial antibodies to this muscle-specific isoform are limited. Some workers, however, have used antibodies that recognize all isoforms of β1 on the assumption that the predominant isoform in muscle is β1D. A secondary reduction of integrin α7β1D occurs when there is a primary defect affecting laminin α2 expression but studies in other forms of CMD are limited by the lack of availability of suitable antibodies. Research studies, however, suggest a secondary reduction in other forms of CMD and that it may occur when α-dystroglycan is hypoglycosylated (Brockington et al 2000, Dr S Brown, personal observations). There is considerable interest in the role of integrins in many cellular mechanisms, in their various isoforms from gene splicing, and in their post-translational modification by glycosylation. It is therefore likely that a wider pathological involvement of integrins will soon be identified.

Congenital muscular dystrophies associated with abnormal glycosylation of α-dystroglycan

Post-translational modification of proteins is common, in particular by phosphorylation or glycosylation. Defects in six genes encoding proven or putative glycosyltransferases, associated with the hypoglycosylation of α-dystroglycan, have been identified (Tables 12.2 and 12.4). Alpha- and β-dystroglycan are widely expressed in various tissues and in muscle they form the central component of the sarcolemmal dystrophin-associated complex (see Fig. 8.1). They are encoded by a single gene on chromosome 3, the product of which is post-translationally cleaved to give rise to the two glycosylated products (Michele and Campbell 2003). Beta-dystroglycan is the transmembrane component, the C-terminus of which directly interacts with dystrophin, and its N-terminus is non-covalently bound to the C-terminus of α-dystroglycan. The core protein of α-dystroglycan has a predicted molecular mass of 72 kDa but variable *N-* and extensive *O-*glycosylation in different tissues increases its mass in muscle to 156 kDa and 120 kDa in brain, and on immunoblots it migrates as a broad band. Alpha-dystroglycan has a serine-threonine rich, mucin-like, domain for multiple *O-*glycosylation, which is believed to be crucial for its binding to ligands such as laminin α2. The epitopes for two commercial antibodies to α-dystroglycan, IIH6 and VIA4-1, probably lie in this region. The antibody IIH6, in particular, is known to inhibit binding of laminin α2 (Ervasti and Campbell 1993, Brown et al 1999). Alpha-Dystroglycan is an *O-*linked glycoconjugate with mannose directly linked to serine or threonine, which is very rare in mammals. Defects in the genes encoding two enzymes involved in *O-*linked mannosylation (POMT1 and POMGnT1) occur in WWS and MEB. As abnormal glycosylation of α-dystroglycan occurs in other forms of CMD and the clinical phenotypes have features in common, the defective proteins are predicted to be involved in some way in *O-*linked mannosylation (Fig. 12.10). The precise function of these putative glycosyltransferases, however, remains to be proven. These CMDs, in which mental retardation and neuronal migration are key features, (FCMD, MEB, WWS, MDC1C and MDC1D), are now often referred to as ***dystroglycanopathies***, reflecting the importance of this secondary alteration in α-dystroglycan in the pathogenetic mechanism. Mutations in the *DAG1* gene itself encoding dystroglycan have not yet been found in humans and may be embryonically lethal, as shown in mice where disruption of the assembly of the early basement membrane (Riechert's membrane) occurs (Williamson et al 1997). A secondary reduction of both α- and β-dystroglycan occurs when dystrophin is reduced in Duchenne muscular dystrophy, but in this group of CMDs it is the hypoglycosylation of α-dystroglycan that is believed to be responsible for the phenotype and β-dystroglycan expression is usually normal. Pathological studies of α-dystroglycan in human samples have made a major contribution to the identification of this key target. Research studies using non-commercial antibodies have shown that reduced sarcolemmal labelling of the core protein of α-dystroglycan also occurs in some dystroglycanopathies (see below), but it is not clear if this is always a reflection of a reduced quantity of protein or if epitope masking may be occurring, as immunoblotting studies with these antibodies are limited.

We summarize here the immunohistochemical abnormalities and current understanding of this newly emerged group of CMDs. The proteins of the six identified genes are proven (POMT1, POMT2, POMGnT1) or putative (fukutin, FKRP) glycosyltransferases, or facilitate proper glycosylation of α-dystroglycan (LARGE). There is considerable clinical and pathological overlap in these disor-

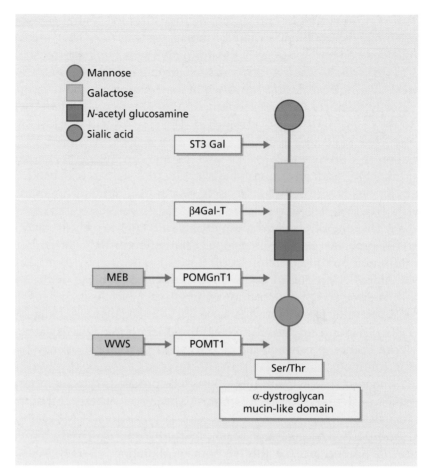

FIG. 12.10 *Schematic representation of the O-mannosyl glycan modification of α-dystroglycan and the position of enzymes responsible for two forms of congenital muscular dystrophies.*

ders and there is undoubtedly further genetic heterogeneity, as cases with phenotypic and pathological similarity to the dystroglycanopathies show no defects in the known genes (in the coding sequences). Interactions between the various proteins involved in glycosylation of α-dystroglycan have been suggested (Michele and Campbell 2003) and may explain the similar clinical and immunohistochemical features found in these CMDs, and make other enzymes involved in this process likely candidates.

Fukuyama CMD (FCMD) (Table 12.2) is caused by defects in the gene encoding a protein named *fukutin* on chromosome 9q31. The disorder is particularly common in Japan where a founder effect has led to a retrotransposon insertion in the 3' untranslated region of the gene. Most cases are heterozygous for this ancestral mutation, together with a deletion or nonsense mutation. Null mutations in mice are lethal but rare human cases have been identified, resulting in a particularly severe phenotype resembling WWS (Silan et al 2003, Beltran-Valero de Barnabe et al 2003). These cases indicate that FCMD can occur outside Japan and that a total absence of fukutin is not necessarily incompatible with life.

Patients with FCMD have severe brain involvement with mental retardation, abnormal eye function and frequently seizures. Generalized weakness is progressive and invariably leads to respiratory failure by the end of the second decade, as well as dilated cardiomyopathy. Serum CK activity is elevated. Severe arthrogryposis is rare but progressive contractures of the hips, knees and ankles and scoliosis are early features. The brain changes are within the type II lissencephaly spectrum, ranging from 'cobblestone' polymicrogyria-pachygyria to complete agyria. Over-migration of neurones beyond the glia limitans disrupts the layering of the cerebral cortex. Cerebellar cysts may also occur and MRI may show a delay in myelination.

A reduction in immunolabelling of laminins (Hayashi et al 1993) was an early observation and, coupled with the identification of the link between dystrophin and the extracellular matrix at the sarcolemma, it alerted Tomé to the possible wider involvement of the extracellular matrix in other disorders and paved the way for the revolution in the CMD field (Muntoni and Sewry 1998). Although the secondary reduction in laminin α2 is usually highlighted, the reduction in FCMD also involves the laminin β1 and γ1 chains of laminin-2 (merosin). There have also been reports of a reduction in dystrophin (Arikawa et al 1991) and β-dystroglycan (Matsumura et al 1993) but some of these early studies have not been substantiated (Arahata et al 1993) and attention has concentrated on the loss of glycosylation of α-dystroglycan (Hayashi et al 2001). Electron microscopy confirms the disruption of the basal lamina in skeletal muscle and the central nervous system (Ishii et al 1997, Yamomoto et al 1997, Saito et 1999). A reduction of a novel protein, P180, has also been reported in FCMD (Sunada et al 2002). Although the function of fukutin is not known, it has homology to the *fringe* family of enzymes that modify glycolipids and glycoproteins, which may relate to the abnormalities in the glycosylation of α-dystroglycan. Localization studies using antibodies to fukutin in muscle have not been reported but *in situ* hybridization and immunohistochemical studies of brain of postnatal and fetal human brain have shown it has a similar localization to POMT1 and POMGnT1 and is reduced in the brain of FCMD cases (Yamamoto et al 2004). These studies also showed reduced glycosylation of α-dystroglycan in the brain, providing further evidence of the pivotal role of glycosylation. *In vitro* studies suggest fukutin resides in the Golgi apparatus and interactions between fukutin and POMT1, POMGnT1 and LARGE have been suggested (Michele and Campbell 2003).

Muscle eye brain disease (MEB) (Table 12.1b) is also a severe form of CMD, first described in Finland by Santavuori and colleagues (Santavuori et al 1977) but with a world wide distribution. In addition to the muscle weakness there is consistent ocular involvement (congenital myopia and glaucoma, retinal dysplasia) and also of the central nervous system, with structural brain abnormalities (pachygyria, flat brain stem, cerebellar hypoplasia, cerebellar cysts), and severe mental retardation. Hydrocephalus and epilepsy are common. Motor ability is variable ranging from the ability to sit unsupported but unable to walk, to those acquiring ambulation for a number of years. The disorder is progressive and life span is diminished. Death may occur before the end of the second decade, although several survive into adulthood. Serum CK activity is always elevated, although it may be normal during the first year of life. With the application of molecular testing the clinical spectrum of MEB has broadened and milder cases have been reported (Haliloglu and Topaloglu 2004).

The gene responsible for MEB encodes the glycosyltransferase POMGnT1 which is responsible for the transfer of *N*-acetylglucosamine to *O*-mannose glycoproteins, including dystroglycan. Mutations identified are missense, nonsense and frame shifting and patients with 5′ mutations are more severe than those with 3′ mutations. There can be diagnostic confusion with WWS (see below) in some of these severe cases. Although antibodies are being developed, localization studies of POMGnT1 in tissues have not been reported in patients, but activity of the enzyme is reduced in those with the common mutation, suggesting the possibility of a diagnostic test (Yoshida et al 2001, Manya et al 2003, Zhang et al 2003).

Immunolabelling of dystrophin and its associated proteins, including β-dystroglycan, is usually normal in MEB but a secondary reduction of laminin α2 may be apparent (Haltia et al 1997). Labelling of the glycosylated epitopes of α-dystroglycan with IIH6 and VIA4-1 shows a marked reduction but with retention of the core protein, in the few cases so far studied.

Walker Warburg syndrome (WWS) is clinically the most severe of the CMDs and death usually occurs within the first few years of like. Features include encephaloceles and severe hydrocephalus, severe ocular and brain involvement, with type II lissencephaly, and abnormal neuronal migration with loss of cortical layering, and pontocerebellar hypoplasia. Prior to the molecular definition of the CMDs, it was uncertain if WWS and MEB were part of a clinical spectrum or genetically separate entities. Identification of mutations in *POMT1* clarified that WWS is a distinct disorder, but it is now apparent that there is considerable genetic heterogeneity associated with the WWS phenotype, as it can result from defects in the genes for POMT1, fukutin or FKRP (see below). This is further complicated by the identification of a milder case intermediate between MEB and WWS with a defect in the *POMT1* gene (Kim et al 2004) and also cases with a presentation resembling a LGMD (Balci et al 2005). Thus the *POMT1* gene is another example of variable clinical phenotypes arising from defects in the same gene (Muntoni 2005). Additional cases with the WWS phenotype remain genetically uncharacterized, suggesting further heterogeneity. POMT1 is a member of a family of glycosyltransferases which are obvious candidates for causative genes; data suggest POMT1 forms a complex with POMT2 and mutations in the gene for this protein have recently been identified (van Reeuwijk et al 2005).

Muscle histology in WWS is again similar to other CMDs with no distinguishing features. Laminin α2 immunolabelling appears normal in WWS in contrast to MEB (Voit et al 1995). There have been reports of reduced laminin β2 in WWS (Wewer et al 1995) but this has to be interpreted with caution as sarcolemmal labelling is weaker in neonatal muscle than in adult muscle, suggesting developmental regulation. Although laminin β2 is thought to have a major role at the neuromuscular junction with enhanced expression, there is also appreciable extrajunctional sarcolemmal laminin β2 in mature muscle (see Ch. 6). Dystrophin and its associated proteins, including β-dystroglycan appear normal.

POMT1 and POMT2 are glycosyltransferases and immunolabelling of the glycosylated epitopes of α-dystroglycan with IIH6 and VIA4-1 is virtually absent in skeletal muscle (Jimenez-Mallebrera et al 2003), in contrast to MEB. Labelling of the core protein in our studies was also not seen but epitope masking has not been excluded, and immunoblot studies suggest that some core protein of α-dystroglycan is retained (Campbell, personal observations). Core protein was also reported to be present in the milder case with a *POMT1* mutation (Kim et al 2004).

Congenital muscular dystrophy 1C (MDC1C) is caused by mutations in the gene encoding FKRP, named after its sequence homology to fukutin (Brockington et al 2001). It was considered a possible candidate for a human disorder after the identification of the equivalent gene in the mouse by Blake (see Brockington et al 2001). Like fukutin and POMGnT1, transfected FKRP is localized to the Golgi and sequence homology suggests it has a glycosyltransferase function, although enzymic activity has not yet been shown. Mutations in the *FKRP* gene are associated with a very wide and variable phenotype ranging from severe cases with or without brain involvement (MDC1C) to milder cases with a limb-girdle presentation (LGMD2I; see Ch. 11; Muntoni and Voit 2004). Some severe cases with brain involvement can resemble MEB or WWS clinically, with ocular abnormalities, whilst others have no apparent ocular involvement and normal brain stem but have mental retardation and structural brain defects with cerebellar cysts. Mutations in the *FKRP* gene are either two missense mutations or a missense plus a null mutation, but the common C826A mutation leading to Leu276Ile that is found in LGMD2I has not been found in any cases of MDC1C. No cases of MDC1C with two null mutations have been identified, suggesting that a complete absence of FKRP may be lethal. Laminin α2 shows a secondary reduction with immunolabelling in the severe forms (MDC1C; Fig. 12.11) but in LGMD2I this may only be seen on immunoblots (Bushby et al 1998). Reduced laminin α2 can also be seen at the epidermal/dermal junction in skin biopsies from MDC1C patients but limited studies show it is normal in fetal chorionic villi in cases with a mutation in the *FKRP* gene. Reduced immunolabelling of α-dystroglycan in muscle is seen in all cases with *FKRP* mutations (Fig. 12.11) and appears to broadly correlate with severity (Brown et al 2004). In MDC1C this reduction is usually pronounced, but is moderate in those with a DMD/Becker muscular dystrophy phenotype and may only be subtle in the clinically milder

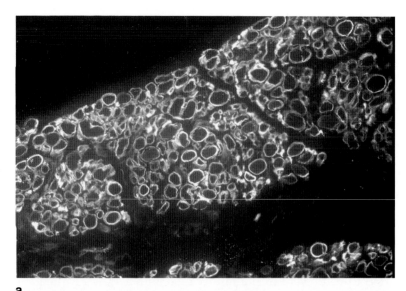

a

b

FIG. 12.11 *Immunolabelling of (a) a mild secondary reduction of laminin α2 and (b) pronounced reduction of the glycosylated epitope of α-dystroglycan in a case of MDC1C with a mutation in the gene for the fukutin-related protein.*

cases of LGMD2I (see Ch. 11). Labelling of β-dystroglycan is usually normal, except on necrotic fibres which lack an intact plasma membrane. Several fibres show neonatal myosin and immaturity has to be taken into account when assessing other reported alterations such as reduced integrin α7β1D (Sabatelli et al 2003). Perlecan has also been reported to be reduced in MDC1C (Sabatelli et al 2003) but this finding has not yet been substantiated.

Congenital muscular dystrophy 1D (MDC1D) is caused by mutations in the *LARGE* gene and was identified as a possible candidate after the mutation in the equivalent gene was found in the spontaneously occurring Large ^{myd} dystrophic mouse (Grewal et al 2001; Longman et al 2003). This form seems to be particularly rare and to date only one patient has been reported, a 17-year-old girl with a missense mutation and a single base pair insertion, who presented with severe mental retardation, white matter changes and subtle structural MRI brain changes. The muscle biopsy again showed reduced labelling of glycosylated α-dystroglycan and a reduced molecular weight on immunoblots. LARGE has recently been shown to interact directly with dystroglycan and facilitate its proper glycosylation (Kanagawa et al 2004).

The locus for *congenital muscular dystrophy 1B (MDC1B)*, on chromosome 1q42, was identified before the *FKRP* gene but the protein responsible is still unknown, and several candidates have been excluded. Muscle biopsies also show reduced glycosylation of α-dystroglycan (S. Brown and T. Voit, unpublished observations), and reduced labelling of laminin α2 and integrin α7β1D, in common with the disorders described above (Brockington et al 2000). This suggests that the unknown protein from this gene may also have a glycosyltransferase function, although there is currently no direct evidence of this. Only two families have been identified that link to this locus and the phenotype is characterized by proximal girdle weakness, generalized muscle hypertrophy, rigidity of the spine, contractures of the Achilles tendons, early respiratory failure due to severe diaphragmatic involvement, and grossly elevated CK activity.

Rigid spine with muscular dystrophy (RSMD1)

The clinical syndrome of rigid spine was designated many years ago (Dubowitz 1973) and is know to be associated with several gene defects, in particular those encoding lamin A/C and emerin, responsible for Emery–Dreifuss forms of muscular dystrophy (see Ch. 13). It is also associated with a form of congenital muscular dystrophy (designated RSMD1) caused by recessive mutations in the gene for SEPN1 on chromosome 1p35-36. Mutations have been found in most of the 13 exons except exon 3 and most lead to a premature stop codon. The function of SEPN1 is not yet fully understood. It is a glycoprotein localized to the endoplasmic reticulum with an N-terminal, membrane-binding domain and is expressed in several tissues, with higher expression in fetal tissues.

The clinical features of RSMD1 (Table 12.3) include axial hypotonia and weakness, spinal rigidity, scoliosis and respiratory insufficiency requiring ventilation. There is usually an overall reduction in muscle bulk and several cases may have nasal speech. Severity is variable but ambulation is usually achieved and maintained into adulthood. Serum CK activity is usually normal or only mildly elevated.

As shown in Fig. 12.1, muscle pathology includes variation in fibre size with a mild increase in endomysial connective tissue. Internal nuclei are not usually a prominent feature, but do occur, and fibre typing is usually maintained. Some cases may show unevenness of oxidative enzyme staining, sometimes affecting both fibre types. These areas may resemble minicores and there is clinical and pathological overlap with some cases classified with multi-minicore disease, in which mutations in SEPN1 also occur. The pathological spectrum associated with SEPN1 mutations also includes Mallory body myopathy (see Ch. 15). Although ultimately these conditions may be thought of as allelic, it appears at the moment that this is another example of defects in one gene resulting in phenotypic variants.

No informative secondary immunohistochemical abnormalities have yet been identified in RSMD1. In keeping with the absence of necrosis and low CK there are usually very few, or no, fibres with neonatal myosin.

CHAPTER 13

Muscular dystrophies and allied disorders IV: Emery–Dreifuss muscular dystrophies and Bethlem myopathy

Although the underlying pathogenesis and inheritance of the Emery–Dreifuss forms of muscular dystrophies and Bethlem myopathy are diverse, they are all characterized by a particular pattern of joint contractures and they share a number of clinical features. In particular, a rigid spine is common in all of them, and early elbow contractures are a typical feature of Emery–Dreifuss muscular dystrophies, and long finger flexor contractures of Bethlem myopathy. Cardiac arrhythmia, however, is a distinguishing feature and occurs in the Emery–Dreifuss muscular dystrophies but not Bethlem myopathy (Table 13.1). Differential diagnosis following clinical examination often includes all of these disorders and muscle pathology can then be helpful.

An X-linked and an autosomal dominant form of Emery–Dreifuss muscular dystrophy have been identified, and both are caused by defects in nuclear envelope proteins (Nagano and Arahata 2000). Bethlem myopathy is an autosomal dominant disorder and is caused by a defect in the extracellular matrix protein collagen VI (Table 13.2; see Fig. 8.1; Jobis et al 1996).

Emery–Dreifuss muscular dystrophies

Emery–Dreifuss muscular dystrophy has been recognized as a separate entity from Duchenne and Becker muscular dystrophy for many years and the first description can be attributed to Cestan and Lejonne in 1902. Following reassessment of a large Virginian family first described by Dreifuss and Hogan (1961), Alan Emery published a seminal description of the X-linked form, now commonly referred to as Emery–Dreifuss muscular dystrophy (Emery and Driefuss 1966, Emery 1989). Description of autosomal dominant cases followed later (Chakrabarti et al 1981, Fenichel et al 1982, Miller et al 1985) and once the underlying pathogenesis relating to nuclear membrane proteins was identified, and the similarity in clinical features recognized, they became linked under the same title of 'Emery–Dreifuss muscular dystrophy'.

TABLE 13.1 *Main features of Emery–Dreifuss muscular dystrophies and Bethlem myopathy*

	Emery–Dreifuss muscular dystrophies	Bethlem myopathy
Clinical features	Onset in childhood, adolescence, or adult life Mild muscle weakness (can be severe in early onset cases) Wasting of upper arms and lower legs Elbow contractures Rigidity of spine Cardiac arrhythmia, also in carriers of the X-linked form	Onset in childhood or within the first two decades of life Mild to moderate muscle weakness of proximal upper and lower limbs Wasting of shoulder girdle and lower legs Contractures of long finger flexors and elbows Ligamentous laxity Hypertrophic scars No cardiac arrhythmia
Ambulation	Usually maintained in X-linked form Lost in first decade in several dominant cases	May be lost in adult life
Creatine kinase	Normal, or slight to moderate elevation	Normal, or mild elevation
Pathology	Mild to moderate myopathic changes Variation in fibre size Internal nuclei Mild fibrosis Atrophic type 1 fibres Absence of emerin from all nuclei (X-linked form) Normal localization of lamins to nuclear envelope Reduced sarolemmal laminin β1	Mild myopathic changes Variation in fibre size Internal nuclei Reduced sarcolemmal laminin β1 Normal collagen VI immunolabelling

The clinical features of the X-linked and autosomal forms are similar but often more severe in the latter (Table 13.2). They both present with muscle weakness and early contractures of the elbow, the Achilles tendons and the spinal extensor muscles. These precede the appearance of cardiac abnormalities, which begin with conduction defects and lead to complete heart block. Most cases show conduction defects before the third decade of life and cardiac problems are frequently more severe in the autosomal form. The contractures are progressive and lumbar lordosis and rigidity of the spine often become marked. Contractures of the wrists and finger flexors can also occur.

Muscle weakness and wasting has a distinct pattern. In the X-linked form it is humero-peroneal, and in the autosomal form, scapulohumero-peroneal. Striking wasting of the upper arms and lower legs is often apparent in both. A particular pattern of muscle involvement is apparent with muscle magnetic

TABLE 13.2 *The genes and protein products responsible for Emery–Dreifuss muscular dystrophies and Bethlem myopathy*

Emery–Dreifuss muscular dystrophies			
Inheritance	Gene	Gene locus	Protein
X-linked	*STA*	Xq28	Emerin
Dominant *de novo* dominant (one recessive case)	*LMNA*	1q21.23	Lamin A/C

Bethlem myopathy			
Inheritance	Gene	Gene locus	Protein
Dominant, some recessive*	*COL6A1*	21q 22.3	α1 Collagen VI
Dominant, some recessive*	*COL6A2*	21q 22.3	α2 Collagen VI
Dominant, some recessive*	*COL6A3*	2q37	α3 Collagen VI

* see text

resonance imaging in each form and can be helpful in differential diagnosis (Mercuri et al 2001, Mercuri et al 2005).

Autosomal dominant Emery–Dreifuss muscular dystrophy is more common than the X-linked form and generally more severe, with earlier onset, even in very early childhood. Ambulation is lost in a significant number of affected patients in the first decade.

Serum creatine kinase levels are usually normal or mildly elevated, up to 10 times the normal level, but never in the high range of Duchenne or Becker muscular dystrophy.

Molecular genetics

The *X-linked* form is caused by a mutation in the *STA* gene on chromosome Xq28 and encodes a protein named emerin (Nagano and Arahata 2000). Emerin is a 34 kDa protein which has a hydrophobic C-terminus anchored in the nuclear membrane and an N-terminal tail projecting into the nucleoplasm (Manilal et al 1996). The *STA* gene has six exons and mutations have been found throughout the gene, with no 'hot-spots'. Most are nonsense or frameshift mutations or occur at splice sites. A list of identified mutations can be found at the Emery Dreifuss website (*http://www.path.cam.ac.uk/emd/*). The majority of mutations result in an absence of protein expression which can be demonstrated with antibodies (Manilal et al 1996, see below). Rare cases have been reported in which emerin expression is reduced (Cartegni et al 1997, di Blasi et al 2000).

Female carriers rarely manifest with muscle weakness but are at risk of cardiac involvement. The absence of emerin in a proportion of nuclei can be detected in carriers (see below).

Autosomal dominant Emery–Dreifuss muscular dystrophy is caused by mutations in the *LMNA* gene on chromosome 1q11-23, which encodes an alternatively spliced protein, lamin A/C, localized to the nuclear envelope (Bonne et al 1999). The gene has 12 exons and alternative splicing produces at least four different RNAs encoding closely related proteins (lamin A, lamin A δ10, lamin C and lamin C2). Lamin A and C are the predominant forms and result from alternative splicing of exon 10; a large part of the protein is therefore common to both (Wilson 2000). Lamin A is the longer and uses the C-terminal exons 11 and 12, while splicing at exon 10 results in the shorter lamin C. Many mutations have been found and are of all types and occur in all exons; but most occur in the common α-helical rod domain of exons 1–10 with a mutation (R453W) in exon 7 being one of the most frequent.

The majority of mutations are dominant, with a striking frequency of *de novo* dominant mutations. These usually result in no detectable alteration in lamin A/C protein localization using immunohistochemistry (Sewry et al 2001a; see below). One rare case, in a consanguineous family, with recessive mutations on both alleles inherited from unaffected parents has been documented (Di Barletta et al 2000).

There is considerable clinical variability, both between and within families with mutations in the *LMNA* gene. The phenotypes attributed to it include not only the autosomal dominant form of Emery–Dreifuss muscular dystrophy and the allelic limb-girdle muscular dystrophy 1B, but also familial partial lipodystrophy, an axonal neuropathy (Charcot–Marie–Tooth type 2B1), mandibuloacral disease, premature ageing disorders and restrictive dermopathy (Mounkes et al 2003, Mounkes and Stewart 2004, Navarro et al 2004). These are now often referred to as 'laminopathies'. Although familial partial lipodystrophy has a distinct phenotype, muscle MRI of autosomal cases of Emery–Dreifuss muscular dystrophy may show a significant reduction of subcutaneous fat (Bonne et al 2002). Similarly, some patients with lipodystrophy may have a rigid spine, cardiac abnormalities and muscle involvement (van der Kooi et al 2002).

Biochemistry

Lamins are a major component of the nuclear envelope, separating the nucleoplasm from the rest of the cell; they are composed of an inner and outer nuclear membrane, joined at nuclear pores, and the nuclear lamina (see Ch. 5). The outer membrane is continuous with the rough endoplasmic reticulum, while the inner membrane contains a number of proteins that bind to lamins and chromatin. Lamins are components of the nuclear lamina and amongst their proposed functions are maintenance of the structural integrity of the nuclear envelope, organization of interphase chromatin and reassembly of the nuclear membrane during mitosis.

There are two main types of nuclear lamins, A and B, which have sequence homology to type V intermediate filaments. Lamin A and C are the two main forms produced by splicing from the *LMNA* gene, while lamin B1 and B2 are encoded by separate genes. A-type lamins, in contrast to ubiquitously expressed B lamins, are believed to be developmentally regulated and are not expressed in embryonic stem cells, early embryonic cells, stem cells in the immune and haematopoietic systems or cells in the neuroendocrine system (Mounkes et al 2003). A direct interaction between lamin A and emerin has been demonstrated (Clements et al 2000), and lamins interact with a group of other integral membrane proteins, including the lamin B receptor, LAP2 and MAN1. These proteins share a LAP2-Emerin-MAN1 (LEM) domain, which binds the barrier-to-autointegration factor (BAF), a protein thought to have an important role in chromatin organization, transcription and efficient retroviral DNA integration (Segura-Totten and Wilson 2004). Lamin B proteins are often studied in parallel with emerin and lamin A/C (see below) and there is considerable interest in other nuclear envelope proteins as candidates for disorders with clinical similarity to the Emery–Dreifuss muscular dystrophies.

Histopathology

The main histological and histochemical features of both X-linked and autosomal dominant Emery–Dreifuss muscular dystrophy are similar and the degree of change varies with the involvement of the muscle sampled. In quadriceps biopsies the abnormal variation in fibre size is not usually marked (Fig. 13.1). Occasional atrophic fibres are common and some fibres may be hypertrophic. Measurement of fibre diameters may be necessary to appreciate this. Internal nuclei may be occasional or numerous, with more than one per fibre (Fig. 13.1).

Necrotic fibres are rare and there is usually only a mild increase in adipose or connective tissue (Fig. 13.1). There are exceptions, however, such as a severely affected boy we assessed prior to the appearance of the characteristic contractures and thought to have a form of limb-girdle muscular dystrophy (Muntoni et al 1998). The pathology resembled a severe limb-girdle type of muscular dystrophy with a wide variation in fibre size, a pronounced increase in connective tissue and necrosis (Fig. 13.2). He was eventually found to lack expression of emerin (see below) and to have a mutation in the *STA* gene, and his mother a carrier. Interestingly this child was also found to have a *LMNA* mutation which is presumed to contribute to his severe phenotype. This case illustrates the importance of considering the possibility of 'double trouble' and a causative mutation in more than one gene, particularly in genes in which mutations are common, like *LMNA*.

We have also noted the presence of small basophilic fibres that may be slightly granular in appearance and show aggregation of NADH-TR stain (Fig. 13.3). These fibres may be regenerating fibres as they show neonatal myosin and desmin (Fig. 13.3). A two fibre type pattern is usually maintained with oxidative enzyme stains and ATPase, with a tendency for the type 1 fibres to be smaller, but not usually to the degree seen in congenital myopathies (Fig. 13.4; see Ch. 15). A predominance of type 1 fibres may also occur. Structural changes such as cores can occur and they were a pronounced feature together with indistinct

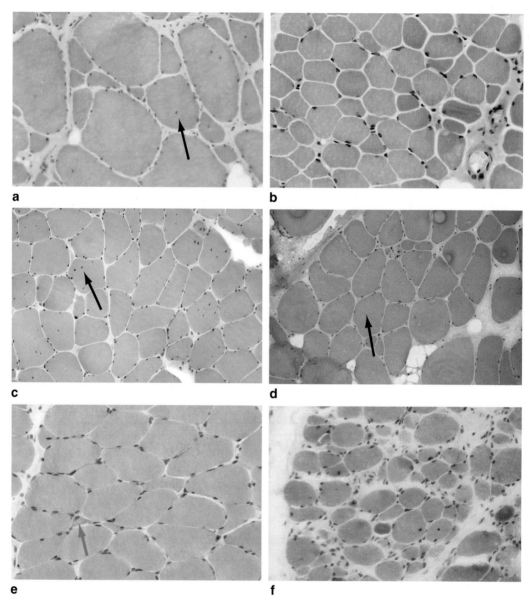

a b c d e f

FIG. 13.1 *Histological features in two cases of X-linked Emery–Dreifuss muscular dystrophy aged 16 and 3 years (a), (b) and four cases of autosomal dominant Emery–Dreifuss muscular dystrophy with a mutation in the lamin A/C gene aged 17, 14, 8 and 4 years (c)–(f). Note the variable degree of fibre size variation with atrophy and hypertrophy in some cases, the increase in internal nuclei (arrows), the small basophilic fibres in (e) (green arrow), the lack of necrosis, and mild endomysial fibrosis which is most extensive in (f) (H&E).*

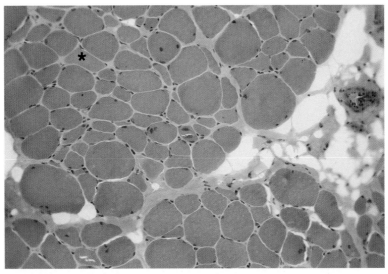

FIG. 13.2 *Quadriceps biopsy from a 4-year-old boy with a mutation in both the gene for emerin and lamin A/C showing dystrophic features with a wide variation in fibre size, a pale necrotic fibre (*), and increased fibrous and adipose tissue (H&E).*

fibre typing in a girl with a *LMNA* mutation that we have observed (Fig. 13.5). A mutation in an additional gene has not been excluded in this child.

Immunohistochemistry

Immunohistochemical studies of emerin easily detect its absence from all nuclei in affected male patients with X-linked Emery–Dreifuss muscular dystrophy (Fig. 13.6). In addition to muscle, the absence can also be shown in skin and buccal cells (Manilal et al 1997, Sabatelli et al 1998; Fig. 13.7). If buccal cells are used it is essential that only viable cells are assessed, to avoid false-negative results in dead buccal cells. Parallel studies of lamins are then a useful control. In carriers of the X-linked form skin biopsies can be used to demonstrate nuclei with and without emerin (Fig. 13.7).

Emerin can be detected by immunofluorescent or enzyme labels such as peroxidase, but if bright field techniques are used it is often easier to assess sections that have not been counterstained with haematoxylin.

In both X-linked and autosomal dominant Emery–Dreifuss muscular dystrophy, labelling of lamins in muscle biopsies shows no detectable difference from normal. Similarly, emerin immunolabelling appears normal when there is a *LMNA* mutation (Fig. 13.8). As in all dominant conditions only one allele is mutated and the normal allele produces a normal product. Only if the abnormal gene product interferes with the normal one (haplo-insufficiency) is any detectable alteration in localization likely to be seen.

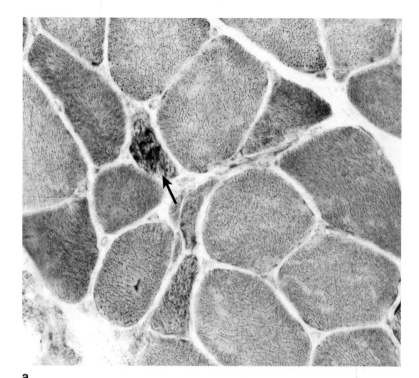

a

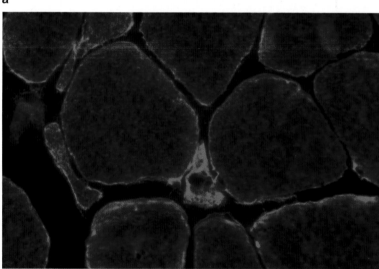

b

FIG. 13.3 *Quadriceps muscle biopsy from an 8-year-old girl with autosomal dominant Emery–Dreifuss muscular dystrophy shown in FIG. 13.1(e). Note in (a) aggregation of NADH-TR staining in a small fibre (arrow) and (b) a high level of desmin in a small fibre.*

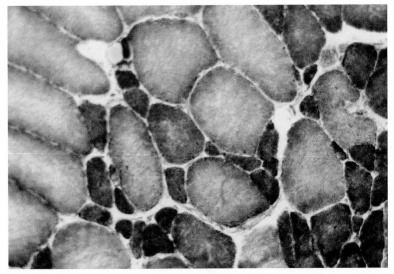

a

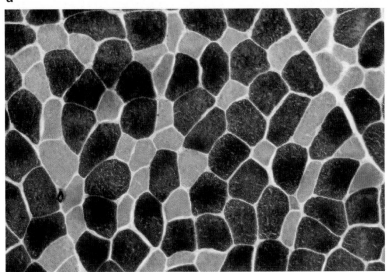

b

FIG. 13.4(a) *Quadriceps biopsy from a case of X-linked Emery–Dreifuss muscular dystrophy aged 16 years stained for NADH-TR and (b) a boy aged 9 years with autosomal dominant Emery–Dreifuss muscular dystrophy stained for ATPase at pH 9.4 showing slightly smaller type 1 fibres in both. Several of the larger fibres in (a) are hypertrophic.*

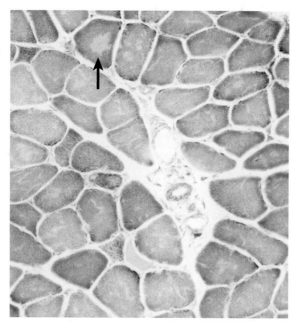

FIG. 13.5 *Quadriceps biopsy from an 8-year-old girl with autosomal dominant Emery–Dreifuss muscular dystrophy showing occasional cores (arrow) and unevenness of stain in several fibres. There is also a predominance of type 1 fibres (NADH-TR).*

Antibodies that specifically detect lamin A show labelling of very few nuclei in mature human muscle with the antibodies currently available (Fig. 13.8) but more labelled nuclei are apparent in fetal muscle. It is not clear if this relates to developmental regulation or to epitope masking. In contrast, antibodies to epitopes common to both lamin A and C show labelling of all nuclei at all stages of development (Fig. 13.8). This difference is thought to be due to epitope masking. Some studies have suggested that there is reciprocal expression of lamin B1 and emerin (Manilal et al 1999), with emerin in myonuclei and lamin B1 in endothelial cell nuclei. Lamin B2 appears to be present in all nuclei and internal nuclei show similar emerin and lamin labelling as peripheral ones (Fig. 13.8).

Immunolabelling of all proteins associated with the sarcolemma is normal in both forms of Emery–Dreifuss muscular dystrophy, with the exception of laminin β1 (Brown et al 2001). Reduced laminin β1 labelling on the sarcolemma may be apparent in some cases but blood vessels, including the capillary network, show a normal intensity (Fig. 13.9). The intensity of laminin α2 and laminin γ1 labelling is similar in these cases and are useful controls. This reduced sarcolemmal laminin β1 labelling is not specific for the Emery–Dreifuss muscular dystrophies and may also be seen in cases of Bethlem myopathy (see below) and in patients with mutations in the fukutin-related protein (FKRP). It is an age related phenomenon and has only been observed in adult and adolescent cases.

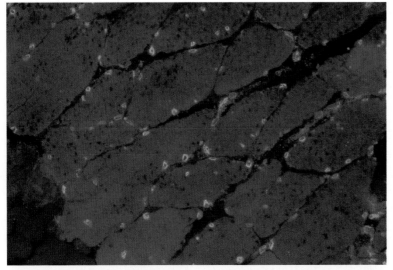

a

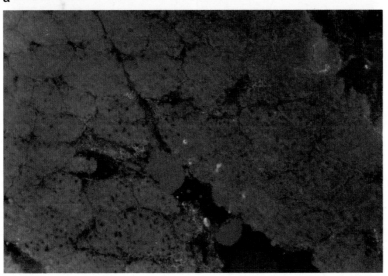

b

FIG. 13.6 *Immunolabelling of emerin in muscle from (a) a control and (b) a case of X-linked Emery–Dreifuss muscular dystrophy with absence of emerin from all nuclei.*

MUSCLE BIOPSY

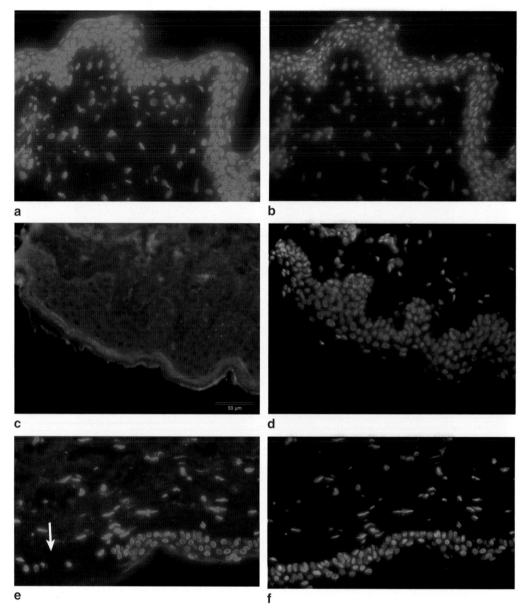

50 μm

FIG. 13.7 *Immunolabelling of emerin in skin in (a) a control, (c) a boy with X-linked Emery–Dreifuss muscular dystrophy and (e) his mother who is a carrier. Note the absence of emerin in all nuclei in (c) and an area of nuclei in the carrier (e) which lack emerin (arrow) alongside those with normal labelling. The panels on the right [(b), (d), and (f)] are of the same fields as (a), (c) and (e) showing labelling of all nuclei with DAPI as control.*

FIG. 13.8 *Immunolabelling of emerin, lamin A, A/C and B2 as shown in a control and a 17-year-old male with autosomal dominant Emery–Dreifuss muscular dystrophy and a mutation in the lamin A/C gene. Note the normal labelling of emerin in both peripheral and internal nuclei, the low level of detectable lamin A in both the control and the case of Emery–Dreifuss muscular dystrophy, and no apparent difference in lamin A/C or B2 labelling.*

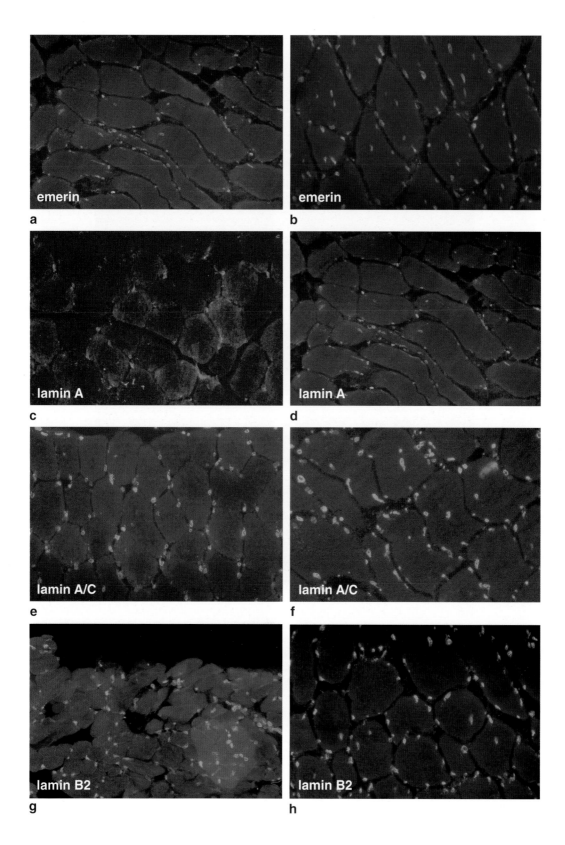

a   emerin

b   emerin

c   lamin A

d   lamin A

e   lamin A/C

f   lamin A/C

g   lamin B2

h   lamin B2

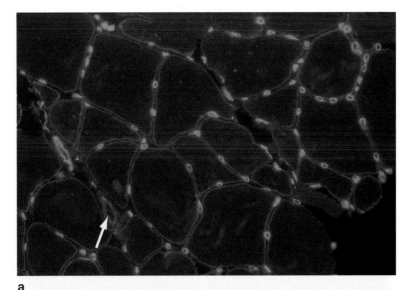

a

b

FIG. 13.9 *Serial areas immunolabelled for (a) laminin β1 and (b) laminin γ1 in a quadriceps biopsy from a 35-year-old male with autosomal dominant Emery–Dreifuss muscular dystrophy showing a reduction of laminin β1 at the sarcolemma but not the blood vessels and normal levels of laminin γ1. Note also the venule that does not show laminin β1 but does label for laminin α1 (arrow; this is a normal finding).*

There are usually only a few fibres present that express neonatal myosin, suggesting that there is little ongoing muscle fibre regeneration. It is not clear if this is a reflection of the lack of necrosis, which precedes regeneration, or if there is some kind of malfunction in the regenerative process that could account for the muscle wasting.

Electron microscopy has shown aggregation of chromatin and lack of attachment of chromatin to the nuclear membrane, as seen in apoptopic nuclei (Brown et al 2001; see Ch. 5). Abnormalities of the nuclear envelope have also been reported in skeletal muscle nuclei and cultured skin fibroblasts (Fidzianska et al 1998, Ognibene et al 1999).

Bethlem myopathy

Bethlem myopathy is an autosomal dominant disorder characterized by mild muscle weakness and contractures, particularly of the long finger flexors (Bethlem and van Wijngaarden 1976) (Table 13.1). Some clinical features also occur in the Emery–Dreifuss muscular dystrophies and sometimes they may not be easy to distinguish clinically. Bethlem myopathy has been regarded in the past as a mainly adult disorder but, with greater awareness of the disorder, it is now apparent that onset is variable and occurs in childhood or may even be congenital. The muscle weakness is often mild. There is progression of the weakness, with a proportion of patients becoming wheelchair bound in adult life, or more rarely in adolescence. Life expectancy, however, is normal and cardiac involvement and respiratory problems are not typical features. Creatine kinase levels are normal, or only mildly elevated.

The weakness is proximal more than distal and muscle atrophy involves the shoulder girdle, upper arms and lower legs. The facial muscles are usually spared. Contractures of the finger flexors are a hallmark of the disorder. In some patients the only obvious sign may be the inability to bring the fingers together in the 'prayer sign'. Elbow and ankle contractures also occur in most patients and torticollis may be present at birth, or develop later in life. Contractures tend to worsen with age but there is no correlation between the contractures and severity of muscle weakness. Hypermobility of the wrists and fingers, evolving later into contractures, may occur in children, and some patients show laxity of the hip joints and dislocation of the patella. Some cases have a rigid spine and scoliosis may also develop (Pepe et al 2000). Hypertrophic scars may also be seen.

Molecular genetics

Bethlem myopathy results from mutations in any of the three genes encoding collagen VI (Table 13.2; Jobis et al 1996, Lamande et al 1998a, b). Collagen VI is composed of three α chains (α1, α2, α3) encoded by three different genes. The three chains assemble intracellularly into a monomer and prior to secretion into

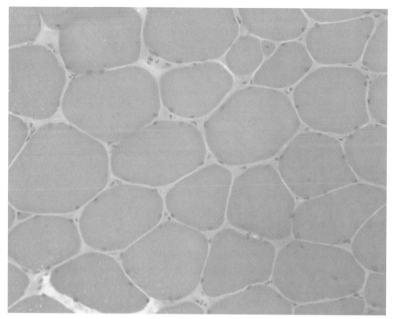

FIG. 13.10 *Quadriceps biopsy from a case of Bethlem myopathy aged 28 years showing mild myopathic features with variation in fibre size and mild fibrosis (H&E).*

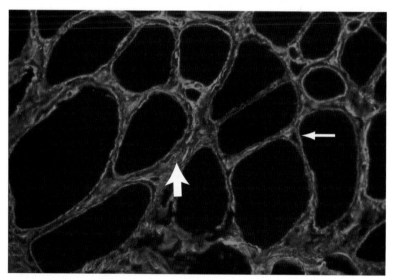

FIG. 13.11 *Immunolabelling of collagen VI in a molecularly proven case of Bethlem myopathy. Note the normal labelling of both the endomysium (large arrow) and the sarcolemma (small arrow).*

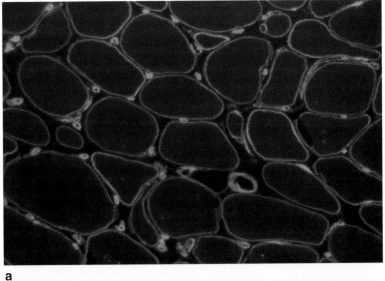

a

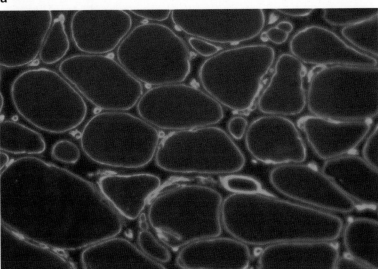

b

FIG. 13.12 *Serial areas immunolabelled for (a) laminin β1 and (b) laminin γ1 in a case of Bethlem myopathy. Note the slight reduced intensity of laminin β1 at the sarcolemma in comparison with normal labelling of blood vessels and of laminin γ1.*

the extracellular space they form antiparallel dimers which then associate into lateral tetramers. In the extracellular matrix the tetramers link end to end and form a microfibrillar network that interacts with other proteins, including fibronectin, decorin, biglycan, perlecan, chondroitin sulphate proteoglycan, NG2 receptor and other collagens such as collagen IV. Collagen VI is present in most connective tissues but patients with mutations in the genes show only muscle weakness and contractures. In normal muscle collagen VI is localized to both the sarcolemma and the endomysial connective tissue (see below and Ch. 6).

Initial molecular studies indicated that the Bethlem myopathy phenotype is associated with dominantly inherited mutations of the collagen VI genes and that the Ullrich form of congenital muscular dystrophy (Ullrich CMD) (see Ch. 16) is associated with recessive mutations (Camacho et al 2001, Lampe and Bushby 2005). This distinction, however, is not universal and some severely affected patients with dominant mutations have been identified, as well as milder cases with recessive mutations (Pan et al 2003, Baker et al 2005, Lampe et al 2005). It is now thought that Ullrich CMD and Bethlem myopathy are part of a clinical spectrum and that severity is determined by the effect of a particular mutation on the production and function of collagen VI.

Histopathology

The features are usually mild and non-specific. Variation in fibre size is mild to moderate, and, as with the Emery–Dreifuss muscular dystrophies, some fibres may be hypertrophic and measurements may be necessary to fully appreciate this. Any increase in connective and adipose tissues is usually mild. A few internal nuclei may be present but they are not usually abundant (Fig. 13.10). A two fibre type pattern is seen with oxidative enzyme and adenosine triphosphatase staining, confirmed with immunolabelling of myosin isoforms. Some cases, however, may show type 1 fibre predominance. Structural changes such as core-like lesions or whorled fibres are not usually seen but some unevenness of oxidative enzyme stain may be apparent.

Immunohistochemistry

Labelling of collagen VI in muscle sections shows no apparent abnormality in Bethlem myopathy (Fig. 13.11). The sarcolemmal labelling is distinct against a background of labelling of the endomysium. This is in contrast to abnormalities that can be seen in some recessive cases of Ullrich CMD (see Ch. 12). As with Ullrich CMD, some research studies suggest that abnormalities in intracellular collagen VI can be detected in cultured skin fibroblasts from patients with Bethlem myopathy but it is not yet clear how universal these changes are (Jiminez-Mallebrera, unpublished observations).

Labelling of sarcolemmal proteins is normal except for a reduction in laminin β1 in adult and adolescent cases, as in the Emery–Dreifuss muscular dystrophies. Labelling of the blood vessels is normal and the reduction only seen on the sarcolemma (Fig. 13.12).

CHAPTER 14

Muscular dystrophies and allied disorders V: Facioscapulohumeral, myotonic and oculopharyngeal muscular dystrophy

Facioscapulohumeral muscular dystrophy, myotonic muscular dystrophy and oculopharyngeal muscular dystrophy are dominantly inherited disorders, all of which have an unusual molecular defect involving nucleotide repeats. Clinically, facial weakness is a prominent characteristic of all of them.

Facioscapulohumeral muscular dystrophy

Facioscapulohumeral muscular dystrophy (FSHD) is one of the most common muscular dystrophies with an estimated prevalence of 1:20 000 and a high frequency of sporadic cases (Tawil and Griggs 2001, Padberg 2002, Thornton 2002). Penetrance based on clinical presentation is age dependent and most cases show clinical signs before the age of 20 years. Infantile cases with onset recognizable before the age of 10 years are seen in some families. Anticipation is also well recognized, although unexplained, with earlier onset in successive generations.

The molecular defect is a deletion of copies of a 3.3 kb DNA repeat fragment in the subtelomeric region of chromosome 4q (D_4Z_4). In normal individuals the fragment varies in size from 35 to 300 kb with 11 or more D_4Z_4 repeats but FSHD patients have 11 or fewer repeats (Tupler and Gabellini 2004, van der Maarel and Frants 2005). There are no transcripts from this repeat region but the deletion is believed to influence the expression of proximally located genes.

The diagnosis of FSHD by molecular analysis is now highly reliable, provided a double digest with *Eco*RI and *Bln*I restriction enzymes is carried out to distinguish the chromosome 4q fragment from the similar fragment on chromosome 10q26, both of which are detectable with the p13E-11 probe. The chromosome 10 fragment contains a *Bln*I restriction site that is absent from the chromosome 4 fragment. Thus these two enzymes completely digest the chromosome 10 fragment leaving the chromosome 4 related fragments. Confusion can arise, however, as interchromosomal exchange of the repeat regions occurs in a few individuals in the normal population, resulting in hybrids of chromosome

4 and 10 fragments. Germ-line mosaicism may also hamper molecular analysis, but the double-digest analysis identifies about 95% of cases. A few families do not link to chromosome 4q but no locus has yet been identified.

Facial and shoulder-girdle weakness are the hallmarks of FSHD, particularly in early stages of the disorder. Facial weakness is detected by the inability to bury the eyelashes, or in whistling, pursing the lips, or puffing out the cheeks. Affected individuals often have a characteristic dimple at the angle of the somewhat pouting mouth, which appears when attempting to smile. Shoulder-girdle weakness results in difficulty in raising the arms and when attempted a characteristic upward drift of the scapulae is seen. Progression is variable and may be slow and minimal in some. In others progression may lead to involvement of the trunk and pelvic muscles, resulting in marked lordosis and loss of ambulation. Weakness of abdominal muscles is also frequently seen in later stages.

Cardiac and intellectual involvement are not features of FSHD. Hearing loss and a retinal vaculopathy, however, often occur. For a recent review of all aspects of FSHD the reader is referred to Upadhyaya and Cooper (2004).

Histology and histochemistry

With the advent of a reliable molecular diagnostic test for FSHD, muscle biopsies are now rarely performed. No specific pathological features have been identified in affected patients, despite extensive studies (Rogers et al 2004). The degree of pathological changes is variable, which may in some cases relate to the site of biopsy (Fig. 14.1). As discussed in Chapter 1 it is important to take a sample from an affected muscle but not one that is so severely affected that there are few muscle fibres to examine. Thus some biopsies from quadriceps muscle in cases where these muscles are relatively less affected may show only very mild changes. Muscles with marked clinical weakness, however, may also show very little pathology. This is another example where clinical severity does not correlate with the degree of pathology.

Changes in fibre size

Increased variability in the size of fibres, with large and small fibres is common, and the mean fibre diameter of both fibre types is often increased. Very small fibres scattered amongst larger fibres are a characteristic feature (Fig. 14.1a). These have often been described as atrophic fibres but the presence of developmentally regulated proteins such as neonatal myosin, MHC class I antigens and desmin, raises other possibilities for their small size, such as regeneration (Fig. 14.2). As in Becker muscular dystrophy, clusters of fibres have been put forward as evidence of denervation but there is no morphological or electrophysiological data to support this. These clusters of small fibres also show the presence of proteins associated with immaturity, including neonatal myosin, suggesting that they may represent attempts at regeneration. (The presence of neonatal myosin, however, does not totally exclude denervation; see Ch. 6.)

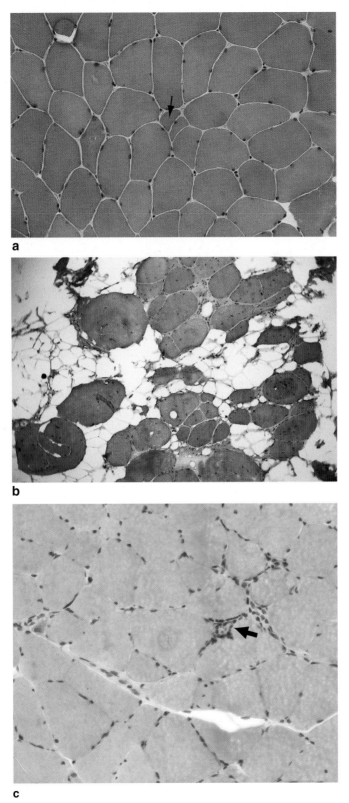

FIG. 14.1 *Biopsies of the quadriceps in three different cases of facioscapulohumeral muscular dystrophy aged 12, 42 and 55 years respectively showing varying degrees of pathology. In (a) note only mild variation in fibre size with a few very small fibres (arrow); in (b) the pronounced proliferation of connective tissue and fat with a wide variation in fibre size and many internal nuclei; and in (c) note the small clusters of inflammatory cells which in some cases may be numerous (arrow).*

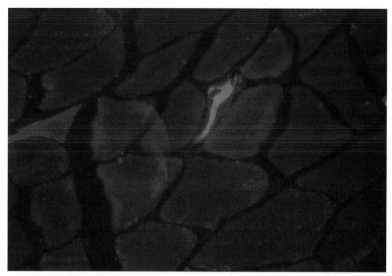

FIG. 14.2 *Immunolabelling of neonatal myosin in an isolated small fibre in a case of facioscapulohumeral muscular dystrophy.*

Changes in distribution

Neither large group atrophy nor type grouping is a feature of FSHD. Fibre type predominance may occur but seems to involve type 2 fibres rather than type 1 fibres, which is common in other muscular dystrophies.

Nuclear changes

Nuclear changes are not a prominent feature of FSHD. Internal nuclei may occasionally be numerous (Fig. 14.1b).

Degeneration

Necrosis can occur but is rare and is not usually a marked feature.

Cellular response

A common finding is an inflammatory response which may vary from mild to profuse (Fig. 14.1c). An increase in fibrous and adipose tissue may also occur (Fig. 14.1b).

Architectural change

The chief architectural change in FSHD is the occurrence of moth-eaten and whorled fibres. These may occur as a separate population of small type 1 fibres among more normal-appearing fibres.

Immunohistochemistry

Although immunohistochemistry has an important role in assessment of biopsies from several neuromuscular disorders, there are no specific abnormalities associated with FSHD that aid diagnosis. Labelling of all the sarcolemmal proteins associated with dystrophin is normal. Labelling of sarcolemmal MHC class I antigens may occur but is not a consistent feature. Sarcolemmal laminin β1 may be reduced in some cases, as in other dominant conditions (Dr Louise Anderson, personal communication), but this is not a consistent feature and we have not observed it.

Myotonic dystrophies

Myotonic dystrophy is also an autosomal dominant disorder characterized by myotonia in association with muscle weakness and wasting and also affecting several other tissues. Two forms of myotonic dystrophy (DM1 and DM2), caused by defects in two different genes, have been identified. DM2 is also known as proximal myotonic myopathy (PROMM). Both are caused by expansion of a nucleotide repeat; DM1 by expansion of a CTG repeat in the 3' untranslated region of a gene on chromosome 19q, and DM2 by a CCTG repeat expansion in the first intron of the *ZNF9* gene on chromosome 3q. The chromosome 19 protein is a putative kinase (DM protein kinase, DMPK) and that from the chromosome 3 gene is a zinc finger protein. Both disorders are believed to result from 'toxic RNA' produced by the expansion, which interferes with other proteins such as muscleblind and SIX5 in the nucleus (Meola 20002, Meola and Moxley 2004).

DM1 is a common disorder with an estimated prevalence of about 1:7400. DM2, in contrast, is relatively rare, and there may be further genetic heterogeneity as not all cases appear to link to either chromosome 9 or 3. There are no reported congenital cases of DM2 but congenital presentation of DM1 is well recognized, with the mother almost invariably carrying the mutant gene, and often only mildly affected. Pathology has an important role in differential diagnosis in these cases (see below).

In normal individuals there are between 4 and 40 CTG repeats in the DMPK gene but in DM1 patients this is increased to 50 or more, sometimes to over 1000. In general, there is a correlation between the size of the repeat and clinical severity and age of onset. Thus those with less than 100 repeats are usually milder than the severely affected congenital cases with more than 1000 repeats. Anticipation in DM1 is common with successive generations being more clinically severe and having more repeats. There is also somatic variability and instability in the size of the repeat expansion with the number being greater and more unstable in muscle than in blood lymphocytes.

In the normal population the number of chromosome 3 CCTG repeats ranges from 10 to 30 but in DM2 patients this is increased to many thousands. Anticipation and somatic variability also appear to occur in DM2 but the correlations are less clear than in DM1 as there are fewer affected families.

Myotonia is common to both DM1 and DM2 but the pattern of muscle weakness is different. In DM2 there is early proximal muscle involvement, in contrast to the distal pattern seen in DM1 (Machuca-Tzili et al 2005). Hence the name of proximal myotonic myopathy (PROMM) commonly attributed to the disorder. Facial weakness is also rare in DM2 but is common in DM1. Ptosis, facial and neck weakness are characteristic features of DM1. Similarly, cardiac malfunction and central nervous system involvement are less common in DM2 than in DM1. Diaphragm weakness leads to respiratory insufficiency and is often a cause of death in DM1. Cataracts occur in both DM1 and DM2, and other associated features of both include frontal balding and gonadal atrophy and cardiac involvement. Molecular analysis of the myotonic dystrophies to confirm a clinical diagnosis is highly reliable and muscle biopsies are now less often performed. Histopathological information on DM2 is limited as relatively few biopsies from molecularly confirmed cases have been studied but there appears to be some differences between DM1 and DM2. The following is a summary of the main histopathological features of the myotonic dystrophies, in particular DM1.

Histology and histochemistry

The most common pathological characteristics of DM1 are multiple internal nuclei (often in long chains), sarcoplasmic masses, and an increased incidence of ring fibres. All of these changes are superimposed on a generally myopathic-looking biopsy.

Changes in fibre size

The earliest change observed in DM1 is a disparity between the size of the type 1 and 2 fibres with atrophy of type 1 fibres and hypertrophy of the type 2 fibres (Fig. 14.3). The type 2 fibre hypertrophy usually involves both subtypes. In patients with more severe disease or those in whom the duration of the illness is longer, this disparity may be less marked. The presence of small angulated fibres has been suggested as evidence of denervation but there is no real evidence of this and no small or large group atrophy. Although type 1 fibre predominance may be present, it is not usually a striking finding, and does not compare to the predominance seen in Duchenne dystrophy. As in other myopathies, type 2B fibre deficiency may occur. In DM2, although there is variation of both fibre types, atrophy appears to affect type 2 fibres more than type 1 fibres in some cases (Vihola et al 2003, Schoser et al 2004).

Nuclear changes

Changes in sarcolemmal nuclei are prominent in both forms. They are an early feature in DM1 and internal nuclei are probably more numerous in myotonic dystrophy than in almost any other disease (Fig. 14.4). In longitudinal section, these nuclei frequently appear in chains. Even cases in which the only other change is in the size of type 1 fibres usually demonstrate internal nuclei. In advanced stages of the illness, all the muscle fibres can be speckled with internal

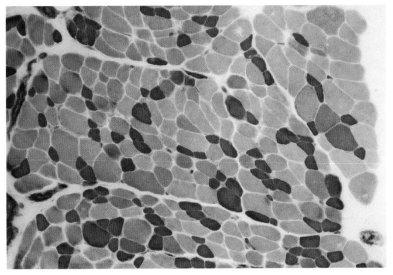

FIG. 14.3 *Myosin ATPase staining with preincubation at pH 4.6 in a quadriceps biopsy of a child with myotonic dystrophy showing atrophy of darkly stained type 1 fibres and hypertrophy of type 2 fibres. Fibre size range approximately 10–70 μm.*

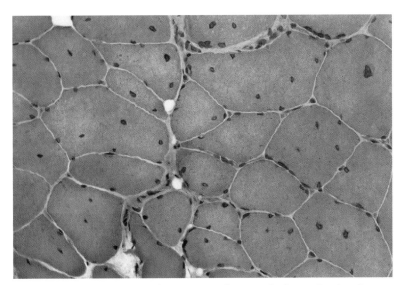

FIG. 14.4 *Quadriceps biopsy from a case of myotonic dystrophy showing variation in fibre size and numerous internal nuclei.*

nuclei. Some nuclei may be pyknotic and form clumps, as seen in other chronic conditions and have been noted as a particular feature of DM2 (Vihola et al 2003, Schoser et al 2004).

In congenital forms the nuclei may be central and there is a striking similarity with myotubular myopathy (see Ch. 15). Thus DM1 should always be molecularly excluded if central nuclei are abundant in a biopsy from a neonate.

Degeneration and regeneration

Degeneration, regeneration and fibrosis may occur in severe cases, but are usually not seen in early stages and rare in DM2. Cellular responses are also not a feature.

Architectural changes

Ring fibres are present in a high proportion of cases of DM1. Although they are a non-specific feature they tend to occur in chronic dystrophies such as myotonic dystrophy. Moth-eaten and whorled fibres may also be present in both forms but not target or targetoid fibres. Sarcoplasmic masses are a typical feature of DM1 and are dark-staining zones which ultrastructurally can be seen to contain disorganized myofibrillar material, free ribosomes and dilated sarcoplasmic reticulum.

Summary

In summary, the changes of DM1 are characteristic. The disease begins with a disparity in the size of type 1 and 2 fibres. There is usually type 1 fibre atrophy and type 2 fibre hypertrophy. However, this disparity may occur in the absence of actual atrophy of the type 1 fibre, in which case type 2 fibre hypertrophy may be the only change. Associated with this early change in fibre size is the presence of multiple internal nuclei. As the disease progresses, more and more myopathic changes make their appearance, together with variability in the size of fibres, fibrosis and architectural changes. In the end stage, the disparity in the size of fibre type may have disappeared but usually the plethora of internal nuclei, together with the abundant number of ring fibres and generally myopathic changes are still obvious.

Immunohistochemistry

Immunohistochemistry with myosin antibodies can be used to study fibre types but adds little additional information to that described above. Little neonatal myosin is present, except in congenital cases, but has not been extensively studied. Studies of DM2 using antibodies to myosin suggested that the fibres with nuclear clumps were type 2 fast fibres (Vihola et al 2003), but the exact properties of these fibres requires clarification as the antibody used (Sigma My-32) also recognizes a neonatal isoform of myosin. The presence of neonatal myosin in these fibres was not studied as only an antibody to a more immature, embryonic isoform was used (Novocastra RNMy2/9D2).

Research studies of transgenic mice and cultured fibroblasts have shown nuclear foci of the nucleotide expansion but they are not abundant in muscle sections and not of practical use to the pathologist (Mankodi et al 2000).

Oculopharyngeal muscular dystrophy

Oculopharyngeal muscular dystrophy (OPMD) is usually transmitted as an autosomal dominant disorder but a few recessive cases have also been reported. Both are caused by short GCG expansions of the first exon of the polyadenylate-binding protein nuclear 1 gene (*PABPN1*) on chromosome 14q11.1 (Brais et al 1998). There are normally six GCG repeats in the first exon of the *PABPN1* gene but in OPMD cases there are an additional two to seven repeats. The disorder has a worldwide distribution but it seems to be particularly prevalent in the French Canadian and Bukhura Jewish populations (Brais et al 1997, Brais 2002).

OPMD is a late onset disorder and the main clinical features are progressive ptosis and dysphagia. Ptosis is an early feature and is usually bilateral, and occasionally asymmetrical. Progression is slow and leads to weakness of several muscles, including those of the face, eyes and limbs, and a nasal voice develops. Cardiac involvement is not a feature of OPMD and creatine kinase activity is usually normal, or occasionally mildly elevated.

Histology and histochemisty

Changes in fibre size

Increased variability in fibre size, particularly of the type 1 fibres, is common and may be accompanied by marked hypertrophy, especially of type 2 fibres. Scattered small angulated fibres, often dark with the oxidative enzyme reaction, may also be present (Fig. 14.5).

Changes in distribution

These are not marked but, as in many disorders, there may be a predominance of type 1 fibres. There is no group atrophy or type grouping, but in some biopsies the distribution of 2A and 2B subtypes may not be random and they may be clustered in some areas. The possibility that this and the small angulated fibres relate to a neural effect associated with ageing has been suggested.

Nuclear changes

Occasional internal nuclei are seen and some biopsies show pyknotic nuclear clumps, particularly in the older patients. The most important nuclear change is seen with electron microscopy (see below).

Degeneration and cellular reactions

Necrosis and inflammatory response are not usually found in OPMD. Increased fibrous connective tissue and deposition of adipose tissue may occur.

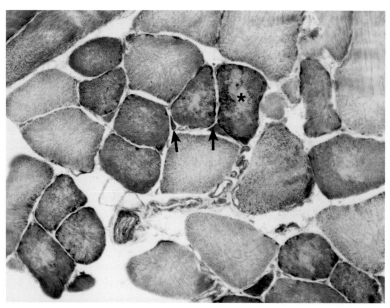

FIG. 14.5 *Muscle from a 77-year-old man with oculopharyngeal muscular dystrophy stained for NADH-TR. Note the wide variation in fibre size (range 15–125 µm) with hypertrophy of pale type 2 fibres and some small dark slightly angular fibres (arrows). Note also the core-like areas devoid of stain (*).*

Architectural changes

A consistent change is the presence of rimmed vacuoles in many fibres (Fig. 14.6). These have the appearance of a sharply punched out areas surrounded by a rim of material staining red with Gomori trichrome and basophilic with H&E (see below for ultrastructure). The vacuoles often contain acid phosphatase and are more common in type 1 fibres than type 2. Although a characteristic of oculopharyngeal myopathy, they are not pathognomonic and can occur in other disorders, such as inclusion body myositis. Electron microscopy is then important (see below). Other architectural changes in OPMD include moth-eaten fibres, core-like areas and whorled fibres (Fig. 14.5). Mitochondrial aggregates, as in lobulated fibres, may be seen and also a few ragged-red fibres and fibres devoid of cytochrome oxidase, reflecting the presence of abnormal mitochondria, may occur. These may be an age-related feature as their occurrence can increase with age.

Electron microscopy

Ultrastructural studies of the rimmed vacuoles show that they are autophagic and contain osmiophilic, membranous, myelin-like whorls and cytoplasmic debris. The characteristic feature of OPMD is the presence of intranuclear tubular filaments. These have an outer diameter of 8.5 nm and an inner diameter of 3 nm and are about 2.5 µm in length. They are unbranched and their orientation

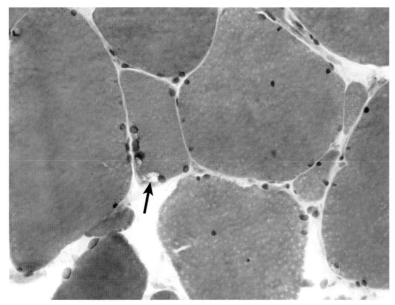

FIG. 14.6 *A rimmed vacuole with red stained material (arrow) in an atrophic fibre in the same case of oculopharyngeal muscular dystrophy as Fig. 14.5 (Gomori trichrome). Diameter of atrophic fibre 25 μm.*

is variable but they often form triangles or palisades. They only occur in muscle nuclei and never in the cytoplasm or nuclei of other cell types, such as satellite cells, endothelial or interstitial cells. In OPMD the nuclear inclusions are distinct from the 15–18 nm filaments seen in inclusion body myositis and distal myopathies with rimmed vacuoles, which can be seen in nuclei and the cytoplasm. The number of affected nuclei in OPMD varies between muscles from 2–5%, but is rarely more than 8%. Similarly, the space occupied by the filamentous inclusions within each nucleus varies. They can be identified as pale or clear areas in semi-thin, toluidine-blue-stained, resin sections.

Other non-specific ultrastructural abnormalities include myofibrillar disruption, Z-line streaming and deposits of lipofuscin, which is a common feature of adult muscle.

Immunohistochemistry

Antibodies to PABPN1 localize to the nuclear inclusions. They do not contain DNA but poly(A) RNA can be detected in them with *in situ* hybridization (Becher et al 2000, Calado et al 2000). The inclusions are also recognized by antibodies to ubiquitin and proteosomal subunits (Askanas et al 1991).

CHAPTER 15

Congenital myopathies

Introduction

The congenital myopathies are a clinically, genetically and pathologically heterogeneous group of muscle disorders defined by the presence of particular histopathological features. They emerged as a group of disorders with the wider application of histochemistry and electron microscopy in the 1950s and 1960s, when abnormal structural defects were identified in association with a particular phenotype. Historically the recognition of this group of disorders probably dates from the description of 'a new congenital non-progressive myopathy' by Magee and Shy (1956), later named central core disease, and the subsequent demonstration of the striking histochemical picture by Dubowitz and Pearse (1960). Presentation of congenital myopathies is often at birth or in early childhood, but some cases may have adult onset and are thus not strictly 'congenital'. It is not yet clear if all of these are parts of clinical spectra or if they are genetically distinct entities, sharing pathological features with congenital cases. Clinically, the congenital myopathies often fall into the 'floppy infant' category with a variable degree of hypotonia (Dubowitz 1969, 1995). Muscle weakness is often, but not always, relatively non-progressive but diaphragmatic weakness and respiratory insufficiency may be disproportionate. Structural abnormalities in the central nervous system or peripheral nerves are absent and congenital myopathies are therefore regarded as primary myopathies.

Advances in molecular analysis have led to the identification of several causative gene mutations associated with the morphological features and this has led to a wider appreciation of the clinical phenotype associated with them. Some of the more common forms are now relatively well defined disorders whilst others are very rare and may be based on very few isolated patients. In these it is not yet clear if all are distinct genetic entities. Few of the pathological features are specific for a particular disorder and all are a secondary consequence of the gene mutation. It is now apparent that there is considerable pathological overlap between the various congenital myopathies and the pathological distinction between them is not always clear. Mutations in different genes can lead to the presence of the same histopathological feature, sometimes as a result of functional association of the gene products, and mutations in the same gene can give rise to a variable clinical phenotype. The pathogenic mechanisms underlying the presence of the structural abnormalities are not fully understood, although several hypotheses have been put forward.

Inheritance may be autosomal recessive, autosomal dominant or X-linked and there is a high incidence of *de novo* dominant mutations.

In this chapter we describe the pathology of the more common congenital myopathies that a pathologist is likely to encounter. We have deliberately steered away from a molecular categorization as it is the pathology in association with the clinical phenotype that usually leads to identification of the causative gene defect. Molecular advances, however, have led to greater knowledge of the range of morphological features that can occur in association with a broad range of clinical phenotypes.

The most common congenital myopathies are central core disease, multi-minicore disease, nemaline myopathy, and myotubular and centronuclear myopathies (see below; Table 15.1; North 2004). Additional rare disorders characterized by other morphological features are also listed in Table 15.1.

Clinical features

In addition to hypotonia, which is usually present at birth or early infancy, there are several additional clinical features that distinguish the various congenital myopathies. Muscle weakness may be predominantly proximal and of girdle distribution, thus resembling muscular dystrophy or mild forms of spinal muscular atrophy, or it may be more generalized. In some, weakness may show marked involvement of the axial muscles and the face and a few may show prominent distal involvement. A long 'myopathic' face is a common feature, particularly in nemaline myopathy, and extraocular involvement occurs in some disorders, such as myotubular myopathy and in some cases with mutations in the ryanodine receptor gene (*RYR1*). Structural abnormalities of the central nervous system or peripheral nerves do not usually occur and intelligence is usually normal. Although generally non-progressive, diaphragmatic involvement may be disproportionate to overall muscle weakness, in particular in some cases of nemaline myopathy and multi-minicore disease.

Arthrogryposis may occur in some severe cases of nemaline myopathy (Lammens et al 1997) and central core disease (Romero et al 2003). Lordosis, spinal rigidity, scoliosis and joint laxity are common and hip dislocation is a particular feature of central core disease.

Investigations

Serum creatine kinase levels are usually normal and electrophysiological studies rarely help in diagnosis. Ultrasound imaging often shows increased echo and

TABLE 15.1 *The congenital myopathies*

Disorders with known gene defects				
	Gene	**Gene locus**	**Inheritance**	**Protein**
Central core disease	*RYR1*	19q.13.1	AD or AR	Ryanodine receptor
Multi-minicore disease	*SEPN1*	1p36	AR	Selenoprotein N1
Nemaline myopathy	*ACTA1*	1q42.1	AD or AR	Skeletal α-actin
	NEB	2q.21.2-22	AR	Nebulin
	TPM3	1q21-q23	AD	α-Tropomyosin
	TPM2	9p13	AD	β-Tropomyosin
	TNNT1	19q13	AR	Slow troponin T
Myotubular myopathy	*MTM1*	Xq28	XL	Myotubularin
Hyaline body myopathy	*MYH7*	14q	AD	Slow myosin heavy chain
Sarcotubular myopathy	*TRIM32*	9q31-34	AR	TRIM32
Fibre type disproportion	*ACTA1*	1q42.1	?	Skeletal α-actin

Disorders with structural defects but unknown gene defects*

Broad A-band disease

Cap disease

Cylindrical spirals myopathy[†]

Cytoplasmic or spheroid body myopathy

Fingerprint body myopathy[†]

Lamellar body myopathy

Myopathy with muscle spindle excess

Reducing body myopathy[†]

Trilaminar fibre myopathy

Tubular aggregate myopathy[†]

Zebra body myopathy

AD, autosomal dominant; AR, autosomal recessive; XL, X-linked; ?, inheritance currently uncertain.
* A genetic basis for some of these is uncertain and only sporadic cases reported.
[†] Familial cases reported.

may reveal differential involvement of muscles. This can be helpful in deciding which muscle to sample. The differential involvement of muscles is clearly seen with magnetic resonance imaging (MRI) and emerging data indicate that particular patterns of selective involvement of thigh and lower leg muscles are associated with mutations in certain genes and are helpful in directing molecular analysis (Jungbluth et al 2004a,b,c). Muscle biopsy, with detailed histochemical studies, supplemented by immunohistochemistry and electron microscopy, is essential for the diagnosis of congenital myopathies and for directing molecular analysis.

Pathological features of congenital myopathies

Hypotrophy of type 1 fibres is seen in several congenital myopathies, and there is often a marked predominance or uniformity of type 1 fibres. Although the fibres appear to be type 1 with stains for oxidative enzymes and for adenosine triphosphatase (ATPase), the intensity of staining is often less than that seen in normal muscle and intermediate between type 1 and 2 fibres. Antibodies to myosin isoforms confirm the slow phenotype of most fibres but again the intensity of labelling may be less than in normal muscle. Necrosis and regeneration are not typical features of congenital myopathies. Scattered, very small fibres containing neonatal myosin, however, are often seen (see Ch. 6), but it is not clear if these represent attempts at regeneration. Fibrosis is also rare in congenital myopathies but can occur (see section on central core disease). Centrally placed nuclei are a particular feature of myotubular and centronuclear myopathies (see below) and we are now aware that they are also common in association with mutations in the *RYR1* gene (see below).

Central core disease

In 1956 Magee and Shy described a 'new congenital non-progressive myopathy' affecting five patients in three generations of the same family, ranging in age from 2 to 65 years. The main clinical features were hypotonia and delay in motor milestones in infancy, and a mild non-progressive weakness, affecting proximal muscles more than distal, and the legs more than the arms. The muscle was characterized by amorphous-looking central areas within the muscle fibres. Greenfield et al (1958) subsequently suggested the name 'central core disease'. A second case documented by Engel et al (1961) was studied histochemically (Dubowitz and Pearse 1960) and the classical histochemical features noted, in particular well delineated areas that ran down a considerable length of the fibres that were devoid of oxidative enzyme stain and phosphorylase. These core areas were not necessarily central and many fibres had multiple cores. In addition, the normal fibre typing was lost and the fibres had a uniform appearance of only type 1 fibres. Electron microscopy showed a virtual absence of mitochondria and sarcoplasmic reticulum in the core region, a marked reduction in the intermyofibrillar space and an irregular pattern (streaming) of the Z lines (Engel et al 1961, Seitelberger et al 1961).

Since these early reports there have been many additional cases with this phenotype associated with the prominent core lesions. With the advent of molecular genetics there has been a greater understanding of the clinical and pathological phenotype of central core disease (Muntoni and Sewry 2003).

The inheritance of most cases is autosomal dominant with variable penetrance; many sporadic *de novo* dominant cases have also been reported and there are also some recessive cases (Jungbluth et al 2002, Ferrerio et al 2002a). Central core disease is one of the most common congenital myopathies. Initial linkage studies assigned a locus to chromosome 19q13.1, and these cases showed a fairly consistent clinical phenotype, presenting with hypotonia and developmental delay. Cases with a severe presentation with features of the fetal akinesia sequence have been reported and some are associated with recessive inheritance (Monnier et al 2003, Romero et al 2003). Most of these severely affected infants require ventilation at birth and follow a downhill course, leading to death in infancy. Other cases, in contrast, may show considerable improvement and it may be possible to wean them off tracheostomy ventilation; one reported child eventually became independently ambulant (Romero et al 2003).

Weakness in most familial cases is pronounced in the hip girdle and in the axial muscle groups and may be associated with muscle wasting. Facial involvement is usually mild and lack of complete eye closure may be the only finding. Orthopaedic complications are common and include congenital dislocation of the hips and scoliosis. Contractures, other than Achilles tendon tightness, are rare, and many affected individuals have marked ligamentous laxity, occasionally associated with patellar instability. Apart from the most severe neonatal cases, and some of those with congenital dislocation of the hips (Manzur et al 1998), most patients achieve independent walking. The course of central core disease is often static, or only slowly progressive, even over prolonged periods of time (Lamont et al 1998). Primary cardiac involvement is rare and respiratory involvement is usually milder than other congenital myopathies, except in the severe neonatal cases. Serum creatine kinase activity is usually normal or only mildly elevated. A striking feature of central core disease is the differential muscle involvement, which can be shown on muscle ultrasound and, more strikingly, with MRI of muscle which reveals a characteristic pattern of selective involvement, even within the quadriceps (Jungbluth et al 2004b). This is helpful when selecting the site for a muscle biopsy and interpreting results.

Histopathology

Fibre size variation occurs but is often mild. Fibre hypertrophy is common, particularly in adults (Fig. 15.1). When fibre typing is retained the cores have a predilection for type 1 fibres but fibre type uniformity is common with most fibres

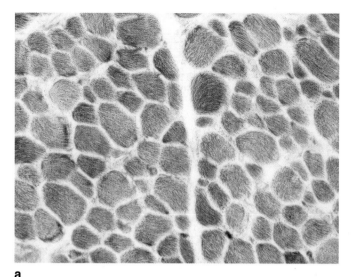

a

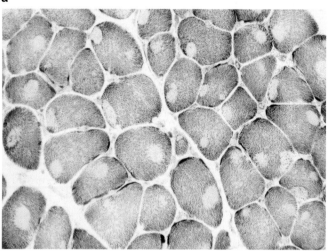

b

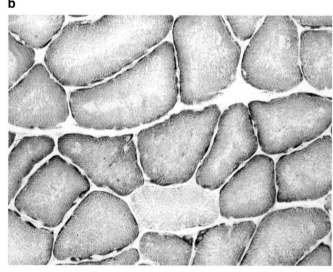

c

staining as type 1 fibres, with the associated properties of slow fibres (Fig. 15.1). A few fibres may co-express fast myosin and there may be a few very small fibres with neonatal myosin scattered through the biopsy. The intensity of stain of the type 1 fibres, however, may not always be as strong as in normal muscle. Classical cores may be central or peripheral, single or multiple, but clearly demarcated cores are not always evident in all cases (Fig. 15.1). Very young cases, in particular, may only show type 1 uniformity or predominance, suggesting there is an age-related development of the cores (Fig. 15.1; Sewry et al 2002). Other cases may show only subtle unevenness in oxidative enzyme stains (Fig. 15.2) or multiple focal areas of disruption, resembling minicores, making a histopathological distinction difficult (Fig. 15.1; Sewry et al 2002; see below). It is important to remember that core formation is a secondary morphological phenomenon and may not itself be the reason for the muscle weakness.

In most cases of central core disease the cores are of the 'structured' type, as they retain a striated myofibrillar pattern and myofibrillar ATPase activity, although myofibrils of the core are often very contracted (Fig. 15.3). In 'unstructured cores' myofibrillar ATPase activity is lost (Fig. 15.4) and there is severe myofibrillar disruption with pronounced accumulation of smeared Z-line material. The length of the cores can be variable but they typically extend down an appreciable length of a fibre. The area devoid of mitochondria may be more extensive than the apparent ultrastructural myofibrillar disruption. Sarcoplasmic reticulum and T tubules may also be reduced in cores but some tubular structures may be apparent within them. Cores are often delineated by a rim of periodic acid-Schiff (PAS) stain (see Ch. 4) and immunohistochemistry shows that desmin may accumulate at their perimeter or within them (Fig. 15.5). Other proteins that have been shown to accumulate in cores are αB-crystallin, γ-filamin, small heat shock proteins and myotilin (Sewry et al 2002, Shröder et al 2003, Bönnemann et al 2003).

Internal nuclei had not been considered a feature of central core disease in studies of early cases but it is now appreciated that they can be an important indicator of central core disease (Fig. 15.6a,d). In some they may be numerous, and several may be in a central position. Similarly, an increase in connective tissue was not considered a feature of 'classical' cases but can occur, and in some samples there may also be extensive adipose tissue (Fig. 15.6d,e). In these samples the separation of fascicles of fibres by adipose tissue and fibrous tissue may cause

---

FIG. 15.1 *Biopsies of the quadriceps from three members of the same family with central core disease with a dominant mutation in the ryanodine receptor gene showing the range of appearance that can be seen with oxidative enzyme stains. (a) Female aged 4 months showing variation in fibre size (fibre diameter range 5–40 μm) and fibre type uniformity but no clear-cut cores; (b) the brother aged 3 years showing mild variation in fibre size (fibre diameter range 15–65 μm), fibre type uniformity and numerous cores of varying size centrally or peripherally; (c) the mother aged 32 years showing hypertrophy of most fibres (fibre diameter range 85–120 μm), type 1 fibre predominance and unevenness of stain or small areas devoid of stain but no pronounced cores.*

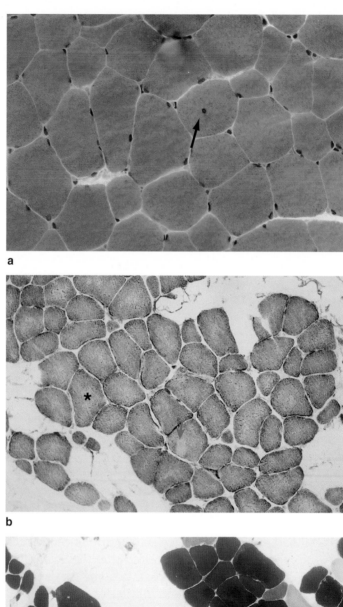

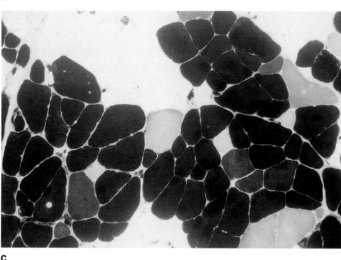

FIG. 15.2 *Quadriceps biopsy from a female aged 28 years with typical clinical features of central core disease and a mutation in the RYR1 gene showing (a) occasional central nuclei (arrow) (Gomori trichrome); (b) indistinct fibre typing and mild unevenness of oxidative enzyme stain (*) and only one core-like area (red arrow) (NADH-TR); but (c) type 1 predominance and variation in size of the dark type 1 fibres (ATPase preincubated at pH 4.6).*

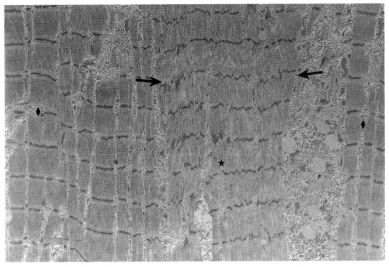

FIG. 15.3 *Electron micrograph of a structured core (arrows) in a case of central core disease showing pronounced contraction of the myofibrils in the core (*) compared with those either side (♦), a little disruption of the Z line and an absence of mitochondria from the core.*

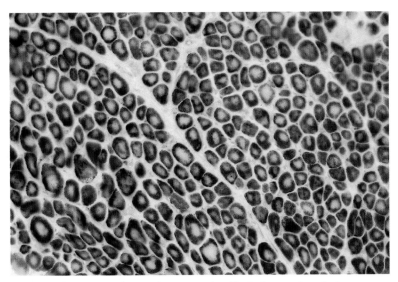

FIG. 15.4 *Unstructured cores in a severely affected case of central core disease showing an absence of ATPase stain in the cores and uniform fibre typing with an intermediate intensity, and a rather brown colour compared with normal (ATPase 9.4).*

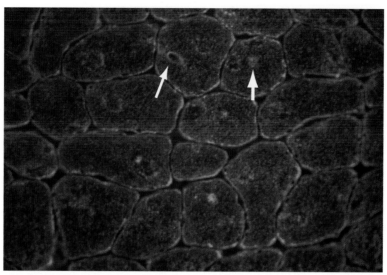

FIG. 15.5 *Immunofluoresent labelling of desmin either within or at the periphery of cores (large and small arrows, respectively) in a proven case of central core disease.*

diagnostic confusion with a muscular dystrophy. Some of these samples may show only subtle unevenness of oxidative enzyme stains, whilst others show large classical cores or multiple small cores (minicores; see Fig. 15.6 b,c,f).

Although cores are the characteristic feature of central core disease caused by mutations in the gene encoding the ryanodine receptor (*RYR1*), core formation can also occur following tenotomy, following neurogenic atrophy (see Ch. 9) and in association with several other gene defects such as the *ACTA1* and *MYH7* genes, encoding skeletal α-actin and β-myosin heavy-chain, respectively (Jungbluth et al 2001, Kaindl 2004, Fananapazir 1993). Cores can also co-exist with rods (Fig. 15.7) and be associated with *RYR1* mutations (Monnier et al 2000). In some cases with *RYR1* mutations only a few fibres may show rods (Fig. 15.8; Jungbluth et al 2002). The coexistence of rods and cores is likely to be genetically heterogeneous as there are examples of cases where linkage to *RYR1* and to the loci of nemaline myopathy (see below) have been excluded.

Molecular genetics

Central core disease is caused by mutations in the gene for the skeletal muscle ryanodine receptor (*RYR1*) on chromosome 19q. The same gene is responsible for malignant hyperthermia, although additional loci are also linked to this. The precise association between central core disease and malignant hyperthermia is not clear but all patients with central core disease are considered at risk and appropriate precautions need to be taken.

The *RYR1* gene contains 106 exons and encodes the skeletal muscle ryanodine receptor protein (RyR1), named after the fact that it binds ryanodine. The receptor is a large transmembrane, tetrameric structure of the sarcoplasmic

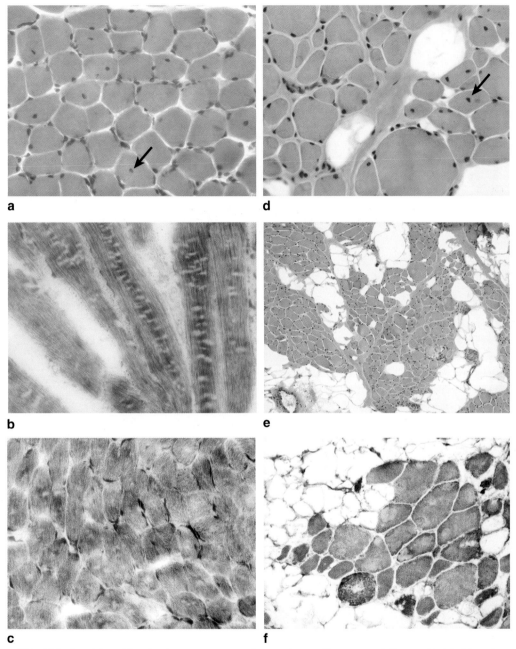

FIG. 15.6 *Quadricep biopsies from two cases of central core disease aged 18 months (a)–(c) and 11 years (d)–(f) with proven mutations in the RYR1 gene. Note the excess internal nuclei, some of which are central, in both cases [arrows; (a), (d)], and the pronounced increase in fat and connective tissue seen at low power in case 2 (e). Case 1 shows multiple cores with oxidative enzyme stains (c) which are particularly apparent in longitudinal section (b), and case 2 shows more classical cores (f) [(a), (d), (e) H&E; (b), (c), (f) NADH-TR. Fibre diameter range (a), (b) 25–40 μm; (d) 10–105 μm; (f) 15–85 μm].*

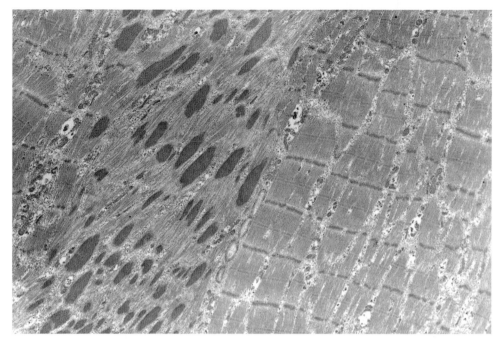

FIG. 15.7 *Electron micrograph showing rods in a central core.*

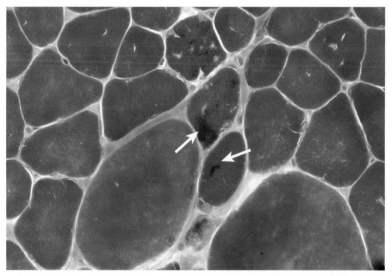

FIG. 15.8 *A few fibres with red-staining rods (arrows) in a case with recessive mutations in the ryanodine receptor gene (Gomori trichrome).*

reticulum and is involved in the regulation of cytosolic calcium levels and excitation–contraction coupling. Genotype–phenotype correlations suggest that mutations in the cytoplasmic N-terminal domain and the cytoplasmic central domain mostly result in malignant hyperthermia susceptibility rather than in central core disease; while mutations affecting the C-terminal exons of the gene commonly result in central core disease (Tilgen et al 2001, Monnier et al 2001).

The majority of mutations in the *RYR1* gene are missense mutations, although small deletions have also been detected.

The large size of the *RYR1* gene makes molecular analysis laborious and, although there appear to be 'hot-spots' for mutations that can help direct analysis (Davis et al 2003), recent data suggest that other regions of the gene are responsible for phenotypic variants. For example cases with ophthalmoplegia are also now known to be caused by *RYR1* mutations. The histopathology in these cases may not show the 'classical' histopathological features of central core and the presence of multi-minicores may cause diagnostic confusion (see below).

In summary the clinical and histopathological spectra associated with mutations in the *RYR1* gene are wide. The use of the term 'central core' disease for all of them may be confusing as some biopsies do not show classical cores. They are linked, however, by common clinical features, and similar patterns of muscle involvement, indicating a spectrum of one disorder. For the histopathologist difficulties in diagnosis may arise if the classical features are not present and because of the histopathological overlap between the various congenital myopathies. In our experience mutations in the *RYR1* gene seem to be particularly common and the features that should alert the pathologist are central nuclei, any unevenness in oxidative enzyme stain, be it marked or subtle, and type 1 fibre uniformity or marked predominance. The coexistence of cores and rods in any fibres also suggests an *RYR1* mutation.

Multi-minicore myopathy

In 1971 Engel et al documented two unrelated children with a benign congenital non-progressive myopathy associated with multifocal areas of degeneration in the muscle fibres and suggested the name 'multicore disease'. Since the original description there have been several reports of cases with a wide range of clinical phenotypes associated with similar histopathological features. The defining histopathological feature is multiple small areas devoid of oxidative enzymes which lack mitochondria and ultrastructurally show disruption of the sarcomeric pattern.

The clinical features of cases with multicores are variable and multiple cores can occur in association with mutations in several genes (see below), and to some extent are a non-specific feature. Four clinical categories of patients with minicores have been identified and molecular defects associated with them are beginning to be identified (Ferrerio et al 2000, Ferrerio and Fardeau 2000, Jungbluth et al 2000). Multi-minicore myopathy is therefore not a single entity and is a name that has been given to several myopathies in which a muscle biopsy shows multifocal areas devoid of oxidative enzyme stains.

Histopathology

The defining feature is multiple focal areas of myofibrillar disruption that lack mitochondria. These can be demonstrated with the oxidative enzyme stains

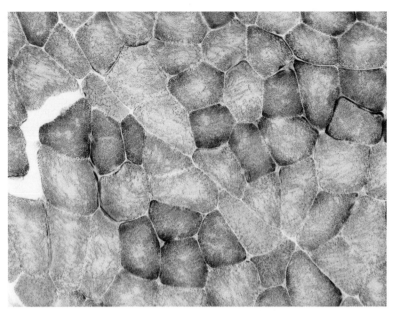

FIG. 15.9 *Areas in both fibre types of varying size and number devoid of oxidative enzyme stain in a quadriceps biopsy from a case of 'multi-minicore disease' aged 11 years with recessive mutations in the SEPN1 gene (NADH-TR). Fibre diameter range 25–55 μm.*

NADH-TR, cytochrome oxidase and succinic dehydrogenase and may appear as punctate or more diffuse areas devoid of stain (Fig. 15.9). The NADH-TR reaction is less specific for absent mitochondria and unevenness of stain can also relate to general disruption of ultrastructure and loss of myofibrils. In some cases the unevenness of oxidative stain may be subtle and difficult to define as abnormal. Ultrastructurally, minicores show a variable degree of focal disruption of myofibrils that affects only a few sarcomeres. In some fibres, only misalignment of the myofibrils compared with surrounding myofibrils may be seen; in others focal Z-line streaming may occur, whilst in others the normal sarcomeric structure may be completely disrupted in a varying number of sarcomeres (see Ch. 5). The common feature, however, is the absence of mitochondria which may extend over a greater area than the disrupted myofibrils. Detailed ultrastructural studies are needed to observe this.

As in central core disease, immunocytochemistry can be helpful in observing the lesions and proteins such as desmin and myotilin that accumulate with them (Bönnemann et al 2003), but there is no specific histopathological method to distinguish the molecular origin of any cores. In contrast to central cores, minicores are not usually delineated by desmin. Immunolabelling of myosin isoforms can be used to assess the proportion of fast and slow fibres and there are usually only a few, or no fibres, containing neonatal myosin in cases with SEPN1 mutations (see below).

Clinical features

The most common phenotype associated with minicores shows marked axial weakness with spinal rigidity, scoliosis, torticollis, and respiratory involvement that is often disproportionate to the overall muscle weakness. They are clinically similar to cases with the rigid spine syndrome and congenital muscular dystrophy (RSMD1) and the two disorders are sometimes considered allelic (Ferreiro et al 2002b). Both are caused by recessive mutations in the gene for selenoprotein N1 (SEPN1) and the spectrum also now includes cases with Mallory bodies (Ferreiro et al 2004; see Chs 5 and 12).

A second clinical group with multiple minicores and with similar proximal and axial weakness also shows partial or complete external ophthalmoplegia. Mutations in the *RYR1* gene have been identified in these patients (Monnier et al 2003, Jungbluth et al 2004a). Mutations in *RYR1* have also been found in a third phenotypic group with similarities to patients with central core disease (Jungbluth et al 2004a; see also Fig. 15.6). The fourth group comprises the rare patients with antenatal onset, generalized arthrogryposis, dysmorphic features and mild to moderate reduction of respiratory function. Primary cardiac malfunction is not a typical feature of any of these groups of patients with multi-minicores, and many of the cases reported in the literature as showing minicores with cardiac involvement are molecularly unsolved and probably heterogeneous.

Inheritance of myopathies with minicores has always been considered as autosomal recessive, distinguishing it from dominantly inherited central core disease. Multi-minicores associated with *SEPN1* mutations are recessively inherited but confusion has arisen as minicores can be a feature of cases with *RYR1* mutations, which can be inherited as an autosomal dominant or recessive trait, or the mutation may be *de novo* dominant. These cases form part of the 'central core' spectrum and are not a separate 'minicore' entity.

Genotype-phenotype correlations

Recent studies have identified additional features that seem to be associated with minicores and a particular gene defect. In cases with a SEPN1 mutation a two fibre type pattern is usually preserved and the minicores can occur in both fibre types (Fig. 15.9). Other myopathic features include variation in fibre size, occasional, or at times, profuse internal nuclei, mild endomysial fibrosis and fat. The SEPN1 gene product is more abundant in fetal muscle and this raises the possibility that muscle repair or regeneration may be influenced by the mutation. There are no studies of its localization in human muscle.

Cases with minicores associated with *RYR1* mutations often have the features described in central core disease (see above), in particular central nuclei and type 1 fibre uniformity or predominance. The pathological features must always be considered together with the clinical phenotype in order to direct molecular analysis.

There have been several reported cases of the presence of minicores in association with an abundance of additional structural defects such as rods or whorled fibres (Afifi et al 1965, Sitz et al 1984, Poumand and Azzarelli 1994). Some have been shown to result from mutations in the *RYR1* gene (Monnier et al 2000, Jungbluth et al 2002) or the *ACTA1* gene (Jungbluth et al 2001) but many of the early cases are still unresolved molecularly.

Nemaline myopathy

In 1963, Shy et al described 'nemaline myopathy, a new congenital myopathy' in a 4-year-old girl who had been a floppy infant and had muscle weakness affecting the upper limbs more than the lower. As they were uncertain whether the rod-like structures in the muscle were separate rods or possibly an undulating thread-like structure, they suggested the name nemaline myopathy (Greek *nema*: thread). Conen et al (1963) independently observed 'myogranules' in the biopsy of a 4-year-old boy with hypotonia and non-progressive muscle weakness. The first description, however, is probably that of Reye in 1958 (Schnell et al 2000) but their significance was uncertain at that time. There have been several subsequent reports of cases with rod-like structures with a wide range of phenotypes and several associated gene defects. The rods may occur in clusters, and stain red with the Gomori trichrome technique.

There is a wide clinical spectrum associated with the presence of rods and six categories have been suggested, based on clinical severity and age of onset (Wallgren-Pettersson et al 1999, Wallgren-Pettersson and Laing 2000, 2001, Wallgren-Pettersson et al 2004). The severe congenital neonatal form is characterized by severe hypotonia and absence of both spontaneous movements and respiration at birth. Some are of antenatal onset within the spectrum of the fetal akinesia sequence (Lammens et al 1997). Patients with an intermediate congenital form have antigravity movement and independent respiration at birth but ambulation is not achieved and respiratory support is subsequently required. The most common form presents with hypotonia in early infancy or childhood, and patients have delayed motor milestones and generalized weakness predominantly affecting facial and axial muscles. They have a low muscle bulk, and feeding and respiratory problems are common. Independent ambulation in these cases is achieved and the disorder is regarded as relatively non-progressive, or mildly progressive. In addition, there are cases with intermediate severity with childhood onset, or those with late or adult onset, or cases in which rods are associated with a variety of other problems (North et al 1997, Sanoudou and Beggs 2001). The distinction between the extremes in this spectrum is obvious but less so between the various milder forms.

Cardiomyopathy has been documented but is not usually considered a feature of nemaline myopathies. Most are adult cases but occasional infantile cases have also been identified (Ishibashi-Ueda et al 1990, Skyllouriotis et al 1999, Muller-Hocker et al 2000, Sanoudou and Beggs 2001).

Histopathology

The defining feature of all nemaline myopathies, regardless of the gene defect, is the red-staining rods seen with the Gomori trichrome stain (Fig. 15.10). In very young cases with very small fibres they may be difficult to observe and oil immersion optics may be required. The rods are often clustered at the periphery of fibres, sometimes near nuclei, but can also be seen within fibres (Fig. 15.10). In a few rare cases rods are restricted to nuclei; in others they occur in nuclei and the cytoplasm (see Ch. 5). In most cases rods are only seen in the cytoplasm. The number of affected fibres varies between muscles and the number of rods per fibre is also variable. There is no correlation between the number of rods and clinical severity. The presence of rods may be accompanied by accumulation of actin filaments (see below).

A wide variation in fibre size may be present, particularly in severe neonatal cases, when the fibres are generally small, but in childhood cases it is often less striking. Type 1 fibre atrophy and/or type 1 fibre uniformity or predominance is common. The type 1 fibre atrophy and the restriction of rods to type 1 fibres in the rare cases with a mutation in the gene for α-tropomyosin may relate to restriction of the protein to type 1 fibres, but type 1 atrophy also occurs when other genes associated with nemaline myopathy are mutated (Fig. 15.11). Fibre hypertrophy may also be apparent (Fig. 15.10b). Internal nuclei, necrosis and fibrosis are not usually seen. Similarly, regeneration is not a feature, although a few very small fibres with neonatal myosin may be scattered through the biopsy in mild cases, suggesting possible attempts at regeneration. Immature fibres with neonatal myosin are often abundant in neonatal cases, and fast and slow isoforms may be co-expressed in a few fibres.

Core-like areas may also occur in association with nemaline rods, again indicating the non-specificity of these structures (Fig. 15.11; Jungbluth et al 2001). Areas with abundant rods lack mitochondria and thus oxidative enzyme stains, and should be distinguished from the type of core-like area described above that have myofibrillar disruption associated with the absence of mitochondria. The presence of more than one type of structural change rarely indicates a separate disease entity but emphasizes the pathological heterogeneity and histopathological overlap within the congenital myopathies.

With electron microscopy, rods are seen as electron dense structures whose shape may be rod-like or sometimes more ovoid. They are often parallel to the longitudinal axis of the sarcomeres, and the appearance of their shape may be dependent on the plane of section (Fig. 15.12). Some rods may be derived from Z lines as they show continuity with them, have a similar lattice structure and contain similar proteins. The major constituent of both rods and Z lines is α-actinin (Fig. 15.13). Rods also contain tropomyosin, and proteins that are anchored in the Z line are also associated with them, such as actin and myotilin. As with Z lines, desmin occurs at the periphery of rods but not within them. Current data suggest that nuclear rods, like cytoplasmic rods, contain α-actinin and actin.

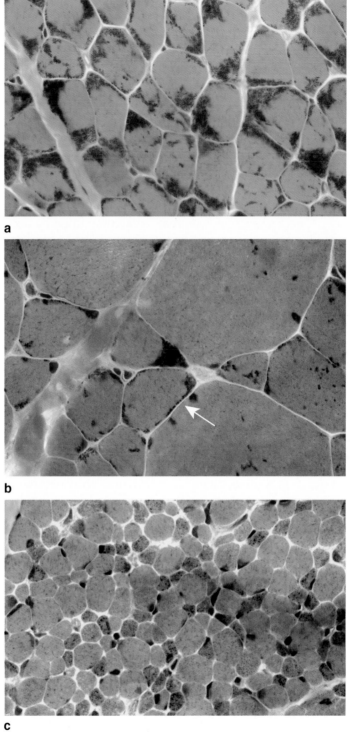

a

b

c

FIG. 15.10 *Biopsies from three cases of nemaline myopathy aged 9 and 17 years (a and b) with dominant mutations in the ACTA1 gene, and (c) 2 month old child with a mutation in the gene encoding nebulin, showing in (a) clusters of red staining rods at the periphery of most fibres and some internal within fibres (fibre diameter range 20–30 μm); in (b) rods in peripheral clusters, in a subsarcolemmal position (arrow) and internally (smallest fibre approximately 35 μm) and in (c) rods scattered through the small fibres which are less than 10 μm in diameter and are type 1 fibres. (Gomori trichrome).*

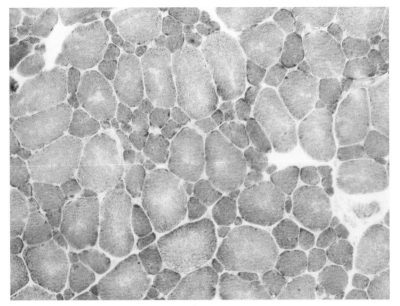

a

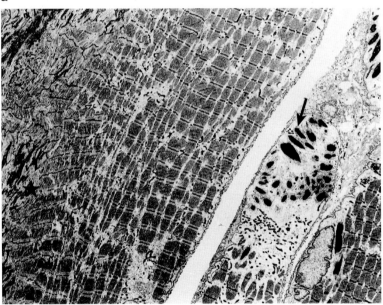

b

FIG. 15.11 *(a) Core-like areas devoid of NADH-TR activity in the case of nemaline myopathy shown in Fig. 15.10 (b). Note also the atrophy of the dark type 1 fibres (diameter range 10–20 μm) compared to the normal sized type 2 fibres (diameter range 40–50 μm). (b) Electron micrograph showing the presence of rods (arrow) and a core region with disrupted myofibrils in an adjacent fibre (*) in the same case.*

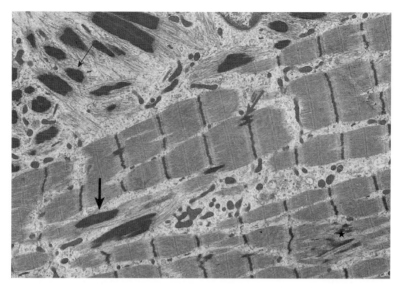

FIG. 15.12 *Electron micrograph showing nemaline rods transversely and longitudinally orientated (small and large arrows, respectively), small rods in continuity with Z lines (green arrow) and smeared Z-line material (*) in a quadriceps biopsy from an 8-year-old boy with mild, non-progressive muscle weakness.*

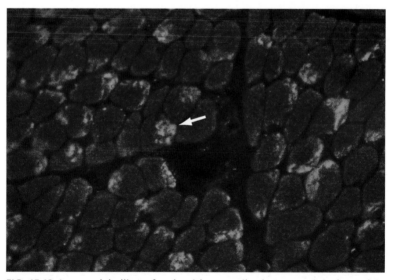

FIG. 15.13 *Immunolabelling of rods with an antibody to α-actinin (arrow) in a case of nemaline myopathy with a mutation in the skeletal α-actin gene.*

Accumulation of actin thin filaments, with or without rods, or in association with various Z-line abnormalities, is seen as pale staining areas with haematoxylin and eosin and with the Gomori trichrome stain (Fig. 15.14).

Various isoforms of α-actinin, a major component of rods have been identified. The isoform encoded by the *ACTN2* gene is present in all fibres but *ACTN3* is restricted to a subset of type 2 fibres (North and Beggs 1996). Rods in general have the same isoform as the myofibrils. Most cases of nemaline myopathy have very few type 2 fibres and only ACTN2 is present, but in a few fibres rods labelled with antibodies to ACTN3 can be seen in addition to the ACTN2 of the myofibrils. These rods therefore have a different isoform from the myofibrils. The reason for this is not known but it may suggest that the rods are very stable structures.

Rod-like structures are not specific to the nemaline myopathies and they can also be found at normal myotendinous junctions, in normal ocular muscles, and occasionally in a variety of neuromuscular disorders. As mentioned above, in some cases with a mutation in the *RYR1* gene they may be a particular feature and be associated with cores (Monnier et al 2000). Confusion regarding disease entities can arise with overlapping pathology and it is important to remember that not all cases with rods are necessarily 'nemaline myopathy' but are better thought of as 'myopathy with rods'.

Molecular genetics

Nemaline myopathy can be inherited as an autosomal recessive or autosomal dominant disorder. There are also a number of *de novo* dominant cases. Mutations in five genes have been found to be associated with an abundance of rods, all of which encode thin filament proteins (Table 15.1; North et al 1999). There is potentially further genetic heterogeneity as some cases do not link to any of the known loci (Wallgren-Pettersson et al 1999; Wallgren-Pettersson and Laing 2000, 2001). Mutations in the *ACTA1* and *NEB* genes, encoding skeletal α-actin and nebulin respectively, are the most common. Mutations in *ACTA1* are mainly dominant or *de novo* dominant with a few rare recessive cases (Sparrow et al 2003, Agrawal et al 2004). In contrast, all reported mutations in the gene for nebulin are recessive. The *NEB* gene is extremely large with 183 exons and several splice sites; searching for mutations is thus tedious and efforts have mostly concentrated on the C-terminus as the C-terminal domain of nebulin is anchored in the Z line, and rods are similar to Z lines (see below). The common childhood type of nemaline myopathy results from mutations in the gene for nebulin, and there is a particular deletion in the Ashkenazi Jewish population (Anderson et al 2004). Mutations in the genes for α- and β-tropomyosin (*TPM3*, *TPM2*) have been identified in a few rare families, and mutations in the gene for tropinin T (*TNNTI*) seem to be restricted to the Amish population in North America (see Table 15.1).

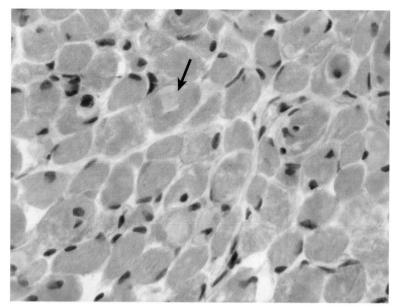

a

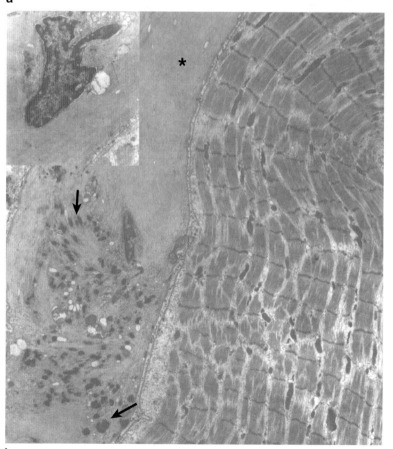

b

FIG. 15.14 *(a) Pale staining areas where actin filaments have accumulated in a quadriceps biopsy of a 1-year-old case of nemaline myopathy (H&E). Fibre diameter range 5–20 μm. (b) Electron micrograph showing actin accumulation, note also the small dense rod-like structures (arrow). Inset shows a higher magnification of the actin filaments adjacent to a nucleus.*

Genotype-phenotype correlations

It is rarely possible to predict the defective gene responsible for the nemaline myopathy from the pathology alone. Mutations in the genes for actin and nebulin are the most common and the pathology must be considered with the clinical phenotype; muscle MRI is also proving to be helpful (Jungbluth et al 2004a,b). An exception to this is the presence of nuclear rods and/or accumulation of actin thin filaments (Fig. 15.14). These seem to be associated only with *ACTA1* mutations, although no *ACTA1* mutations have been found in a few cases with accumulations of actin filaments. Research studies using a non-commercial antibody to the SH3 domain of nebulin suggested that its absence could help identify a mutation in the nebulin gene in severe cases (Sewry et al 2001a, Wallgren-Pettersson et al 2002). Subsequently, however, secondary changes in nebulin have also been identified in severe *ACTA1* cases (Ilkovski et al 2004).

Myotubular myopathies

In 1966 Spiro et al suggested the name 'myotubular myopathy' for the histological changes observed in the biopsies from a 12-year-old boy, because of the striking resemblance to the myotubes of fetal muscle. On biopsy of the gastrocnemius, the muscle fibres were normal in size, but in about 85% of fibres there were one to four centrally placed nuclei, surrounded by an area devoid of myofibrils. Similar changes were noted in about 45% of fibres in a second biopsy. Histochemical studies showed normal oxidative enzyme activity in unaffected fibres, but in affected fibres there was a central zone either devoid of enzyme activity or with increased enzyme activity. Phosphorylase and PAS activity also showed either an increase or a decrease in the central zone of respective fibres. The ATPase reaction, on the other hand, showed a consistent absence of activity in these central areas. On electron microscopy, the perinuclear zone contained aggregates of mitochondria and myelin figures, which may have resulted from prior freezing of the muscle. There were no ribosomal aggregates. Spiro et al (1966) considered these abnormal fibres to be comparable to the myotubes of developing muscle and postulated an arrest in the development of the muscle at a cellular level.

Sher and her colleagues (1967) subsequently observed similar pathological changes in the muscle of two Negro sisters, aged 18 and 16 years, and their symptom-free mother. The first sister had delay in early motor milestones, generalized atrophy of the musculature, a slowly progressive weakness of the skeletal muscles, ptosis, external ophthalmoplegia and facial weakness. The clinical photograph with the long, thin face showed a striking resemblance to the case of Spiro et al (1966) and also to the 'dysmorphic' features of some reported cases of nemaline myopathy. The younger sister, who had not been floppy as an infant and had no delay in motor milestones, showed a fairly diffuse wasting and weakness of the limbs and bilateral ptosis, but no facial weakness or ophthalmoplegia.

Biopsy of the rectus femoris and gastrocnemius in both sisters showed central nuclei in the majority of fibres. In the mother's gastrocnemius, about a third of the fibres had internal nuclei. Fibre diameter was normal in all three. Histochemical study showed both type 1 and 2 fibres. Oxidative enzyme activity was either concentrated or absent in the central zones of the fibres with central nuclei. Phosphorylase and glycogen showed an intracellular distribution similar to the dehydrogenases. Myofibrillar ATPase was lacking in the central zones. Electron microscopy confirmed the presence of central nuclei and showed other relatively non-specific changes in the central region of the fibres. Sher et al (1967) were not convinced of the pathogenesis of the condition and suggested the alternative descriptive title 'centronuclear myopathy' rather than 'myotubular'. The term 'myotubular' is firmly entrenched in the literature and will probably persist in spite of the possibly erroneous premise for its choice.

Since these early descriptions many cases with prominent central nuclei have been identified. They are clinically heterogeneous with neonatal, childhood or adult onset, and an X-linked form and autosomal forms have been identified. The X-linked form usually has a severe neonatal presentation and the term 'myotubular' is now often restricted to these cases, whilst the more descriptive term of 'centronuclear' is applied to the autosomal cases. We have adhered to this distinction, although not universally applied by all, as the severe X-linked neonates are an identifiable group for which a molecular test is now available, whilst those with autosomal inheritance are heterogeneous and defined by the descriptive 'centronuclear' term.

X-linked myotubular myopathy

This is a severe condition with onset in utero. Pregnancy is complicated by polyhydramnios and there is often a history of miscarriages and neonatal death in the maternal line. There is marked neonatal hypotonia, a variable degree of external ophthalmoplegia, feeding difficulties and respiratory failure at birth which is often fatal. Some severely affected infants may survive if the respiratory problems in the neonatal period can be overcome (Herman et al 1999, McEntagart et al 2002). The molecular defect is a mutation in the *MTM1* gene on the X-chromosome, encoding a protein named myotubularin (see below).

Histopathology

The key feature is the large centrally placed nuclei (Fig. 15.15a). In longitudinal section these are regularly spaced down the fibre (Fig. 15.15b), thus the plane of section influences the number of central nuclei observed in transverse section. The number of central nuclei can vary between muscles and they may not always be numerous, or be apparent at birth (Sasaki et al 1989, Helliwell et al 1998). Central nuclei occur in both fibre types.

A striking feature associated with the central nuclei is the dark-staining areas with oxidative enzyme stains and PAS, reflecting aggregation of

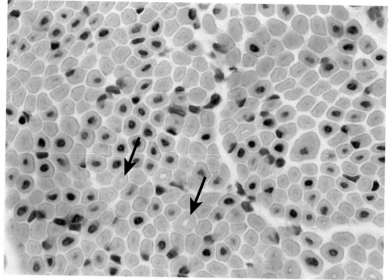

a

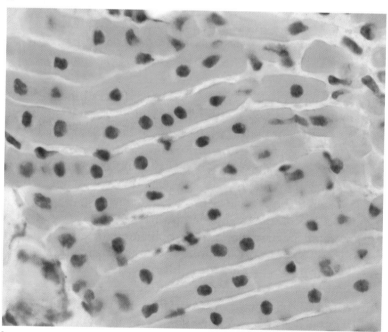

b

FIG. 15.15 *Quadriceps biopsy from a case of X-linked myotubular myopathy aged 8 months showing large central nuclei in several fibres in (a) transverse and (b) longitudinal section; in longitudinal section note the widely spaced nuclei which affects the number seen in transverse section and in transverse section note the central holes devoid of myofibrils (arrows) (H&E). Most fibres are less than 10 μm in diameter.*

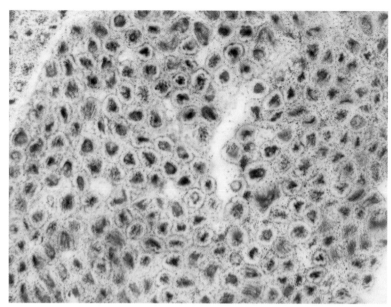

FIG. 15.16 *Accumulation of oxidative enzyme stain in the centre of fibres and pale peripheral halos in a quadriceps biopsy from a male aged 8 months with myotubular myopathy (NADH-TR). Most fibres are less than 10 µm in diameter.*

mitochondria and glycogen (Fig. 15.16). These areas around the nuclei are devoid of myofibrils and appear as holes with ATPase staining or myosin immunolabelling, and are also apparent with H&E (see Fig. 15.15a). Oxidative enzyme staining, in addition to the dark centres may also show pale subsarcolemmal peripheral halos round many fibres. Such halos can also be observed in other conditions and it is not clear if they may be an age-related phenomenon. They are also observed in autosomal centronuclear cases (see below).

As in many congenital myopathies type 1 fibres may be predominant, and most fibres are small in diameter (hypotrophic and/or atrophic), particularly type 1 fibres. Necrosis and fibrosis are not typical features of X-linked myotubular myopathy, but it is not known if this may develop with age. Similarly, architectural features such as whorled or split fibres are not usually seen.

Ultrastructural studies reveal the central accumulation of mitochondria and glycogen, and absence and disorganization of myofibrils. We have also noted collections of dense tubules, of unknown origin, in some severe cases (Heckmatt et al 1985).

Immunohistochemistry

Some fibres show more abundant desmin and vimentin than normal. As these occur in immature fibres this has been put forward as evidence of a developmental defect (Sarnat 1990), but it is not a feature of all fibres with central nuclei. Fibres with neonatal myosin are common in neonates and its presence in these cases is to be expected. Labelling of myosin isoforms generally indicates, however, that maturation at least with regard to myosin isoforms, does occur in myotubular myopathy and fibres with central nuclei have the fast or slow isoform of mature muscle (Fig. 15.17; Sewry 1998). Expression of neural cell adhesion molecule (N-CAM), utrophin and laminin α5 has also been observed (Helliwell et al 1998), and, although these are associated with immaturity, they are a non-specific finding.

Studies of antibodies to the gene product, myotubularin, fail to detect endogenous protein in muscle sections but immunoprecipitation has identified a reduction or absence in most patients studied (Laporte et al 2001).

Female carriers of myotubular myopathy

Female carriers with *MTM1* mutations may manifest and in some this has been shown to relate to skewed X-inactivation (Dahl et al 1995, Tanner et al 1999, Jungbluth et al 2003). The clinical severity in MTM1 carriers is variable and ranges from mild, with mild facial weakness, to severe with hypotonia from birth and inability to stand or walk (Jungbluth et al 2003). A mutation in the *MTM1* gene should therefore be considered in any female showing abundant central nuclei in a muscle biopsy.

Differential diagnosis

An essential differential diagnosis in neonatal cases with central nuclei is congenital myotonic dystrophy. The pathological features are identical and no histopathological way of distinguishing them has yet been found. Thus molecular exclusion of an expansion of the *DM1* gene should always be performed. It has been suggested that the expansion of the *DM1* gene may interfere with processing of other proteins and it is interesting to note that RNA from a gene with homology to the myotubularin gene (the myotubularin-related protein 1 gene, *MTMR1*) may be a target for abnormal splicing in congenital myotonic dystrophy (Buj-Bello et al 2002).

Molecular genetics

X-linked myotubular myopathy is caused by mutations in the gene encoding myotubularin (*MTM1*) on chromosome Xq28 (Laporte et al 2000). Myotubularin belongs to a family of proteins and is expressed in most tissues. It is a dual specificity phosphatase that dephosphorylates phosphatidylinositol 3-phosphate and phosphatidylinositol (3,5)-bisphosphate. Its exact function is not clear but some evidence suggests it may have a role in signalling pathways involved in growth and development. Preliminary studies indicated that myotubularin was localized to nuclei (Cui et al 1998) but later studies show it is essentially cytoplasmic (Mandel et al 2002). Despite extensive efforts, antibodies to myotubularin fail to detect endogenous myotubularin in muscle sections. The large number of different mutations are distributed throughout the gene and may be point mutations, small or large deletions, insertions, or missense, nonsense or splice site mutations.

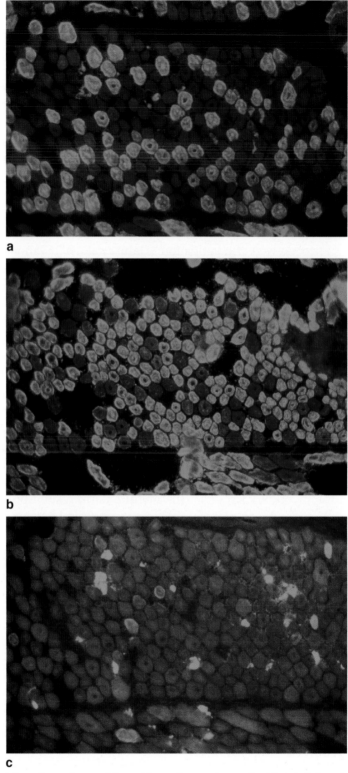

FIG. 15.17 *Serial sections of a quadriceps biopsy from a 4-month old male infant with myotubular myopathy immunolabelled with antibodies to (a) fast, (b) slow and (c) neonatal isoforms of myosin heavy chains. Note that the central nuclei (seen as holes) are present in fibres with fast or slow myosin but they do not show neonatal myosin, indicating that the fibres have matured, at least to some extent.*

The *MTM1* gene is part of a family with at least nine members that share sequence homology. These genes are clearly candidates for other disorders and the myotubularin-related protein 2 and myotubularin-related protein 13/SBF2 genes are mutated in forms of Charcot–Marie–Tooth neuropathy (Bolino et al 2000, Senderek et al 2003, Azzedine et al 2003).

Autosomal centronuclear myopathy

Several cases not linked to Xq28 with central nuclei have been identified (Wallgren-Pettersson and Thomas 1994, Wallgren-Petterson 2000, Bertini et al 2004). Some are clearly familial, others sporadic and they are very likely to be molecularly heterogeneous. Inheritance may be recessive or dominant. Onset is generally later than in the X-linked form and the clinical phenotype is also heterogeneous.

Histopathology

The main morphological features are similar to X-linked cases with central nuclei, some peripheral nuclei, and type 1 fibre atrophy and/or predominance. Central areas again show accumulation of mitochondria and sometimes an absence of myofibrils (Fig. 15.18). There may also be a spoke-like effect radiating from the centre of the fibres that is seen with oxidative enzyme stains and the PAS technique for glycogen. Subsarcolemmal peripheral halos are also commonly seen with oxidative enzymes (Fig. 15.18). Some fibres may also show core-like areas devoid of oxidative enzymes.

A few fibres may show neonatal myosin but, as in X-linked cases, fibres with central nuclei do not show neonatal myosin and most fibres have either fast or slow myosin (Fig. 15.19). Fibres with slow myosin (type 1 fibres) tend to be smaller in diameter and may be more predominant (Fig. 15.19).

Molecular analysis of cases with abundant central nuclei is in progress. The similarity of some features, in particular central nuclei and core-like areas, to those seen in cases with *RYR1* mutations was recently discussed at a European NeuroMuscular Centre (ENMC) workshop on myotubular myopathies (Bertini et al 2004), and the consortium agreed that in all cases of centronuclear myopathy both the *DM1* and *RYR1* genes should be excluded. The large size of the latter, however, makes this difficult. We have recently identified a mutation in the *RYR1* gene in a female previously considered to be an autosomal case of centronuclear myopathy (Fig. 15.20). A second biopsy taken during orthopaedic surgery revealed clear core-like areas, in addition to numerous central nuclei, but core lesions had been much less apparent in her original biopsy taken at 2 years of age.

Recently, mutations in 11 families with an autosomal dominant disorder characterised histopathologically by central nuclei, have been identified in the gene encoding dynamin 2 (*DNM2*) on chromosome 19q13.2 (Bitoun et al 2005). Dynamin 2 is involved in endocytosis and membrane trafficking, actin assembly and centrosome cohesion (Thompson et al 2004).

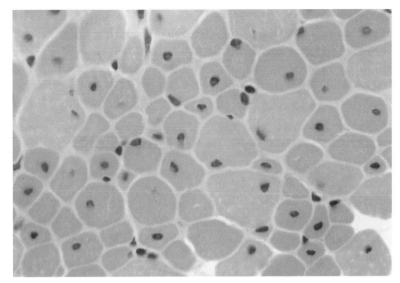

a

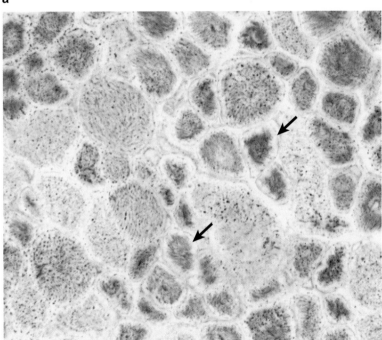

b

FIG. 15.18 *Quadriceps biopsy from a male case of autosomal centronuclear myopathy aged 18 months in whom a mutation in the myotubularin gene has been excluded showing in (a) many central nuclei, particularly in the small fibres (H&E), and (b) small type 1 fibres with dark centres and pale peripheral halos (arrows) (NADH). Diameter of type 1 fibres 10–20 μm and type 2 up to 30 μm.*

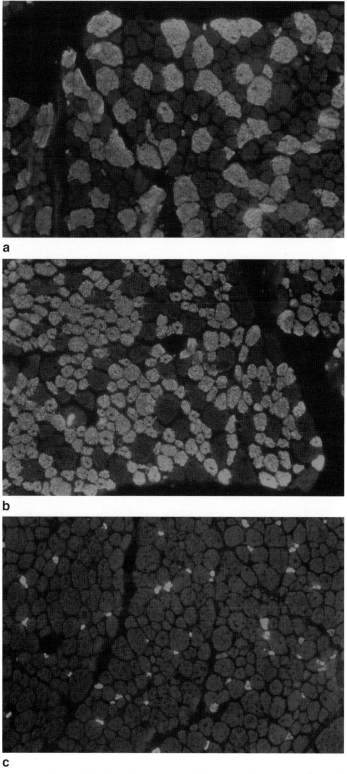

FIG. 15.19 *Immunolabelling of (a) fast, (b) slow and (c) neonatal isoforms of myosin in the same case as Fig. 15.18 showing many small slow (type 1) fibres and larger fast fibres but very little neonatal myosin, indicating that the fibres have matured with regard to their myosin expression.*

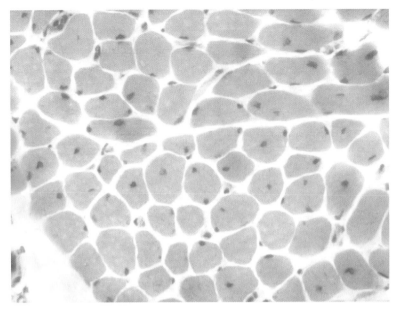

a

b

FIG. 15.20 *Muscle biopsy from a 9-year-old girl with autosomal centronuclear myopathy. Note in (a) numerous central nuclei (H&E) and (b) core-like areas devoid of cytochrome oxidase activity (fibre diameter range 10–25 µm). A mutation in the myotubularin gene was excluded but a mutation in the ryanodine receptor gene (RYR1) has been identified.*

Hyaline body myopathy

This rare disorder has been described with other congenital myopathies and the original patients described presented at birth with hypotonia. The molecular basis of this disorder has recently been identified as a mutation in the gene encoding slow/β-cardiac myosin (*MYH7*). It can therefore be considered as a myofibrillar myopathy and will be discussed further in Chapter 16. Pathologically the muscle is characterized by accumulations of areas of granular material that stain for myosin ATPase and myosin.

Sarcotubular myopathy

In 1973 Jerusalem and co-workers described a congenital myopathy in two Hutterite brothers in whom a proportion of muscle fibres showed focal dilation of the sarcoplasmic reticulum. Two further German cases were also described (Muller-Felber et al 1999). A mutation in the *TRIM32* gene has recently been found in these families (Schoser et al 2005). The same mutation in *TRIM32* causes limb-girdle muscular dystrophy 2H (see Ch. 11), which is restricted to the Hutterite population. Schoser et al (2005) have suggested that sarcotubular myopathy and LGMD2H are the same disorder.

Congenital fibre type disproportion

In the course of their histographic analysis of muscle biopsies, Brooke and Engel (1969d) suggested that children's biopsies could be classified into five categories according to their histographic characteristics. It was noted that in most normal children, the type 1 and type 2 fibres were of roughly equal size and had a variability coefficient which was less than 250. Children suffering from neurogenic disease were usually found to have histograms characterized by one population of large fibres and another of small fibres, thus giving a 'twin-peaked' appearance to the histogram of an individual fibre type (see Ch. 4). Biopsies from myopathic patients were found to exhibit an increased variability in the size of fibres, without a twin-peaked appearance in the histogram. Thus, the histogram maintained its bell-shaped appearance. A large number of children were seen in whom the type 2 fibres were smaller than the type 1 fibres and this was found in conditions as varied as simple disuse and mental retardation. Some of the biopsies, however, were characterized by the fact that the type 1 fibres were smaller than type 2 fibres, and in 10 of these children a relatively non-progressive weakness was found which was usually present at birth. Brooke (1973) subsequently delineated a fairly consistent clinical picture based on a further 12 cases, and suggested the name 'congenital fibre type disproportion'.

All of the children were floppy babies, the condition being noted at or shortly after birth. In 50% of the cases, contractures of various muscles of either the hands or feet were noted. One patient had a torticollis due to a contracted ster-nomastoid. Congenital dislocation of the hip, either bilaterally or unilaterally, was also found in 50% of the patients. The degree of weakness varied quite considerably. It seemed to involve all the muscles of the trunk and extremities, although in some patients the legs seemed to be more involved than the arms. It was so severe in one patient that little voluntary movement of the arms or legs was possible until almost 2 years of age. In other cases, the weakness was mild enough to cause only a delay in the development of the motor milestones, rather than any obvious paralysis. In some, there appeared to be an initial progression of the weakness during the first year of life, but in no case was there any pro-gression once the child had attained 2 years of age. As the child grew older, the disease became static or improvement took place.

Recurrent respiratory infections were frequently a problem during the first year of life. There was an associated abnormality in stature, and most patients were below the third percentile in weight, even though the birth weight was normal in most cases, and below the tenth percentile in height. Commonly occur-ring anomalies included a high arched palate, kyphoscoliosis and deformities of the feet – either flat feet or occasionally high arched feet.

Although the genetics of this disease was not clear cut, about half of the patients had a relative with a similar clinical condition. In some, there were affected siblings only, suggesting an autosomal recessive pattern of inheritance, but one patient had both a father and brother affected, suggesting a dominant mechanism.

A similar histochemical pattern was documented in female siblings with a non-progressive congenital myopathy (see Dubowitz 1980) and in the cases reported by Caille et al (1971). Several reports have subsequently documented further cases, including a number of familial ones (see Clarke and North 2003).

The pathological criterion for determining fibre type disproportion that is often quoted is the presence of type 1 fibres that are at least 12% smaller in diameter than type 2 fibres and the absence of any other pathological feature, but Brooke acknowledged subsequently that this is too narrow a distinction and agreed to at least 25%.

Small type 1 fibres are a feature of several disorders and it is important to exclude other conditions such as congenital myotonic dystrophy, and the various congenital myopathies mentioned above. It is also important to restrict the diag-nosis to 'pure' cases with no change histologically other than the variation in fibre size.

There has been a long debate on whether fibre type disproportion is a disease entity or if it is 'pathology in search of a disease'. Recent molecular data, however has thrown some light on this and mutations in the *ACTA1* gene have been found in a small proportion of cases that only showed small type 1 fibres (Fig. 15.21; Laing et al 2004). The clinical phenotype in the cases identified to date is variable and the absence of a detectable mutation in additional cases suggests further genetic heterogeneity.

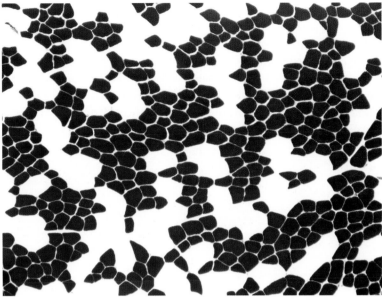

FIG. 15.21 *Muscle biopsy from a case of fibre type disproportion in whom a mutation in the skeletal actin gene has been found. The only apparent pathology in this case was the small size of the dark-staining type 1 fibres and type 1 fibre predominance (ATPase preincubated at pH 4.3). Fibre diameter 25–70 µm.*

Congenital myopathies with ultrastructural abnormalities

A number of rare cases have been reported in which a biopsy has been characterized by, and the disorder named after, the presence of a particular ultrastructural abnormality (see Table 15.1). It is not clear if all are genetic entities as some are sporadic, non-familial cases (Goebel and Anderson 1999, Taratuto 2002). The clinical presentation of these cases is variable and not all may fall into the 'congenital myopathy' category, and are perhaps more strictly 'myopathies with structural abnormalities'. Many of the structures are highlighted by the Gomori trichrome stain and stains that use a tetrazolium salt. Examples of the ultrastructure of several of these structures are shown in Chapter 5.

The morphological structures that have given their name to a disorder that may have a genetic basis include *fingerprint bodies* (Engel et al 1972, Fardeau et al 1976, Curless et al 1978), *cylindrical spirals* (Carpenter et al 1979, Bove et al 1980), *tubular aggregates* (de Groot and Ants 1982, Rohkman et al 1983, Cameron et al 1992) and *reducing bodies* (Brooke and Neville 1972, Dubowitz and Brooke 1973, Sahgal and Sahgal 1977, Nomiizu et al 1992, Bertini et al 1994). *Tubular aggregates* are a non-specific finding which often occur in cases with periodic paralyses where they are restricted to type 2 fibres. In familial tubular aggregate myopathy, they occur in both fibre types. *Reducing bodies* are intracytoplasmic bodies that are non-reactive for oxidative enzymes and ATPase, but are able to reduce nitroblue tetrazolium directly when mediated by menadione – hence the suggested name of 'reducing-body' myopathy.

Other structures that have given their name to a myopathy have been seen in rare sporadic cases and a genetic basis is far from clear (see Table 15.1). These include *cap disease* (Fidzianska et al 1981), characterized by crescent-shaped granular areas at the periphery of several fibres; and *zebra body myopathy* (Lake and Wilson 1975).

CHAPTER 16

Myofibrillar myopathies

Over the years a number of disorders with various types of inclusions have been described, such as spheroid bodies (Goebel et al 1978), sarcoplasmic bodies (Edström et al 1980), cytoplasmic bodies (Goebel et al 1981) and granulomatous material (Fardeau et al 1978b). More recently it has been appreciated that these disorders share similar histopathological features, in particular accumulation of several proteins, especially desmin. This led to the use of terms such as 'desminopathies' or 'desmin-related myopathies'. Several other proteins also accumulate; several of which are also seen in inclusion body myositis (see Ch. 22) and the terms 'hereditary inclusion body myopathy' or 'protein surplus myopathies' have been suggested (Goebel and Borchet 2002). The more general term of 'myofibrillar myopathies' has been applied to encompass all these disorders (de Bleecker et al 1996) and their molecular basis is gradually being determined. The term 'myofibrillar myopathy' is sometimes restricted to conditions in which proteins of the Z line, or associated with it, are implicated, but we also include here disorders caused by sarcomeric proteins, in particular myosin, as they also have characteristic histopathological inclusions. Disorders related to other sarcomeric proteins such as actin, nebulin and tropomyosin have been discussed in Chapter 15 on congenital myopathies, and telethonin and titin in Chapter 11 on limb-girdle muscular dystrophies (see also Ch. 6).

Inheritance in the majority of cases where it can be determined is autosomal dominant, although rare recessive mutations in the desmin gene have been identified (Goldfarb et al 1998, Munoz-Marmol et al 1998). Defects have so far been found in the genes for myosin (*MYHC2A* and *MYH7*), desmin, αB-crystallin, myotilin and ZASP (Z line alternatively spliced PDZ protein) and γ-filamin (Vicart et al 1998, Martinson et al 2000, Bohlega et al 2004, Meredith et al 2004, Tajsharghi et al 2002, 2003, Selcen and Engel 2003, 2004, 2005, Vorgerd et al 2005). Loci with unmapped genes have been identified on chromosome 2q24–31, 10q23 and 12q. No causative gene mutations have been found in several patients with the clinical and pathological phenotype of a myofibrillar myopathy and proteins that interact with Z-line proteins or play a role in maintaining myofibrillar integrity are likely candidates.

Clinical features

With identification of the various molecular defects, the spectrum of clinical features associated with myofibrillar myopathies is emerging and expanding. Age of onset is variable, with most identified cases of adult onset, often late. In the series of 63 patients studied at the Mayo clinic, onset was from 7 to 77 years of age, with only four cases presenting before the age of 20 years (Selcen et al 2004). Cases with mutations in the myosin IIa gene (*MYHC2A*) may present at birth. The number of identified childhood cases may increase with better ascertainment.

Muscle weakness is slowly progressive and may be proximal, or more frequently, distal. Muscle weakness may be accompanied by muscle wasting, stiffness or aching, cramps and sensory symptoms. Facial weakness is uncommon. A particular feature associated with *MYHC2A* mutations is external ophthalmoplegia. Evidence of peripheral neuropathy is present in a significant proportion of patients and cardiomyopathy is common, but less so in cases with mutations in myosin genes (see below). Cardiomyopathy may be a presenting feature, for example in cases with a mutation in the desmin gene. Serum creatine kinase activity is usually normal or mildly elevated.

Cataracts are a feature associated with mutations in the αB-crystallin gene and can be a useful clinical distinction from cases with a mutation in the desmin gene in which the pathology is very similar.

Histopathology

Fibre size variability with atrophy and hypertrophy is present in most biopsies (Fig. 16.1). Some fibres may look basophilic and granular (Fig. 16.1a). Other myopathic features include fibre splitting, excess internal nuclei, and proliferation of endomysial connective tissue and adipose tissue. A few inflammatory cells may be present and necrosis and regeneration may occur but are not usually extensive.

The Gomori trichrome stain is particularly useful for assessing myofibrillar myopathies and reveals areas within fibres that are more darkly stained than the surrounding myofibrils (Fig. 16.2). These may have a more bluish colour with the trichrome, and with haematoxylin and eosin they are eosinophilic (Figs 16.1 and 16.2). Some inclusions may be stained red with the Gomori trichrome and are cytoplasmic bodies (Fig. 16.3). The dark areas lack mitochondria and therefore do not stain for oxidative enzymes. They are also congophilic indicating the presence of β-amyloid. The Congo red stain is best viewed under fluorescence, using an excitation filter in the red range, as for rhodamine or Texas Red (Fig. 16.4).

Vacuoles rimmed by basophilia with H&E or red material with Gomori trichrome are a particular feature (Fig. 16.5) but may not be present in all cases (see Fig. 16.1a).

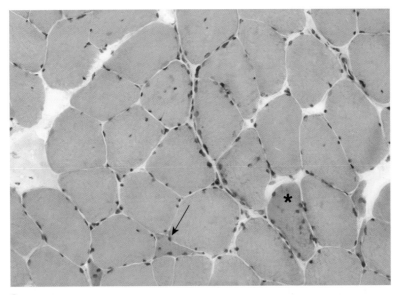

a

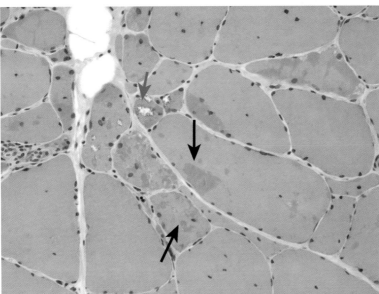

b

FIG. 16.1 *Quadriceps biopsies from (a) a male aged 38 years with a mutation in the gene encoding desmin and (b) a 69-year-old male with a molecularly unresolved myofibrillar myopathy. Note in both the fibre size variability, the increase in internal nuclei and eosinophilic areas which are particularly pronounced in (b) (large arrows); (a) also shows small slightly basophilic fibres (small arrow) and a granular fibre (*) and in (b) there are atrophic fibres with rimmed vacuoles (green arrow) (H&E). Fibre diameter range (a) 35–95 μm; (b) 10–105 μm.*

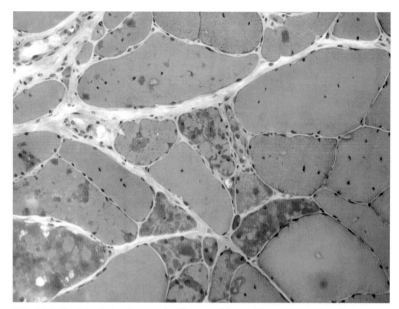

FIG. 16.2 *Darkly stained areas in the quadriceps biopsy from the 69-year-old case shown in Fig. 16.1b (Gomori trichrome). Fibre diameter range 10–105 μm.*

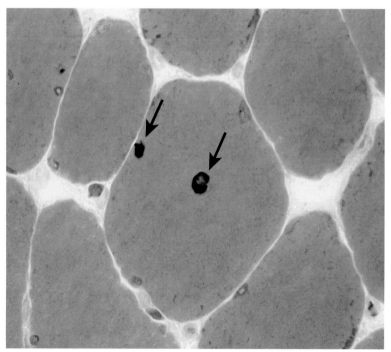

FIG. 16.3 *Red-stained cytoplasmic bodies (arrows) in a quadriceps biopsy from a 28-year-old male with a molecularly unresolved myofibrillar myopathy (Gomori trichrome). Fibre diameter range 25–50-μm.*

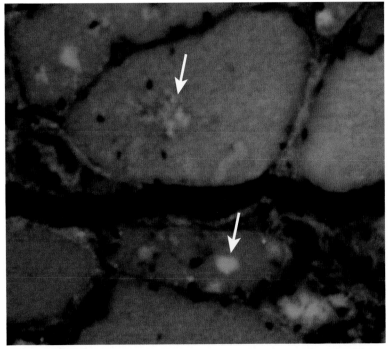

FIG. 16.4 *Congo red staining viewed with fluorescence using a 545–580-nm excitation filter in the biopsy from the case shown in Fig. 16.1b. Note the bright fluorescent areas (arrows).*

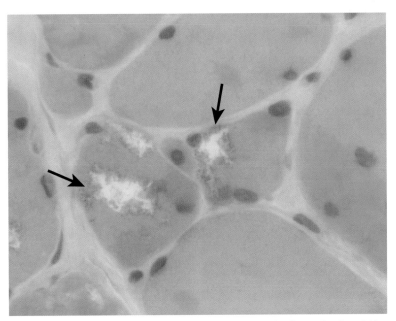

FIG. 16.5 *Quadriceps biopsy from the 69-year-old male shown in Fig. 16.1b showing prominent vacuoles with basophilic granules at the periphery which are myelin-like whorls (arrows) (H&E).*

Fibre type grouping and groups of atrophic fibres of both types may be present, consistent with a peripheral neuropathy, and nerves may show loss of myelin and increased fibrosis (see Ch. 4). A predominance of type 1 fibres may occur in some cases.

Unevenness of oxidative enzyme staining and minicore-like lesions, particularly in type 2A fibres (Martinsson et al 2000) occurs in association with *MYHC2A* mutations and the 2A fibres may be smaller in diameter.

Immunohistochemistry

The abnormal fibres contain an accumulation of several proteins and immunohistochemistry is useful for assessing them. The proteins detected in the abnormal fibres include desmin, αB-crystallin, syncoilin, ubiquitin, myotilin, γ-filamin, dystrophin, β-amyloid precursor protein, filamentous actin (as shown with phalloidin), gelsolin, neural cell adhesion molecule (N-CAM) and prion protein (Fig. 16.6). Some of these proteins are also seen in inclusion body myositis and heredi-

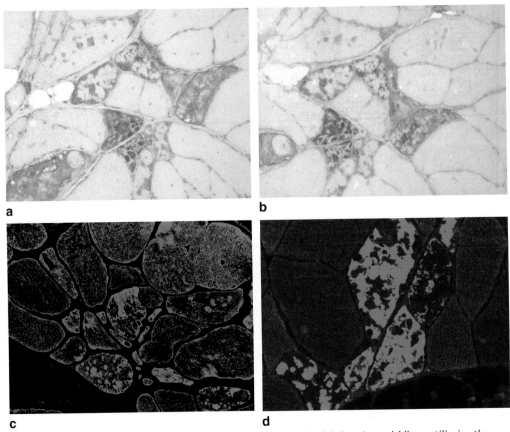

a

b

c

d

FIG. 16.6 *Immunolabelling of (a) ubiquitin, (b) αB-crystallin, (c) desmin and (d) myotilin in the biopsy of a molecularly unresolved myofibrillar myopathy showing accumulation of all these proteins in several fibres.*

tary inclusion body myopathy caused by defects in the *GNE* gene (UDP-*N*-acetylglucosamine 2-epimerase/*N*-acetylmannosamine kinase; see Ch. 22) and rimmed vacuoles may also be seen in other myopathies with distal involvement. This may cause diagnostic confusion, but in inclusion body myopathy caused by GNE mutations, dystrophin and desmin accumulation are not usually associated with the vacuolated fibres. In cases with mutations in myosin genes (see below) the hyaline structures contain myosin.

Electron microscopy

Electron microscope reveals various degrees of myofibrillar disruption with Z-line streaming, accumulation of Z-line material, accumulation of characteristic granulomatous material, and inclusions of various types (Selcen et al 2004; see Figs 5.41 and 5.42). Cytoplasmic bodies with a halo of filaments radiating from them are common, as are myelin-like whorls and autophagic debris. In cases with a mutation in the fast myosin *MYHC2A* gene 15–20 nm tubulofilamentous cytoplasmic and nuclear inclusions are present.

It is rarely possible to predict the molecular defect from the histopathological pattern but, as with all neuromuscular disorders, an indication may be obtained when considered with the clinical assessment.

Molecular defects

The defective genes that have been identified are shown in Table 16.1. The number of cases with an identified mutation is still small but is likely to rise with greater awareness of the myofibrillar myopathies. Nevertheless they are rare. Mutations in the gene for **desmin** were the first identified (Goldfarb et al 1998) and most are dominant, although a few recessive cases have also been reported (Goldfarb et al 1998, Munoz-Marmol et al 1998). Desmin is a highly conserved intermediate filament of skeletal, cardiac and smooth muscle. It is localized to the periphery of the Z line and the subsarcolemmal cytoskeleton and the filaments are 10 nm in diameter, intermediate between actin and myosin. Desmin is linked to the Z line by plectin and associates with other intermediate filaments to link the myofibrils to each other, to the sarcolemma, and to mitochondria and nuclei. The various mutations identified impair assembly of the desmin filaments.

αB-crystallin is a cytoplasmic small heat shock protein that has a chaperone role in protecting the intermediate filament network from stress induced damage (Perng et al 2004). Mutations in the αB-crystallin gene interfere with this chaperone function. Two α-crystallin forms (A and B), encoded by different genes, have been identified and both are abundant in the lens where they prevent the formation of cataracts. The presence of cataracts is a distinguishing feature of cases with a mutation in the αB-crystallin gene that is not found in the other myofibrillar myopathies.

TABLE 16.1 *Features of myofibrillar myopathies caused by known gene defects*

Popular name	Locus	Gene symbol	Protein	Inheritance	Cardiac involvement	Peripheral neuropathy	Other features
Desminopathy	2q35	DES	Desmin	AD (rare AR)	Yes	Yes	–
αB-crystallinopathy	11q-22.3	CRYAB	αB-crystallin	AD	Yes	Possibly	Cataracts
Myotilinopathy	5q31	MYOT (TTID)	Myotilin	Possibly AD	Yes	Yes	–
–	10q22.3	LDB3	ZASP	AD	Yes	–	–
–	7q32.1	FLNC	γ-filamin	AD	Not reported	–	–
Inclusion body myopathy	17p13	MYHC2A	Fast myosin heavy chain IIa	AD	Not reported	Yes	Ophthalmoplegia
Hyaline body myopathy and myosin storage myopathy	14q11	MYH7	Slow myosin heavy chain	AD	No Occasional arrhythmias		

AD, autosomal dominant; AR, autosomal recessive; ZASP, Z line alternatively spliced PDZ protein.

Mutations in the *myotilin* gene not only cause a myofibrillar myopathy (Selcen and Engel 2004) but also a form of limb-girdle muscular dystrophy (LGMD1A; see Ch. 11). All identified mutations occur in the serine-rich N-terminal domain and identical mutations apparently give rise to the different phenotypes. The reason for this is not clear but the effect of a modifying gene has been suggested (Karpati and Sinnreich 2004). As only a few cases with mutations in myotilin gene have been identified it is possible that LGMD1A and the myofibrillar myopathy are not separate entities. Biopsies from both show some similarities.

Dominant mutations in two genes encoding *myosin isoforms* have been found, *MYHC2A* and *MYH7* encoding *fast myosin type IIa* and *slow myosin* heavy chain of type 1 fibres, respectively. The disorder associated with *MYHC2A* mutations has been referred to as an hereditary inclusion body myopathy as rimmed vacuoles, tubulofilamentous inclusions 15–20 nm in diameter, and accumulation of similar proteins to those seen in inclusion body myositis are present (Tajsarghi et al 2002). The ophthalmoplegia that occurs in this disorder is thought to result from the fact that myosin IIa is a major constituent of extraocular muscles.

The dominant disorder caused by mutations in the *MYH7* gene has been referred to as hyaline body myopathy because of the characteristic inclusions, often peripheral, that stain for myosin adenosine triphosphatase (ATPase), and contain slow myosin (Tajsharghi et al 2003). Mutations in the same gene, but in different exons, are responsible for another disorder with predominantly distal muscle involvement and rimmed vacuoles, Laing myopathy (Meredith et al 2004), and for familial hypertrophic cardiomyopathy (Seidman and Seidman 2001, Richard et al 2003). Interestingly, cardiac involvement in Laing myopathy and hyaline body myopathy is minimal. Disorders with similar hyaline bodies to those caused by *MYH7* mutations are linked to chromosome 3p22.2 and 12q13.3–q15 but the genes responsible have not yet been found.

CHAPTER 17

Metabolic myopathies I: Glycogenoses

There has been a dramatic increase in the understanding of disorders that affect the metabolism of muscle, particularly with regard to their biochemistry and molecular basis. A large number of clinical syndromes related to glycogen and lipid metabolism, mitochondrial function, and ion channels are now known but only in some is muscle pathology helpful. In the follow chapters we shall concentrate on conditions where pathological studies are helpful rather than attempting to give a detailed review of the biochemistry.

Glycogenoses

The breakdown of glycogen is an important source of energy in muscle. Defects in any step in the glycolytic pathway can cause muscle fatigue, cramps or rhabdomyolysis, which is an important indicator of several metabolic problems. The discovery by Cori and Cori of deficient glucose-6-phosphatase in von Gierke's disease (Cori and Cori 1952) opened the way for the recognition of a number of inborn errors of glycogen metabolism. The numerical classification suggested by Cori (1958) has found wide acceptance and they are numbered approximately in the order they were discovered (with some variation in the later forms). Of the 11 established types to date muscle symptoms are apparent in several, in particular exercise intolerance, cramps and fatigue, and other organs and tissues are also affected (Table 17.1). Inheritance of glycogenoses is usually autosomal recessive.

On muscle biopsy there will often be an excessive deposition of glycogen, sometimes in vacuoles, but glycogen can easily be lost from the fibres and an excess may not always be apparent. The degree of pathological change can vary considerably from a striking vacuolar myopathy with marked disruption of the muscle structure, as shown in most cases of type II glycogenosis, to a fairly normal histological pattern with very little structural change, as seen in some cases of types III and V glycogenosis. In phosphorylase (type V) and phosphofructokinase (type VII) deficiency the absence of the enzyme can readily be

TABLE 17.1 *Features of glycogenoses that affect muscle*

Type	Enzyme deficiency	Eponymous or other names	Clinical features	Other tissues/systems affected
Type II	α-1,4-Glucosidase (acid maltase)	Pompe's disease	(a) Severe form: resembles SMA (b) Milder forms: resemble LGMD	Heart, nervous system, leukocytes, liver, kidneys
Type III	Amylo-1,6-glucosidase (debrancher enzyme)	Forbes' disease Cori's disease	Infantile hypotonia Mild weakness	Hepatic hypoglycaemia, ketosis, leukocytes, heart
Type IV	Amylo (1,4 → 1,6) transglucosidase (branching enzyme)	Amylopectinosis	Usually no muscle symptoms, muscle wasting in some	Liver, heart
Type V	Myophosphorylase	McArdle's disease	Exercise intolerance, cramps, fatigue, myoglobinuria	None
Type VII	Phosphofructokinase	Tarui's disease	Exercise intolerance, cramps, fatigue, myoglobinuria	Haemolytic anaemia
Type VIII	Phosphorylase *b* kinase		Exercise intolerance, muscle stiffness, muscle weakness	Liver, heart
Type IX	Phosphoglycerate kinase		Exercise intolerance, cramps, fatigue, myoglobinuria	Haemolytic anaemia, CNS
Type X	Phosphoglycerate mutase		Exercise intolerance, cramps, fatigue, myoglobinuria	
Type XI	Lactate dehydrogenase		Exercise intolerance, cramps, fatigue, myoglobinuria	

demonstrated histochemically (Bonilla and Schotland 1970). The confirmation of the specific enzyme deficiency rests on accurate biochemical study of the muscle biopsy, in addition to the histological, histochemical and electron microscopic investigations.

Type II glycogenosis (acid maltase deficiency)

There are three main clinical types associated with acid maltase deficiency; a severe infantile form (Pompe's disease), a juvenile form and adult onset form.

Pompe's disease is the most severe form of glycogenosis and is usually fatal in infancy. It is a generalized disease, with involvement not only of liver, heart and skeletal muscle, but also many other tissues such as the central nervous system and kidneys. Affected infants present either with severe hypotonia and weakness, or with symptoms of cardiac or respiratory failure. The muscle weakness is due either to direct involvement of the muscle itself or to the involvement of the anterior horn cells of the spinal cord. These severely affected infants may look very similar clinically to cases of infantile spinal muscular atrophy (SMA) but can be distinguished by the associated diaphragmatic and cardiac involvement which does not occur in SMA.

The amount of glycogen deposition in different tissues may vary considerably and in some cases cardiac involvement may be minimal or completely absent. The accumulation of glycogen is due to a deficiency of acid maltase (α-1,4-glucosidase) which hydrolyses maltose, linear oligosaccharides and the outer chains of glycogen to glucose. Muscle biopsies have a pronounced vacuolar appearance and periodic acid-Schiff (PAS) staining shows large deposits of glycogen in most fibres (Fig. 17.1). The glycogen is digested by diastase but some resistant material remains. The enzyme is present in lysosomes and there is consequently abundant acid phosphatase activity (Fig. 17.2). In addition, discrete areas of glycogen accumulation can be shown in lymphocytes and is a very simple diagnostic test. The standard PAS technique is performed on celloidin-coated lymphocytes spun down from whole blood, and smeared on a slide (see Ch. 2). Ultrastructurally, glycogen is characteristically seen in membrane bound areas in muscle fibres, as well as in large lakes of freely dispersed granules (Fig. 17.3 and see Fig. 5.70). In some cases very few myofibrils may remain and the fibres are so disrupted that only the sarcolemma is left (Fig. 17.1). Glycogen may be lost during processing for electron microscopy and the excessive amount is therefore not always apparent. Although overall a biopsy may look very disrupted and abnormal, sarcolemmal labelling of proteins such as dystrophin and β-spectrin is preserved.

The clinical picture in the milder cases is variable. Some cases may present with respiratory failure, and some may resemble a limb-girdle dystrophy. Cardiac involvement is a less consistent feature. The muscle pathology in milder cases is also variable. The vacuolation may be extensive, or minimal, or may only be apparent in some fibres, mainly type 1 fibres (Figs 17.4 and 17.5) or sometimes both fibre types. Increased areas of acid phosphate activity, however, are always

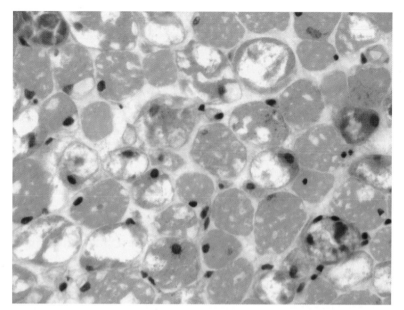

a

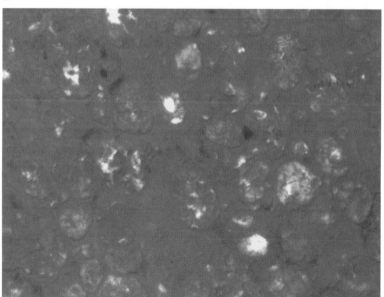

b

FIG. 17.1 *Biopsy from the quadriceps of a 9-month-old infant with type II glycogenosis (Pompe's disease) showing in (a) pronounced vacuolation of many fibres, some with very little red-staining myofibrillar material (H&E), and in (b) intense PAS staining of accumulated glycogen. Fibre diameter range 5–30 μm.*

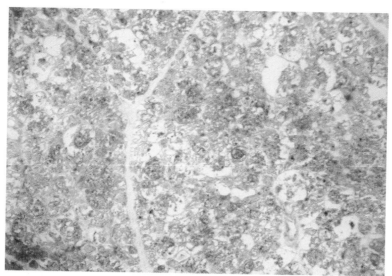

FIG. 17.2 *Biopsy from the quadriceps from a 3-month-old infant with type II glycogenosis (Pompe's disease) showing high red acid phosphatase activity associated with the vacuolated fibres.*

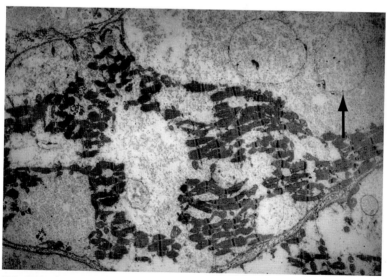

FIG. 17.3 *Electron micrograph of a quadriceps biopsy from a 3-month-old infant with type II glycogenosis (Pompe's disease) showing extensive loss of myofibrils and accumulation of glycogen, some of which is membrane bound (arrow).*

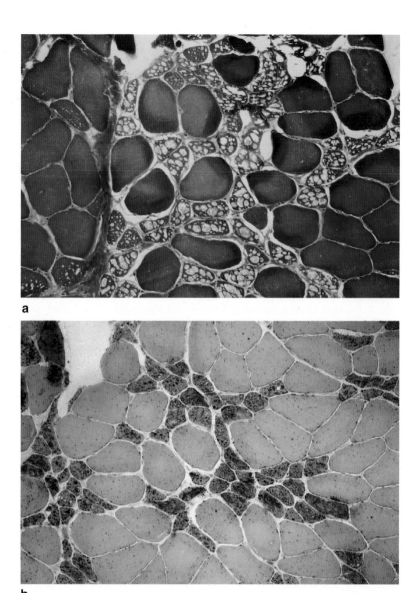

FIG. 17.4 *Biopsy from the quadriceps of a mild case of childhood onset acid maltase deficiency (type II glycogenosis) aged 11 years showing pronounced vacuolation and excess glycogen in a population of fibres that stained as type I fibres with ATPase(a), Gomori trichrome; (b), acid phosphate.*

apparent and this is one of the most useful applications of the technique (Figs. 17.4 and 17.5). Increased glycogen is also usually apparent (Fig. 17.5).

The vacuoles may be surrounded by dystrophin and spectrin but not by laminins, although indentations of the sarcolemma show laminins and may appear like vacuoles in transverse section. There is also abundant MHC class I labelling associated with the vacuoles and on the sarcolemma of some fibres (Fig. 17.6). Vacuoles without sarcolemmal proteins and the absence of labelling of

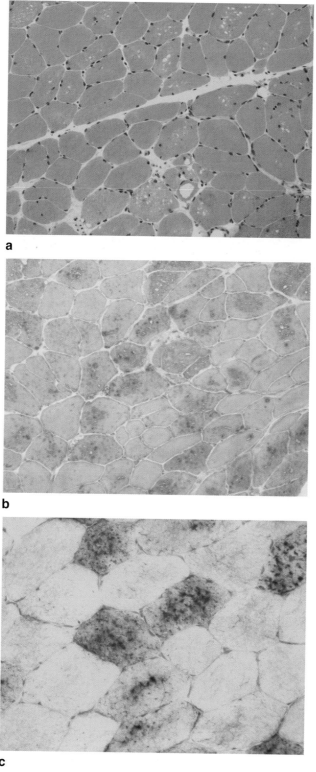

a

b

c

FIG. 17.5 *Biopsy from the quadriceps of a male aged 40 years with adult onset acid maltase deficiency. Note in (a) the variation in fibre size, excess internal nuclei and the vacuoles in several fibres (H&E), in (b) high acid phosphatase activity in the vacuoles, and in (c) glycogen accumulation (PAS). The non-vacuolated fibres do not show excess glycogen. Fibre diameter range (a) and (b) 20–74-μm; (c) 45–70-μm.*

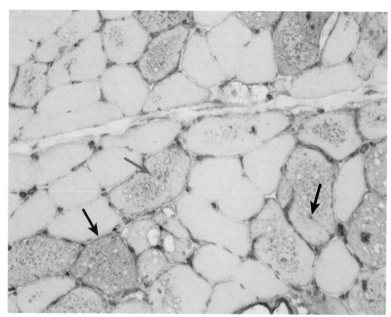

FIG. 17.6 *Immunolabelling of MHC class I in the same case of adult onset acid maltase deficiency as shown in Fig. 17.5 showing labelling inside fibres associated with the vacuoles (green arrow) and on the sarcolemma (blue arrow). Note also a few labelled capillaries that appear to be inside fibres and have grown into indentations of the sarcolemma (black arrow).*

certain lectins helps to distinguishing vacuoles caused by defects in the gene for the lysosomal associated membrane protein 2 (LAMP-2), responsible for Danon's disease (Usuki et al 1994), and those seen in X-linked myopathy with excessive autophagy (XMEA; see Fig. 6.16 and below).

Type III glycogenosis (debrancher enzyme deficiency, Cori-Forbes disease)

In 1952, Illingworth and Cori discovered an abnormal glycogen with very short side chains (limit dextrin) in the liver and muscle of the 12-year-old girl recorded by Forbes (1953). They postulated that the deficient enzyme was probably amylo-1,6-glucosidase (the debrancher enzyme) and this was subsequently confirmed (Illingworth et al 1956, Hers 1959).

Type III glycogenosis is more benign than early onset type II (Pompe's) but also affects both liver and skeletal muscle, and sometimes cardiac muscle. Skeletal muscle is usually only mildly affected in type III glycogenosis, which can present with hypotonia and weakness, but a proportion of cases show only liver involvement with no muscle-specific symptoms. This may relate to differential expression of the six spliced forms produced from the single gene. The enzyme, in concert with phosphorylase, influences the number of glucose molecules of the glycogen and the enzyme deficiency results in glycogen with short side

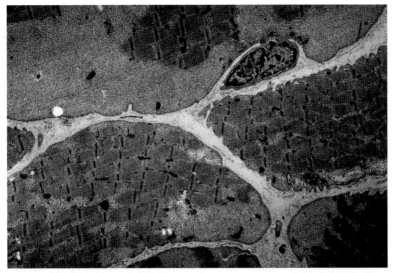

FIG. 17.7 *Electron micrograph of a biopsy from a 4-month-old case of type III glycogenosis (debrancher enzyme deficiency) showing extensive areas of myofibrillar loss and accumulated non-membrane bound glycogen.*

chains (limit dextrin). This contrasts with the structurally abnormal glycogen (amylopectin) that occurs in type IV glycogenosis (branching enzyme deficiency).

Muscle biopsies in type III show a vacuolar change with glycogen accumulation often at the periphery of fibres (Fig. 17.7). In some cases, however, there may be only mild variation in fibre size with very little vacuolation or excess glycogen (Dubowitz 1995a).

Type V glycogenosis (McArdle's disease)

In contrast to the above glycogenoses, type V glycogenosis is entirely restricted to striated muscle. In 1951, McArdle demonstrated the failure of blood lactic acid to rise after ischaemic exercise in a 30-year-old man suffering from muscle cramps on exertion, and he postulated an enzyme defect in the glycolytic pathway. It was not until 8 years later that the deficient enzyme was shown to be phosphorylase in two separately studied cases (Schmid and Mahler 1959, Pearson et al 1961).

There are two interesting historical aspects of McArdle's disease. It is the first myopathy which proved to be due to a single enzyme defect and thus presumably resulting from a defect in a single gene. It also helped to settle a longstanding controversy among biochemists as to the action of phosphorylase in vivo. The presence of excess glycogen in the muscle in McArdle's disease, in the absence of myophosphorylase, proved that this enzyme is only responsible for the breakdown of glycogen.

Clinical features

The main clinical features of McArdle's disease are cramps on exertion, but these may not be present in the early stages. Schmid and Mahler (1959) recognized three phases of symptoms in their 52-year-old patient. In childhood and adolescence, the only symptom was easy fatigability. From the age of 20, there were severe cramps and weakness on exertion and transient myoglobinuria. Subsequently, he developed weakness and wasting of proximal muscles. There is, however, marked variation in severity from one patient to another. Cardiac muscle does not appear to be affected, although electrocardiogram (ECG) changes have been recorded (Ratinov et al 1965).

The weakness and wasting may be progressive and the exercise induced cramps may be accompanied by myoglobinuria. Elevated creatine kinase levels are common.

Following ischaemic exercise, there is no rise in the blood lactate or pyruvate levels, in contrast to a two- to fivefold elevation in a normal subject. This in itself is not specific to phosphorylase deficiency since a similar result could be produced by absence of other enzymes along the glycolytic pathway.

Many McArdle's patients experience a 'second wind phenomenon' in which exercise can be better endured after a short pause.

Biochemistry

There are three forms of phosphorylase encoded by different genes:

- a liver form encoded on chromosome 14;
- a brain form encoded on chromosome 20 and also expressed in fetal muscle; and
- the muscle form encoded on chromosome 11.

Only the muscle form is defective in McArdle's disease and results in an absence of enzyme activity (see below). There is also a concomitant absence of immunoreactive protein (McConchie et al 1990). Fetal muscle utilizes the isoform from chromosome 20 and regenerating fibres and myotubes in culture show phosphorylase activity with the histochemical technique used (see Ch. 2; Meinehofer et al 1977, Sato et al 1977, DiMauro et al 1978). If spindle fibres are present these will also show activity as they have several properties in common with fetal fibres. Although several different mutations in the chromosome 11 gene have been found, the R50X (previously known as R49X) is the most common in the Caucasian population.

Pathology

In contrast to the striking pathological changes in the muscle in type II glycogenosis, the muscle biopsy in type V glycogenosis may show relatively little change on light microscopy. The histological picture is variable. There may be some degenerating or necrotic fibres, accompanied by regeneration, but the most consistent finding is the presence of subsarcolemmal vacuoles or blebs, which may contain PAS-positive glycogen granules (Fig. 17.8). Excess glycogen on PAS staining may be visible but it may not be striking and may only be apparent at the periphery of the fibre. It is more apparent at the ultrastructural level (see below).

The absence of phosphorylase can readily be demonstrated with the histochemical reaction but must always be performed with a positive control to avoid false-negative results. The end product of the reaction fades if mounted in aqueous mountants but can be preserved using alcohol dehydration and resin mountants (see Ch. 2). The result is unequivocal and McArdle's disease is the only disorder to show this complete absence of enzyme activity (Fig. 17.9).

Electron microscopy reveals a striking excess of glycogen, with aggregation particularly in the subsarcolemmal regions, corresponding to the subsarcolemmal blebs seen under light microscopy, and also between myofibrils and myofilaments (Fig. 17.10). The glycogen may sometimes be between the plasma membrane and the basal lamina (see Fig. 5.4). Other changes have been inconsistent and have included mitochondrial changes, the presence of lysosomes in relation to the subsarcolemmal glycogen collections, and breaks in continuity of the sarcolemma, which may be an artefact. The sarcoplasmic reticulum and transverse tubular system are essentially normal, apart from some observations of dilatation of the sarcoplasmic reticulum.

As in other glycogenoses, immunolabelling of sarcolemmal proteins is normal.

Type VII glycogenosis (Tarui's disease, phosphofructokinase deficiency)

Phosphofructokinase (PFK) catalyses the conversion of fructose-6-phosphate to fructose-1,6-diphosphate and its absence completely inhibits the utilization of glucose via the Embden–Meyerhof pathway. The glycogenosis associated with PFK deficiency was first identified by Tarui et al (1965) in three siblings, a female of 20 years and her 23- and 27-year-old brothers, with clinical features identical to McArdle's syndrome. All three had experienced easy fatigability and intolerance of exercise since childhood. Vigorous exertion produced marked weakness and stiffness. In the ischaemic exercise test there was no rise in venous lactate. Muscle biopsy showed raised glycogen levels in all three. The glycogen was normal in structure. Phosphorylase activity was normal but PFK was practically zero (1–3% of normal) in all three. The levels of PFK in the parents, who were first cousins, were normal. Tarui et al (1965) also observed a lowered level of PFK in the erythrocytes of their three patients, and a slight but definite reduction in the presumptively heterozygote mother. The inheritance thus conformed to an autosomal recessive pattern.

A further case, with identical features, was described by Layzer et al in 1967. This 18-year-old male had also been intolerant of exercise since childhood but his two siblings were normal. Ischaemic exercise produced contracture of the

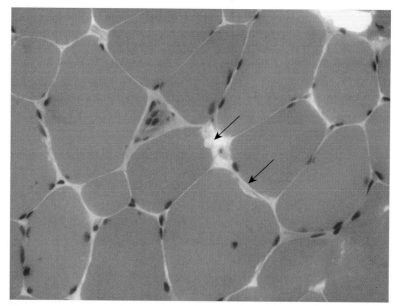

a

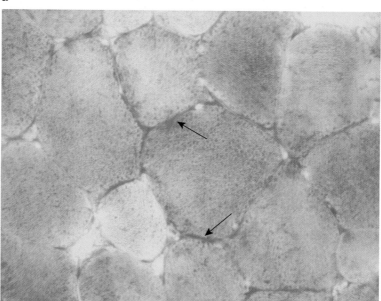

b

FIG. 17.8 *Biopsy from the quadriceps of a case of type V glycogenosis (McArdle's disease) aged 13 years showing (a) variation in fibre size, occasional internal nuclei and small sarcolemmal vacuolated areas (arrows) (H&E) and (b) blebs that contain glycogen and are more intensely stained with PAS (arrows) (fibre diameter range 30–90-μm). In some cases the sarcolemmal 'blebs' may be very conspicuous and there may be more overall excess glycogen than shown here.*

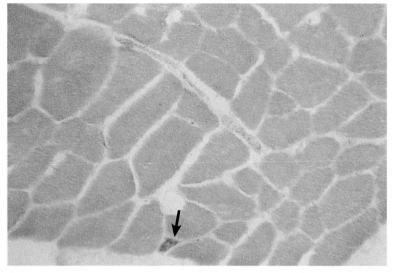

a

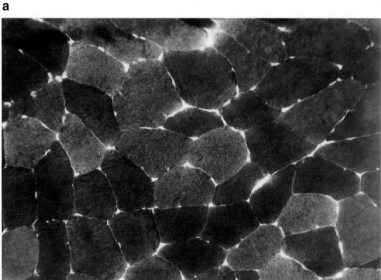

b

FIG. 17.9 *(a) Biopsy from the quadriceps of a 52-year-old case of type V glycogenosis (McArdle's disease) stained for phosphorylase showing a total absence of activity except in one very small regenerating fibre (arrow), compared with (b) a normal two-fibre pattern in a control sample.*

forearm muscles and no rise in venous lactate or pyruvate. On muscle biopsy, the PFK was practically zero (less than 2%) and immunological studies, using an antibody to purified normal human muscle PFK, failed to reveal the presence of a structurally related but inactive protein, thus confirming the absence of PFK. The small amount of activity of PFK present in this and the previous patients is compatible with contamination of the muscle by blood and other non-muscle tissues. As in Tarui's cases, there was a marked reduction in the PFK of the

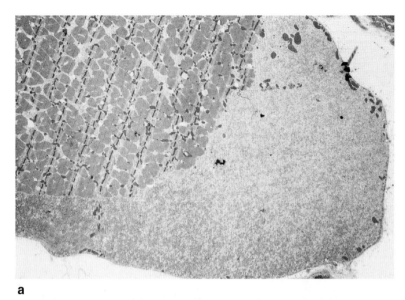

FIG. 17.10 *Electron micrographs of quadriceps biopsies showing accumulation of glycogen in type V glycogenosis (McArdle's disease) which in (a) is prominent beneath the sarcolemma, corresponding to the subsarcolemmal 'blebs' [Fig. 17.8(a)], and in (b) is more diffuse between the myofibrils.*

erythrocytes in this case and also a similar reduction in both parents. Muscle biopsy was not performed on the parents.

Additional cases conforming to the typical clinical pattern have been documented and the absence of the muscle isoenzyme in erythrocytes probably accounts for the commonly associated mild haemolytic anaemia (Tarui et al 1969, Dupond et al 1977, Tarui et al 1978), a feature one does not see in McArdle's disease. The 'second wind phenomenon' is also rare in PFK deficiency.

An adult case with PFK deficiency and atypical features has also been reported (Serratrice et al 1969) and there are also a number of severe infantile cases that have been diagnosed (Guibaud et al 1978). Muscle biopsies showed non-specific changes on light microscopy and excessive glycogen at the electron microscopic level. Biochemical studies confirmed an increased glycogen content, absence of PFK and a reduction in phosphorylase *b* kinase to about 30% of normal.

Other glycogenoses

There have been several reports in the literature of muscle disorders associated with glycogen storage that are not caused by a defect in an enzyme of the glycolytic pathway. Analysis of muscle biopsies reveals several features of interest in these cases.

Lysosomal glycogen storage with normal acid maltase (Danon's disease)

Danon et al (1981) reported two unrelated 16-year-old boys with mental retardation, cardiomegaly and proximal myopathy, whose muscle showed a vacuolar myopathy similar to that in acid maltase deficiency but with normal acid maltase levels and no other demonstrable enzyme deficiency associated with glycogen storage. Since then a number of similar cases have been reported (Morisawa et al 1998, Muntoni et al 1994b, Verloes et al 1997). All affected cases were male and most mothers had late-onset cardiomyopathy, which suggested X-linked inheritance. The gene responsible has been mapped to Xq24 and encodes *LAMP-2* (Nishino et al 2000). Not all cases show glycogen storage and the disorder is frequently now referred to as 'X-linked vacuolar myopathy' or 'Danon's disease'. Onset is in childhood and is characterized by a severe hypertrophic cardiomyopathy, a mild and relatively stable myopathy, and mental retardation of variable degree. Creatine kinase levels are elevated, even in preclinical cases. Muscle weakness and atrophy affect the shoulder and neck muscles, but there may also be distal involvement. In addition to the heart and skeletal muscle, other organs may also be involved, such as the liver.

Pathology

Muscle biopsies show abnormal variation in fibre size, with atrophy of both histochemical fibre types. Necrosis is rare. The striking feature is the presence of vacuoles in several fibres. These stain for glycogen with PAS, although in some cases this may be minimal, and often appear as basophilic areas with haematoxylin and eosin staining. In contrast to the vacuoles in acid maltase deficiency, acid phosphatase in the vacuoles is reported to be minimal or absent (Muntoni et al 1994b). This is somewhat surprising in view of the function of the affected protein in lysosomes. The vacuoles are lined by a membrane that shows dystrophin, β-spectrin and laminin chains and other sarcolemmal proteins.

Acetylcholinesterase activity and non-specific esterases have also been demonstrated in the vacuoles. Some vacuoles show laminins, some only plasma membrane proteins, and invaginations of the sarcolemma are common (see Ch. 6). Labelling of lectins has shown that the membrane and content of the vacuoles are labelled with some lectins such as wheat germ agglutinin, UEA-1 and *Limas flavus* agglutinin (Usuki et al 1994). This can help distinguish the vacuoles from those seen in acid maltase deficiency which show little or no labelling with lectins. With the electron microscope basal lamina is seen on the inner surface of some vacuoles which contain abundant amounts of granular, osmiophilic debris (see below).

Immunohistochemistry and immunoblots show a virtual absence of LAMP-2 protein, indicating that immunohistochemistry would be useful for assessment of muscle biopsies (Nishino et al 2000). Commercial antibodies have just become available (Abcam) but have not been evaluated yet.

The pathology in Danon's disease is remarkably similar to that in XMEA, first described by Kalimo et al (1988), with numerous vacuoles showing sarcolemmal proteins (see Fig. 6.16). The two disorders are not allelic and XMEA maps to Xq28. Clinically they are different, and no cardiac involvement or mental retardation occurs in XMEA. In XMEA some vacuoles stain for acid phosphatase. The sarcolemma of affected fibres and some vacuoles show calcium deposits and complement C5-9 (membrane attack complex; Villanova et al 1995). Ultrastructurally the vacuoles are similar in the two disorders (see Fig. 5.82) but in XMEA there is abundant duplication of the basal lamina and debris occurs between the plasma membrane and basal lamina. The presence of complement and duplication of the basal lamina may distinguish the two disorders.

CHAPTER 18

Metabolic myopathies II: Lipid related disorders and mitochondrial myopathies

Skeletal muscles use not only glycogen as a source of energy but also lipid. The oxidation of lipids occurs in the mitochondria and involves a series of enzymatic reactions. Defects in these pathways and in the pathways of oxidative phosphorylation in the mitochondria lead to a heterogeneous group of muscle disorders (Fig. 18.1; see Fig. 18.6).

Fatty acid metabolism

The oxidation of fatty acids is a major source of energy and a heterogeneous group of disorders are caused by defects in the β-oxidation metabolic pathway.

The first association of a myopathy with a disorder of lipid metabolism was the report by Engel et al (1970b) who suggested the possibility in 18-year-old identical twin sisters, who from childhood had muscle cramps associated with myoglobinuria, at times occurring some hours after exercise. Carbohydrate metabolism was normal. Attacks could be provoked by prolonged fasting or by a high fat, low carbohydrate diet. Muscle biopsy was histologically normal but showed excess lipid droplets on oil red O staining. They postulated a defect in the utilization of long-chain fatty acids. In a prophetic annotation in the same journal, Bressler (1970) predicted a deficiency of either carnitine or carnitine palmitoyl transferase (CPT) to account for this lipid storage myopathy. Engel and Angelini (1973) were subsequently able to demonstrate carnitine deficiency in the muscle of a 24-year-old woman with weakness all her life and progression from the age of 19. Muscle biopsy showed a vacuolar myopathy filled with lipid droplets on histochemical staining. In the same year, DiMauro and DiMauro (1973) reported a 29-year-old man with episodic cramps and myoglobinuria of 16 years' duration but no muscle weakness. Muscle biopsy showed no excess of lipid but a deficiency of the enzyme CPT.

In the ensuing 10 years, many more cases with carnitine or CPT deficiency have contributed to the definition of the various clinical syndromes, and several other disorders caused by defects in other members of the fatty acid β-oxidation

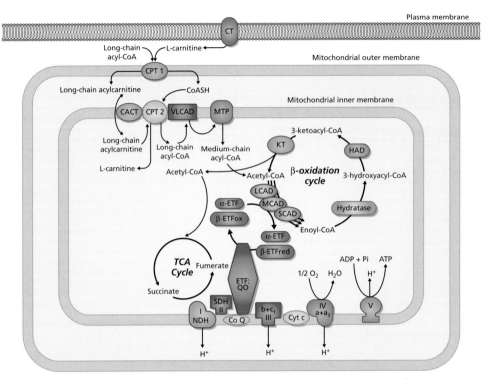

FIG. 18.1 *Schematic representation of the functional and physical organization of FA β-oxidation enzymes in mitochondria. CT, plasma membrane high-affinity sodium-dependent carnitine transporter (OCTN2); CPT 1, carnitine palmitoyltransferase 1; CACT, carnitine/acylcarnitine translocase; CPT 2, carnitine palmitoyltransferase 2; VLCAD, LCAD, MCAD, SCAD, very-long-, long-, medium-, and short-chain acyl-CoA dehydrogenase, respectively; MTP, mitochondrial trifunctional protein; Hydratase, 2-enoyl-CoA hydratase; HAD, L-3-hydroxyacyl-CoA dehydrogenase; KT, 3-ketoacyl-CoA thiolase; ETF, electron transfer flavoprotein (ox, oxidized; red, reduced); ETF:QO, ETF:coenzyme Q oxidoreductase; I, respiratory chain complex I (NDH, NADH:coenzyme Q reductase); II, respiratory chain complex II (SDH, succinate dehydrogenase); CoQ, coenzyme Q; III, respiratory chain complex III (b, cytochrome b; c_1, cytochrome c_1); Cyt c, cytochrome c; IV, respiratory chain complex IV (cytochrome c oxidase) (a, cytochrome a; a_3, cytochrome a_3); V, respiratory chain complex V (ATP synthase). Enzymes which use FAD as a coenzyme are indicated in red colour. Reprinted by kind permission from Di Donata and Taroni 2002 in: Karpati G (ed) Structural and molecular basis of skeletal muscle disease. ISN Neuropathology Press, Basel, p189–201.*

pathway identified (Di Donato and Taroni 2002, 2003). Most of the genes involved have now been identified (see OMIM *http://www.ncbi.nlm.nih.gov/omim*), and there is now a greater understanding of the biochemical pathogenesis. The contribution of muscle pathology has diminished in these disorders with advances in molecular analysis and biochemical assays.

Morphological aspects

The triglycerides are stored in muscle in the form of lipid droplets. Under the light microscope they are readily revealed by stains for neutral fat such as oil

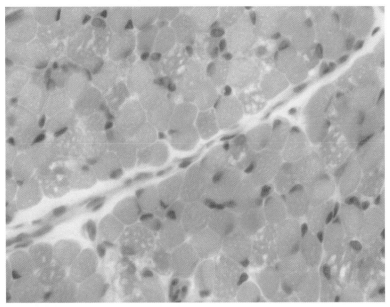

FIG. 18.2 *Biopsy from the quadriceps of a 5-week-old infant with carnitine deficiency showing a vacuolar appearance of many fibres due to the accumulation of lipid (H&E). Fibre diameter range 10–15 μm.*

red O or Sudan black. The droplets are more numerous in the type 1 fibres and tend to be concentrated more at the periphery of the fibre. The presence of excess lipid can give a very vacuolated appearance with routine histological stains such as haematoxylin and eosin and may be more marked in type 1 fibres (Figs 18.2 and 18.3). Under the electron microscope, the lipid droplets appear as empty, rounded spaces of uniform size and do not have a limiting membrane. They are located between the myofibrils and under the sarcolemma and are often adjacent to mitochondria. An excess of lipid, as in carnitine deficiency, shows as a striking increase in the number and size of the droplets under light microscopy, as well as on electron microscopy, and may be associated with structural abnormalities in the mitochondria (Fig. 18.3). In cases with CPT deficiencies, however, the amount of lipid may not appear particularly increased, and in other enzyme defects it varies with the metabolic state of the patient.

Biochemical aspects

Carnitine

Carnitine (β-hydroxy-α-trimethylaminobutyric acid) is the indispensable carrier of medium- and long-chain fatty acids across the inner mitochondrial membrane into the mitochondrion, where they undergo β-oxidation. There are two sources of carnitine – diet and synthesis. The synthesis of carnitine (which is dependent on two essential amino acids, lysine and methionine) takes place predominantly,

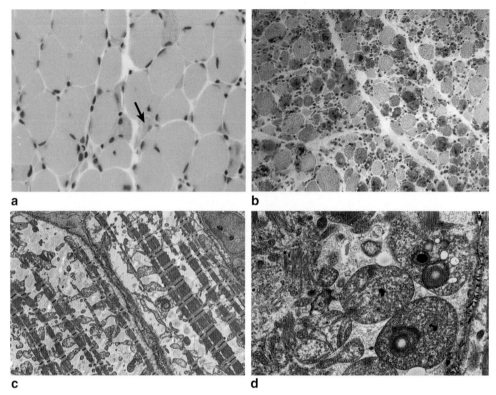

FIG. 18.3 *Biopsy from the quadriceps of a 21-month-old infant with carnitine deficency showing (a) a vacuolar appearance in some fibres (arrow) (H&E); fibre diameter range 5–30 μm; (b) accumulation of lipid in several fibres (oil red O); (c) the accumulation of fat between myofibrils seen with the electron microscope; and (d) ultrastructurally abnormal mitochondria in the same case.*

if not exclusively, in the liver and it is then transported by the blood to other tissues. The highest concentration of free carnitine is in muscle, followed by liver with about half the concentration, and the heart which is lower still. The concentration of carnitine in muscle is about 40 times that in serum, suggesting an active transport system. The excretion of carnitine takes place mainly in an unchanged form in the urine.

Carnitine deficiency could arise from: (a) defective biosynthesis, (b) abnormal degradation, (c) altered transport into and/or out of cells, or (d) abnormal renal handling.

In a study of two children with primary systemic carnitine deficiency and three healthy adult controls, Rebouche and Engel (1981) were unable to detect any defective biosynthesis or abnormal degradation of carnitine. In a separate study of four children with systemic carnitine deficiency, two of their mothers, one case of muscle carnitine deficiency and seven controls, Engel et al (1981) concluded that a renal defect could not fully account for primary systemic carnitine deficiency but might contribute to the carnitine depletion.

Carnitine palmitoyl transferase

Carnitine palmitoyl transferase (CPT) is an enzyme which catalyses the reversible reaction of carnitine and long-chain fatty acyl groups. It exists in two forms, CPTI and CPTII. CPTI is located on the inner side of the outer mitochondrial membrane, whereas CPTII is on the inner side of the inner mitochondrial membrane.

Clinical syndromes associated with abnormalities in fatty acid metabolism

The clinical features of lipid disorders of muscle fall into two broad groups: those in which muscle symptoms are the predominant abnormality and those in which muscle involvement is part of a more general systemic illness. In those patients in whom the muscle involvement is the major or only clinical feature, the presenting symptoms and signs may be proximal or diffuse muscle weakness, or muscle pain, particularly on prolonged exertion, which may be associated with muscle necrosis and myoglobinuria. The muscle symptoms seen in children in whom muscle involvement is part of a systemic illness are predominantly hypotonia and generalized muscle weakness. In some, the symptoms may resolve as the clinical condition improves; in others, the hypotonia and muscle weakness persist, and recovery may take several months.

Carnitine deficiency

A decreased content of free carnitine in muscle may result from: (a) deficient dietary supply, (b) decreased hepatic synthesis, (c) defective transport into the muscle, (d) increased excretion; or (e) abnormally high proportion of esterified to free carnitine. These may in turn be due to a primary and isolated disorder of carnitine metabolism or transport, or may be secondary to a variety of other disorders (Rebouche and Engel 1981). Two distinct clinical syndromes have been delineated in association with decreased free carnitine in the muscle; a myopathic form confined to muscle, and a systemic form affecting multiple systems.

Myopathic carnitine deficiency

Myopathic carnitine deficiency is characterized by weakness, a lipid storage myopathy, and a decreased concentration of carnitine in the muscle but not in the serum. DiMauro et al (1980) reviewed the nine cases documented in the literature up to that time. Five were female and four male. There was generalized weakness, usually starting in childhood and affecting proximal limb and trunk muscles, but sometimes also facial and pharyngeal muscles. The weakness was usually slowly progressive, but worsened rapidly in two adult women and in one adolescent boy. Cardiac involvement was suggested by abnormal electro-, echo- and vector-cardiography in one patient and by death from cardiac failure in one 2-year-old child. No other case died.

The serum carnitine level was normal or only slightly decreased. Serum creatine kinase was variably raised in all but one case. Electromyography showed myopathic features.

Muscle biopsy showed striking accumulation of lipid droplets affecting type 1 more than type 2 fibres. On electron microscopy, the lipid spaces, which were not membrane bound, were often adjacent to mitochondria, which showed no major change in size or number but did show occasional structural changes.

The inheritance seemed to follow an autosomal recessive pattern. Although only one case had an affected sibling as well as consanguineous parents, the muscle carnitine concentration was decreased in the parents and maternal aunt of one patient and in the mother and father of two others. The relatives had no clinical or histological abnormality.

Because of the normal serum carnitine level, it was suggested that the primary defect may lie in the active transport of carnitine into muscle. However, more than one mechanism may be responsible since Willner et al (1979) documented a case with muscle carnitine deficiency that did not respond to oral replacement therapy. In addition, the carnitine uptake of the muscle in vitro was normal and the addition of carnitine did not correct the impaired fatty acid oxidation in muscle homogenates.

Systemic carnitine deficiency

In addition to the lipid storage myopathy and muscle weakness usually starting in childhood, these patients may also have recurrent episodes of acute hepatic encephalopathy, with nausea, vomiting, confusion or coma (reminiscent of Reye's syndrome) and, in some, associated hypoglycaemia, and a metabolic acidosis caused by increased levels of lactate and ketoacids.

Of the eight cases reviewed by DiMauro et al (1980), six had died from cardiorespiratory failure, five of them before the age of 20 years. In two patients, the weakness worsened towards the end of pregnancy or after delivery.

The serum carnitine concentration was markedly reduced in all patients tested. The serum CK was elevated in some but not in others and electromyography showed a myopathic pattern.

Muscle biopsy showed severe lipid storage, similar to the myopathic form of carnitine deficiency. A liver biopsy in one case showed only proliferation of endoplasmic reticulum, but in two others there was lipid accumulation and three cases studied at autopsy showed lipid storage in the liver, heart and tubular epithelium of the kidney. Muscle carnitine was deficient in all cases. The liver carnitine level was 12% of normal in one biopsy specimen and ranged from 14 to 55% of normal in three autopsy cases.

The decreased carnitine in liver, serum and muscle suggested a primary defect in hepatic biosynthesis, with resultant inadequate carnitine supply for tissues from dietary sources alone. In one study of a liver biopsy, the third stage in carnitine synthesis by the enzyme α-butyrobetaine hydroxylase was shown to be normal (Karpati et al 1975), and Rebouche and Engel (1981) were unable to pinpoint any defective biosynthesis in their isotopic studies of two cases and three controls.

With the low level of serum carnitine and the suggestion of defective synthesis by the liver, replacement therapy with oral carnitine would seem potentially more logical and therapeutically beneficial than in the myopathic form. Indeed, some cases have responded well (Karpati et al 1975), but surprisingly the carnitine concentration in the liver or muscle did not rise in spite of the blood level becoming normal. Other patients have apparently not responded to the same therapy (Cornelio et al 1977, Cruse et al 1984), suggesting once again possible varying types of biochemical deficit. Perhaps the tissue carnitine receptors are defective in these cases. Di Donato et al (1984) documented a 20-year-old woman with systemic carnitine deficiency who had a dramatic improvement in her clinical state, accompanied by resolution of the lipid myopathy and elevation of the muscle carnitine from low to normal levels. They suggested the possibility of three distinct clinical variants of systemic carnitine deficiency, depending on the presence or absence of a response to replacement therapy and the associated resolution of the tissue deficit in responsive cases.

Mixed forms of carnitine deficiency

While the muscle and systemic forms of carnitine deficiency seem fairly distinct, there are some cases that are not easily compartmentalized and may share features of either form. Thus they may have the clinical features of systemic carnitine deficiency but normal serum carnitine levels, or they may have consistently low serum carnitine but no evidence of hepatic involvement.

Carnitine palmitoyltransferase deficiency (CPT deficiency)

A deficiency of either CPTI or CPTII can result in a myopathic problem (Bonnefont et al 1999).

CPT deficiency is characterized by recurrent myoglobinuria, often precipitated by prolonged exercise, fasting or a combination of the two. DiMauro et al (1980) reviewed 16 cases from the literature and added three of their own plus two others in which they had studied the biopsies. All but one of the 21 cases were male, including three pairs of affected brothers.

Most patients recalled recurrent muscle pains since childhood but they did not seem to have cramps during exercise, which act as warning signals in patients with phosphorylase or phosphofructokinase (PFK) deficiency to stop using their muscles. This may explain the earlier onset as well as the greater frequency of myoglobinuria in CPT deficiency than in phosphorylase or PFK deficiency. By the time patients with CPT deficiency experienced muscle stiffness or pain, it was usually too late to avoid myoglobinuria. The myoglobinuria usually followed vigorous exercise of a few hours' duration, such as a long hike or a football game, and fasting before exercise was recognized by most patients as a precipitating factor. Five of the 21 had renal failure. In about one-third of cases, there was no apparent precipitating cause for at least some of the episodes of myoglobinuria.

During attacks, affected muscles became swollen, tender and weak. Respiratory muscles were often severely involved and three cases needed assisted ventilation. Between attacks, patients were usually normal and did not show residual weakness. In 19 of the 21 cases the diagnosis was established between 15 and 30 years of age.

Serum CK was normal between attacks and blood lactate rose normally after ischaemic exercise. Plasma lipids were abnormal in four cases, with increased triglyceride and cholesterol in three and slightly increased triglycerides in one.

Muscle biopsies taken during the quiescent phase between attacks were normal in about two-thirds of the reported cases. When lipid storage was present, this was usually less marked than in carnitine deficiency, and in two reports was only noted in one out of two biopsies on the patients. Areas of necrosis noted in the limb muscle of one patient and the intercostal muscle of another were probably related to a recent episode of myoglobinuria. Liver biopsy in one case showed no lipid storage but some abnormality of mitochondria, and the morphology of leukocytes was normal in two cases. In general, muscle biopsies rarely show significant pathological changes in CPT deficiencies and levels of lipid within fibres appear normal. If a sample is taken soon after an episode of myoglobinuria, however, necrosis and fibre regeneration will be apparent.

The biochemical abnormality was first demonstrated by DiMauro and DiMauro (1973) in two brothers with recurrent myoglobinuria but no demonstrable defect in glycogen metabolism. CPT activity by three different assays was less than 20% of normal. The enzyme deficiency has been confirmed in all subsequent cases. CPT activity may be undetectable by colorimetric analysis but with the more sensitive radioactive assays there is usually some residual activity, varying from 5 to 24% of the normal mean.

The diagnosis of CPT deficiency should be considered in any patient with recurrent myoglobinuria, particularly if precipitated by prolonged exercise or fasting. Two clinical criteria are helpful in distinguishing it from phosphorylase or PFK deficiency: (a) there is no intolerance to vigorous exercise of short duration and no 'second-wind' phenomenon, and (b) cramps are unusual and contracture is not induced by ischaemic exercise.

Confirmation of the metabolic block can be provided by dietary and exercise studies. The respiratory quotient, normally close to 0.7 at rest, may be higher in patients due to abnormal dependence on carbohydrate metabolism. Prolonged fasting without exercise may cause a rise in serum CK and the appearance of myoglobin in the urine (Bank et al 1975). In one study, depletion of glycogen was produced by a combination of exercise and a ketogenic diet, following which only a few minutes of exercise produced myalgia and tachycardia (Layzer et al 1980). In another patient, prolonged exercise on a normal diet produced an abnormal increase in serum CK (Carroll et al 1978).

Although the marked preponderance of affected males suggested a possible X-linked inheritance, both CPTI and CPTII are encoded by autosomal genes on chromosomes 11 and 1, respectively.

Whilst myoglobinuria is a feature of CPT deficiency, it can also occur in other metabolic disorders, such as glycogen storage disorders (see Ch. 17), as a result of a toxic insult (see Ch. 23), or in association with malignant hyperthermia (see Ch. 20).

Clinical features associated with other specific defects of lipid metabolism

A number of additional clinical syndromes have been identified in relation to specific defects in the metabolism of fatty acids (Di Donata and Taroni 2003).

Biochemistry

Before the β-oxidation of fatty acids can occur, they have to be converted first to their coenzyme A (CoA) thioesters, which is catalysed by the acyl-CoA synthetases, of which there are at least four types, classified according to their chain lengths as short-chain, medium-chain, long-chain and very long-chain. Long-chain acyl-CoA synthetase acts on the outer mitochondrial membrane, whilst very long-chain acyl-CoA synthetase is in the inner mitochondrial membrane and the short-chain and medium-chain acyl-CoA synthetases in the mitochondrial matrix (Fig. 18.1).

Acyl-CoA dehydrogenase deficiency

Defects of the acyl-CoA dehydrogenases are the most frequently identified abnormalities of fatty acid oxidation.

Short-chain acyl-CoA dehydrogenase deficiency

This deficiency has been described in two different clinical situations: a myopathic form in which the defect is limited to muscle and presenting with a slowly progressive muscle weakness and exercise-induced pain (Turnbull et al 1984), and a systemic form with hepatomegaly and microcephaly (Amendt et al 1987, Coates et al 1988). The 16-year-old girl documented by Tein et al (1991) had recurrent myoglobinuria, hypoketotic hypoglycaemia, encephalopathy and an associated cardiomyopathy.

Medium-chain acyl-CoA dehydrogenase deficiency

This may be one of the most commonly inherited metabolic disorders, with an incidence of 1 in 5000 to 10 000 live births (Roe and Coates 1989). It usually presents in infancy with an episodic illness in which muscle symptoms and signs are not prominent (Stanley et al 1983). The clinical presentations include sudden infant death, Reye's syndrome and hypoglycaemic episodes. Some cases, however, present in later life and exercise-induced muscle pain may be a feature, and yet others are asymptomatic and are detected only when the disorder is diagnosed in another family member (Duran et al 1986). Medium-chain acyl-CoA dehydrogenase deficiency is inherited in an autosomal recessive pattern, with intermediate enzyme activity in fibroblasts from the parents (Coates et al 1985).

Long-chain acyl-CoA dehydrogenase deficiency

These defects can be divided into three different clinical phenotypes (Hale et al 1990), one group presenting in early life (under 6 months) with a severe illness with cardiac involvement and often death (Hale et al 1985); the second with coma associated with fasting (those surviving this initial insult have no cardiac involvement or muscle weakness); and a third group of children with a later onset with muscle pain when stressed as a prominent feature (Naylor et al 1980, Amendt et al 1988), accompanied by myoglobinuria and increased plasma CK. Between episodes there is no evidence of muscle disease. Long-chain acyl-CoA dehydrogenase deficiency seems to be inherited as an autosomal recessive disorder (Hale et al 1985).

Several children and adults have also been documented with multiple acyl-CoA dehydrogenase deficiency with a combined defect of the acyl-CoA dehydrogenases. Muscle pain and weakness were prominent features in these patients (Turnbull et al 1988b, Di Donato et al 1989).

Very long-chain acyl-CoA dehydrogenase (VCLAD) deficiency

Following the discovery of VCLAD in 1992 it became apparent that some patients thought to have a long-chain acyl-CoA dehydrogenase deficiency in fact had VCLAD deficiency (Wanders et al 1999). Three phenotypes are associated with this deficiency: (a) a severe, often lethal, childhood form with early onset, cardiomyopathy and hypoglycaemia, (b) a milder childhood form with hypoglycaemia and dicarboxylic aciduria, and (c) a form resembling CPTII deficiency with rhabdomyolysis and myoglobinuria.

Most patients suffer from the severe cardiomyopathic form (Di Donato and Taroni 2002). Muscle pathology associated with VCLAD deficiency is mild, with variation in fibre size and maintenance of a normal fibre typing pattern (Fig. 18.4). A mild increase in lipid staining may be seen.

Mitochondrial trifunctional protein deficiency

This protein is a hetero-octomer of four α-subunits with long-chain 2-enoyl CoA hydratase and long-chain L-3-hydroxylacyl-CoA dehydrogenase activities, and four β subunits with long-chain 3-ketoacyl-CoA thiolase activity. The majority of affected patients have a deficiency of long-chain 3-hydroxyacyl-CoA dehydrogenase (Wanders et al 1999). Age of onset ranges from neonatal to early childhood, and clinical manifestations include recurrent episodes of non-ketotic hypoglycaemia, sudden infant death, cardiomyopathy and myopathy. Muscle weakness is prominent in some children and associated with myoglobinuria and respiratory failure. Distinctive features of long-chain 3-hydroxyacyl-CoA dehydrogenase deficiency are progressive pigmentary retinopathy and peripheral neuropathy.

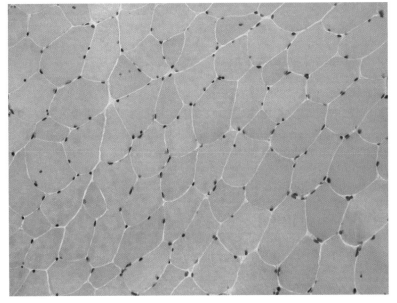

a

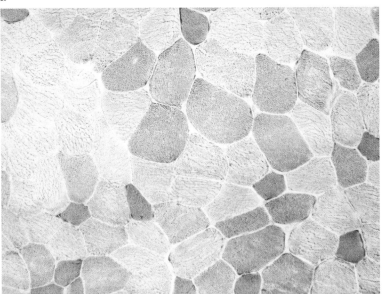

b

FIG. 18.4 *Biopsy from the quadriceps of a female aged 35 years with very long chain acyl-CoA dehydrogenase deficiency (VCLAD) showing in (a) only mild variation in fibre size and occasional fibres with internal nuclei (H&E), and in (b) a normal distribution of fibre types (NADH-TR). Fibre diameter range 30–70 μm.*

In a small group of patients all subunits of the mitochondrial trifunctional protein are deficient. Clinical features are similar to those described above, and although usually more severe a few benign cases with recurrent exercise-induced rhabdomyolysis have been reported (Tyni et al 1999).

Riboflavin-responsive multiple acyl-CoA dehydrogenase deficiency (also known as glutaric aciduria type II)

This complex disorder, associated with electron transfer flavoprotein and electron transfer flavoprotein ubiquinone oxidoreductase deficiency, has different clinical presentations. Some patients present in infancy with renal cystic dysplasia and other congenital anomalies, and usually death occurs in the first few weeks (Yamaguchi et al 1991); other infants and children develop episodic hypoglycaemia, acidosis and hepatomegaly (Loehr et al 1990); and a third group present with muscle weakness (Turnbull et al 1988a). Morphological changes in muscle have been observed in all three clinical groups. The child described by Turnbull et al (1988a) presented with severe muscle weakness at 6 months and responded well to treatment with a low-fat diet, riboflavine, carnitine and glycine. Her brother had died at 3 months, probably with the same condition.

Genetics

Most of the genes encoding the enzymes involved in mitochondrial fatty acid metabolism have been identified and this has greatly assisted diagnosis (see OMIM database). Some genes, for example the gene for CPTII, have common mutations. The gene structure of several has been determined and the number of exons ranges from 5 to 20. Inheritance, where known, is autosomal recessive.

Mitochondrial myopathies

The mitochondrial myopathies are a complex and heterogeneous group of neuromuscular disorders in which abnormalities in mitochondrial metabolic function may be associated with structural abnormalities in the mitochondria. Defects in enzymes encoded by nuclear genes or those of the mitochondrial genome can cause a myopathy. In addition, defects in some enzymes of the fatty acid pathway discussed above can cause secondary structural abnormalities in mitochondria.

During recent years the field of mitochondrial myopathies has mushroomed on a number of fronts – the clinical, with recognition of an ever-increasing variety of presenting disorders, often with overlap of features between different syndromes; the genetic, with recognition of a maternal pattern of inheritance in some syndromes and an autosomal dominant or recessive pattern in others; the biochemical, with identification of specific biochemical abnormalities within the various complexes of the respiratory chain; and the molecular, with recognition of certain specific mutations in relation to the mitochondrial and nuclear genome. The situation has been further compounded by the fact that the same molecular abnormality may produce very divergent clinical features and, in addition, there can also be a wide range in the severity of expression of a mutation within a single family.

Histopathology

Mitochondrial myopathies may be overlooked on routine histological stains of muscle but may be suspected by the presence of disrupted, red-staining fibres on the Gomori trichrome stain, the so-called '**ragged-red fibres**' (Fig. 18.5). Mitochondrial proliferation occurs in the mitochondrial myopathies and it may sometimes be difficult to distinguish abnormal peripheral aggregates of mitochondria from those that occur to varying degrees in normal muscle. The term 'ragged red' was introduced by King Engel to describe the very disrupted fibres seen with the Gomori trichrome. These fibres may be more basophilic and granular with H&E and they react intensely with succinic dehydrogenase and NADH-TR and may lack cytochrome oxidase activity (Fig. 18.6). Fibres which show increased red stain restricted to the periphery of fibres, due to mitochondrial proliferation, are also referred to as 'ragged red'. Although they lack the overall disrupted appearance of the classical ragged-red fibre they also show enhanced SDH and NADH-TR activity and may lack COX. Careful assessment of the three oxidative enzyme reactions is required and combining the demonstration of SDH with COX on the same section can be helpful in identifying fibres devoid of COX, as they appear blue (see Ch. 4).

Ragged-red fibres and fibres devoid of COX are not seen in all cases of mitochondrial myopathy and are more commonly associated with mutations in mitochondrial DNA rather than the nuclear genes (see below). It must also be remembered that ragged-red fibres may occur as a secondary change in other disorders, such as muscular dystrophies and inflammatory myopathies.

The number of affected fibres with abnormal mitochondria is variable, ranging from numerous to few, irrespective of the degree of clinical involvement. Their presence is confirmed on electron microscopy, and at times a careful search for isolated affected fibres may be required. The changes may affect the number of mitochondria, their size and shape, with bizarre and giant forms, and also the patterns of the cristae and the presence of crystalline or osmiophilic inclusions (see Ch. 5). All these individual changes are not related to any particular clinical syndrome or a particular molecular defect. The presence of the disrupted 'ragged-red fibres' invariably implies ultrastructural abnormalities in the mitochondria but the cristae of clusters of proliferated mitochondria may look normal. An increase in intracellular lipid and glycogen may also be seen with lipid droplets of variable size and number.

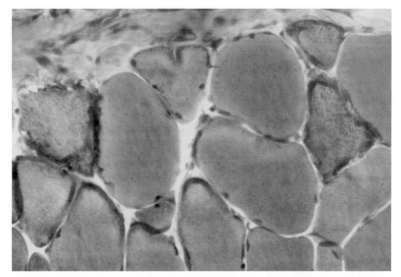

a

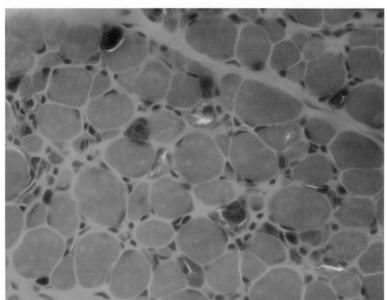

b

FIG. 18.5 *Examples of ragged-red fibres stained with Gomori trichrome in (a) a male aged 30 years with an undefined mitochondrial myopathy (fibre diameter range 30–80 μm) and (b) 22-month-old infant with lipid storage as well as abnormal mitochondria. Fibre diameter range 5–30 μm.*

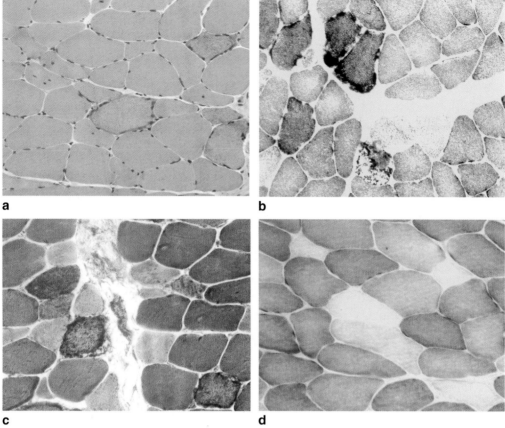

a

b

c

d

FIG. 18.6 *Biopsy from the quadriceps of a male aged 30 years with an undefined mitochondrial myopathy showing variation in fibre size, occasional internal nuclei and fibres with basophilic rims and slight granularity (a) (H&E). These fibres show intense SDH (b) and NADH-TR (c) activity and are devoid of cytochrome oxidase activity and appear white (d). Fibre diameter range 20– 100 μm.*

Clinical syndromes

Mitochondrial diseases are clinically heterogeneous. Age of onset may be from birth to adulthood; the course may be rapidly progressive, static, or even reversible; and distribution of weakness may be generalized with respiratory failure, or proximal more than distal, and may involve facial muscles with associated ptosis and progressive external ophthalmoplegia.

The common indicators of a mitochondrial myopathy are muscle weakness, ptosis, ophthalmoplegia, exercise intolerance, fatigue, raised serum lactate levels, and signal abnormalities on brain magnetic resonance imaging.

The overlapping symptoms and signs of the mitochondrial disorders have made classification difficult but with the identification of molecular defects it has been possible to attribute certain features to particular mutations. The classification of DiMauro (1993) links the clinical features with defects in either nuclear encoded proteins or those from the mitochondrial genome and then disorders caused by defects of communication between the two genomes. Each group is then subdivided on the basis of their clinical and biochemical features.

Genetics

Both the nuclear and mitochondrial genome are required for assembly and maintenance of the enzyme complexes involved in oxidative phosphorylation. The respiratory chain is composed of five multimeric complexes, plus two electron carriers, coenzyme Q10 and cytochrome *c*, with a total of over 80 proteins. Thirteen of these are encoded by mitochondrial DNA, and all others by nuclear DNA. In addition, mitochondrial DNA also encodes for 22 transfer RNAs (tRNA) and two ribosomal RNAs (rRNA) required for the translation of these mitochondrial enzymes. Numerous mutations in these genes have been identified with some being more common (see gene table in Neuromuscular Disorders volume 16:1, 2006).

Mitochondrial DNA is a circular, double-stranded molecule. Its entire sequence is known and it contains no introns (Fig. 18.7). It is maternally inherited and sperm mitochondrial DNA (mtDNA) that enters the zygote is inactivated. Thus inheritance of mitochondrial myopathies related to mtDNA is maternal, whilst those affecting nuclear genes are autosomal dominant or recessive or sporadic. Each cell, including the oocyte, contains many copies of mtDNA which are randomly distributed when a cell divides. The effect of a particular mutation depends on the relative proportion of mutant to wild type. Thus, several organs are affected, and the phenotypic expression of a mutation is a threshold effect determined by the ratio of mutant to wild-type mitochondria. Mutations may not, therefore, always be identified in lymphocyte DNA, requiring studies of DNA extracted from muscle or cultured skin fibroblasts. In addition, there is in muscle a segmental distribution of the mutant mitochondria and only part of a fibre may be affected. Although the mutant DNA is transmitted maternally, both males and females are affected and the severity of subsequent generations is determined by the threshold effect and the number of mutant mitochondria per cell. The threshold levels vary between tissues, depending on the relative importance of oxidative metabolism.

Disorders of mitochondrial DNA

The main types of mutations in mtDNA are large-scale rearrangements (deletions or duplications), point mutations in the tRNAs or rRNAs, or point mutations in the protein coding genes (Fig. 18.7). The first two affect protein translation whilst the latter results in enzyme deficiencies.

Mitochondrial DNA rearrangements

Most large-scale rearrangements occur in sporadic cases. Deletions are mainly confined to an 11-kb region of the mitochondrial genome with an identical

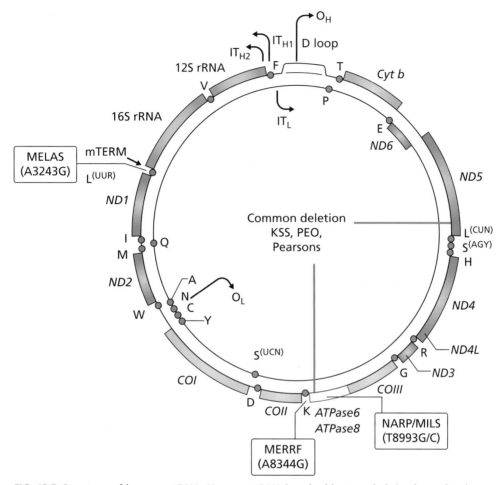

FIG. 18.7 *Structure of human mtDNA. Human mtDNA is a double-stranded circular molecule of 16,659 base pairs. The two strands are termed heavy (outer circle) and light (inner circle) because of their behaviour in alkaline cesium chloride gradients. The genome codes for 13 polypeptides, two rRNAs and 22 tRNAs, which are indicated on the strand containing the coding sequence. The genes coding for polypeptides and rRNAs are depicted as coloured segments on the circle as follows: ND genes of complex I (blue); Cytb gene of complex III (purple); CO genes of complex IV (orange); ATP genes of complex V (white); rRNA genes (green). The tRNA genes are shown in the single letter amino acid code. O_H and O_L represent the replication origins of heavy and light strand replication and IT_H and IT_L the transcription initiation sites on each strand. The D loop is a triple stranded, non-coding structure that contains several regulatory sequences and a nascent heavy strand. mTERM indicates a binding site for a transcription termination factor that regulates the relative rates of transcription of the rRNA genes and the rest of the genes coded on the H-strand. The sites of the most common mtDNA mutations associated with neuromuscular disease are indicated on the figure. Reprinted with kind permission from Shoubridge and Molnar in: Karpati G (ed) Structural and molecular basis of skeletal muscle disease. ISN Neuropathology Press, Basel, p 202–213.*

'common deletion' in 30–40% of cases. The three main clinical syndromes caused by a large-scale deletion are Kearns–Sayre syndrome (KSS), progressive external ophthalmoplegia (PEO) with ragged-red fibres, and Pearson marrow/pancreas syndrome. These sporadic syndromes differ in severity, according to the proportion of mutant mitochondria in each tissue. All are slowly progressive, probably reflecting the slow increase in mitochondria with mutant mitochondria in post-mitotic tissues like muscle.

Kearns-Sayre syndrome

Kearns-Sayre syndrome (KSS), named after the two clinicians who first described it (Kearns and Sayre 1958), is the most severe variant and recognized by a triad of features: retinitis pigmentosa, progressive external ophthalmoplegia (PEO) and heart block. Onset is before 20 years of age. Additional features have been added to these and include progressive eye signs such as ptosis, restricted eye movements and pigmentary retinopathy. Neurological symptoms include incoordination, cerebellar involvement, mental retardation and episodic coma. Seizures are infrequent, and usually associated with concomitant hypoparathyroidism. Complete heart block may lead to sudden death. The cardiac abnormality begins with left anterior fascicular heart block, occasionally in combination with right bundle branch block. Insertion of a pacemaker may be life saving. Short stature and sensorineural hearing loss are common in KSS, as in other mtDNA-associated conditions. Endocrine disturbances are common in patients with mtDNA duplication and include diabetes mellitus, hypoparathyroidism, and isolated growth hormone deficiency. Prognosis is poor; even after provision of a pacemaker, and most patients die in the third or fourth decade.

Elevated lactate and pyruvate values are found in plasma and in cerebrospinal fluid (CSF). Cranial computed tomography and MRI may demonstrate lesions in the cerebral white matter. Calcification of the basal ganglia is also a feature, particularly in patients with hypoparathyroidism.

Muscle pathology

The characteristic morphological change in the muscle is the presence of typical ragged-red fibres with the Gomori trichrome stain, which may look granular or disrupted with H&E and are devoid of COX (see Figs 18.5 and 18.6). Additional fibres not showing ragged-red features may also lack COX. The ragged-red fibres may be isolated and infrequent and constitute not more than 5% or less of the biopsy, or may be much more numerous and also occur in clusters. They involve mainly type 1 fibres but may also affect type 2 fibres.

With the SDH and NADH-TR oxidative reactions, there are either aggregations of more intensely reactive granules, usually subsarcolemmal in distribution (see Fig. 18.6), or there may be disruption with splits which may balloon out, with loss of stain surrounded by a more intensely staining rim. Some affected fibres may be more strikingly disrupted throughout the fibre. These abnormal fibres may also show excessive lipid and glycogen accumulation on the corresponding stains.

The overall distribution of fibre types is usually normal. There may be associated atrophy of fibres affecting particularly the type 2 fibres. There is usually not much proliferation of connective tissue or adipose tissue. The characteristic accumulations of mitochondria with structural changes are readily apparent on electron microscopy.

Progressive external ophthalmoplegia (PEO) with ragged-red fibres

PEO with ragged-red fibres may be sporadic, but is frequently inherited. It is clinically relatively benign condition characterized by ophthalmoplegia, ptosis and proximal limb weakness. Onset is usually in adolescence or early adult life, and the course is slowly progressive and compatible with a relatively normal life. Muscle biopsy, as in KSS, shows ragged-red fibres and COX-negative fibres.

Pearson marrow/pancreas syndrome

Pearson marrow/pancreas syndrome is a non-neurological disease of childhood, characterized by refractory sideroblastic anaemia, vacuolization of marrow precursors and exocrine pancreatic dysfunction, and is usually fatal in early childhood, from sepsis secondary to bone marrow failure (Pearson et al 1979, Rotig et al 1990). The overlap with KSS has been established in a few exceptional patients with Pearson syndrome who survived into adolescence, and developed symptoms and signs of KSS (Larsson et al 1990, McShane et al 1991). The clinical improvement of the blood dyscrasia in these patients is probably due to a gradual decrease of the number of mtDNA deletions in blood cells, whereas the muscle, in contrast, on repeated biopsies in a patient who developed KSS, showed an increase in the proportion of deletions with time (Larsson et al 1990).

Point mutations in mitochondrial tRNA

The two best known main syndromes caused by point mutations in mitochondrial tRNA are myoclonic epilepsy with ragged-red fibres (MERRF) and mitochondrial encephalopathy, lactic acidosis and stroke-like episodes (MELAS), which is more common.

Myoclonic epilepsy with ragged-red fibres (MERRF)

MERRF is a multisystem disorder characterized by myoclonic seizures, mitochondrial myopathy, and cerebellar ataxia. Additional, less common signs include dementia, hearing loss, optic atrophy, peripheral neuropathy and spasticity. Onset can be in childhood or in adult life. Blood lactate and pyruvate levels are elevated and brain MRI may show brain atrophy and calcification. About 80% of cases are caused by the same A8344G mutation in the tRNA[Lysine] gene and a smaller percentage has a T8356C mutation in the same gene.

Muscle pathology

All cases show ragged-red fibres with the Gomori trichrome stain and histochemistry reveals numerous COX-negative fibres. Correlation with immunohistochemistry shows the presence of two populations of mitochondria in individual muscle fibres: one with normal COX activity, the other with decreased activity, but both being immunoreactive for subunit II (Lombes et al 1989).

Mitochondrial encephalopathy, lactic acidosis and stroke-like episodes (MELAS)

This is one of the most common respiratory chain disorders and is characterized by sudden onset, stroke-like episodes. Onset is usually under the age of 45 years and recurrent migraine-like headaches are common. Additional features may include myopathy, cardiomyopathy, ataxia, diabetes mellitus, retinitis pigmentosa and renal dysfunction. Most cases have lactic acidosis and ragged-red fibres in muscle biopsies but in contrast to other situations they show COX activity. About 80% of cases are caused by an A3243G point mutation in the tRNA Leu (UUR) gene. A few other point mutations in this gene have been found as well as a few in other tRNA genes.

Point mutations in mitochondrial protein coding genes

These are less common than mutations of mitochondrial tRNA and the syndromes related to them and include Leber hereditary optic neuroretinopathy (LHON), neuropathy, ataxia and retinitis pigmentosa (NARP) and Leigh syndrome.

Mutations in ND4 (complex I) were the first identified and associated with *Leber hereditary optic neuroretinopathy (LHON)*. In the majority of cases only optic nerve pathology is seen and there is little change in the muscle. Ragged-red fibres are not present, although some increase in oxidative enzyme stains may be seen.

Cases with overlapping features of LHON and MELAS with mutations in ND5 have been reported to show ragged-red fibres.

Neuropathy, ataxia and retinitis pigmentosa (NARP) and maternally inherited Leigh syndrome (MILS) are caused by mutations in the *ATP6* gene, causing a deficiency in complex V. These syndromes are phenotypic variants resulting from variations in the ratio of wild type to mutant mtDNA (heteroplasmy). Leigh syndrome is the more severe and sometimes referred to as necrotizing encephalomyelopathy and a similar phenotype can also arise from mutations in nuclear encoded mitochondrial proteins (see below). Muscle pathology is usually not informative in NARP or MILS, and they do not show ragged-red fibres.

Mutations in *cytochrome b, other complex I, complex III and complex IV (COX) subunits* encoded by mitochondrial DNA have also been identified. In some cases occasional ragged-red fibres are seen which may be COX positive or negative.

Mitochondrial disorders with mutations in nuclear DNA

Several phenotypes are associated with mutations in nuclear genes encoding mitochondrial enzymes. Several of these have a Leigh syndrome phenotype which can also be associated with defects in mtDNA. Disorders caused by defects in nuclear encoded mitochondrial proteins can be classified according to the area of mitochondrial metabolism affected.

Defects of substrate transport

The better known defects of mitochondrial substrate transport affect lipid metabolism and are due to carnitine palmitoyltransferase deficiency and carnitine deficiencies, both primary and secondary (see previous section).

Defects of substrate oxidation

Specific enzyme defects have been identified at several steps in the β-oxidation pathway. Defects of the pyruvate dehydrogenase complex (PDHC) can affect each of the three catalytic components of PDHC, E_1 (pyruvate decarboxylase), E_2 (dihydrolipoyl transacetylase), or E_3 (dihydrolipoyl dehydrogenase), as well as either of the two regulatory components, PDH-kinase, which inactivates the enzyme, and PDH-phosphatase, which activates it. Most of the disorders associated with these enzymes affect the central nervous system, with little 'muscle' component, apart from associated hypotonia in some of the infantile syndromes.

Defects of the Krebs cycle

There are three known defects in the Krebs cycle, involving α-ketoglutarate dehydrogenase, fumarase and aconitase. Once again these enzyme deficiencies affect predominantly the central nervous system.

Defects of the respiratory chain

Respiratory chain defects resulting from genetic errors in nuclear DNA are as follows.

Complex I deficiency

NADH-coenzyme Q (CoQ) reductase, the largest complex of the respiratory chain, contains at least 40 different polypeptides (seven of which are encoded by the mtDNA) and several non-protein components, including flavin mononucleotides (FMN), eight nonheme iron-sulphur clusters, and phospholipid.

Three broad clinical categories associated with complex I deficiencies can be identified:

- a fatal infantile multisystem disorder characterized by severe congenital lactic acidosis, psychomotor delay, diffuse hypotonia and weakness, cardiopathy and cardiorespiratory failure;
- a myopathy with childhood or adult onset and exercise intolerance followed by fixed weakness;
- an encephalomyopathy with onset in childhood or adult life, ophthalmoplegia, seizures, dementia, ataxia, neurosensory hearing loss, pigmentary retinopathy, sensory neuropathy and involuntary movements.

Complex II deficiency

Biochemical documentation of complex II deficiency has been based on defects of succinate-cytochrome c reductase activity in five reported patients with encephalomyopathy (Sengers et al 1983, Behbehani et al 1984, Riggs et al 1984, Sperl et al 1988). Further evidence, accompanied by complete lack of SDH stain in muscle biopsies, was documented by Haller et al (1991) in a case with exercise intolerance and exercise-related myoglobinuria.

Coenzyme Q_{10} (CoQ_{10}) deficiency

Coenzyme Q_{10}, or ubiquinone, transfers electrons derived from complex I and II, and the oxidation of fatty acids and branched-chain amino acids to complex III. It also has a role in membrane stabilization and antioxidation.

Myoglobinuria is a feature and is associated with exercise intolerance, muscle weakness, seizures, ataxia and mental retardation. Muscle biopsies show excessive accumulation of lipid droplets and ragged-red fibres.

Diagnosis is important as the condition is treatable.

Complex III deficiency

Complex III is composed of 11 subunits, and a block at the level of complex III should impair utilization of both NAD-linked and FAD-linked substrates. Enzymatic analyses show defects of both succinate cytochrome c reductase and NADH-cytochrome c reductase, whereas cytochrome oxidase activity is normal.

Clinical presentation is heterogeneous, but falls into two major groups: multisystem disease (encephalomyopathy) and tissue-specific defects such as myopathy or cardiopathy.

Complex IV (COX) deficiency

Complex IV (COX), the last component of the respiratory chain, catalyses the transfer of reducing equivalents from cytochrome c to molecular oxygen. The apoprotein is composed of 13 polypeptides; the three largest subunits (I, II and III) are encoded by mtDNA and are synthesized in mitochondria; the 10 smaller subunits (IV, Va, Vb, VIa, VIb, VIc, VIIa, VIIb, VIIc and VIII) by nuclear DNA and synthesized in the cytoplasm. Full-length complementary DNAs (cDNA) have been obtained for all subunits of human COX and Northern analysis using these cDNAs as probes has shown that only subunits VIa and VIIa are tissue-specific (DiMauro et al 1990).

Clinical phenotypes

The clinical phenotypes associated with complex IV deficiency fall into two groups: one characterized by myopathy, the other involving multiple tissues with predominantly encephalopathy (DiMauro et al 1990).

Myopathy Two forms of myopathy have been described, both presenting soon after birth with severe diffuse weakness, respiratory distress and lactic acidosis but with very different outcomes.

- *Fatal infantile myopathy.* This causes respiratory insufficiency and death before 1 year of age. Heart, liver and brain are clinically spared, but many patients have renal disease with DeToni–Fanconi syndrome. Pedigree analysis in informative families suggests autosomal recessive transmission. The muscle biopsy shows ragged-red fibres and absence of COX staining, but normal staining of spindle fibres and blood vessels. Immunohistochemistry and immunoassay can demonstrate decreased amount of enzyme in muscle (Bresolin et al 1985, Tritschler et al 1991).
- *Benign infantile myopathy.* These infants also have severe weakness, which can be life threatening, and often need assisted ventilation and tube feeding early in life, but then improve spontaneously and are usually normal by 2 or 3 years of age (DiMauro et al 1983, Zeviani et al 1987, Nonaka et al 1988, Servidei et al 1988).

Muscle biopsies from children with this benign COX deficiency lack both subunit VIIa and subunit II, and histochemically muscle biopsies show a virtual absence of COX except in spindle fibres and blood vessels. The spontaneous recovery in these children is associated with a gradual return of COX activity in the muscle, which can be demonstrated both histochemically and biochemically (DiMauro et al 1983). The defect probably involves a nuclear DNA-encoded COX subunit that is not only tissue-specific but also developmentally regulated. Mutations of a fetal or neonatal muscle isozyme would be corrected when the mature isozyme starts to be expressed.

A different clinical presentation, probably not related genetically to the fatal infantile myopathy, is characterized by the association of *myopathy and cardiopathy* with cytochrome oxidase deficiency (Zeviani et al 1986, Hart and Chang 1988).

Encephalomyopathies COX deficiency is the most common biochemical abnormality in Leigh syndrome (DiMauro et al 1990) and is genetically heterogeneous, involving proteins with a role in COX assembly (Shoubridge 2001). Mutations in the SURF-1, SCO1, SCO2 and COX10 genes have been identified (Zhu et al 1998, Tiranti et al 1998, Papadopoulou et al 1999, Valnot et al 2000a,b).

COX deficiency has also been found by Prick et al (1983) in muscle biopsy specimens from two unrelated cases of poliodystrophy (Alpers' disease) and by Bardosi et al (1987) in three patients with MNGIE syndrome (myoneurogastrointestinal disorder and encephalopathy), characterized by PEO limb weakness, peripheral neuropathy, gastroenteropathy with chronic diarrhoea and intestinal pseudo-obstruction, leukodystrophy, lactic acidosis and ragged-red fibres. MNGIE is caused by mutations in the thymidine phosphorylase gene on chromosome 22q (Nishino et al 1999, Spinazzola et al 2002). Simon et al (1990) suggested the acronym POLIP (polyneuropathy, ophthalmoplegia, leukoencephalopathy and intestinal pseudo-obstruction) for their four cases. Partial COX deficiency was found in muscle and liver of the original patient (Bardosi et al 1987) and in muscle biopsy specimens from two other patients (Suomalainen and Kaukonen 2001).

Defects of oxidation/phosphorylation coupling

Complex V deficiency

Complex V (ATP synthase) converts the transmembrane proton gradient generated in the respiratory chain into chemical energy by synthesizing adenosine triphosphate (ATP) from adenosine diphosphate (ADP) and inorganic phosphorus (Pi). It is composed of 12 to 14 subunits, two of which (subunits 6 and 8) are encoded by mtDNA (Hatefi 1985). Defects of ATPase were demonstrated indirectly by polarographic analysis of isolated muscle mitochondria in two patients with a different clinical phenotype. One was a 37-year-old woman with congenital, slowly progressive myopathy, ragged-red fibres, and paracrystalline inclusions in virtually all mitochondria (Schotland et al 1976), the other a 17-year-old boy with a multisystem disorder characterized by weakness, ataxia, retinopathy, dementia and peripheral neuropathy (Clark et al 1983) resembling the affected members of a family with a maternally inherited multisystem disorder and a mutation in subunit 6 of complex V (Holt et al 1990) (see below).

Defects of mitochondrial protein transport

Schapira et al (1990) described a 14-year-old girl with congenital myopathy whose muscle biopsy showed increased lipid droplets, scattered COX-negative fibres, and complete lack of the SDH histochemical reaction, but no ragged-red fibres. Biochemical analysis showed combined defects of the respiratory chain, with a specific defect of both the 27.7-kD iron–sulphur protein of SDH and the Rieske protein of complex III. Because the Rieske protein was present both in muscle homogenate and in the cytosol, but not in isolated mitochondria, it was suggested that the primary defect in this patient involved mitochondrial protein import.

Defects of the inner membrane

The inner mitochondrial membrane has a high proportion of the phospholipid, cardiolipin. Evidence suggests cardiolipin is essential for the correct assembly and function of the respiratory chain. Barth syndrome, characterized by mitochondrial myopathy, cardiomyopathy and cyclic neutropenia, is caused by defects in the G4.5 gene on Xq28 that encodes a protein, tafazzin that influences the incorporation of cardiolipin. Muscle biopsies in Barth syndrome show ragged-red fibres and biochemically show a reduction of various respiratory enzymes.

CHAPTER 19

Endocrine disorders

Many hormones have an important role in maintaining normal muscle function. Myopathies have been described in association with several endocrine disorders, either an excess or deficiency, in particular those affecting thyroid, parathyroid, glucocorticoid, growth hormone and insulin levels. In most cases the muscle involvement is an incidental feature of the disorder, and may even be subclinical and only revealed by special investigations, such as serum enzyme levels, electromyography and biopsy, in the course of study of these disorders. In other instances, the muscle symptoms may be the presenting features and may lead to the diagnosis of the underlying disorder, e.g. thyrotoxicosis. In many cases the muscle weakness is disproportional to the degree of muscle wasting.

There have been relatively few recent detailed histochemical or electron microscopic studies on the muscles in these various disorders and estimation of the hormone levels is the primary diagnostic tool. Many of the reported studies from the pioneering days of muscle pathology show that in general, only non-specific myopathic changes accompany changes in hormone levels. These relate mainly to changes in fibre size (atrophy or hypertrophy) and fibre type proportions.

Disorders of the thyroid
Hyperthyroidism

There are four different neuromuscular disorders associated with hyperthyroidism:

- thyrotoxic myopathy;
- myasthenia gravis;
- thyrotoxic periodic paralysis; and
- exophthalmic ophthalmoplegia.

Thyrotoxic myopathy

The most common myopathy in association with thyrotoxicosis is a chronic form which may be generalized or confined mainly to proximal muscles. Although commonly seen in females, particularly after the age of 50 years, males can also be affected (Rose and Griggs 2002). At times, it may precede other signs of thyrotoxicosis. The electromyogram shows abnormality, usually of a myopathic type, in about 90% of cases of hyperthyroidism, but histological changes occur in only about 50% (Havard et al 1963, Ramsay 1966).

The muscle biopsy may show no abnormality on light microscopy or varying degrees of fibre atrophy and fatty infiltration. Ultrastructural studies have revealed a number of relatively non-specific changes (Engel 1966, 1972). These include mitochondrial hypertrophy, focal loss of mitochondria, focal myofibrillar degeneration beginning at the Z line, focal dilatations of the transverse tubular system, subsarcolemmal glycogen deposits and papillary projections of the surface of the muscle fibres, probably resulting from fibre atrophy.

Acute thyrotoxic myopathy may involve bulbar and extraocular muscles and is probably due to associated myasthenia rather than being a separate entity.

Myasthenia gravis

The association of myasthenia and thyrotoxicosis is well documented (see Ch. 21; Millikan and Haines 1953, Silver and Osserman 1957, Simpson 1968). The incidence of hyperthyroidism in the course of myasthenia is in the region of 5%, whereas that of myasthenia in the course of hyperthyroidism is much lower, being less than 0.5% (Kissel et al 1970). The association of the two diseases is perhaps not surprising since both are recognized to have an autoimmune origin.

Thyrotoxic periodic paralysis

The clinical pattern of the paralytic attacks is very similar to the idiopathic type of hypokalaemic periodic paralysis. The attacks usually subside after treatment of the hyperthyroidism. The condition appears to be more common in oriental races (Okinaka et al 1957, McFadzean and Yeung 1967) and there is a marked preponderance of affected males.

The biopsy may show vacuolation, as in idiopathic hypokalaemic periodic paralysis, but at times may be practically normal in appearance (Resnick et al 1969).

Exophthalmic ophthalmoplegia

Although usually looked upon as a complication of thyrotoxicosis, many cases do not have associated hyperthyroidism at the time of its development. Overproduction of thyroid-stimulating hormone, long-acting thyroid stimulator, or a specific exophthalmos-producing factor have been invoked, but the mechanism still remains unknown (Havard 1972). Mullin et al (1977) suggested a delayed hypersensitivity response directed against the orbital contents as a result of the development of antibodies to thyroglobulin.

Hypothyroidism

Muscle cramps or aching are common in hypothyroidism and there may be associated weakness. Movements as well as reflexes tend to be sluggish ('myotonic reflexes'). Some cases may show ridging of the muscle on percussion (myoedema). There may be increased muscle bulk but others have muscle atrophy. In childhood, hypothyroidism may cause hypertrophy in association with slowness of movements, fatigability and myotonic tendon reflexes. The creatine kinase is usually elevated, even in the absence of overt muscle weakness. In addition, there is delayed myelination of the peripheral nerves, with slow nerve conduction velocity (Moosa and Dubowitz 1971).

The rare syndrome of 'hypertrophia musculorum vera' in children was first described by Kocher in 1892 (Debré and Semelaigne 1935) and the term was popularized by Debré and Semelaigne (1935) who stressed the relation with hypothyroidism. This syndrome has been described in congenital cases and in children of all ages with hypothyroidism, and also following surgical or radioactive ablation of the thyroid. The hypertrophy is completely reversible by treatment of the hypothyroidism.

The so-called Hoffmann syndrome occurring in adults is another form of hypothyroid myopathy with myotonia-like features but no muscle hypertrophy.

Muscle biopsy in hypothyroid patients has revealed relatively non-specific changes such as fibre atrophy or enlargement, type 1 fibre predominance, increased internal nuclei, glycogen and mitochondrial aggregates, dilated sarcoplasmic reticulum and proliferating T-system profiles, and focal myofibrillar loss (Norris and Panner 1966, Afifi et al 1974, Emser and Schimrigk 1977). Khaleeli et al (1983) studied needle biopsies before and several months after treatment in 11 adult hypothyroid patients aged 51 to 71 years with associated muscle weakness. Abnormalities were found in 8 of the 11 biopsies, the commonest being type 2 fibre atrophy. After treatment, resolution of the changes was slow and 50% of the patients had persistent abnormalities.

Hypothyroidism during pregnancy can affect the expression of myosin isoforms and fibre typing in the fetus (Butler-Browne et al 1990).

Disorders of the parathyroids and osteomalacia

Muscle weakness can occur in the course of primary and secondary hyperparathyroidism and in osteomalacia. In addition, disorders which lead to osteomalacia, such as vitamin D deficiency, renal tubular acidosis and chronic renal failure, are associated with secondary hyperparathyroidism.

Vicale (1949) drew attention to myopathy affecting mainly the proximal muscles, with associated pain and fatigability, a waddling gait and hyper-reflexia, in two cases of primary hyperparathyroidism and one of osteomalacia associated with renal tubular acidosis. This association of myopathy with primary or secondary hyperparathyroidism has been well substantiated in many subsequent reports (Bischoff and Esslen 1965, Prineas et al 1965, Smith and Stern 1967, Frame et al 1968, Cholod et al 1970, Dastur et al 1975, Schott and Wills 1975, Mallette et al 1975, Skaria et al 1975, Serratrice et al 1978). Muscle biopsy in many of these patients showed relatively minor changes even in the face of fairly severe clinical weakness. These have included non-specific fibre atrophy, selective type 2 fibre atrophy, minor vacuolar changes and degeneration of isolated fibres.

Treatment of the underlying cause, particularly in primary hyperparathyroidism, has led to resolution of the associated neuromuscular involvement.

Hypoparathyroidism

Myopathy is not a feature of hypoparathyroidism, the main manifestations of which are tetany and carpopedal spasms.

Disorders of the pituitary and adrenals
Hyperpituitarism

In acromegaly there is a general hypertrophy of muscle, especially in the early phases, but later there may be muscle weakness. In a study of eight cases, Lundberg et al (1970) detected EMG changes of a myopathic nature (small polyphasic potentials), but the muscle histology in six cases biopsied was apparently normal. However, no histographic analysis of fibre diameter and no histochemical studies were done. Mastaglia et al (1970) found mild proximal weakness in 6 of their 11 cases of acromegaly and elevation of serum CK in five. EMG in all of them showed a shorter mean action potential duration than controls and there was histological abnormality in five of the biopsies taken. These comprised segmental necrosis of single muscle fibres and proliferation of sarcolemmal nuclei. The histochemical pattern was normal, but there was an increase in size of both type 1 and 2 fibres. There was no apparent correlation of histological change with clinical weakness. In a more detailed analysis of the muscle biopsies from nine of these patients, Mastaglia (1973) found hypertrophy of type 1 and 2 fibres in two subjects, hypertrophy of type 1 fibres only in two subjects, atrophy of both fibre types in two and atrophy of type 2 fibres only in four. Isolated fibre necrosis or vacuolar degeneration was present in three biopsies and an increase in internal nuclei in five.

Pickett et al (1975) found clinical and electromyographic evidence of myopathy in 9 of their 17 acromegaly cases and a frequently associated carpal tunnel syndrome but no abnormalities in the muscle biopsies from three patients.

In a detailed histographic analysis of needle biopsies of the quadriceps from 18 cases, Nagulesparen et al (1976) found that the most frequent changes were hypertrophy of type 1 fibres (nine cases) and atrophy of type 2 fibres (2A and/or 2B, nine patients). Only two showed atrophy of type 1 fibres and four had hypertrophy of type 2A and/or 2B fibres. There was no apparent direct correlation of the degree of change with the level of growth hormone.

The two cases of pituitary gigantism reported by Lewis (1972) had an associated peripheral neuropathy. However, the muscle biopsy done in one of them showed a marked variation in fibre size and proliferation of connective tissue, thought to be 'myopathic' in appearance, in addition to some group atrophy and selective type 2 fibre atrophy.

Hypopituitarism

In children with hypopituitarism there is poor muscle development and reduced muscle mass in parallel with the deficit in skeletal growth, but no evidence of any associated myopathy.

Hyperadrenalism (Cushing's syndrome) and steroid myopathy

Proximal weakness, especially of the lower limbs, is a well recognized complication of Cushing's syndrome (Müller and Kugelberg 1959) and probably occurs in more than 50% of cases.

Myopathy as a result of steroid therapy was first documented in the same year as Cushing's myopathy (Perkoff et al 1959, Williams 1959) and many reports have followed, especially since the introduction of the 9α-fluorosteroids (dexamethasone, triamcinolone) which appear to be even more toxic to muscle than the non-fluorinated drugs (cortisone, prednisone).

The onset of steroid-induced myopathy is partly dependent on the dosage and the duration, but there is considerable variation in individual susceptibility and the onset may occur within weeks rather than months (Askari et al 1976). In Cushing's syndrome itself, the onset is usually insidious.

While the diagnosis of steroid myopathy may be readily apparent in the steroid treatment of conditions that are not associated with muscle weakness, it can be extremely difficult in muscle disorders such as dermatomyositis being treated with steroids. Moreover, the superadded steroid myopathy in some of these cases may be more responsible for the patient's disability than the underlying myositis (Dubowitz 1976, Miller et al 1983).

The most consistent change in the muscle biopsies, both from Cushing's syndrome (Pleasure et al 1970) as well as in steroid myopathy, is selective type 2 fibre atrophy, usually the 2B fibres (see Ch. 4). This has also been produced in some of the experimental studies in animals. On electron microscopy, enlargement, proliferation and degeneration of mitochondria, dilatation of the sarcoplasmic reticulum, thickening of the basal lamina, loss of myofibrils, and increase in lipid droplets and subsarcolemmal glycogen have been described (Engel 1966, Afifi et al 1968).

Prineas et al (1968) described a severe myopathy developing in patients who had undergone adrenalectomy for Cushing's syndrome. There was associated pigmentation of the skin and the muscle contained excessive lipid deposit, especially in the type 1 fibres.

Hypoadrenalism (Addison's disease)

Muscle weakness is a common symptom in Addison's disease but there has been no record of any underlying myopathy. The weakness probably has a biochemical basis in relation to the fluid and electrolyte changes and responds rapidly to treatment of the disorder.

Hyperaldosteronism

When Conn (1955) first described primary aldosteronism, he drew attention to the associated periodic attacks of weakness, presumably related to the hypokalaemia. In a subsequent review of 145 cases (Conn et al 1964), muscular weakness was one of the most common presenting features, occurring in 73% of their cases. Sambrook et al (1972) documented a case, including detailed studies of a muscle biopsy. There was necrosis of isolated muscle fibres and also the presence of small angulated fibres, strongly reactive with NADH-TR, similar to those associated with denervation. Atsumi et al (1979) also documented a myopathy in association with primary aldosteronism in two adult patients. There was necrosis and vacuolation of muscle fibres on light microscopy and at electron microscopic level the necrotic areas were characterized by dissolution of myofilaments and degenerative vacuoles.

Insulin associated disorders

Primary muscle weakness is not a feature of diabetes or hypoglycaemia but may result secondarily from a neuropathy. This is painful and asymmetrical and may be accompanied by muscle tenderness and swelling. Muscle biopsies show no distinctive features but thickening of capillary basal lamina may be seen with electron microscopy, even in prediabetics (see Ch. 5).

Muscle pain, cramps and fatigue, without weakness, may be associated with insulin-resistant diabetes.

CHAPTER 20

Ion channel disorders

Action potentials in muscle, initiated by depolarization by a nerve impulse, and depolarization of the muscle fibre, require the rapid movement of inorganic ions through transmembrane ion channels. The action potential results in the release of calcium ions from the sarcoplasmic reticulum (SR), leading to contraction of the myofibrils. Mutations in the genes encoding the proteins of these ion channels of the sarcolemma, SR and T tubules disrupt the normal transport of ions, in particular sodium, potassium, chloride and calcium ions (Davies and Hanna 2001, Jurkat-Rott et al 2002). They are associated with a number of clinically overlapping syndromes and defects in the same gene can give rise to varying phenotypes (Fig. 20.1, Table 20.1). The clinical manifestations of a particular mutation are often determined by its functional effect, which may be either a gain or loss of function. The ion channel proteins are multidomain, transmembrane glycoproteins and numerous mutations in several genes have now been identified.

There are a number of diverse syndromes involving skeletal muscle which are associated with abnormalities in ion channels which clinically fall into two main groups: those with myotonia; or those with periodic paralysis. There have been major advances in the understanding of the molecular basis of many of them with the identification of several gene defects in proteins that encode ion channels (Table 20.1). In addition, malignant hyperthermia is caused by defects in a calcium channel, and Brody's disease by disturbances in a calcium pump of the SR. There are also syndromes affecting the heart (long QT syndromes) and various disorders of the central nervous system, such as periodic ataxias that are caused by defects in ion channels (Wullner 2003).

Syndromes with myotonia

Myotonia is a state of delayed relaxation, or sustained contraction, of skeletal muscle. It may manifest after a voluntary muscle contraction, so-called *active myotonia*, and the patient may be aware of difficulty in relaxing the grip after

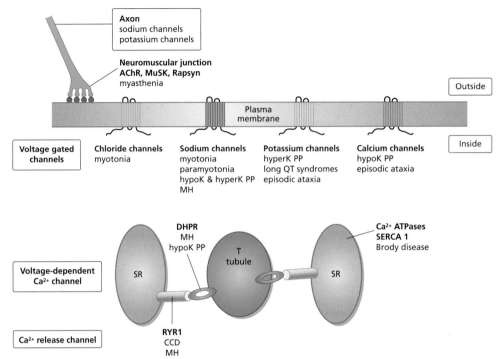

FIG. 20.1 *Diagram showing the disorders of ion channels and those caused by disturbances in ionic balance (CCD = central core disease, MH = malignant hyperthermia, hypoK PP = hypokalemic periodic paralysis; hyperK PP = hyperkalemic periodic paralysis, SR = sarcoplasmic reticulum)*

TABLE 20.1 *Ion channel disorders of skeletal muscle*

Clinical syndrome	Type of ion channel	Gene	Locus	Inheritance
Myotonia congenita (Becker)	Chloride channel	CLCN1	7q35	Recessive
Myotonia congenita (Thomsen)	Chloride channel	CLCN1	7q35	Dominant
Potassium-aggravated myotonia	Sodium channel	SCN4A	17q23	Dominant
Paramyotonia congenita	Sodium channel	SCN4A	17q23	Dominant
Hyperkalaemic periodic paralysis	Sodium channel	SCN4A	17q23	Dominant
Hypokalaemic periodic paralysis	Calcium channel Sodium channel	CACNA1S SCN4A	1q32 17q23	Dominant Dominant
Hyperkalaemic or hypokalaemic periodic paralysis (Andersen's syndrome)	Potassium channel	KCNJ2	17q	Dominant
Malignant hyperthermia	Calcium channel Calcium channel	RYR1 CACNA1S	19q13 1q32	Dominant Dominant

grasping something. With repetition of the same movement, the myotonia gradually becomes less and then disappears (warm-up phenomenon), and may be accompanied by transient muscle weakness. If the myotonia becomes worse with exercise, instead of improving, the term *paradoxical myotonia* or *paramyotonia* is used. In addition, in congenital paramyotonia the muscle stiffness is often profoundly worse with cold environments.

In infants the first manifestation of myotonia may be delayed opening of the eyes after their closure with crying. In some patients the myotonia may be fairly localized to only some muscle groups; in others there may be a more general 'stiffness' during the bouts of myotonia.

Myotonia may also be elicited by percussion of a muscle, so-called *percussion myotonia*. This can usually be demonstrated clinically by percussion with a finger of sites such as the tongue, thenar eminence, or the deltoid, brachioradialis or gluteal muscles, which give a local contraction dimple.

Both myotonia and paramyotonia show characteristic patterns with electromyography due to repetitive firing of action potentials and imbalances in sodium or chloride ions. With the use of the concentric needle, there is increased activity and irritability of the muscle as the needle is inserted and spontaneous myotonic bursts may be produced. The myotonic bursts can also be elicited if the muscle is tapped with a finger in the vicinity of the needle, or when the patient voluntarily contracts the muscle. These myotonic bursts consist of a prolonged series of rhythmical activity, initially of high frequency (around 20–80-Hz) and high amplitude, and then gradually waning in amplitude and also slowing down. The burst may continue for several seconds and an acoustic amplification gives a characteristic sound, likened to a 'dive-bomber' or a motor cyclist taking off at speed and disappearing into the distance. The individual elements of the myotonic discharge usually resemble either positive sharp waves or fibrillation potentials, and represent action potentials from single muscle fibres.

'Pseudomyotonia' is sometimes noted on electromyogram in other neuromuscular disorders such as type II glycogenosis. The bursts are usually shorter and less striking than true myotonia and do not show the characteristic decrement. Clinical myotonia cannot be elicited in these patients.

Muscle pathology

Despite the essential role of ions in muscle function, muscle architecture is rarely altered to a significant degree. Muscle biopsy is then used for exclusion of other disorders and diagnosis relies on thorough clinical and neurophysiological examination.

Many of the pathological descriptions of syndromes now known to relate to ion channel malfunction were reported several years ago before their molecular basis had been determined (Jurkat-Rott et al 2002). The features are non-specific and usually mild. They include variation in fibre size, with atrophy and hypertrophy, and an increase in internal nuclei. In chloride channel myotonias there may be hypertrophy of type 2A fibres, and there may be a reduction in the proportion of this fibre type. In myotonias due to potassium-aggravated sodium channel malfunction, in addition to non-specific variation in fibre size, subsarcolemmal vacuolation relating to dilatation of the T tubules and disruption of myofibrils may be seen with electron microscopy. In paramyotonia congenita, caused by defects in the voltage-gated sodium channel *SCN4A* gene, tubular aggregates may also occur.

Genotype-phenotype correlations of the myotonias

These disorders can be divided into those related to chloride or to sodium channels and include Thomsen and Becker myotonias, potassium-aggravated myotonia and paramyotonia (Table 20.1). Inheritance is generally autosomal dominant, except in Becker's myotonia. ***Thomsen and Becker myotonias*** are caused by mutations in the gene encoding the voltage-gated chloride channel, *CLCN1*, on chromosome 7q35. The division into dominant mutations in Thomsen's disease and recessive mutations in Becker is now less clear and a particular mutation can be inherited in either a dominant or recessive pattern (Davies and Hanna 2001). The clinical features associated with both disorders are similar and both show classical myotonia on EMG and a 'warm-up' phenomenon, with improvement on activity. Both can present in childhood, and onset is usually later in Becker's myotonia. In Becker, the myotonia is greater in the lower limbs than in the face and arms and may be associated with transient weakness.

Defects in the voltage-gated sodium channel gene (*SCN4A*) on chromosome 17q23 are associated with two clinically overlapping syndromes with myotonia, ***potassium aggravated myotonia and paramyotonia congenita***. They also cause hyper- and hypokalaemic periodic paralysis syndromes (see below). All these disorders are inherited as an autosomal dominant trait. As the name suggests, potassium ingestion provokes the myotonia in potassium-aggravated myotonia and it may be painful. Paramyotonia congenita shows a characteristic worsening of the muscle stiffness with activity (paradoxical myotonia) and with cold, and particularly affects the muscles of the face and hands. On EMG the myotonia is similar to that seen in chloride channel disorders but the effect of cold immersion is an important distinction, with a marked reduction in the evoked compound muscle action potential amplitude.

The mutations in the *SCN4A* sodium channel gene are distributed throughout the various domains of the channel but there appears to be a hot spot for paramyotonia congenita in the voltage-sensing region (S4) of domain IV. Many of the mutations lead to a gain in function of the sodium channel, and most lead to impairment of fast inactivation of the channel.

Periodic paralysis syndromes

Episodes of weakness or periodic paralysis characterize some disorders associated with disturbances in serum potassium levels, both hypo- and hyperkalaemia.

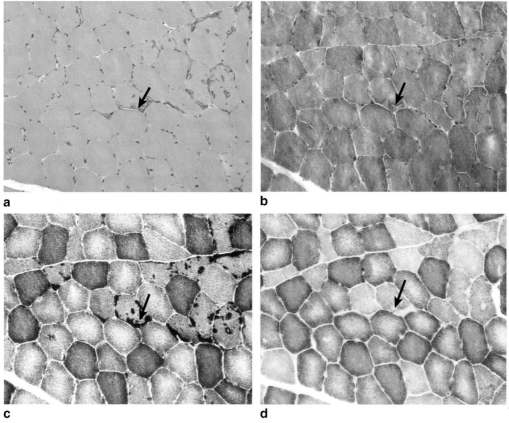

FIG. 20.2 *Biopsy from the quadriceps of a man aged 27 years showing tubular aggregates in serial sections (arrows) that are basophilic with H&E (a), red with Gomeri trichrome (b), intensely stained in type 2 fibres with NADH-TR but negative for COX activity (d). Note also the loss of oxidative enzyme activity in the centre of many fibres. Fibre diameter range 50–85 μm.*

Muscle pathology

The familial forms and thyrotoxic hypokalaemia may be associated with proliferation and dilation of the T-tubular and SR systems. This is identified at the light microscope level as vacuoles or as red-stained areas with Gomori trichrome, which are aggregates of tubules (see Figs 5.67 and 5.68). The vacuolation is thought to appear in a sequence ranging from focal dilation of the SR to large mature membrane bound vacuoles (Engel 1970). The dilated SR may contain amorphous granular material, cell debris and myelin-like whorls. The vacuolar areas stain for NADH-TR and acid phosphatase, and immunolabelling shows the presence of dystrophin and β-spectrin, but not laminin, on the membrane (De Bleecker et al 1993).

Tubular aggregates, in addition to the red staining with Gomori trichrome, are basophilic with haematoxylin and eosin and show reactivity for NADH-TR but not succinic dehydrogenase or menadione-linked α-glycerophosphate dehydrogenase (Fig. 20.2). Tubular aggregates are thought to be derived from the SR but there are examples in which they stain for enzymes thought to be specific for mitochondrial enzymes, such as cytochrome oxidase and ubiquinone, and this has not been explained (Pearse and Johnson 1970). Tubular aggregates also stain for myoadenylate deaminase, non-specific esterase and other enzymes such as phosphofructokinase. They are often restricted to type 2 fibres and do not show adenosine triphosphatase activity as they contain no myofibrils. With immunohistochemistry the tubular aggregates have been shown to label with antibodies to the SERCA1-ATPase, heat shock proteins, dysferlin and emerin (Martin et al 1991, Ikezoe et al 2003, Manta et al 2004).

Tubular aggregates are not specific for ion channel disorders but may be seen frequently in periodic paralysis (Morgan-Hughes 2001). They may also be seen in paramyotonia congenita caused by defects in the same gene (see below).

Genotype-phenotype correlations in periodic paralysis

These disorders fall into two main groups, hyper- and hypokalaemic periodic paralysis and result from defects in the genes for a sodium (SCN4A), or calcium (CACNA1S) channel (Table 20.1). It will be noted in Table 20.1 that defects in the same genes can be associated with different phenotypes. The episodes of weakness are often triggered by rest after a period of exercise or stress. Hypokalaemic periodic paralysis is characterized by more prolonged (days/weeks) and more severe (four limb) bouts of weakness. Attacks in hyperkalaemic periodic paralysis can last for only a few minutes or hours and may be remarkably focal. They show autosomal dominant inheritance and onset is usually in childhood or early adolescence.

Patients with hyperkalaemic periodic paralysis overlap clinically with potassium-aggravated myotonia and paramyotonia congenita caused by mutations in the gene for the same sodium channel (SCN4A) on chromosome 17q. The same gene can also cause hypokalaemic periodic paralysis. The phenotypic difference is believed to relate to a gain (hyperkalaemic) or loss (hypokalaemic) of function of the ion channel caused by the different mutations. Hypokalaemic periodic paralysis, however, is more commonly caused by mutations in the calcium channel gene CACNA1S on chromosome 1q32. Two particular mutations account for most cases.

Mutations in the KCNE3 gene on chromosome 11q13–14 have been described in two rare families, one with a phenotype consistent with hypokalaemic periodic paralysis, the other with hyperkalaemic periodic paralysis. Recent studies have failed to demonstrate mutations within this gene in many families with periodic paralysis and it may be that mutations in KCNE3 may modify other ion channel functions rather than cause the condition directly.

In 1971 Andersen described a syndrome characterized by periodic paralysis, ventricular arrhythmia and mild dysmorphism (Andersen et al 1971). Most cases experience hypokalaemic attacks but hyperkalaemic periodic paralysis has also been described in a minority of cases with this syndrome (Sansone et al 1997) and the cause has been shown to be mutations in the *KCNJ2* gene on chromosome 17q (Plaster et al 2001) that encodes the inward rectifying potassium channel Kir 2.1.

Malignant hyperthermia (MH)

This dramatic and often fatal condition was first described in 1960 by Denborough and Lovell in an Australian family in which there had been 10 deaths after anaesthesia. It is now a well recognized complication of anaesthesia and an attack can be precipitated by almost any anaesthetic agent, but halogenated hydrocarbons, such as halothane, and succinylcholine are the ones most frequently involved (Hogan 1998). It is characterized by a rapid and sustained rise in temperature during general anaesthesia (often as rapid as 1°C every 5 minutes and going up to 43°C or higher), accompanied by generalized muscle rigidity, tachycardia, tachypnoea and cyanosis. There is also a severe respiratory and metabolic acidosis. Extensive muscle necrosis follows, with subsequent myoglobinuria and renal shutdown. The serum creatine kinase is grossly elevated (up to 50.000 IU/L or more), as is the serum potassium (McLennan 1992).

The condition is inherited as an autosomal dominant trait and family members are at risk if a patient has a reaction to anaesthesia. Identifying those at risk can be difficult, even in those known to carry the genetic defect, although some tests are available (see below). The reaction of individuals with the genetic trait is variable, and a reaction may not occur at each exposure.

Serum CK and an abnormal EMG occur in some relatives at risk but normal findings do not exclude the risk of MH. The *in vitro* contracture test was developed to identify those at risk but this requires a large fresh muscle biopsy. It is based on measuring the muscle tension of the sample when exposed to halothane and caffeine. Although the test can identify most susceptible cases, the results can be equivocal (Ording et al 1997).

Muscle pathology

The histological changes in the muscle, both at light and electron microscopic level, are non-specific. Harriman (1988) reviewed the histological changes in a series of 200 patients investigated for MH, both by *in vitro* testing of muscle strips as well as by light and electron microscopy of motor point biopsies. He compared biopsies from 'susceptible' patients (80) with a positive *in vitro* test, with those in whom the *in vitro* test was negative (120) and were considered 'controls'. In the biopsies from 35 of the 80 malignant hyperthermia-susceptible group there were myopathic changes; the remainder were considered normal. Histological changes were also found in 61 of the 120 'control' biopsies. Fourteen of these control patients had actually suffered a malignant hyperpyrexia episode under anaesthesia, although results from the *in vitro* contraction test were interpreted as normal. This highlights the unreliability of the *in vitro* contracture test, although improvements to the technique have been made since these studies.

The presence of myopathic changes in the biopsies from MH-susceptible patients does not necessarily relate to a previous episode of MH following anaesthesia, and, conversely, patients who have previously had a reaction to anaesthesia can still have a normal biopsy. Muscle biopsies taken immediately after an episode of MH show the expected changes of rhabdomyolysis (fibre destruction and regeneration), whereas biopsies taken before or some months following an episode may show only minor non-specific changes, such as scattered smaller fibres and fibres with central nuclei. Thus, the routine evaluation of muscle biopsy is not necessarily of value in diagnosing the disorder or in predicting the potential susceptibility to MH.

Molecular genetics

Several chromosome loci have been linked to MH susceptibility (Loke and MacLennan 1998, Jurkat-Rott et al 2000) and two genes identified, *RYR1* and *CACNA1S* on chromosome 19q13.1 and 1q32, respectively. The *RYR1* gene codes for the calcium release channel, the ryanodine receptor, and was identified as a candidate following studies of the 'porcine stress syndrome', an animal model for MH (Mitchell and Heffron 1982, Fujii et al 1991). Mutations in humans were subsequently identified (Quane et al 1993). The same gene is also responsible for central core disease (see Ch. 15 and below) and, although the association of MH in central core disease is not clear, all patients with central core disease are considered at risk for MH. The *RYR1* gene is large with 106 exons, 2 of which are alternatively spliced to produce two isoforms of proteins. Four subunits of *RyR1* protein assemble to form the Ca^{2+} release channel in the junctional cisternae of the SR. The C-terminal domain of the protein is transmembrane whilst the large cytoplasmic domain interacts with sequences in the L-type voltage dependent Ca^{2+} channel, the dihydropyridine receptor. Although mutations in the *RYR1* gene are known to occur across the gene, many of them are clustered in three regions: (i) exons 2–18, (ii) exons 39–46, and (iii) exons 100–104.

Mutations associated with central core disease are often, but not exclusively, in the C-terminal exons, whilst those associated with MH are often in the cytoplasmic domain (Tilgen et al 2001, Monnier et al 2001).

The dihydropyridine receptor, the voltage-dependent L-type calcium channel of the T tubule, is composed of various subunits encoded by different genes. The α1-subunit is encoded by the *CACNA1S* gene and transmembrane domains of the protein form both the voltage sensor of the dihydropyridine receptor and the Ca^{2+} channel pore. Sequences in the cytoplasmic domain interact with the ryanodine receptor and mutations in this domain are associated with MH. Mutations in the same region also give rise to hyopkalaemic periodic paralysis (see above).

Linkage to chromosome 17q in several MH-susceptible families makes the sodium channel gene *SCN4A* a possible candidate for MH (Levitt et al 1992).

Association of malignant hyperthermia with other disorders

Denborough et al (1973) drew attention to a possible link between malignant hyperpyrexia and central core disease after discovering the presence of cores in more than 50% of the type 1 fibres of a patient with malignant hyperpyrexia. There was, however, no type 1 predominance in the biopsy, a feature often present in central core disease (see Ch. 15). It was not clear whether the presence of cores in the fibres merely reflected one of the various relatively non-specific changes found in muscle in MH or whether patients with the dominantly inherited central core disease are more susceptible to malignant hyperpyrexia. A child subsequently documented by Eng et al (1978) seemed to have had a genuine association of both disorders, and this has been reinforced by the molecular genetic revelations (see below). Additional families have also been reported in which presentation of both MH susceptibility and central core disease occur (Romero et al 1993).

In 1973 the syndrome now commonly known as King–Denborough's syndrome was described (King and Denborough 1973a,b). This syndrome is characterized by the association of a slowly progressive myopathy in young boys with short stature, pectus carinatum, cryptorchidism, kyphoscoliosis and distinctive facial features, with known susceptibility to MH. Elevation of serum CK has been noted in a large proportion of patients with King–Denborough syndrome, though this finding is not invariable. It is still unclear whether the association of MH with the King–Denborough syndrome is coincidental or is part of a multiple congenital anomalies syndrome characterized by a primary myopathy with secondary deformities. The syndrome appears to be sporadic rather than familial, though variability of associated clinical findings may result in underdiagnosis of the syndrome. All patients with known King–Denborough syndrome should be treated as MH susceptible, and evaluation of other family members is recommended.

Patients with Duchenne and Becker muscular dystrophy are also at risk of a reaction to anaesthetics and sudden cardiac arrest. Post-anaesthetic skeletal muscle breakdown has also been reported. Published reports of MH-like episodes in patients with Duchenne muscular dystrophy may over-emphasize the risk of this association, as rhabdomyolysis and cardiac abnormalities could be ascribed to the underlying muscle disorder rather than a hypermetabolic response. However, it is prudent to treat all patients with Duchenne muscular dystrophy as possibly MH susceptible and to avoid triggering anaesthetics.

Bush and Dubowitz (1991) documented a case of cardiac arrest during anaesthesia in a 7-year-old boy with a mild Becker muscular dystrophy and a deletion of exons 3–7 in the gene. They reviewed the differences between the delayed onset of bradycardia and cardiac arrest, usually without hyperthermia, occurring in these Duchenne/Becker cases, and the classical MH reaction.

There have been a large number of reports in the literature suggesting the association of other neuromuscular diseases with MH-like clinical findings or positive *in vitro* contracture testing (Wedel 1992, Kingler et al 2005). These include myoadenylate deaminase deficiency, Schwartz–Jampel syndrome, the Fukuyama type of congenital muscular dystrophy, limb-girdle dystrophy, facioscapulo-humeral dystrophy, periodic paralysis, myotonia congenita, mitochondrial myopathy and minimal change myopathy. It has also been suggested that there may be an association with sudden infant death (Denborough et al 1982). It is difficult to know whether the occurrence in these situations is mere chance or whether in some disorders there is an inter-relationship.

Some cases of so-called 'hyperCKaemia' with unexplained high serum CK on screening, who do not turn out to be Becker muscular dystrophy or other forms of muscular dystrophy, may possibly be latent cases of malignant hyper-thermia (Wedel 1992).

Many of the signs and symptoms of heatstroke are similar to those seen in MH, including muscle damage, which can result in rhabdomyolysis. Case reports of heat- and exercise-induced hyperthermia and muscle breakdown often bear striking resemblance to intraoperative fulminant MH episodes (Denborough et al 1984). Investigators have also described heat- and exercise-induced, mild MH-like episodes in individuals who are known to be MH susceptible, the symptoms of which respond to oral doses of dantrolene (Gronert et al 1980).

Myoglobinuria/rhabdomyolysis

The appearance of myoglobin in the urine reflects an acute necrosis of muscle, with severe damage and increased permeability of the muscle fibre membrane. In addition to MH, myoglobinuria may be a feature of metabolic disorders such as the glycogenoses or CPT deficiency (see Chs 17 and 18), inflammatory myopathies (see Ch. 22), and of toxic myopathies (see Ch. 23). Being a relatively small protein molecule (molecular mass 17,000 daltons), myoglobin has a low renal threshold and is readily cleared by the kidney. Renal shutdown can occur in severe cases. In metabolic disorders there is often a history of preceding muscle cramps and the muscles involved are frequently contracted and painful as well as firm and tender to palpation. There may also be localized oedema. Myoglobinuria will usually occur within 24 hours of the acute episode. Large quantities of myoglobin produce mahogany-coloured urine, resembling vinegar or Coca-Cola.

There is an associated leak of enzymes from the damaged muscle, with grossly elevated serum CK levels. Other constituents such as glycogen, potassium and creatine will also be released. The associated hyperkalaemia may produce life-threatening cardiac arrhythmia.

Other disturbances in calcium ions

Calcium concentrations required for contraction are regulated by ion channels of the SR and T tubules, the ryanodine and dihydropyridine receptors. The calcium released must then be rapidly removed to prevent the deleterious effects of high calcium concentrations. This removal is achieved by the sarco(endo) plasmic ATPases (SERCAs), by the plasma membrane calcium ATPases and mitochondria. These are calcium pumps rather than multimeric ion channels.

The *ATP2A1* gene on chromosome 16p21.1p12.2 encodes SERCA1 which is confined to fast (type 2) fibres (see Ch. 6). Mutations throughout the gene are responsible for Brody's disease (Odermatt et al 1998), a recessive disorder characterized by painless cramps and impairment in muscle relaxation (Brody 1969). Muscle contraction is normal but the relaxation phase becomes increasingly slow during exercise. An absence of SERCA1 from fast fibres can be detected with immunohistochemistry in some patients with an *ATP2A1* mutation. Thus the presence of SERCA1 does not exclude Brody's disease. Patients with some features in common with Brody's disease, but with no mutations in the *ATP2A1* gene, are described as having Brody's syndrome. Inheritance of this can be dominant or recessive and various candidate genes have been excluded, including the *ATP2A2* gene, encoding SERCA 2 in slow fibres.

CHAPTER 21

Myasthenic syndromes

There have been major advances in the understanding of the underlying causes of the various myasthenic syndromes, all of which involve abnormalities related to the neuromuscular junction (Fig. 21.1). Their characteristic feature is muscle fatigue. Myasthenia gravis is an acquired autoimmune disorder caused by antibodies to the acetylcholine receptors, or to a tyrosine kinase receptor, muscle specific kinase (MuSK), both of which are on the post-synaptic membrane of the neuromuscular junction. Most congenital forms of myasthenia are caused by mutations in genes encoding various key pre- or post-synaptic players in neuromuscular transmission (Fig. 21.1; Table 21.1). In addition, neonates of mothers with autoantibodies may show transient myasthenia (see below). Antibodies to voltage-gated calcium channels on the pre-synaptic membrane cause Lambert–Eaton syndrome, and neuromyotonia results from antibodies to a pre-synaptic voltage-gated potassium channel (not discussed in this chapter).

Myasthenia is usually suspected on clinical history, and abnormal fatigability may be demonstrated by the inability to sustain a particular movement such as upward gaze, or speech, or holding out the arms, in addition to characteristic features such as the myasthenic snarl. Confirmation is usually provided by pharmacological tests such as the response to acetylcholinesterase inhibitor, either intravenous edrophonium, tensilon, or a trial of oral pyridostigmine, by electrophysiological studies, such as the response decrement of the motor action potential to repetitive stimulation of a nerve, or by the presence of 'jitter' on single fibre electromyography, or by the finding of serum antibodies to acetylcholine receptors or MuSK. Routine muscle biopsy usually has very little diagnostic role to play, although pathological features may be present, and specialized studies of the nerve terminals and the neuromuscular junction have contributed substantially to our understanding of the pathophysiology.

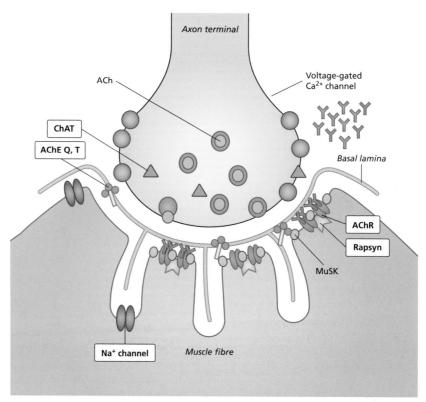

FIG. 21.1 *Diagram of the neuromuscular junction showing the defects that are associated with various myasthenic syndromes. The different coloured Y symbols represent autoantibodies to AChR and MuSK, responsible for myasthenia gravis, and to the voltage-gated calcium channel responsible for Lambert–Eaton syndrome (After Hantai et al 2004). ACh, acetylcholine; ChAT, choline acetyltransferase; AChE Q, T, the collagen Q tail attached to T globular subunits of acetylcholinesterase; AChR, acetylcholine receptor; MuSK, muscle specific kinase.*

Myasthenia gravis

This autoimmune disorder is caused by circulating antibodies to acetylcholine receptors (AChR) or to MuSK, and has a higher prevalence in females than males (6 : 4). The majority of cases are due to antibodies to AChR and most of those previously described as 'seronegative' have antibodies to MuSK (Palace et al 2001). In addition to antibodies to AChR, antibodies to various muscle proteins also occur, including myosin, actin, α-actinin, titin, filamin, vinculin, tropomyosin and the ryanodine receptor (Engel and Hohlfeld 2004).

A significant proportion of cases with AChR autoantibodies have a thymoma, and thymectomy, immunosuppression and plasma exchange are the main therapeutic approaches. The muscle weakness and fatigability are generalized, with weakness of the ocular muscles and ptosis being the most common presenting

TABLE 21.1 *Congenital myasthenic syndromes and known gene defects*

Location of defect	Protein	Gene	Locus	Inheritance
Pre-synaptic (7%)*				
Defects in ACh resynthesis	ChAT	*CHAT*	10q11.2	AR
Paucity in synaptic vesicles		?		
Lambert–Eaton-like congenital myasthenia		?		
Synaptic (14%)				
Endplate AChE deficiency	Collagen tail of AChE	*COLQ*	3p24.2	AR
Post-synaptic (79%)				
Fast channel syndromes	ACh receptor α subunit	*CHRNA1*	2q24-q32	AR
	ACh receptor δ subunit	*CHRND*	2q33-q34	AR
	ACh receptor ε subunit	*CHRNE*	17p13	AR
Slow channel syndromes	ACh receptor α subunit	*CHRNA1*	2q24-q32	AD
	ACh receptor β subunit	*CHRNB1*	17p11-p12	AD
	ACh receptor δ subunit	*CHRND*	2q33-q34	AD
	ACh receptor ε subunit	*CHRNE*	17p13	AD, AR
ACh deficiency	ACh receptor β subunit	*CHRNB1*	17p11-p12	AR
	ACh receptor δ subunit	*CHRND*	2q33-q34	AR
	ACh receptor ε subunit	*CHRNE*	17p13	AR
Abnormalities in clustering of ACh receptors	Rapsyn MuSK	*RASPN* *MUSK*	11p11 9q31.3–q32	AR AR
Anomaly of muscle sodium channel	Sodium channel α-subunit	*SCN4A*	17q23	AR

*Prevalence figures from Engel et al 2003; ACh, acetylcholine; AChE, acetylcholinesterase; AD, autosomal dominant; AR, autosomal recessive; ChAT, choline acetyltransferase.

symptoms. Ocular involvement occurs in the majority of cases eventually, and in a proportion of patients the weakness remains isolated to the ocular muscles and eyelids. The weakness characteristically worsens with sustained exertion and during the course of the day. Spontaneous remissions of variable length can occur.

The clinical features associated with antibodies to MuSK are less well defined than those associated with antibodies to AChR but there is prominent bulbar involvement, respiratory problems and relative sparing of the limb muscles.

There is a high incidence of miscarriages in females with myasthenia gravis. Transient neonatal myasthenia affects about one in seven infants born to myasthenic mothers and may produce life-threatening weakness requiring urgent treatment. The infant is usually affected at birth but the symptoms may sometimes be delayed for some days. The infant is usually floppy, with general hypotonia and weakness, and there may be associated swallowing and breathing problems. The condition is self-limiting with gradual recovery, usually within 2–4 weeks.

Pathology

Few, if any, abnormalities are seen in muscle biopsies, except at the neuromuscular junction. If present, the changes may be focal and are usually non-specific. They include atrophy of type 2 fibres, and sometimes atrophy of type 1 fibres, which may be accompanied by the presence of small dark angulated fibres with the oxidative enzymes, suggestive of denervation. Although lymphorrhages have been reported in myasthenia gravis, they are not a consistent feature.

The pioneering studies of AG Engel have made a major contribution to our understanding of the pathogenesis of myasthenia gravis (Engel et al 1976, 1977). The folds of the junction are reduced, or absent, and debris from them accumulates between the nerve and the muscle membrane. Complement (C3, C9 and the membrane attack complex) and immune complexes can be demonstrated on the post-synaptic membrane and binding of the autoantibodies in the serum from affected patients to neuromuscular junctions can be demonstrated.

Neuromuscular junctions are only occasionally present in a muscle biopsy, unless a motor point sample is specifically taken. In practice, the diagnosis of myasthenia is usually made without the need for a muscle biopsy, from clinical and electrophysiological examinations, and a response to acetylcholinesterase inhibitors and AChR and MuSK antibody estimation.

Pathogenesis

The nerve impulse results in the release of acetylcholine which binds to its receptor on the peak of the post-synaptic folds of the muscle fibre, which induces depolarization of the muscle membrane, the release of calcium, and results in an action potential. The AChRs in skeletal muscle are formed from five homologous subunits organized round a central ion channel, two α1, a β1, the ε or γ, and the δ subunits. In fetal muscle the γ subunit is present and is replaced by 34 weeks' gestation by the ε subunit. Denervated muscle reverts to the fetal type, with the γ subunit. In myasthenia gravis the anti-AChR antibodies bind mainly to one site on an extracellular region of the α1 subunit. This is referred to as the main immunogenic region and is distinct from the cholinergic binding site. The bound antibodies cross link AChRs, as well as inducing receptor loss due to complement mediated lysis. The net result is a reduction in the number of functional AChRs and disruption of the structure of the post-synaptic membrane. Weakness and fatigue become obvious when a threshold number of affected receptors is exceeded.

Sera from patients with myasthenia gravis often also react with fetal muscle, suggesting that the γ subunit of AChR is also involved. It has been suggested, but not substantiated, that the involvement of the extraocular muscles might relate to the presence of this subunit in these muscles. Ocular muscles express several proteins found in fetal muscle. Rare patients, who show no symptoms of myasthenia gravis, have been identified in whom antibodies to the γ subunit cross the placenta and severely affect the fetus, causing death or arthrogryposis multiplex congenita (Riemersma et al 1996).

Autoantibodies to MuSK affect the clustering of AChRs. The activation of MuSK by agrin causes a cascade of signalling events through rapsyn, leading to clustering of AChR (Sanes and Litchman 2001). It has been proposed that MuSK is also important in the clustering of acetylcholinesterase by the formation of a complex with perlecan and the collagen Q tail of acetylcholinesterase (Cartaud et al 2004).

Lambert-Eaton syndrome

The characteristic features of Lambert–Eaton myasthenic syndrome are weakness and fatigability, principally of the limb muscles. Bulbar and ocular muscles are usually spared. Many patients also present with varying degrees of autonomic dysfunction and there is strong association with lung neoplasms. It can be distinguished from myasthenia gravis by the augmentation in strength following voluntary contraction, due to pre-synaptic facilitation, and by depressed tendon reflexes. It results from immunoglobulin G (IgG) antibodies to voltage-gated calcium channels which reduce their number and impair the calcium-dependent release of acetylcholine (Lang and Vincent 2002).

Pathology

Pathological studies of muscle biopsies show only mild non-specific changes, such as a reduction of type 1 fibres and a progressive type 2 fibre predominance

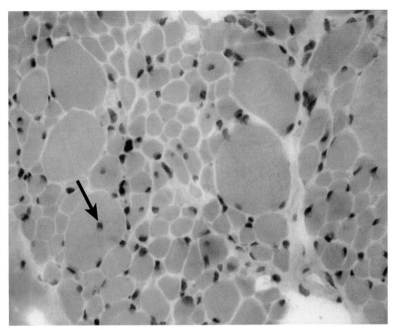

FIG. 21.2 *Biopsy from the quadriceps of a 16-month-old boy with congenital myasthenia (molecularly unresolved) showing many atrophic fibres and hypertrophic fibres. Note also the occasional central nucleus (arrow). Fibre diameter range 5–50 μm (H&E).*

(Squier et al 1991). Freeze fracture electron microscopy of the pre-synaptic membrane shows a reduction in the number of active zone particles, which are believed to represent the voltage-gated calcium channels, and abnormalities in their distribution (Fukunaga et al 1982).

Congenital myasthenic syndromes

The congenital myasthenic syndromes are a heterogeneous group of inherited disorders caused by mutations in the genes encoding various proteins involved in neuromuscular transmission (Fig. 21.1; Engel et al 2003, Hantai et al 2004). Classification of these disorders is based on the location of the defective protein, pre-synaptic, the synapse basal lamina, or post-synaptic (Table 21.1). As with autoimmune myasthenia, diagnosis is based on family history, careful clinical examination, particularly with regard to observing the weakness and fatigability, electrophysiology and the response to acetylcholinesterase inhibitors (edrophonium; Tensilon test). A negative response to acetylcholinesterase inhibitors does not exclude a diagnosis of congenital myasthenia. A particular feature of cases with a deficiency of choline acetyltransferase (ChAT) is sudden episodes of severe dyspnoea and bulbar and respiratory muscle weakness.

area 1　　　　　　　　　　area 2

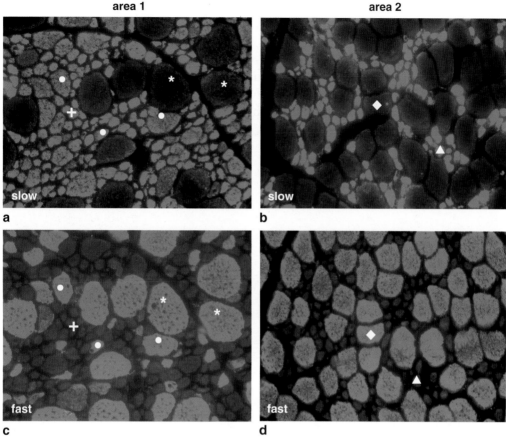

FIG. 21.3 *Serial sections from two areas of the same biopsy as shown in Fig. 21.2 immunolabelled with antibodies to (a), (b) slow and (c), (d) fast myosin. Area 1 shows many atrophic fibres (+) that mainly contain slow myosin, and hypertrophic fibres with fast myosin (*). Some fibres of varying size show both fast and slow myosin (•). Area 2 shows atrophic fibres with only slow myosin (▲) and only fast myosin (♦) in fibres of normal size. Fibre diameter range (a), (c) 5–50 μm; (b), (d) 3–30 μm.*

Pathology

Most of the recorded morphological features relate to abnormalities of the neuro-muscular junction, which are not routinely available for study in muscle biopsies. The features observed include small synaptic vesicles (choline acetyltransferase deficiency), small endplates with an absence of acetylcholinesterase (acetylcho-linesterase deficiency), and destruction of the junctional folds (slow-channel syndromes). In some congenital myasthenias there are no morphological changes in the endplate.

Routine histological and histochemical studies of muscle biopsies in the slow-channel syndrome show variation in fibre size, endomysial fibrosis, small groups of atrophic fibres of both fibre type, type 1 predominance and tubular aggregates (Engel 2004).

We have recently observed marked pathology in the muscle biopsy of a case of congenital myasthenia (currently not molecularly resolved). There was pronounced atrophy of type 1 fibres throughout the sample, accompanied by hypertrophy of type 2 fibres in some areas. Some areas showed a marked predominance of atrophy of type 1 fibres with slow myosin and there was a striking variation between fascicles (Figs 21.2 and 21.3). This pattern had some resemblance to that seen in congenital myopathies (see Ch. 15) but the clinical examination and response to acetylcholinesterase inhibitors confirmed the diagnosis. Type 1 fibre predominance and disproportion have been noted in other cases of congenital myasthenia (Gurnett et al 2004).

CHAPTER 22

Inflammatory myopathies

There is a large and heterogeneous group of acquired disorders that have been grouped together collectively as inflammatory myopathies. They include polymyositis, adult and juvenile dermatomyositis and inclusion body myositis, as well as those of bacterial, parasitic, viral or toxic origin (see Ch. 23). Although hypotheses for pathogenesis have been proposed, the underlying causes are not clear, and some disorders approximate more closely to the connective tissue group of disorders.

The histological features which these conditions have in common are the presence of inflammatory cell infiltrates together with various degenerative changes in the muscle fibres. In addition, major histocompatibilty class I antigens (MHC-I) can be detected by immunohistochemistry on the sarcolemma of muscle fibres, irrespective of the presence of inflammatory cells. Detection of CD8+ T lymphocyte cells is now also recognized as an important diagnostic criterion (see below; Dalakas and Hohlfeld 2003, Dalakas 2004). From a diagnostic point of view, it is important to note that infiltrates of inflammatory cells, particularly round cells, are fairly commonly seen in the muscular dystrophies, particularly in relation to necrotic fibres, and conversely the absence of any inflammatory infiltrates in a biopsy does not exclude an inflammatory myopathy, as for example in acute dermatomyositis in childhood. The presence of MHC-I can also occur in some muscular dystrophies, such as Duchenne and limb-girdle muscular dystrophy 2B, caused by mutations in the gene encoding dysferlin, all which may show infiltration of inflammatory cells. Although cases of facioscapulohumeral muscular dystrophy may also show inflammatory cells, sarcolemmal MHC-I is not usually seen (see Ch. 14). The distinction between these disorders relies on the clinical presentation.

Recognizing the form of inflammatory myopathy is important as many respond well to drug therapy. Therapy regimes, however, are variable and although the use of corticosteroids is common and beneficial in a number of situations, side-effects have to be monitored and not all cases are responsive. For example, patients with inclusion body myositis frequently show no response to corticosteroids.

Polymyositis and dermatomyositis

Polymyositis may present as an isolated disorder, with the clinical signs and symptoms restricted to the muscle, or it may have associated skin manifestations (dermatomyositis). Both polymyositis and dermatomyositis may also occur in association with other disorders, the commonest being neoplasms and collagen disorders, such as systemic lupus erythematosus, periarteritis nodosa and rheumatoid arthritis. Polymyositis is rare in children and the childhood form of dermatomyositis (juvenile dermatomyositis) is a separate condition. It is not associated with malignancy and responds much better than the adult forms to corticosteroid and immunosuppressive therapy (see below).

For many years the papers of Bohan and Peter (1975a,b) provided the basis and clinical criteria for the classification of polymyositis and dermatomyositis. With increasing knowledge these have been modified (Dalakas and Hohlfeld 2003). The main categories, however, remain:

- isolated polymyositis;
- isolated dermatomyositis;
- myositis associated with malignancy;
- juvenile dermatomyositis; and
- polymyositis or dermatomyositis associated with features of connective tissue disorders (overlap syndromes).

Clinical features

The onset of polymyositis or dermatomyositis in adults is often associated with aching pains in the shoulders or hips or other sites, accompanied by some degree of weakness. The weakness may be proximal and symmetrical, as in limb-girdle dystrophy, or may be asymmetrical and have varying distribution. The weakness does not show the selectivity seen in the muscular dystrophies. It may be rapidly progressive, and may result in severe weakness, with the patient being confined to bed, or be relatively mild and chronic. There may be accompanying tenderness and swelling of muscle, but some 30–40% of patients may have no muscle pain, even in the presence of quite severe inflammatory disease.

In the most acute cases there may be profound generalized weakness developing over a few days, together with marked necrosis of muscle and associated gross elevation of creatine kinase and other serum enzymes. There may also be myoglobinuria which may be severe enough to cause renal failure. Rhabdomyolysis and myoglobinuria, however, are relatively rare in dermatomyositis. The majority of cases tend to follow a more insidious subacute or chronic course.

The association with malignancy has been known for some time (Bohan and Peter 1975a,b) with a link to dermatomyositis rather than polymyositis (Sigurgeirsson et al 1992, Hill et al 2001). The tumour and myopathy usually present within a short time of each other, but in occasional cases the myopathy may precede diagnosis of the tumour by months or even years.

Dysphagia may also be associated with the illness, and this can become severe enough to necessitate feeding by nasogastric tube. Some patients may also have respiratory symptoms, either from intercostal or bulbar weakness, or rarely because of direct involvement of the lung parenchyma.

In dermatomyositis, there are the additional changes in the skin. Frequently, there is a heliotrope or violaceous rash, particularly over the eyes and malar regions of the face. There is an erythema around the nail beds and over the knees and elbows. In severe cases, the skin changes become generalized and the entire skin becomes tight, shiny and reddened. In intractable cases, the development of ulcers over the pressure points may be a severe problem. In juvenile cases calcinosis is a particular feature (see below).

Serum CK activity is frequently, but not invariably, elevated. A normal level does not exclude a diagnosis of myositis. Electromyography shows a fairly characteristic pattern, with a combination of spontaneous fibrillation potentials similar to those seen in denervation, and polyphasic, short duration potentials on voluntary contraction as in myopathies.

Other laboratory investigations that may be helpful are a raised erythrocyte sedimentation rate (ESR), detection of serum autoantibodies and measurement of serum or urinary compounds such as myoglobin, hyaluronate, manganese superoxide dismutase, neopterin and quinolinic acid. The ESR is raised in only a proportion of cases, however, and there is no correlation with weakness. Similarly, serum autoantibodies are not detected in all cases. Amongst the ones most often assessed are antinuclear antibodies, anti-RNA antibodies such as Jo-1, and anti-signal recognition particle antibodies (Miller 1993).

Magnetic resonance imaging of muscle shows increased signal in relation to oedema and inflammatory changes in subcutaneous fat (Lovitt et al 2004). The changes are not specific, however, but MRI may be useful for selecting the site of muscle biopsy or monitoring therapy.

There is considerable evidence that certain haplotypes are associated with certain myositic conditions. For example in Caucasians, juvenile dermatomyositis and polymyositis are associated with HLA-B8, both of which are associated with HLA-DR3. Juvenile dermatomyositis is also associated with HLA-DQA1 allele DQA1*0501. Studies of other ethnic groups suggest an association of HLA-B7 and HLA-DRw6 in polymyositis.

The majority of cases respond to steroid therapy, although recovery may at times be slow and incomplete. Azathioprine, cyclophosphamide, cyclosporin and methotrexate are also used in the treatment of these conditions. It can be extremely difficult in a case of chronic polymyositis, with apparent deterioration or lack of response to 'adequate' or often very high doses of steroids, to decide whether the persistent weakness is a reflection of a superadded steroid myopathy or continuing activity of the underlying polymyositis itself. Certainly in the childhood groups, many of the problems in chronic cases seem to reflect complications of the drug treatment, particularly over treatment with too high dosage of corticosteroids, or lack of supportive and rehabilitative care, rather than the underlying disease which has already become quiescent.

The childhood form of dermatomyositis, *juvenile dermatomyositis,* differs from the adult form in a number of respects. It is always an 'idiopathic' condition and is not associated with malignancy. Although muscle weakness is an invariable accompaniment of the condition, its degree may be extremely variable and, in some early cases, readily missed. Children with dermatomyositis usually have associated general symptoms, such as malaise, listlessness and lethargy, which may be the presenting feature. As there are no other neuromuscular disorders which present with these general symptoms in addition to weakness, it is a useful rule of thumb in paediatric practice that 'misery + muscle weakness = dermatomyositis' until proved otherwise.

The associated skin manifestation may at times be florid and readily apparent over the face or other sites, but at times may be minimal and no more than a violaceous discolouration of the eyelids, or erythema or telangiectasia over the knuckles, malleoli of the ankle or other pressure points (Dubowitz 1995).

Calcinosis is another complication peculiar to childhood dermatomyositis and occurs particularly in the more chronic cases. The calcium is deposited in the subcutaneous tissue and in the supportive connective tissue within the muscle but not in the muscle fibres themselves. It may be extensive and not necessarily related to the degree of weakness.

Pathology

Although the underlying pathogenesis of polymyositis and dermatomyositis is different, which influences some of the pathological features, they have several features in common; in particular, muscle fibre necrosis and the presence of inflammatory cells. Some biopsies, however, may show very little change and no inflammation, and immunohistochemistry is then particularly useful.

Abnormalities of fibre size are often present but hypertrophy is less pronounced, or absent, compared with muscular dystrophies (Fig. 22.1). Small or large group atrophy, or fibre type grouping, are not seen. Internal nuclei are common, and vesicular nuclei are present in almost all biopsies, particularly in basophilic fibres, when present. Moth-eaten fibres or fibres with core-like areas are also frequent (see Fig. 22.3) and fibre splitting may occur but is not often a prominent feature of polymyositis.

Perifascicular atrophy is a particular feature of dermatomyositis that is not seen in polymyositis (Fig. 22.2). Histochemically these perifascicular fibres are of both types with staining for ATPase, but often show intense and aggregated NADH-TR activity (Fig. 22.3). Many of these small fibres express a number of proteins associated with immaturity (see below), and differentiating them from regenerating fibres is then difficult. Some may represent attempts at regeneration rather than being atrophic but the presence of heat shock proteins in these perifascicular fibres is consistent with a response to injury.

Necrosis and regeneration are common, and there is a characteristic vacuolar degeneration which can be extensive (Fig. 22.4). Some of these vacuolated, degenerate fibres may be unstained with most reactions and have been termed 'ghost

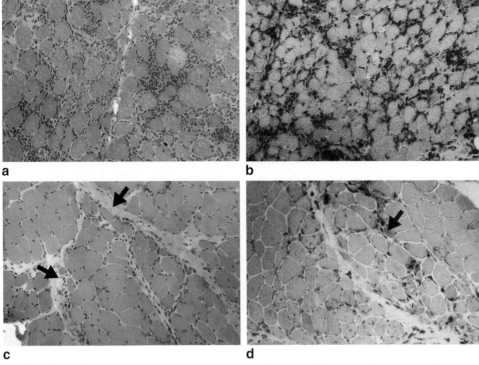

a   b

c   d

FIG. 22.1 (a and b) *Biopsy from the quadriceps of a 59-year-old female with polymyositis showing variation in fibre size and abundant endomysial inflammatory cells (a) (H&E) which are intensely stained with acid phosphatase (b).* **(c and d)** *Quadriceps biopsy from a male aged 43 years with dermatomyositis showing perifascicular atrophy (black arrows) but very few inflammatory cells (c) (H&E) and high internal acid phosphatase activity in several fibres in the perifascicular region (d) (blue arrow).*

fibres'. Macrophages and T cells invade the fibre after it becomes necrotic. The necrosis may be segmental and may involve single muscle fibres or clusters of fibres. In dermatomyositis areas of infarction with groups of pale-staining fibres may be seen. There is frequently a granular change, which is basophilic with haematoxylin and eosin stain and red on the trichrome. Basophilic regenerating fibres are also present and necrotic fibres may show a peripheral basophilic regenerative cuff (Fig. 22.5). These cuffs are rarely seen in the muscular dystrophies.

Inflammatory changes are the hallmark of polymyositis and dermatomyositis, but the extent is variable, and some biopsies show no inflammatory infiltration (Fig. 22.1). The inflammatory cells consist of lymphocytes, plasma cells and histiocytes and they occur in the perimysial and endomysial regions and are often perivascular (Fig. 22.6). Eosinophils are not a feature of polymyositis and dermatomyositis. The proportion and distribution of the various inflammatory cell types differs in polymyositis and dermatomyositis (see below). Acid phosphatase activity is associated with the inflammatory cells and is also increased in the muscle fibres (Fig. 22.1). Basophilic, regenerating fibres, however, also show high acid phosphatase activity (Neerunjun and Dubowitz 1977).

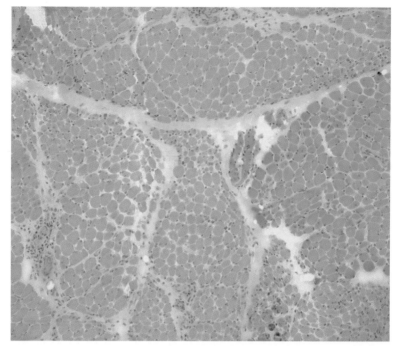

a

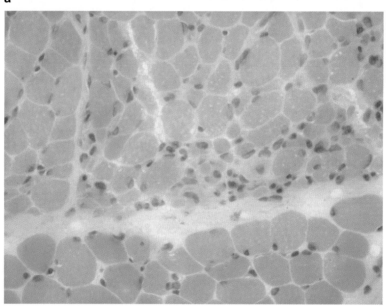

b

FIG. 22.2 *Quadriceps biopsy from a 5-year-old girl with juvenile dermatomyositis showing perifascicular atrophy in low power (a) and high power (b) views (H&E). Fibre diameter range 5–20 μm.*

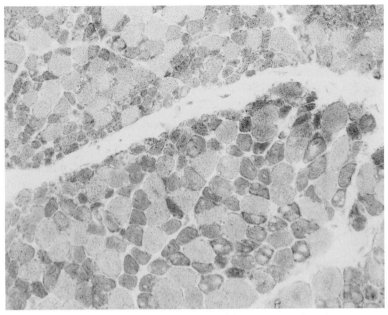

FIG. 22.3 *Same biopsy as in Fig. 22.2 stained for NADH-TR showing more intense activity in several of the perifascicular fibres and in vacuolated fibres.*

Fibrosis is frequently seen and there may be a loose oedematous separation of the muscle fibres with interspersed fibrous tissue (Fig. 22.4).

Blood vessels in dermatomyositis often have thickened walls (Fig. 22.6), the capillaries may be enlarged, and with electron microscopy endothelial cells show tubuloreticular inclusions (see Fig. 5.90). The number of capillaries is also reduced in dermatomyositis (see below).

Immunohistochemistry

The most important application of immunohistochemistry in the study of all inflammatory myopathies is the localization of MHC class I antigens and this has significantly increased the value of muscle biopsy in the assessment of inflammatory myopathies. In normal muscle MHC class I antigens can only be detected on the blood vessels but in all inflammatory myopathies there is appreciable expression on the sarcolemma and also internally in several fibres (Appleyard et al 1985, McDouall et al 1989; Fig. 22.7). In the majority of cases all fibres show sarcolemmal MHC-I but occasionally some areas may be normal (Fig. 22.7d). It is seen in the absence of cellular infiltrates and when the sample shows no, or minimal, pathology (Topaloglu et al 1996).

Sarcolemmal MHC-I is not specific to inflammatory myopathies and can also be seen in Duchenne and Becker muscular dystrophy and limb-girdle dystrophy 2B, with a defect in the gene for dysferlin (Karpati et al 1988, Fanin and Angelini

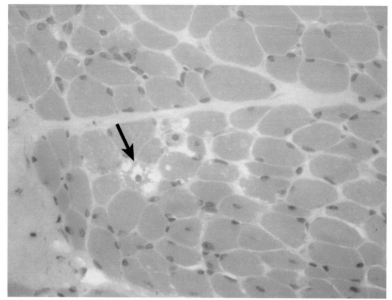

a

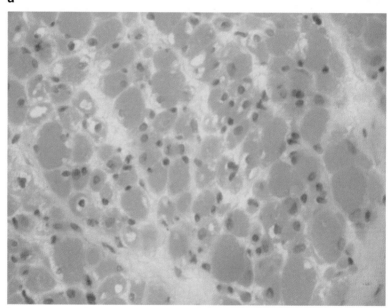

b

FIG. 22.4 *Two areas from the biopsy of the child with juvenile dermatomyositis shown in Figs 22.2 and 22.3 showing in (a) a focal area of vacuolated fibres (arrow) and in (b) several vacuolated fibres separated by oedematous connective tissue. Note also the frequent number of internal nuclei (H&E).*

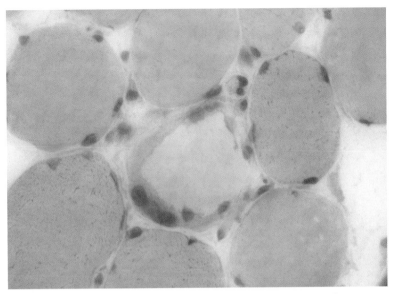

FIG. 22.5 *Biopsy from the quadriceps of a 63-year-old female with polymyositis showing a pale necrotic fibre surrounded by a basophilic rim of a regenerating myotube (H&E). Fibre diameter range 50–65-μm.*

2002, Confalonieri et al 2003). Some expression may also occasionally be seen in neonates and in a variety of undefined conditions, but the reason is unknown. Regenerating fibres in all disorders show sarcolemmal and internal labelling of MHC-I, and it is important to distinguish this normal phenomenon from the abnormal labelling on mature fibres by the use of a marker for immaturity, such as neonatal myosin.

As MHC-I is present on all blood vessels it can be used to assess the number of capillaries but this is more easily seen with markers such as the lectin *ulex europaeus* or laminin α5 as the capillaries are highlighted against the negative (ulex) or weak (laminin α5) labelling of the sarcolemma. In normal muscle there is a capillary adjacent to every fibre, although in normal neonatal muscle the capillary network is less developed and fewer capillaries are seen. In both adult and juvenile dermatomyositis there is a depletion of capillaries and this is an early feature that can be seen in the absence of other pathology (Fig. 22.8).

Blood vessels in adult and juvenile dermatomyositis also show deposits of immune complexes and the terminal component of the complement pathway, the membrane attack complex C5b-9 (MAC) (Fig. 22.9). Complement and immune complexes, immunoglobulin G (IgG) and immunoglobulin M (IgM), are also seen in necrotic fibres (Fig. 22.9b).

Immunolabelling of myosin isoforms reveals the pattern of different fibre types and there may be a predominance of fibres with slow myosin and co-expression of more than one isoform in several fibres (Fig. 22.10). In dermatomyositis the small fibres at the periphery of the fascicles often show neonatal myosin (Fig. 22.10). Some of this may represent attempts at regeneration but as

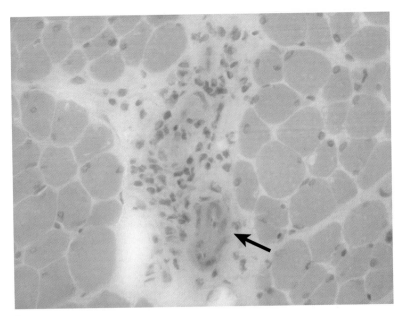

a

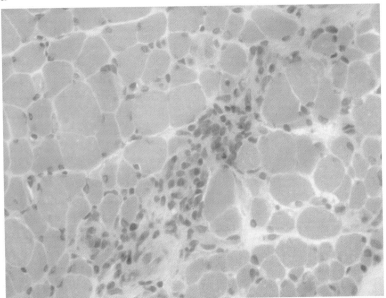

b

FIG. 22.6 *Two areas of the biopsy of the child with juvenile dermatomyositis shown in Figs 22.2, 22.3 and 22.4 showing in (a) an area of inflammatory cells in the perimysium by a blood vessel with a thickened wall (arrow) and in (b) a collection of endomysial inflammatory cells associated with early stages of muscle fibre regeneration (H&E).*

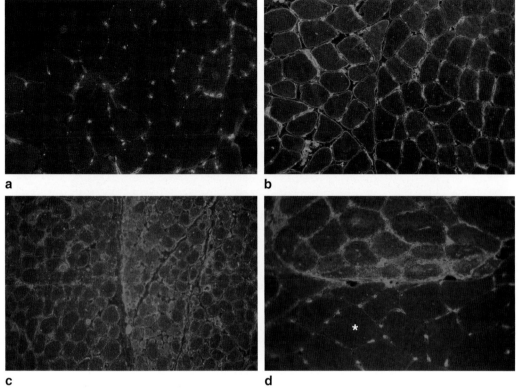

a   b

c   d

FIG. 22.7 *Immunolabelling of MHC class I antigens in (a) a control, showing labelling of the blood vessels only, in (b) a case of polymyositis, showing intense labelling of the sarcolemma of all fibres, in (c) a case of juvenile dermatomyositis, showing labelling of the sarcolemma of all fibres and internal labelling of several fibres particularly those in the perifascicular region, and in (d) an adult with dermatomyositis, showing normal labelling restricted to the blood vessels in one area (*) and abnormal sarcolemmal labelling in the adjacent area.*

neonatal myosin is not a specific marker for regeneration and they have also been shown to express proteins related to stress, as well as showing degenerative features, they are considered to be atrophic, damaged fibres.

The principal cell types in the infiltrate cells are T lymphocytes, B cells, dendritic cells and macrophages, which can be identified with specific antibodies to their surface molecules, the cluster of differentiation markers (CD markers). In polymyositis the infiltrate is predominately endomysial, with a high number of CD8[+] T lymphocytes. These are seen to surround and invade non-necrotic muscle fibres but this is not a feature of dermatomyositis. B cells, in contrast, are predominantly perivascular and are very rare in the endomysium in polymyositis. In dermatomyositis the cells are predominantly perivascular and perimysial, although some may be endomysial (see Fig. 22.6) and there is a higher proportion of B cells and CD4[+] cells, some of which are T cells, but many are dendritic cells (Greenberg et al 2005).

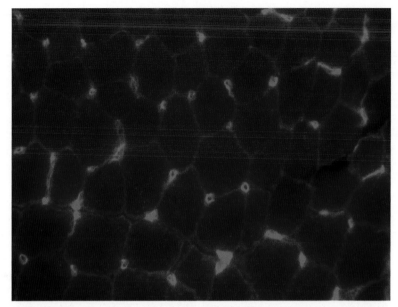

a

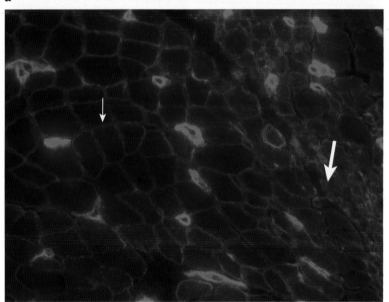

b

FIG. 22.8 *Two areas of a biopsy from the quadriceps of a 5-year-old child with juvenile dermatomyositis immunolabelled with antibodies to laminin α5 showing in (a) a normal distribution of capillaries round most fibres, the sarcolemma of which shows weak labelling, and in (b) areas where there has been loss of capillaries and not all fibres have a capillary adjacent to them (small arrow). Note also the absence of capillaries in the perifascicular region (large arrow).*

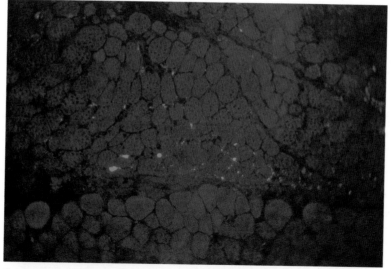

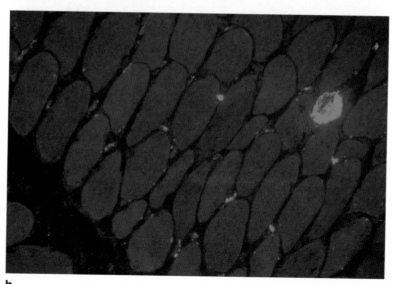

FIG. 22.9 *Immunolabelling of C9 of the membrane attack complex in biopsies from (a) a 30-year-old female with dermatomyositis and (b) a 45-year-old male with dermatomyositis showing complement on the capillaries, in both cases.*

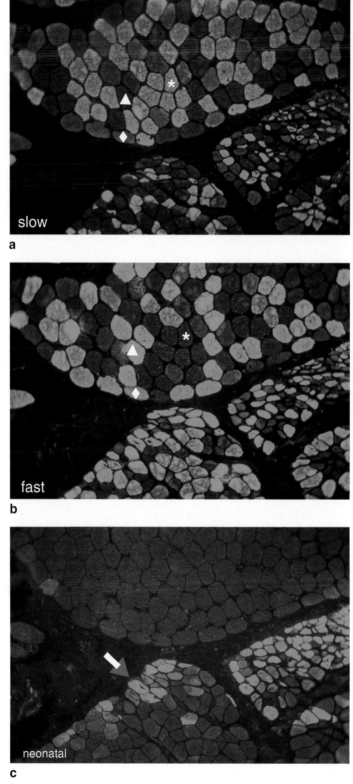

FIG. 22.10 *Serial sections of a biopsy from the quadriceps of a 3-year-old boy with juvenile dermatomyositis immunolabelled with antibodies to (a) slow myosin heavy chain, (b) fast myosin heavy chains and (c) neonatal myosin. Note that some fibres only show slow myosin (*), some only show fast myosin (▲) and some show intermediate intensity of slow myosin and co-express fast myosin (♦). Several fibres in the perifascicular area show neonatal myosin (arrow) and co-express fast and/or slow myosin.*

In summary, the muscle biopsy from patients with polymyositis or dermatomyositis may show unequivocal features with an inflammatory response and necrosis and a distinctive perifascicular atrophy in dermatomyositis. Frequently, however, the pathologist is faced with a sample with only mild non-specific changes and no pronounced cellular infiltrate. It is then that it is important to look for MHC-I expression and to look closely for any changes in blood vessels, in particular complement deposition and loss of capillaries. These features, in conjunction with the clinical features and laboratory data are often sufficient to arrive at a diagnosis and the detailed studies described above may not be necessary.

Pathogenesis

Polymyositis is believed to be T-cell mediated, whereas dermatomyositis is thought to be predominantly mediated by humoral factors (Dalakas 2004). In polymyositis evidence indicates that there is antigen-directed and MHC-I-restricted cytotoxicity, mediated by CD8[+] T cells. The T cells, which are mainly in the endomysium, cross the basal lamina of the muscle fibres and release a variety of substances that induce necrosis, such as perforin. In dermatomyositis there is activation of complement which leads to the deposition of the MAC on the capillaries, resulting in lysis of the endothelial cells and loss of capillaries. The resulting ischaemia leads to necrosis, infarcts and the characteristic perifascicular atrophy. It is still unclear what the initial trigger is in either disorder.

Inclusion body myositis

Sporadic inclusion body myositis (IBM) is one of the most common acquired disorders in patients over the age of 50 years and is more common in males than females. Although usually sporadic, a few familial cases have been reported. There are also hereditary disorders that share some of the same pathological features as IBM but lack the inflammatory component and have been termed hereditary inclusion body *myopathies*. The underlying gene defects in some of these inherited forms have been identified (see Ch. 17). IBM is distinguished from polymyositis or dermatomyositis by a more insidious onset, and there is usually a different pattern of weakness. In cases that lack the classical pathological features (see below), differentiating between IBM and polymyositis may be difficult. Re-evaluation of some cases thought to have polymyositis has sometimes later shown them to have IBM, with the presence of the typical pathological features in repeat biopsies. In contrast to polymyositis and dermatomyositis, IBM is usually unresponsive to corticosteroid therapy and this often alerts the clinician to the possibility of IBM.

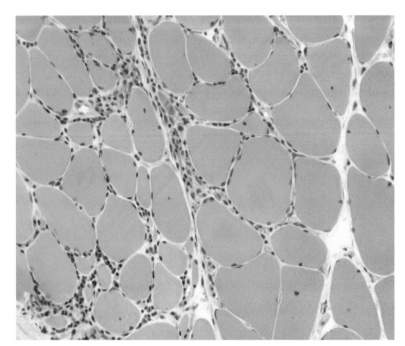

FIG. 22.11 *Biopsy from a 71-year-old male with inclusion body myositis showing pronounced variation in fibre size, some internal nuclei and a marked inflammatory response (H&E). Fibre diameter range 10–55 μm.*

Clinical features

Muscle weakness is proximal and distal, with prominent weakness and wasting of the quadriceps. Weakness of the wrist, finger flexor muscles and of ankle dorsiflexion are common features. The muscle involvement is often asymmetrical, and dysphagia is common. The rate of progression is slow but can lead to severe disability. Serum CK levels may be normal, or elevated up to 10 times the normal limit.

There is an association between IBM and other autoimmune disorders, and it is strongly associated with the MHC antigens HLA-DR3, DR52 and B8. There may also be an association with mutations in the gene encoding transthyretin, a protein known to sequester β-amyloid (Askanas and Engel 2003).

Pathology

Fibre sizes are variable, with both atrophy and hypertrophy (Fig. 22.11). There may be small angulated fibres scattered through the biopsy, or in clusters, but there is no perifascicular atrophy. There is often an increase in internal nuclei, and in endomysial connective tissue. Necrosis, with invasion of the fibre by phagocytes, and basophilic regenerating fibres are common. Cytoplasmic bodies, stained red with the Gomori trichrome stain, may also be seen and can be confirmed with electron microscopy.

The characteristic feature is fibres with vacuoles rimmed by basophilic granules which also stain red with the Gomori trichrome stain (Fig. 22.12). The number of fibres with rimmed vacuoles is variable. Similarly, the extent of the inflammatory response is variable. This is composed mainly of lymphocytes and macrophages. The predominant T cell type is CD8$^+$ which invades non-necrotic fibres. Enzyme histochemistry shows high acid phosphatase activity in some vacuoles, disruption of the myofibrillar pattern with core-like areas lacking NADH-TR activity, and a higher than expected number of fibres devoid of cytochrome oxidase, bearing in mind that the number of these fibres increases with age. Electron microscopy identifies structurally abnormal mitochondria, and deletions in mitochondrial DNA have been found in a high proportion of cases of IBM. The abnormal mitochondria correspond to ragged-red areas, additional to the rimmed vacuoles that are seen with the Gomori trichrome technique.

The inclusions in IBM are congophilic, which is best viewed with a fluorescence microscope fitted with an excitation filter suitable for rhodamine or Texas red (Fig. 22.13). The inclusions reflect the presence of β-amyloid, which can be demonstrated with antibodies (see below).

Electron microscopy reveals the presence of filamentous inclusions in the cytoplasm, nuclei or both. The filaments are 15–20 nm in diameter and may be arranged in parallel or haphazardly (see Fig. 5.50). Myelin-like whorls are also common, as are cytoplasmic bodies.

Immunohistochemistry

As with polymyositis and dermatomyositis, there is sarcolemmal labelling of MHC-I, irrespective of the presence of inflammatory cells. This may be a distinguishing feature from the hereditary myopathies with rimmed vacuoles but existing data on this is limited, and MHC-I is not specific to the myositic conditions.

A large number of proteins have been shown to be associated with the vacuoles. These include β-amyloid, β-amyloid precursor protein, ubiquitin, presenilin-1, apolipoprotein E, α-synuclein, prion protein, phosphorylated tau and survival motor neurone protein (SMN; Fig. 22.14; Oldfors and Fyhr 2001, Askanas and Engel 2001). Many of these are found in the brain of patients with Alzheimer's disease which has led to the idea that similar ageing mechanisms may be involved in both disorders. In particular, β-amyloid precursor may have a role in inducing a cascade of events leading to cell degeneration and misfolding of proteins (Askanas and Engel 2001, 2003).

Hereditary inclusion body myopathies

This is a heterogeneous group of disorders with progressive muscle weakness, and mutations in various genes have been shown to be associated with them. Many of them are of late onset, like IBM, but some congenital and childhood

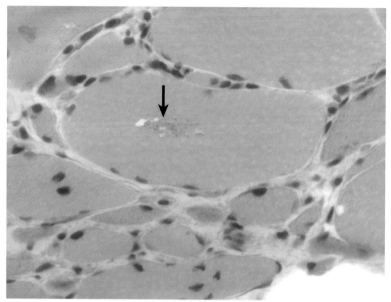

a

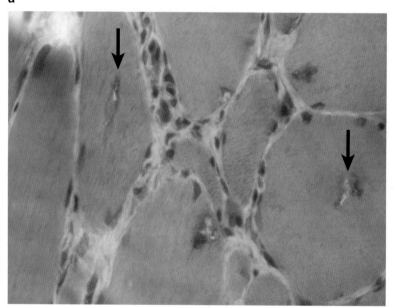

b

FIG. 22.12 *Rimmed vacuoles in the case of inclusion body myositis shown in Fig. 22.11. (a) H&E, (b) Gomori trichrome. Fibre diameter range 10–60 μm.*

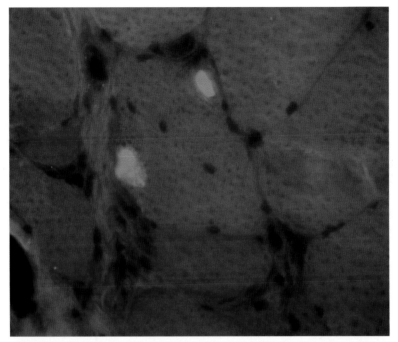

FIG. 22.13 *Biopsy from the quadriceps of a case of inclusion body myositis stained with Congo red and viewed with a 545–580 nm excitation filter for Texas Red, showing discrete areas of congophilia reflecting the presence of β-amyloid.*

cases have been reported. The pathological features of these myopathies are remarkably similar to those seen in IBM, in particular with regard to the presence of rimmed vacuoles and fibres with accumulation of the proteins mentioned above, the 15–20 nm filamentous inclusions and congophilia. The distinguishing feature, however, is the lack of lymphocytic inflammatory cells and this led to the introduction of the name by Askanas and Engel 'inclusion body *myopathy*', in contrast to inclusion body *myositis*. The similarity in titles has inevitably led to confusion, and the similarity in pathological features has raised the possibility of a common pathogenic mechanism for their formation in all these disorders.

Another pathological distinction has been shown using two different antibodies to phosphorylated tau (Mirabella et al 1996). These authors suggested that the monoclonal antibody SM-310, in contrast to another monoclonal antibody, SM-31, only labels the inclusions in sporadic IBM and not in the myopathic conditions. In IBM the inclusions are labelled by both antibodies. Studies of α-dystroglycan also suggest a reduction in glycosylation may be seen (Huizing et al 2004) but are not a consistent finding (Broccolini et al 2005).

Genetics

One form of hereditary inclusion body myopathy is characterized by sparing of the quadriceps, in contrast to the pronounced involvement in IBM. The disorder

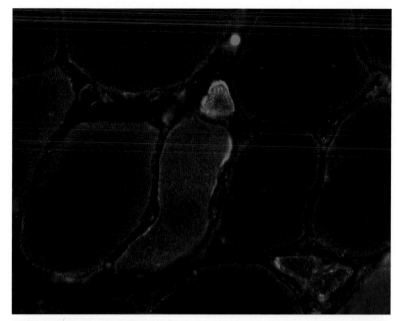

a

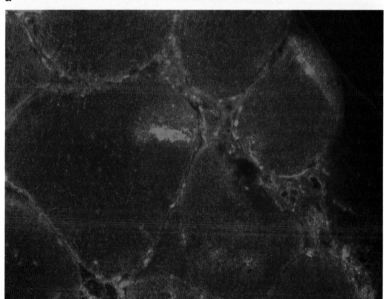

b

FIG. 22.14 *Immunolabelling of (a) phosphorylated tau and (b) ubiquitin in two cases of inclusion body myositis.*

is recessive and the defect is in the gene on chromosome 9p12-13 encoding UDP-N-acetylglucosamine 2-epimerase/N-acetylmannosamine kinase (GNE). This enzyme is involved in the synthesis of sialic acid and abnormalities are thought to impair sialic acid production (Huizing et al 2004). The disorder was first identified in patients of Jewish ancestry but it is now apparent that it is allelic to the 'distal myopathy with rimmed vacuoles', described by Nonaka in the Japanese population, and can also occur in other ethnic groups (Nonaka et al 2005).

Amongst other disorders considered as inclusion body myopathies because of the presence of rimmed vacuoles are oculopharyngeal muscular dystrophy, caused by defects in the poly(A) binding protein 2 gene (PABP2; see Ch. 14), Welander distal myopathy linked to chromosome 2p13, and tibial muscular dystrophy linked to 2q31 (the locus for titin), and the disorder caused by defects in the myosin heavy chain IIa gene on chromosome 17p13 (see Ch. 16). There is considerable pathological overlap with disorders classified as 'myofibrillar myopathies' (see Ch. 16). All these disorders are dominantly inherited.

Summary

The similarity of pathological features of inclusion body myositis and myopathies may cause diagnostic confusion in isolated cases with no family history, especially in sporadic cases with rimmed vacuoles and an absence of inflammation, and the distinction may not be clear. Biopsies showing rimmed vacuoles should be studied with a panel of techniques that should include the Gomori trichrome stain, Congo red viewed with fluorescence, antibodies to phosphorylated tau (SM-31, SM-310), ubiquitin and MHC-I. Additional antibodies can then be used to study the inclusions further, especially if a myofibrillar myopathy is suspected. It must be remembered that rimmed vacuoles, like so many pathological features in diseased muscle, are not specific to the inclusion body disorders and may be secondary to a number of gene defects.

CHAPTER 23

Toxic and drug-induced myopathies

Russell Lane

In addition to the many inherited disorders already described in this book, a wide range of drugs and toxins can also affect nerves and muscle. It is important that the pathologist is aware of these and is able to recognize them, since withdrawal of the culpable agent usually allows full recovery. Otherwise, the consequences can be serious or even fatal.

Some drug-related myopathies, such as those caused by steroids and alcohol, are common, while others are very rare. The widespread use of statins has resulted in these drugs becoming probably the commonest cause of myalgia and hyperCKaemia in clinical practice. Drugs and toxins have also provided useful paradigms of muscle disease and have helped to elucidate cellular mechanisms. For example, zidovudine, used in the treatment of AIDS, threw light on mitochondrial DNA turnover. A number of reviews have been published on drug-induced and toxic myopathies (including Lane and Mastaglia 1978, Khan 1995, Lane 1996a, Argov and Squier 2002, Bannwarth 2002, Barnes & Hilton-Jones 2003, Guis et al 2003).

Classification

As with muscle diseases in general, it is possible to classify drug and toxic effects on skeletal muscle in a number of ways: based on clinical features, the action of the drug, or the pathology produced. Within the general context of this book, this chapter concentrates on the pathology, which is discussed under seven main categories:

- Focal myopathy
- Necrosis and rhabdomyolysis
- Inflammation (lymphocytic, eosinophilic, macrophagic)
- Mitochondrial damage/depletion
- Myosin heavy chain loss
- Type 2 fibre atrophy
- Vacuolar myopathy

The clinical presentation resulting from toxic effects may be acute, such as an episode of rhabdomyolysis; subacute, with proximal weakness, variable degrees of myalgia and elevated serum creatine kinase; or chronic, typically resulting in a painless proximal myopathy with a normal CK level. However, some drugs can cause a variety of pathological changes and clinical presentations. For example, alcohol can cause an acute or subacute painful myopathy and may precipitate rhabdomyolysis, but paradoxically more often produces a slowly progressive painless myopathy.

Focal myopathy

Focal myopathy results from intramuscular injections. In the Western World, it is most often encountered in connection with opiate abuse, while in the Third World, particularly the Indian sub-continent and South America, antibiotic injections are the chief cause, with the deltoid and quadriceps commonly being affected. Focal myopathy can produce disabling muscle contractures but excision of the affected areas can restore function. The characteristic pathological features are of dense focal fibrosis, with scattered fibre necrosis and variable inflammatory infiltration (Fig. 23.1).

'Needle myopathy' is the commonest cause of focal myopathy in hospitals. The discovery of a raised CK level in a patient who has had intramuscular injec-

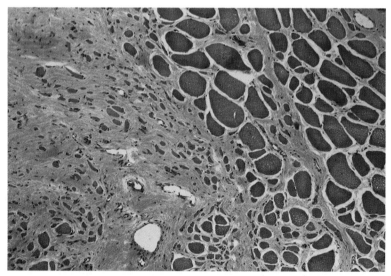

FIG. 23.1 *Typical pathology of focal myopathy, taken from an area of contracture. This biopsy was from a patient who repeatedly injected himself with pentazocine, an opiate derivative. The few remaining bundles of fibres show both atrophy and hypertrophy and there is pronounced replacement of muscle with fibrous tissue. There is little inflammatory response in this chronic lesion (H&E).*

tions or an electromyogram (EMG) can sometimes precipitate a fruitless search for evidence of muscle disease or myocardial infarction. Such iatrogenic trauma can also cause difficulties for the pathologist, if a biopsy is taken from a site where an EMG needle has been probing. Focal necrosis and accumulations of inflammatory cells may be seen.

Intramuscular injections of drugs and toxins cause injury by several mechanisms, including direct trauma to the fibres, bleeding, secondary infection, and through histamine release from damaged lysosomes. The pH and osmolarity of the agents are also thought to be important. Intramuscular injections of opiates, lidocaine and benzodiazepines can all cause focal myonecrosis.

Snake venoms also produce focal myonecrosis, with immediate local effects as well as more widespread damage (see below).

Necrosis and rhabdomyolysis

Several drugs and toxins can precipitate muscle fibre necrosis of varying degree, resulting in an acute or subacute painful myopathy, characterized by generalized myalgia and muscle tenderness, especially in proximal muscles, and marked increase in CK levels. Toxicity may result from the direct myotoxic action of drugs, through immune reaction resulting in inflammation, or by causing severe hypokalaemia (Table 23.1). The precise mechanisms of direct action vary, and some are unknown. In addition to necrosis, phagocytosis and fibre regeneration, non-specific changes such as variation in fibre size and an increase in internal nuclei can occur.

Rhabdomyolysis is acute necrosis resulting in the dissolution of many muscle fibres. It can be induced by most of the drugs or toxins that cause an acute or subacute painful myopathy (Lane and Phillips 2003). Alcohol and opiates (particularly heroin and cocaine) and other drugs of abuse are common culprits. Statins have been frequently implicated in the recent past but less so since their potential myotoxicity has been recognized. Anaesthetic agents can also cause rhabdomyolysis, and some snake venoms have widespread toxic effects in addition to those that result in only focal necrosis.

Agents causing acute rhabdomyolysis generally do so by precipitating metabolic failure of muscle fibres, with acute breakdown of sarcolemmal membranes. This may result in a massive leakage of intracellular contents such as myoglobin and CK, and an influx of calcium causing further cellular disruption. Depending on when or where the biopsy is performed, pronounced fibre necrosis may be seen but it is not uncommon to see surprisingly little pathology in the muscle, even with a CK over a 1000 times the normal limit.

Alcohol is a common cause of muscle injury, damaging the muscle membranes, probably through the action of acetaldehyde and free radicals. This is reflected in increases in sarcoplasmic reticulum calcium adenosine triphosphatase activity and cholesterol metabolites (Adachi et al 2003). Although alcohol can induce necrosis and rhabdomyolysis, a much more common effect is type 2 fibre atrophy or a chronic neuropathy (see below).

TABLE 23.1 *Pathological classification of toxic and drug-induced myopathies*

Dominant pathology	Mechanism	Drugs commonly implicated
Fibrosis, necrosis	Myotoxicity, fibre trauma, infection, lysosomal rupture	Intramuscular injection of opiates and antibiotics
Necrosis, macrophages	Myotoxicity Ischaemia Hypokalaemia (acute) Microvascular thrombosis Impaired protein and energy metabolism	Alcohol, statins, fibrates Opiates Diuretics, liquorice derivatives EACA Emetine (ipecac), retinoids
Inflammation Lymphocytic Eosinophilic Macrophagic	Immune mediated	D-penicillamine, procainamide L-tryptophan Aluminium-based vaccines
Mitochondrial damage or depletion (ragged-red fibres, COX-negative fibres, EM abnormalities)	Inhibition of mitochondrial γ DNA polymerase	Zidovudine
Myosin heavy chain loss	Ionic imbalance leading to filament disaggregation?	Steroids in association with neuromuscular blockade
Type 2 fibre atrophy	Reduced protein synthesis	Alcohol (chronic), drug induced hypokalaemia
Vacuoles	Lysosomal inhibition	Amiodarone, chloroquine, perhexilene
Myeloid bodies Spheromembranous bodies	Inhibition of microtubular polymerization	Colchicine, vincristine Amphotericin
Featureless	Hypokalaemia (chronic)	Diuretics, liquorice derivatives

COX, cytochrome oxidase; EACA, ε-aminocaproic acid; EM electron microscopy.

Drugs of abuse, particularly opiates, are also common causes of necrosis but are more often implicated in drug-induced rhabdomyolysis. Stimulant drugs, such as phencyclidine (PCP, 'Angel Dust') are thought to induce necrosis through extreme motor hyperactivity.

Statins [HMG-CoA (3-hydroxy-3-methylglutaryl-coenzyme A) reductase inhibitors] and *fibrates* reduce cholesterol synthesis and lower low density lipoprotein (LDL) cholesterol levels in the blood. As an adverse consequence, however, they also affect cholesterol metabolism in cell membranes. Adverse reactions involving skeletal muscle are the commonest side-effects of these drugs and have been reported in 1–7% of cases (Evans and Rees 2002a), although it is unclear to what extent this reflects the true extent of myotoxicity. Myalgia, raised CK and

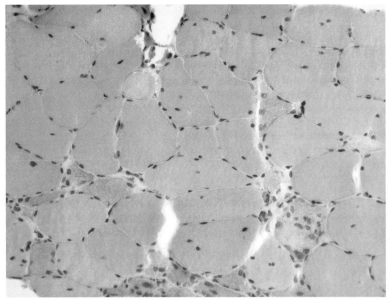

FIG. 23.2 *Quadriceps biopsy from a 71-year-old male showing necrosis and regeneration thought to have been induced by statins. The patient had a very high CK (20 000 IU/L) but very low sarcolemmal MHC class I, suggesting that he did not have a myositis (H&E).*

sometimes proximal weakness probably occur in about 1 in 1000 cases (Evans and Rees 2002b), but this is usually rapidly reversible on withdrawing the offending drug. In rare instances (1 per million prescriptions), rhabdomyolysis develops, and has caused fatalities (Lane and Phillips 2003).

Myotoxicity appears to result from injury to muscle membrane systems, including the sarcolemma and mitochondria. Membrane damage allows an influx of calcium, resulting in cycles of fibre necrosis. Experimental studies have shown accumulation of sub-sarcolemmal autophagic lysosomes, with degeneration of mitochondria and the sarcoplasmic reticulum, followed by marked necrosis and regeneration with macrophage infiltration (Waclawik et al 1993, Nakahara et al 1998; Ucar et al 2000; Fig. 23.2).

The statins vary in their propensity to cause myonecrosis. For example, cerivastatin was withdrawn because the incidence of rhabdomyolysis was orders of magnitude greater than other statins, owing to its high lipophilicity and bioavailablity, and there are currently concerns about rosuvastatin. Low constitutional cytochrome P450 activity may be a risk factor for statin myotoxicity, and may explain why it is much more likely to occur when these drugs are used in concert with other myotoxic drugs which are catabolized by this pathway, particularly fibrates, nicotinic acid and cyclosporin.

There are analogies between statin myopathy and the myopathy of selenium deficiency, and it has been suggested that these drugs might inhibit selenium metabolism in muscle (Moosmann and Behl 2004). Another interesting observation is that inhibition of mevalonate kinase, but not enzymes more distal in the cholesterol synthesis pathway, causes muscle fibre damage. This enzyme is essential for isoprenylation, which is vital for optimal function of a number of muscle membrane proteins, including lamin A/C and the dystroglycans. Statins might exert their myopathic effects by depleting the isoprenoid pool, through the inhibition of β-hydroxy-β-methylglutaryl CoA reductase, upstream of mevalonate kinase (Baker 2005).

Although myopathic symptoms generally resolve on withdrawing the statin, examples of more chronic myopathy have been reported, with pathological changes including ongoing necrosis, inflammation, fibre vacuolation and ragged-red fibres (Gambelli et al 2004, Carvalho et al 2004).

Fibrates are usually implicated when used in conjunction with statins but may occasionally cause fibre injury independently by up-regulation of lipoprotein lipases. Clofibrate may also cause myotonia through its effects on membrane function, as also observed experimentally with lovastatin (Waclawik et al 1993).

Steroids generally cause a slowly progressive painless myopathy with atrophy of type 2 fibres (see below), but large doses of intravenous hydrocortisone can precipitate myonecrosis. Intravenous steroids can also cause an acute quadriplegic myopathy, although in that situation the pathology and pathogenesis is different (see 'Myosin loss' below).

The anti-fibrinolytic *ε-aminocaproic acid* (EACA) causes a dramatic multifocal myonecrosis (Lane et al 1979), possibly as a result of capillary thrombosis and fibre ischaemia (Kennard et al 1980) (Fig. 23.3).

The amoebicide *emetine* (the active component of *ipecac*) may also cause this syndrome, as can large doses of *vitamin E* and vitamin A derivatives such as *etretinate* and *isotretinoic acid*, used in the treatment of acne and other skin disorders.

With regard to toxins, *organophosphates* inhibit acetylcholinesterase at the neuromuscular junction, causing excessive acetylcholine accumulation and calcium influx into muscle cells, resulting in myonecrosis. A muscle biopsy will generally show a mixed picture of ongoing fibre necrosis with macrophage activity, together with regeneration, but relatively little inflammatory infiltration.

Severe hypokalaemia can also lead to necrosis and an acute painful myopathy. This has been reported in association with alcohol (often with accompanying hypomagnesaemia), diuretics (particularly long acting agents such as chlorthalidone), purgatives, amphotericin B (which causes renal potassium loss) and glycyrrhizic acid derivatives (liquorice, carbenoxolone). A sustained fall in serum potassium to around 1–2-mM, with severe hypochloraemic alkalosis, can cause a profound flaccid, areflexic weakness but with florid changes on electromyography, reflecting muscle fibre necrosis and membrane damage. Scattered fibre necrosis may be seen in the biopsy, but typically this is an acute-on-chronic presentation and there are also changes of more longstanding damage, such as type 2 fibre atrophy. Vacuole-like structures, possibly derived from T tubules, may also be present (Fig. 23.4).

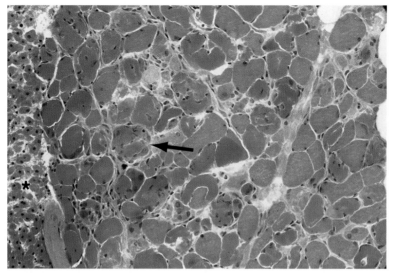

FIG. 23.3 *Acute necrotizing myopathy induced by ε-aminocaproic acid, showing multifocal fibre necrosis and macrophage activity, and marked regenerative response shown by many small basophilic areas around necrotic fibres (arrow). There is little lymphocytic infiltration but macrophages are abundant (*) (H&E).*

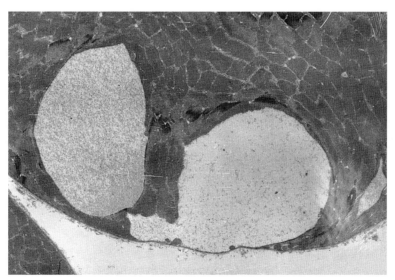

FIG. 23.4 *Liquorice (glycyrrhizinic acid) myopathy; electron microscopy of vacuole-like structures believed to be derived from T tubules.*

Inflammation

A few drugs can induce an inflammatory myopathy resembling polymyositis, and rarely dermatomyositis, as described in Chapter 22, although whether there is expression of MHC class I on muscle fibres in drug-induced myositis is not known. Inflammatory myopathy has been reported most often in connection with *d-penicillamine* treatment for rheumatoid disease, scleroderma and systemic sclerosis, Wilson's disease and cystinuria. Recovery follows withdrawal of the drug, although steroids may be required. Fatal myocarditis has also been reported. It should be noted that this drug more commonly precipitates antibody-positive myasthenia gravis.

Other drugs reported to induce inflammatory myopathy include *L-dopa*, *phenytoin, procainamide, leuprolide, propylthiouracil* and *cimetidine*. Polymyositis has also been reported with *α-interferon* treatment for chronic viral hepatitis, although in some reports it is unclear whether the drug or hepatitis C virus precipitates this. *Ciguetera* poisoning may also cause inflammatory myopathy.

Eosinophilic myofasciitis was reported with the use of *L-tryptophan* in the 1980s and early 1990s, but this was eventually shown to be due to adulterants in batches of the drug from certain US manufacturers.

An unusually high incidence of *macrophagic myofasciitis* was reported from France at the end of the 1990s. This appears to have been due to *aluminium* in certain vaccination products. Cases are still emerging, however, and this should be considered when focal macrophage accumulation is observed in the presence of an otherwise normal muscle biopsy (Fig. 23.5). Electron microscopy reveals dense spicular osmiophilic material, containing aluminium, which can be identified with electron microscopy X-ray analysis techniques.

Mitochondrial damage/depletion

Drugs such as *azidothymidine* (AZT; zidovudine), used in the treatment of HIV infection, cause mitochondrial damage by inhibiting the mitochondrial γ DNA polymerase. Accumulation of mitochondria, ragged-red fibres and ultrastructurally abnormal mitochondria can be seen (Lane et al 1993; Fig. 23.6). The relationship of AZT to muscle disease in patients with HIV infection is of interest. HIV infection can itself cause a number of muscle diseases and pathologies. These include a wasting syndrome, a classical inflammatory myopathy (with myalgia, weakness and raised CK level), a necrotizing myopathy with vacuolation and variable inflammation (presenting with fatigue, myalgia, proximal weakness and usually a raised CK level), and non-specific pathological changes such as nemaline rod formation and type 2 atrophy (Lane 1996b). Prior to the introduction of AZT treatment, muscle disease was reported in less than 1% of HIV cases, but subsequently up to a third of cases taking around 1-g AZT daily developed an acute or subacute painful myopathy. HIV patients taking AZT with no evidence of weakness and normal CK levels usually show no pathological abnormalities on muscle biopsy (Lane et al 1993).

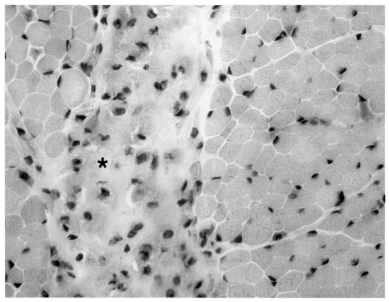

FIG. 23.5 *Macrophagic fasciitis induced by vaccination showing many macrophages in the perimysium (*). The muscle fibres show variation in size (range 5–25 μm) but there is no other pathological feature (child aged 7 months at time of biopsy; H&E).*

The microvacuolation appearance in AZT myopathy is due to swollen mitochondria, while in HIV myopathy it is caused by dilated sarcoplasmic reticulum (Lane et al 1996). Abundant endothelial tubuloreticular inclusions, seen in viral and immune mediated diseases such as dermatomyositis, are usually evident in biopsies from clinically myopathic cases but less commonly in non-myopathic cases. Tubuloreticular inclusions probably reflect generation of interferons and are an early manifestation of HIV infection in several tissues (Lane et al 1993).

Cyclosporin has also been shown to cause a myopathy with ragged-red fibres, by inhibiting mitochondrial respiration. This is a rare complication, largely confined to patients who have undergone renal transplantation. The mechanism is unclear, although cyclosporin-related hypomagnesaemia may play a role. This drug also increases the propensity of statins to induce muscle necrosis (see above).

Germanium-based elixirs and dietary supplements, which have become popular in a number of Western countries, are potentially highly toxic and can cause a myopathy, among other ills. Ragged-red fibres, fibres devoid of cytochrome oxidase activity and ultrastructural damage to mitochondria are seen. These mitochondrial changes are associated with marked vacuole-like appearance and lysosomal activation.

Senna (cassia) intoxication in cattle results in muscle disease with features of a mitochondrial cytopathy. Senna is widely used as a purgative but no instances of this pathology have been published in man, although a case seen by the authors of this book had abundant cytoplasmic bodies.

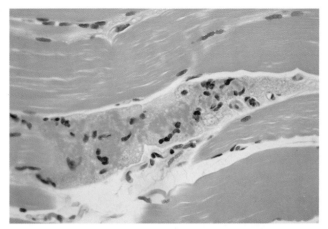

a

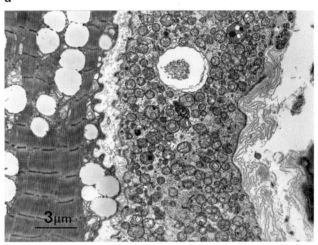

b

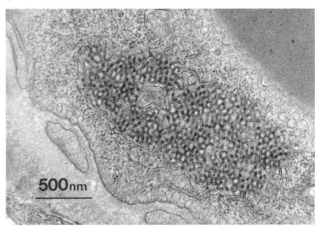

c

FIG. 23.6 *AZT myopathy in HIV infection showing (a) a fibre sectioned longitudinally undergoing degeneration (H&E), and electron micrographs of (b) abnormal mitochondria and (c) tubuloreticular inclusions in an endothelial cell. (Electron micrographs kindly supplied by Dr J Moss.)*

Myosin heavy chain loss

Severely ill patients in a high dependency or intensive care unit setting may develop neuromuscular dysfunction which may be neurogenic or myopathic, often referred to as *critical care* or *critical illness neuropathy* or *myopathy*. Critical illness neuropathy is a mild, distal, symmetrical and self-limiting axonal polyneuropathy of unknown cause. More severe and protracted instances of neuromuscular dysfunction in this situation are usually myopathic.

Critical care myopathy most often occurs with high doses of intravenous *steroids* given during mechanical ventilation under neuromuscular blockade with pancuronium or related drugs. When the paralysing agent is withdrawn, the patient is found to have a severe myopathic quadriplegia with depressed or absent tendon reflexes. The CK may be very high at the outset but falls rapidly and the patient generally recovers after a number of weeks. Rarely, recurrent attacks of this type can occur.

As noted, high dose intravenous steroids can induce a necrotizing myopathy, but in critical care myopathy there is selective loss of myosin thick filaments from the A bands, affecting both fibre types equally (Fig. 23.7). Occasional fibres with A-band loss can occur in several disorders (see Ch. 5, Fig. 5.15) but in critical care myopathy they are numerous. It is thought that the myosin monomers composing the filaments disaggregate, possibly as a result of ionic imbalance in the sarcoplasm. Myosin ATPase staining is markedly reduced, while myosin heavy chain immunohistochemistry is less affected, although disruption is visible (Fig. 23.7), suggesting that the disaggregated myosin monomers are retained but have no enzyme activity (Karpati 2002). The pathology can be reproduced experimentally in denervated muscles, and in rats given high doses of steroids.

Type 2 fibre atrophy

This is associated with a number of drug-induced chronic painless proximal myopathies. Clinically these myopathies are usually slowly progressive, with symmetrical proximal weakness and wasting. Several of the drugs that can cause acute or subacute painful myopathy more often produce myopathy of this type. While the more acute forms are characterized by myalgia and increased CK levels, in the chronic painless forms of myopathy, CK is usually normal or only mildly increased. Electromyography may reveal myopathic changes but without the increased insertional and spontaneous activity often seen in the acute situation. Stopping the offending agent usually allows some recovery but the time course and progress mirror the chronicity of the presentation.

The two commonest causes of chronic painless myopathy causing type 2 fibre atrophy are *alcohol* and *steroids*. The type 2B fibres are particularly affected (see Fig. 4.9). Chronic *alcohol*-related neuromyopathy is the most common neuromuscular disorder in the world (Rajendram et al 2003). Chronic myotoxicity often occurs on a background of alcohol-related neuropathy. The incidence of alcoholic myopathy (40–60% of alcoholics) is about twice as high as cirrhosis,

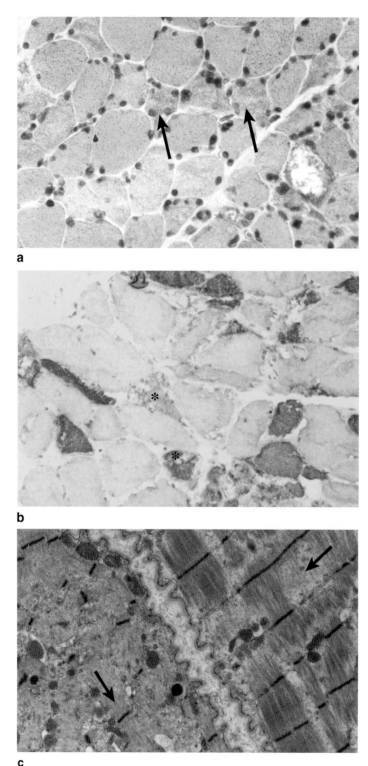

FIG. 23.7 *Critical care myopathy showing (a) several fibres with abnormal H&E stain (arrows); (b) disruption of fast myosin immunolabelling (*) and (c) electron micrograph showing varying degrees of selective A-band loss (arrows). (Electron micrograph kindly provided by Dr J Moss).*

polyneuropathy or cardiomyopathy. However, the condition evolves insidiously and the symptoms are often relatively mild, so many cases go unrecognized. Although the CK level is typically normal in the chronic form of alcohol-related myopathy, ingestion of alcohol by the patient will usually result in a rapid increase in CK level (Lane and Radoff 1981).

Steroids act at the nuclear level, interfering with protein metabolism, with an overall catabolic effect. A common difficulty is in distinguishing steroid myopathy from an underlying myopathy related to the condition being treated e.g. inflammatory myopathy. In the latter, inflammatory cells in the muscle biopsy are often apparent, and sarcolemmal expression of MHC class I is increased; although the effect of steroid therapy on MHC class I expression is not clear. Typical EMG changes of fibre injury and increased CK are also more likely in an inflammatory myopathy.

Vacuolar myopathies

Two forms of vacuolar change may be seen in drug-induced chronic progressive proximal myopathies:

- accumulation of autophagic vacuoles of lysosomal origin, associated with whorled membranous 'myelinoid' or spheromembranous bodies, derived from the sarcoplasmic reticulum; and
- vacuoles induced by chronic hypokalaemia, thought to be derived from T tubules.

Amphiphilic cationic drugs induce the lysosomal type of vacuolar myopathy. The drugs most often implicated are *anti-malarial drugs* (e.g. chloroquine, mepacrine), *amiodarone* and *perhexilene maleate*. These have lipid soluble hydrophobic regions and a primary or substituted amine group bearing a net positive charge, which allows these molecules to insert into membrane structures. These membranes undergo autodigestion by lysosomal enzymes, resulting in the accumulation of autophagic vacuoles and fibre degeneration. There is increased acid phosphatase staining due to increased lysosomal activity. This process occurs in many tissues, notably peripheral nerves, and the resulting polyneuropathy may be more significant than effects on muscle. The vacuoles occur in both fibre types and necrosis may also occur. In some cases of chloroquine-induced myopathy, the vacuoles are not abundant at the light microscope level but curvilinear bodies may be seen with the electron microscope (Fig. 23.8).

Whorled membranous bodies and spheromembranous bodies occur in the vacuolar myopathy associated with *colchicine* and *vincristine* (Fernandez et al 2002). Spheromembranous bodies are believed to be derived from the sarcoplasmic reticulum. These drugs inhibit microtubule polymerization, which is thought to result in impaired lysosomal transport along the microtubules. Colchicine can also cause a subacute painful myopathy with raised CK levels but more often

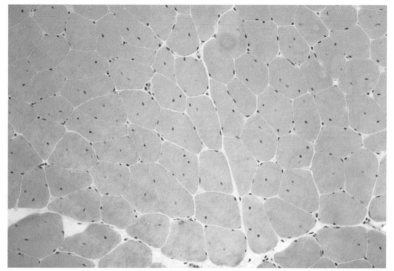

a

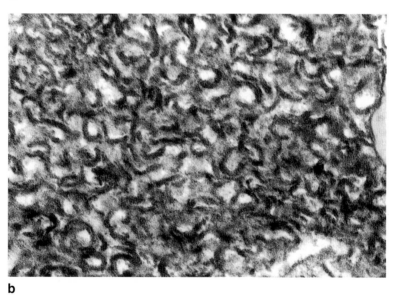

b

FIG. 23.8 *Pathological changes induced by chloroquine showing (a) mild variation in fibre size and an increase in internal nuclei but no prominent vacuoles (H&E); (b) electron micrograph from the same case showing curvilinear bodies.*

induces a chronic painless myopathy. About 80% of the drug is catabolized in the liver, and the kidneys excrete free drug, so myopathy is most likely to occur in patients with renal and hepatic disease, but myopathy can also occur in patients with normal renal function.

Vincristine is a vinca alkaloid used in chemotherapy. This drug was shown to cause spheromembranous degeneration of muscle in experimental studies in the 1960s, but in practice is more likely to induce a neuropathy.

A chronic vacuolar myopathy can also be induced by the same drugs that cause acute hypokalaemic painful necrotizing myopathy, notably diuretics, laxatives and liquorice derivatives (see above). These vacuoles are thought to originate from the T tubules, and type 2 atrophy is also a feature.

References

Adachi J, Asano M, Ueno Y et al 2003
Alcoholic muscle disease and biomembrane
perturbations. Journal of Nutrition and
Biochemistry 14:616–625

Afifi AK, Bergman RA, Harvey JC 1968
Steroid myopathy: clinical histologic and
cytologic observations. John Hopkins
Medical Journal 123:158–173

Afifi AK, Najjar SS, Mire-Salman J et al 1974
The myopathy of the Kocher-Debre-
Semelaigne syndrome. Electro-myography
light and electron-microscopic study.
Journal of the Neurological Sciences
22:445–470

Afifi AK, Smith JW, Zellweger H 1965
Congenital nonprogressive myopathy.
Central core and nemaline myopathy in
one family. Neurology 15:371–381

Agrawal PB, Strickland CD, Midgett C et al
2004 Heterogeneity of nemaline myopathy
cases with skeletal muscle alpha-actin gene
mutations. Annals of Neurology 56:86–
96

Amendt BA, Green C, Sweetman L et al 1987
Short-chain acyl-coenzyme A
dehydrogenase deficiency: clinical and
biochemical studies in two patients.
Journal of Clinical Investigation 79:1303–
1309

Amendt BA, Moon A, Teel L et al 1988 Long-
chain acyl-coenzyme A dehydrogenase
deficiency: biochemical studies in
fibroblasts from three patients. Pediatric
Research 23:603–605

Andersen ED, Krasilnikoff PA, Overvad H
1971 Intermittent muscular weakness,
extrasystoles, and multiple developmental
anomalies. A new syndrome? Acta
Paediatrica Scandinavica 60:559–564

Anderson LVB, Davison K 1999 Multiplex
Western blotting system for the analysis of
muscular dystrophy proteins. American
Journal of Pathology 154:1017–1022

Anderson LVB, Harrison RM, Pogue R et al
2000 Secondary reduction in calpain 3
expression in patients with limb girdle
muscular dystrophy type 2B and Miyoshi
myopathy (primary dysferlinopathies).
Neuromuscular Disorders 10:553–559

Anderson LVB, Davidson K, Moss JA et al
1998 Characterisation of monoclonal
antibodies to calpain 3 and protein
expression in muscle from patients with
limb-girdle muscular dystrophy type 2A.
American Journal of Pathology 153:1169–
1179

Anderson LVB, Davidson K, Moss JA et al
1999 Dysferlin is a plasma membrane
protein and is expressed early in human
development. Human Molecular Genetics
8:855–861

Anderson SL, Ekstein J, Donnelly MC et al
2004 Nemaline myopathy in the Ashkenazi
Jewish population is caused by a deletion
in the nebulin gene. Human Genetics
115:185–190

Appleyard ST, Dunn MJ, Dubowitz V et al
1985 Increased expression of HLA ABC
class I antigens by muscle fibres in
Duchenne muscular dystrophy,
inflammatory myopathy and other
neuromuscular disorders. Lancet i:361–363

Arahata K, Engel AG 1984 Monoclonal
antibody analysis of mononuclear cells on

myopathies I. Quantitation of subsets according to diagnosis and sites of accumulation and demonstration and counts of muscle fibers invaded by T cells. Annals of Neurology 16:193–208

Arahata K, Engel AG 1988a Monoclonal antibody analysis of mononuclear cells in myopathies IV: Cell-mediated cytotoxicity and muscle fibre necrosis. Annals of Neurology 23:168–173

Arahata K, Engel AG 1988b Monoclonal antibody analysis of mononuclear cells in myopathies V: Identification and quantitation of T8+ cytotoxic and T8+ suppressor cells. Annals of Neurology 23:493–499

Arahata K, Hayashi YK, Mizuno Y et al 1993 Dystrophin associated protein and dystrophin in FCMD. Lancet 342:623–624

Argov Z, Gardner-Medwin D, Johnson M A et al 1980 Congenital myotonic dystrophy. Fibre type abnormalities in two cases. Archives of Neurology (Chicago) 37:693–696

Argov Z, Soffer D 2002 Hereditary inclusion body myositis. In: Karpati G (ed) Structural and molecular basis of skeletal muscle diseases. ISN Neuropathology Press, Basel, pp 274–276

Argov Z, Squier W 2002 Toxic and iatrogenic disorders. In: Karpati G (ed) Structural and molecular basis of skeletal muscle diseases. ISN Neuropathology Press, Basel, pp 246–249

Arikawa E, Ishihara T, Nonaka I et al 1991 Immunocytochemical analysis of dystrophin in congenital muscular dystrophy. Journal of Neurological Sciences 105:79–87

Arikawa-Hirasawa E, Le AH, Nishino I et al 2002 Structural and functional mutations of the perlecan gene cause Schwartz-Jampel syndrome, with myotonic myopathy and chondrodysplasia. American Journal of Human Genetics 70:1368–1375

Askanas V, Engel WK 2001 Inclusion body myositis: new concepts of pathogenesis and relation to aging and Alzheimer disease. Journal of Neuropathology and Experimental Neurology 60:1–14

Askanas V, Engel WK 2003 Unfolding story of inclusion-body myositis and myopathies: role of misfolded proteins, amyloid-beta, cholesterol, and aging. Journal of Child Neurology 18:185–190

Askanas V, Engel WK, Alvarez RB 1993 Enhanced detection of Congo red positive amyloid deposits in muscle fibres of inclusion body myositis and brain of Alzheimer disease using fluorescence technique. Neurology 43:1265–1267

Askanas V, Serdaroglu P, Engel WK et al 1991 Immunolocalization of ubiquitin in muscle biopsies of patients with inclusion body myositis and oculopharyngeal muscular dystrophy. Neuroscience Letters 130:73–76

Askari A, Vignos PJ, Moskowitz RW 1976 Steroid myopathy in connective tissue disease. American Journal of Medicine 61:485–492

Asmus F, Zimprich A, Tezenas Du Monteel S et al 2002 Myoclonus-dystonia syndrome: epsilon-sarcoglycan mutations and phenotype. Annals of Neurology 52:489–492

Atsumi T, Ishikawa S, Miyatake T et al 1979 Myopathy and primary aldosteronism: electron microscopic study. Neurology 29:1348–1353

Azzedine H, Bolino A, Taieb T et al 2003 Mutations in MTMR13, a new pseudophosphatase homologue of MTMR2 and Sbf1, in two families with an autosomal recessive demyelinating form of Charcot–Marie–Tooth disease associated with early-onset glaucoma. American Journal of Human Genetics 72:1141–1153

Baghdiguian S, Martin M, Richard I et al 1999 Calpain 3 deficiency is associated with myonuclear apoptosis and profound perturbation of the I kappa3 alpha/NF-kappa B pathway in limb-girdle muscular dystrophy type 2A. Nature Medicine 5:503–511

Baker SK 2005 Molecular clues into the pathogenesis of statin-mediated muscle toxicity. Muscle and Nerve 31:572–580

Balci B, Uyanik G, Dincer P et al 2005 An autosomal recessive limb girdle muscular dystrophy (LGMD2) with mild mental retardation is allelic to Walker-Warburg syndrome (WWS) caused by a mutation in the POMT1 gene. Neuromuscular Disorders 15:271–275

Bank WJ, DiMauro S, Bonilla E et al 1975 A disorder of muscle lipid metabolism and myoglobinuria: absence of carnitine palmityl transferase. New England Journal of Medicine 292:433–449

Banker BQ 1975 Dermatomyositis of childhood. Ultrastructural alterations of muscle and intramuscular blood vessels. Journal of Neuropathology and Experimental Neurology 34:46–75

Bannwarth B 2002 Drug-induced myopathies. Expert Opinion on Drug Safety 1:65–70

Bansal D, Campbell KP 2004 Dysferlin and the plasma membrane repair in muscular dystrophy. Trends in Cell Biology 14: 206–213

Banwell BL, Russel J, Fukudome T et al 1999 Myopathy, myasthenic syndrome, and epidermolysis bullosa simplex due to plectin deficiency. Journal of Neuropathology and Experimental Neurology 58:832–846

Bardosi A, Creutzfeldt W, DiMauro S et al 1987 Myo-, neuro-, gastrointestinal encephalopathy (MNGIE syndrome) due to partial deficiency of cytochrome c oxidase. Acta Neuropathologica 74:248–258

Barka T, Anderson PJ 1963 Histochemistry: theory, practice and bibliography. Hoeber, New York

Barker D, Banks RW 1986 The muscle spindle. In: Engel AG, Banker AQ (eds) Myology basic and clinical. McGraw-Hill, New York, pp 309–337

Barnes PRJ, Hilton-Jones D 2003 Toxic and endocrine myopathies. In: Barnes PRJ, Hilton-Jones D (eds) Myopathies in clinical practice. Martin Dunitz, London, pp 139–146

Barohn RJ, Griggs RC 2001 Distal myopathies. In: Karpati G, Hilton-Jones D, Griggs RC (eds) Disorders of voluntary muscle, 7th edn. Cambridge University Press, Cambridge, pp 471–487

Barohn RJ, Brumback RA, Mendell JR 1994a Hyaline body myopathy. Neuromuscular Disorders 4:257–262

Barohn RJ, Jackson CE, Kagan-Hallet KS 1994b Neonatal nemaline myopathy with abundant intranuclear rods. Neuromuscular Disorders 4:513–520

Bartoccioni E, Gallucci S, Scuderi F et al 1994 MHC class I, MHC class II and intercellular adhesion molecule (ICAM-1) expression in inflammatory myopathies. Clinical and Experimental Immunology 95:166–172

Bashir R, Britton S, Strachan T et al 1998 A gene related to *Caenorhabditis elegans* spermatogenesis factor fer-1 is mutated in limb-girdle muscular dystrophy type 2B. Nature Genetics 20:37–42

Becher MW, Kotzuk JA, Davis LE et al 2000 Intranuclear inclusions in oculopharyngeal muscular dystrophy contain poly(A) binding protein 2. Annals of Neurology 48:812–815

Becker PE, Kiener F 1955 Eine neue X-chromasomale Muskeldystrophie. Archiv für Psychiatrie und Nervenkrankheiten 193:427–448

Beckmann JS, Fardeau M 1999 Limb girdle muscular dystrophies. In: Emery AEH (ed) Neuromuscular disorders: clinical and molecular genetics. Wiley, New York, pp 123–156

Behan WM, Cossar DW, Madden HA et al 2002 Validation of a simple, rapid, and economical technique for distinguishing type 1 and 2 fibres in fixed and frozen skeletal muscle. Journal of Clinical Pathology 55:375–380

Behbehani AW, Goebel H, Osse G et al 1984 Mitochondrial myopathy with lactic acidosis and deficient activity of muscle succinate-cytochrome c oxidoreductase. European Journal of Pediatrics 143:67–71

Bergström J 1962 Muscle electrolytes in man determined by neutron activation analysis on needle biopsy specimen: a study in normal subjects, kidney patients, and patients with chronic diarrhoea. Scandinavian Journal of Clinical and Laboratory Investigation 14(suppl 68):1–110

Bertini E, Salviati G, Apollo F et al 1994 Reducing body myopathy and desmin storage in skeletal muscle: morphological and biochemical findings. Acta Neuropathologica 87:106–112

Bertini E, Giusti T, Brunelli P et al 1998 Characterisation of COL6 mutations in two Italian families with Bethlem myopathy. Neuromuscular Disorders 8:249

Bertini E, Biancalana V, Bolino A et al 2004 118th ENMC International Workshop on Advances in Myotubular Myopathy 26–28 September 2003, Naarden, The Netherlands, 5th workshop of the International Consortium on Myotubular Myopathy. Neuromuscular Disorders 14:387–396

Bertran-Valero de Bernabe D, van Bokhoven H, van Beusekom E et al 2003 A homozygous nonsense mutation in the *Fukutin* gene causes a Walker-Warburg syndrome phenotype. Journal of Medical Genetics 40:845–848

Bethlem J, van Wijngaarden GK 1976 Benign myopathy, with autosomal dominant inheritance. A report on three pedigrees. Brain 99:91–100

Bethlem J, van Wijngaarden GK, de Jong J 1973 The incidence of lobulated fibres in the facioscapulohumeral type of muscular dystrophy and the limb-girdle syndrome. Journal of the Neurological Sciences 18:351–358

Betz RC, Schoser BG, Kasper D et al 2001 Mutations in CAV3 cause mechanical hyperirritability of skeletal muscle rippling muscle disease. Nature Genetics 28:218–219

Bischoff A, Esslen E 1965 Myopathy with primary hyperparathyroidism. Neurology 15:64–68

Bitoun M, Maugenre S, Jeannet PY et al 2005 Mutations in dynamin 2 cause dominant centronuclear myopathy. Nature Genetics 37:1207–1209

Blake DJ, Martin-Rendon E 2002 Intermediate filaments and the function of the dystrophin-protein complex. Trends in Cardiovascular Medicine 12:224–228

Blake DJ, Weir A, Newey SE et al 2002 Function and genetics of dystrophin and dystrophin-related proteins in muscle. Physiological Reviews 82:291–329

Bohan A, Peter JB 1975a Polymyositis and dermatomyositis. New England Journal of Medicine 292:344–347

Bohan A, Peter JB 1975b Polymyositis and dermatomyositis. New England Journal of Medicine 292:403–407

Bohlega S, Abu-Amero SN, Wakil SM et al 2004 Mutation of the slow myosin heavy chain rod domain underlies hyaline body myopathy. Neurology 62:1518–1521

Bolino A, Muglia M, Conforti FL et al 2000 Charcot–Marie–Tooth type 4B is caused by mutations in the gene encoding myotubularin-related protein-2. Nature Genetics 25:17–19

Bonavaud S, Agbulut O, Nizard RR et al 2001 A discrepancy resolved: human satellite cells are not preprogrammed to fast and slow lineages. Neuromuscular Disorders 11:747–752

Bonilla E, Schotland DL 1970 Histochemical diagnosis of muscle phosphofructokinase deficiency. Archives of Neurology (Chicago) 22:8–12

Bonne G, Di Barletta MR, Varnous S et al 1999 Mutations in the gene encoding lamin A/C cause autosomal dominant Emery-Dreifuss muscular dystrophy. Nature Genetics 21:285–288

Bonne G, Gisèle J, Capeau J 2002 82nd ENMC International Workshop, 5th International Emery–Dreifuss Muscular Dystrophy (EDMD) Workshop, 1st Workshop of the MYO-CLUSTER project EUROMEN, 15–16 September 2000, Naarden, The Netherlands. Neuromuscular Disorders 12:187–194

Bonnefont JP, Demaugre F, Prip-Buus C et al 1999 Carnitine palmitoyltransferase deficiencies. Molecular Genetics and Metabolism 68:424–440

Bönnemann CG, Finkel RS 2002 Sarcolemmal proteins and the spectrum of limb-girdle muscular dystrophies. Seminars in Pediatric Neurology 9:81–99

Bönnemann CG, Laing NG 2004 Myopathies resulting from mutations in sarcomeric proteins. Current Opinion in Neurology 17:529–537

Bönnemann CG, Modi R, Noguchi S et al 1995 Beta-sarcoglycan (A3b) mutations cause autosomal recessive muscular dystrophy with loss of sarcoglycan complex. Nature Genetics 11:266–276. Erratum in: Nature Genetics12:110

Bönnemann CG, Cox GF, Shapiro F et al 2000 A mutation in the alpha 3 chain of type IX collagen causes autosomal dominant multiple epiphyseal dysplasia with mild myopathy. Proceedings of the National Academy of Sciences of the United States of America 97:1212–1217

Bönnemann CG, Thompson TG, van der Ven PF et al 2003 Filamin C accumulation is a strong but nonspecific immunohistochemical marker of core formation in muscle. Journal of Neurological Sciences 206:71–78

Booth FW, Baldwin KM 1996 Muscle plasticity: energy and supply processes. In: Rowell LB, Shepperd JT (eds) Handbook of physiology, section 12: Exercise regulation and integration of multiple systems. Oxford University Press, New York, pp 1075–1123

Bourne GH, Golarz MN 1959 Human muscular dystrophy as an aberration of the connective tissue. Nature (London) 183:1741–1743

Bove KE, Jannaccone ST, Hilton PK et al 1980 Cylindrical spirals in a familial neuromuscular disorder. Annals of Neurology 7:550–556

Bowman W 1840 On the minute structure and movements of skeletal muscle. Philosophical Transactions of the Royal Society of London 457–501

Brais B 2002 PABPN1 dysfunction in oculopharyngeal muscular dystrophy. In: Karpati G (ed) Structural and molecular basis of skeletal muscle diseases. ISN Neuropathology Press, Basel pp 115–118

Brais B, Bouchard JP, Gosselin F et al 1997 Using the full power of linkage analysis in 11 French Canadian families to fine map the oculopharyngeal muscular dystrophy gene. Neuromuscular Disorders 7:70–74

Brais B, Bouchard JP, Xie YG et al 1998 Short GCG expansions in the PABP2 gene cause oculopharyngeal muscular dystrophy. Nature Genetics 18:164–167. Erratum in Nature Genetics 19:404 (Korcyn AD corrected to Korczyn AD)

Bresolin N, Zeviani M, Bonilla E et al 1985 Fatal infantile cytochrome oxidase deficiency: decrease of immunologically detectable enzyme in muscle. Neurology 35:802–812

Bressler R 1970 Carnitine and the twins (Editorial) New England Journal of Medicine 282:745–746

Briggs MD, Chapman KL 2002 Pseudoachondroplasia and multiple epiphyseal dysplasia: mutation review molecular interactions, and genotype to phenotype correlations. Human Mutation 19:465–478

Broccolini A, Gliubizzi C, Pavoni E et al 2005 alpha-Dystroglycan does not play a major pathogenic role in autosomal recessive hereditary inclusion-body myopathy. Neuromuscular Disorders 15:177–184.

Brockington M, Sewry CA, Hermann R et al 2000 Assignment of a form of congenital muscular dystrophy with secondary merosin deficiency to chromosome 1q42. American Journal of Human Genetics 66:428–435

Brockington M, Blake DJ, Prandini P et al 2001a Mutations in the fukutin-related protein gene (FKRP) cause a form of congenital muscular dystrophy with secondary laminin alpha2 deficiency and abnormal glycosylation of alpha-dystroglycan. American Journal of Human Genetics 69:1198–1208

Brockington M, Yuva Y, Prandini P et al 2001b Mutations in the fukutin-related protein gene (FKRP) identify limb-girdle muscular dystrophy 2I as a milder allelic variant of congenital muscular dystrophy MDC1C. Human Molecular Genetics 10:2851–2859

Brockington M, Brown SC, Lampe A et al 2004 Prenatal diagnosis of Ullrich congenital muscular dystrophy using haplotype analysis and collagen VI immunocytochemistry. Prenatal Diagnosis 24:440–444

Brody IA 1969 Muscle contracture induced by exercise. A syndrome attributed to decreased relaxing factor. New England Journal of Medicine 281:187–192

Brooke MH 1973 Congenital fiber type disproportion. In: Kakulas BA (ed) Clinical Studies in Myology, Proceedings of the Second International Congress on Muscle Diseases, Perth, Australia, November 1971. ICS No. 295. Excerpta Medica, Amsterdam, pp 147–159

Brooke MH, Engel WK 1969a The histographic analysis of human muscle biopsies with regard to fiber types. 2. Diseases of the upper and lower motor neurons. Neurology 19:221–233

Brooke MH, Engel WK 1969b The histographic analysis of human muscle biopsies with regard to fiber types. 1. Adult male and female. Neurology 19:378–393

Brooke MH, Engel WK 1969c The histographic analysis of human muscle biopsies with regard to fiber types. 3. Myotonias, myasthenia gravis, and hypokalemic periodic paralysis. Neurology 19:469–477

Brooke MH, Engel WK 1969d The histographic analysis of human muscle biopsies with regard to fiber types. 4. Children's biopsies. Neurology 19:591–605

Brooke MH, Kaiser KK 1970 Muscle fibre types: how many and what kind? Archives of Neurology (Chicago) 23:369–379

Brooke MH, Neville HE 1972 Reducing body myopathy. Neurology 22:829–840

Brooke MH, Williamson E, Kaiser KK 1971 The behavior of four fiber types in developing and reinnervated muscle. Archives of Neurology (Chicago) 25: 360–366

Brown SC, Lucy JA 1997 Dystrophin: gene, protein and cell biology. Cambridge University Press, Cambridge

Brown SC, Fassati A, Popplewell L et al 1999 Dystrophic phenotype induced in vitro by antibody blockade. Journal of Cell Science 112:209–216

Brown SC, Muntoni F, Sewry CA 2001 Non-sarcolemmal muscular dystrophies. Brain Pathology 11:193–205

Brown SC, Torelli S, Brockington M et al 2004 Abnormalities in α-dystroglycan expression in MDC1C and LGMD21 muscular dystrophies. American Journal of Pathology 164:727–737

Buckingham ME 1985 Actin and myosin multigene family: their expression during the formation of skeletal muscle. Essays in Biochemistry 20:77–109

Buj-Bello A, Furling D, Troncere H et al 2002 Muscle-specific alternative splicing of myotubularin-related 1 gene is impaired in DM1 muscle cells. Human Molecular Genetics 11:2297–2307

Buller AJ, Eccles JC, Eccles RM 1960 Interactions between motor neurones and muscles in respect of the characteristic speeds of their responses. Journal of Physiology 150:417–439

Burck U, Goebel HH, Kuhlendahl HD et al 1981 Neuromyopathy and vitamin E deficiency in man. Neuropediatrics 12:267–278

Burghes AH, Logan C, Hu X et al 1987 A cDNA clone from the Duchenne/Becker muscular dystrophy gene. Nature 328:434–437

Burke RE, Levine DN, Tsiaris P et al 1973 Physiological types and histochemical profiles in motor units of cat gastrocnemius. Journal of Physiology 234:723–748

Burkin DJ, Wallace GQ, Nicol KJ et al 2001 Enhanced expression of the alpha 7 beta 1 integrin reduces muscular dystrophy and restores viability in dystrophic mice. Journal of Cell Biology 152:1207–1218

Burton EA, Tinsley JM, Holzfeind PJ et al 1999 A second promoter provides an alternative target for therapeutic up-regulation of utrophin in Duchenne muscular dystrophy. Proceedings of the National Academy of Sciences of the United States of America 96:14025–14030

Bush A, Dubowitz V 1991 Fatal rhabdomyolysis complicating general anaesthesia in a child with Becker muscular dystrophy. Neuromuscular Disorders 1:201–204

Bushby KM 1999 Making sense of the limb-girdle muscular dystrophies. Brain 122:1403–1420

Bushby KM, Anderson LVB 2001 Methods in molecular medicine – the muscular dystrophies. Humana Press, Totowa

Bushby K, Anderson LV, Pollitt C et al 1998 Abnormal merosin in adults. A new form of late onset muscular dystrophy not linked to chromosome 6q2. Brain 121:581–588

Butler-Browne GS, Barbet JP, Thornell LE 1990 Myosin heavy and light chain expression during human skeletal muscle development and the precocious accumulation of the adult heavy chain isoforms by thyroid hormone. Anatomy and Embryology 181:513–522

Caille B, Fardeau M, Harpey JP, Lafourcade J 1971 Hypotonie congénitale avec atteinte sélective des fibres musculaires de type 1. Archives Françaises de Pédiatrie 28:205–220

Calado A, Tomé FM, Brais B et al 2000 Nuclear inclusions in oculopharyngeal muscular dystrophy consist of binding protein 2 aggregates which sequester poly(A) RNA. Human Molecular Genetics 9:2321–2328

Camacho Vanegas O, Bertini E, Zhang RZ et al 2001 Ullrich scleroatonic muscular dystrophy is caused by recessive mutations in collagen type VI. Proceedings of the National Academy of Sciences of the United States of America 98:7516–7521

Cameron CH, Allen IV, Patterson V et al 1992 Dominantly inherited tubular aggregate myopathy. Journal of Pathology 168:397–403

Cancilla PA, Kalyanaraman K, Verity MA 1971 Familial myopathy with probable lysis of myofibrils in type 1 fibers. Neurology 21:579–585

Capanni C, Sabatelli P, Mattioli E et al 2003 Dysferlin in a hyperCKaemic patient with caveolin 3 mutation and in C2C12 after p38 MAP kinase inhibition. Experimental and Molecular Medicine 35:538–544

Carbone I, Bruno C, Sorgia F et al 2000 Mutation in the CAV3 gene causes partial caveolin-3 deficiency and hyperCKemia. Neurology 54:1373–1376

Carpenter S 2001a Muscle pathology on semithin resin sections. In: Karpati G, Hilton-Jones D, Griggs RC (eds). Disorders of voluntary muscle, 7th edn. Cambridge University Press, Cambridge, pp 283–295

Carpenter S 2001b Electron microscopy in the study of normal and diseased muscle. In: Karpati G, Hilton-Jones D, Griggs RC (eds) Disorders of voluntary muscle, 7th edn. Cambridge University Press, Cambridge, pp 296–318

Carpenter S, Karpati G 1979 Duchenne muscular dystrophy. Plasma membrane loss initiates muscle cell necrosis unless it is repaired. Brain 102:147–161

Carpenter S, Karpati G 2001 Pathology of skeletal muscle, 2nd edn. Oxford University Press, New York

Carpenter S, Karpati G, Rothman S et al 1976 The childhood type of dermatomyositis. Neurology 26:952–962

Carroll JE, Brooke MH, De Vivo DC et al 1978 Biochemical and physiologic consequences of carnitine palmityltransferase deficiency. Muscle and Nerve 1:103–110

Cartaud A, Strochlic l, Guerra M et al 2004 MuSK is required for anchoring acetylcholinesterase at the neuromuscular junction. Journal of Cell Biology 165:505–515

Cartegni L, di Barletta MR, Barresi R et al 1997 Heart-specific localization of emerin: new insights into Emery–Dreifuss muscular dystrophy. Human Molecular Genetics 6:2257–2264

Carvalho AA, Lima UW, Valiente RA 2004 Statin and fibrate associated myopathy: study of eight patients. Arqiv Neuropsiquiatric 62:257–261

Cashman NR, Covault J, Wollman RL 1987 Neural cell adhesion molecule in normal, denervated, and myopathic muscle. Annals of Neurology 21:481–489

Cestan R, Lejonne S 1902 Une myopathie avec rétractions familialles. Nouvelle Iconographie de la Salpetriere15:37–52

Chakrabarti A, Pearce JM 1981 Scapuloperoneal syndrome with cardiomyopathy: report of a family with autosomal dominant inheritance and unusual features. Journal of Neurology Neurosurgery and Psychiatry 44:1146–1152

Chalmers RA, Johnson M, Pallis C et al 1969 Xanthinuria with myopathy. Quarterly Journal of Medicine 38:493–512

Chen YJ, Spence HJ, Cameron JM et al 2003 Direct interaction of beta-dystroglycan with F-actin. Biochemical Journal 15:329–337

Chevessier F, Marty I, Paturneau-Jouas M et al 2004 Tubular aggregates are from whole sarcoplasmic reticulum origin: alterations in calcium binding protein expression in mouse skeletal muscle during aging. Neuromuscular Disorders 14:208–216

Cholod EJ, Haust MD, Hudson AJ et al 1970 Myopathy in primary familial hyperparathyroidism: clinical and morphologic studies. American Journal of Medicine 48:700–707

Chou SM 1968 Myxovirus-like structures and accompanying nuclear changes in chronic polymyositis. Archives of Pathology 86:649–658

Clark JB, Hayes DJ, Byrne E et al 1983 Mitochondrial myopathies: defects in mitochondrial metabolism in human skeletal muscle. Biochemical Society Transactions 11:626–627

Clarke NF, North KN 2003 Congenital fiber type disproportion – 30 years on. Journal of Neuropathology and Experimental Neurology 62:977–989

Clemens PR, Ward PA, Caskey CT et al 1992 Premature chain termination causing Duchenne muscular dystrophy. Neurology 42:1755–1782

Clements L, Manila S, Love DR et al 2000 Direct interaction between emerin and lamin A. Biochemistry Biophysics and Research Communications 267:709–714

Clerk A, Rodillo E, Heckmatt JZ et al 1991 Characterisation of dystrophin in carriers of Duchenne muscular dystrophy. Journal of the Neurological Sciences 102:197–205

Clerk A, Dubowitz V, Sewry CA 1992a Characterisation of dystrophin in foetuses at risk for Duchenne muscular dystrophy. Journal of the Neurological Sciences 111:82–91

Clerk A, Strong PN, Sewry CA 1992b Characterization of dystrophin during development of human skeletal muscle. Development 114:395–402

Clerk A, Morris GE, Dubowitz V et al 1993 Dystrophin-related protein, utrophin, in normal and dystrophic human foetal skeletal muscle. Histochemical Journal 25:554–561

Coates PM, Hale DE, Stanley CA et al 1985 Genetic deficiency of medium-chain acyl-coenzyme A dehydrogenase: studies in cultured skin fibroblasts and peripheral mononuclear leukocytes. Pediatric Research 19:671–676

Coates PM, Hale DE, Finocchiaro G et al 1988 Genetic deficiency of short-chain acyl-coenzyme A dehydrogenase in cultured fibroblasts from a patient with muscle carnitine deficiency and severe skeletal muscle weakness. Journal of Clinical Investigation 81:171–175

Cohn RD, Campbell KP 2000 Molecular basis of muscular dystrophies. Muscle and Nerve 23:1456–1471

Cohn RD, Herrmann R, Wewer UM 1997 Changes of laminin beta 2 chain expression in congenital muscular dystrophy. Neuromuscular Disorders 7:373–378

Cohn RD, Mayer U, Saher G et al 1999 Secondary reduction of alpha7B integrin in laminin alpha2 deficient congenital muscular dystrophy supports an additional transmembrane link in skeletal muscle. Journal of the Neurological Sciences 163:140–152

Colling-Saltin A 1978 Enzyme histochemistry on skeletal muscle of the human foetus. Journal of the Neurological Sciences 39:169–185

Conen PE, Murphy EG, Donohue WL 1963 Light and electron microscopic studies of 'myogranules' in a child with hypotonia and muscle weakness. Canadian Medical Association Journal 89:983–986

Confalonieri P, Oliva L, Andreetta T et al 2003 Muscle inflammation and MHC class 1 up-regulation in muscular dystrophy with lack of dysferlin: an immunopathological study. Journal of Neuroimmunology 14:130–136

Conn JW 1955 Primary aldosteronism: a new clinical syndrome. Journal of Laboratory and Clinical Medicine 45:661–664

Conn JW, Knopf RF, Nesbit RM 1964 Clinical characteristics of primary aldosteronism from an analysis of 145 cases. American Journal of Surgery 107:159–172

Conte G, Gioja L 1836 Scrofola del sisterna muscolare. Annali Clinici dell'Ospedale degl'Incurabili (Napoli) 2:66–79

Cori GT 1958 Biochemical aspects of glycogen deposition disease. In: Hottinger A, Hauser F, Berger H (eds) Modern Problems in Paediatrics. Vol 3. Bibliotheca Paediatricia, Fascicle No. 66. Karger, Basel, pp 344–358

Cori GT, Cori CF 1952 Glucose-6-phosphatase of the liver in glycogen storage disease. Journal of Biological Chemistry 199:661–667

Cornelio F, Di Donato S, Peluchetti P et al 1977 Fatal cases of lipid storage myopathy with carnitine deficiency. Journal of Neurology, Neurosurgery and Psychiatry 40:170–178

Crosbie RH, Heighway J, Venzke DP et al 1997 Sarcospan, the 25-kDa transmembrane component of the dystrophin-glycoprotein complex. Journal of Biological Chemistry 272:31221–31224

Crosbie RH, Yamada H, Venzke DP et al 1998 Caveolin-3 is not an integral component of the dystrophin glycoprotein complex. FEBS Letters 427:279–282

Cruse RP, Di Mauro S, Towfighi J et al 1984 Familial systematic carnitine deficiency. Archives of Neurology (Chicago) 41:301–305

Cui X, De V, Slany I et al 1998 Association of SET domain and myotubularin-related proteins modulates growth control. Nature Genetics 18:331–337

Cullen MJ, Fulthorpe JJ 1975 Stages in fibre breakdown in Duchenne muscular dystrophy. An electron microscopic study. Journal of the Neurological Sciences 24:179–200

Cullen MJ, Fulthorpe JJ 1982 Phagocytosis of the A band following Z line and I band loss. Its significance in skeletal muscle breakdown. Journal of Pathology 138:129–143

Cullen MJ, Mastaglia FL 1982 Pathological reactions of skeletal muscle. In: Mastaglia FL, Walton J (eds) Skeletal muscle pathology. Churchill Livingstone, London, pp 88–139

Cullen MJ, Weightman D 1975 The ultrastructure of normal human muscle in relation to fibre type. Journal of the Neurological Sciences 25:43–56

Curless RG, Payne CM, Brinner FM 1978 Fingerprint myopathy: a report of twins. Developmental Medicine and Child Neurology 20:793–798

Cusco I, Barcelo MJ, del Rio E et al 2004 Detection of novel mutations in the SMN Tudor domain in type 1 SMA patients. Neurology 13:146–149

Dahl N, Hu LJ, Chery M et al 1995 Myotubular myopathy in a girl with a deletion at Xq27-

q28 and unbalanced X inactivation assigns the MTM1 gene to a 600-kb region. American Journal of Human Genetics 56:1108–1115

Dalakas 2004 Inflammatory disorders of muscle: progress in polymyositis, dermatomyositis and inclusion body myositis. Current Opinion in Neurology 17:561–567

Dalakas MC, Hohlfeld R 2003 Polymyositis and dermatomyositis. Lancet 362:971–982

Dakalas MC, Park KY, Semino-Mora, C et al 2000 Desmin myopathy, a skeletal myopathy with cardiomyopathy caused by mutations in the desmin gene. New England Journal of Medicine 342:770–780

Dalkilic I, Kunkel LM 2003 Muscular dystrophies: genes to pathogenesis. Current Opinion in Genetics and Development 13:231–238

Danon MJ, Carpenter S 1991 Myopathy with thick filament (myosin) loss following prolonged paralysis with vecuronium during steroid treatment. Muscle and Nerve 14:1131–1139

Danon MJ, Oh SJ, DiMauro S et al 1981 Lysosomal glycogen storage disease with normal acid maltase. Neurology 31:51–57

Dastur DK, Gagrat BM, Wadia NH et al 1975 Nature of muscular change in osteomalacia: light and electron microscope observations. Journal of Pathology 117:211–228

Davies NP, Hanna MG 2001 The skeletal muscle channelopathies: basic science, clinical genetics and treatment. Current Opinion in Neurology 14:539–551

Davis MR, Haan E, Jungbluth H et al 2003 Principal mutation hotspot for central core disease and related myopathies in the C-terminal transmembrane region of the RYR1 gene. Neuromuscular Disorders 13:151–157

Dawson TP, Neal JW, Llewellyn L et al 2003 Neuropathology techniques. Hodder Arnold, London

De Bleecker JL, Engel AG, Winklemann JC 1993 Localization of dystrophin and beta-spectrin in vascular myopathies. American Journal of Pathology 143:1200–12008

De Bleecker JL, Engel AG, Ertl BB 1996 Myofibrillar myopathy with abnormal foci of desmin positivity. II. Immunocytochemical analysis reveals accumulation of multiple other proteins.

Journal of Neuropathology and Experimental Neurology 55:563–577

de Groot JG, Arts WF 1982 Familial myopathy with tubular aggregates. Journal of Neurology 227:35–41

de Paula F, Vainzof M, Bernardino AL et al 2001 Mutations in the caveolin-3 gene: When are they pathogenic? American Journal of Medical Genetics 99:303–307

Debré R, Semelaigne G 1935 Syndrome of diffuse muscular hypertrophy in infants causing athletic appearance: its connection with congenital myxedema. American Journal of Diseases of Children 50:1351–1361

Demir E, Sabatelli P, Allamand V et al 2002 Mutations in COL6A3 cause severe and mild phenotypes of Ullrich congenial muscular dystrophy. American Journal of Human Genetics 70:1446–1458

Denborough MA, Lovell RRH 1960 Anaesthetic deaths in a family. Lancet ii:45

Denborough MA, Dennett S, Anderson RM 1973 Central core disease and malignant hyperpyrexia. British Medical Journal 1:272–273

Denborough MA, Galloway GJ, Hopkinson KC 1982 Malignant hyperpyrexia and sudden infant death. Lancet 2:1068–1069

Denborough MA, Collins S, Hopkinson KC 1984 Rhabdomyolysis and malignant hyperpyrexia. British Medical Journal 288:1878

Deodata F, Sabatelli M, Ricci E et al 2002 Hypermyelinating neuropathy, mental retardation and epilepsy in a case of merosin deficiency. Neuromuscular Disorders 12:392–398

di Blasi C, Morandi L, Raffaele di Barletta MR et al 2000 Unusual expression of emerin in a patient with X-linked Emery–Dreifuss muscular dystrophy. Neuromuscular Disorders 10:567–571

Di Donato S, Pelucchetti D, Rimoldi M et al. 1984 Systemic carnitine deficiency: clinical, biochemical, and morphological cure with L-carnitine. Neurology 34:157–162

Di Donato S, Gellera C, Peluchetti D et al 1989 Normalization of short-chain acyl-coenzyme A dehydrogenase after riboflavin treatment in a girl with multiple acylcoenzyme A dehydrogenase-deficient myopathy. Annals of Neurology 25:479–484

Di Donato S, Taroni F 2002 Defects in fatty acid metabolism. In: Karpati G (ed)

Structural and molecular basis of skeletal muscle diseases. ISN Neuropathology Press, Basel, pp 189–201

Di Donato S, Taroni F 2003 Disorders of lipid metabolism. In: Rosenberg RN, Prusiner SB, DiMauro S, Barchi RL, Nestler EJ (eds) The molecular and genetic basis of neurological and psychiatric disease. Butterworth and Heinemann, Boston, pp 591–601

DiMauro S 1993 Mitochondrial encephalomyopathies. In: Rosenberg RN, Prusiner SB, DiMauro S et al (eds) The Molecular and Genetic Basis of Neurological Disease. Butterworth-Heinemann, Boston, pp 665–694

DiMauro S, DiMauro PM 1973 Muscle carnitine palmityl-transferase deficiency and myoglobinuria. Science 182:929–931

DiMauro S, Hartlage PL 1978 Fatal infantile form of muscle phosphorylase deficiency. Neurology 28, 1124–1129

DiMauro S, Trevisan C, Hays AP 1980 Disorders of lipid metabolism in muscle. Muscle and Nerve 3:369–388

DiMauro S, Nicholson JF, Hays AP et al 1983 Benign infantile mitochondrial myopathy due to reversible cytochrome c oxidase deficiency. Annals of Neurology 14: 226–234

DiMauro S, Lombes A, Nakase H et al 1990 Cytochrome c oxidase deficiency. Pediatric Research 28:536–541

Dobyns WB, Pagon RA, Armstrong D et al 1989 Diagnostic criteria for Walker-Warburg syndrome. American Journal of Medical Genetics 32:195–210

Donner K, Ollikainen M, Ridanpaa M et al 2002 Mutations in the beta-tropomyosin (TPM2) gene – a rare cause of nemaline myopathy. Neuromuscular Disorders 12:151–158

Draeger A, Weeds AG, Fitzsimons RB 1987 Primary, secondary and tertiary myotubes in developing skeletal muscle: a new approach in the analysis of human myogenesis. Journal of the Neurological Sciences 81:19–43

Dreifuss FE, Hogan GR 1961 Survival in X-chromosomal muscular dystrophy. Neurology 11:734–737

Duance VC, Stephens HR, Dunn MJ et al 1980 A role for collagen in the pathogenesis of muscular dystrophy. Nature (London) 284:470–472

Dubowitz V 1965 Enzyme histochemistry of skeletal muscle. Part II. Developing human muscle. Journal of Neurology, Neurosurgery and Psychiatry 28:519–524

Dubowitz V 1966 Enzyme histochemistry of skeletal muscle. Part III. Neurogenic muscular atrophies. Journal of Neurology, Neurosurgery and Psychiatry 29:23–28

Dubowitz V 1967 Pathology of experimentally re-innervated skeletal muscle. Journal of Neurology, Neurosurgery and Psychiatry 30:99–110

Dubowitz V 1969 The floppy infant. Clinics in developmental medicine No. 31. Spastics International/Heinemann, London

Dubowitz V 1973 Rigid spine syndrome: a muscle syndrome in search of a name. Proceedings of Royal Society of Medicine 66:219–220

Dubowitz V 1976 Treatment of dermatomyositis in childhood. Archives of Disease in Childhood 51:494–500

Dubowitz V 1980 The Floppy Infant, 2nd edn. Clinics in Developmental Medicine, No. 76. Spastics International Medical Publications. Blackwell, Oxford; Lippincott, Philadelphia

Dubowitz V 1991 Chaos in classification of the spinal muscular atrophies of childhood. Neuromuscular Disorders 1:77–80

Dubowitz V 1994 22nd ENMC sponsored workshop on congenital muscular dystrophy held in Baarn, The Netherlands, 14–16 May 1993. Neuromuscular Disorders 4:75–81

Dubowitz V 1995a Muscle disorders in childhood, 2nd edn. WB Saunders, London

Dubowitz V 1995b Chaos in the classification of SMA: a possible resolution. Neuromuscular Disorders 5:3–5

Dubowitz V 1996 41st ENMC International Workshop on Congenital Muscular Dystrophy, 8–10 March, Naarden, The Netherlands. Neuromuscular Disorders 6:295–306

Dubowitz V 1997 50th ENMC International Workshop on Congenital Muscular Dystrophy, 28 February–2 March 1997, Naarden, The Netherlands. Neuromuscular Disorders 7:539–547

Dubowitz V 1999 68th ENMC International Workshop on Congenital Muscular Dystrophy, 9–11 April 1999, Naarden, The Netherlands. Neuromuscular Disorders 9:446–454

Dubowitz V, Brooke MH 1973 Muscle Biopsy: A Modern Approach. WB Saunders, London

Dubowitz V, Fardeau M 1994 Proceedings of the 27th ENMC sponsored workshop on congenital muscular dystrophy 22–24 April 1994, The Netherlands. Neuromuscular Disorders 5:253–258

Dubowitz V, Pearse AGE 1960a A comparative histochemical study of oxidative enzyme and phosphorylase activity in skeletal muscle. Histochemie 2:105–117

Dubowitz V, Pearse AGE 1960b Oxidative enzymes and phosphorylase in central core disease of muscle. Lancet ii:23–24

Dubowitz V, Pearse AGE 1960c Reciprocal relationship of phosphorylase and oxidative enzymes in skeletal muscle. Nature (London) 185:701–702

Dubowitz V, Pearse AGE 1961 Enzymic activity of normal and diseased human muscle: a histochemical study. Journal of Pathology and Bacteriology 81:365–378

Dubowitz V, Daniels RJ, Davies KE 1995 Olivopontocerebellar hypoplasia with anterior horn cell involvement (SMA) does not localize to chomosome 5q. Neuromuscular Disorders 5:25–29

Duchenne GBA 1861 De l'Electrisation Localisée et son Application à la Pathologie et à la Thérapeutique, 2nd edn. Baillière et Fils, Paris

Duchenne GBA 1868 Recherches sur la paralysie musculaire pseudohypertrophique ou paralysie myosclerosique. Archives Générales de Médecine 11:5, 179, 305, 421, 552

Dupond JL, Roberts M, Carbillet JP et al 1977 Glycogenose musculaire et anemie hemolytique par deficit enzymatique chex deux permains. Forme familiale de maladise de Tarui, par deficit en phosphofructokinase musculaire et erythrocytaire. Nouvelle Presse Medicale 6:2665–2668

Duran M, Hofkamp M, Rhead WJ et al 1986 Sudden child death and healthy affected family members with medium-chain acyl-coenzyme A dehydrogenase deficiency. Pediatrics 78:1052–1057

Dyck PJ, Thomas PK, Griffin JW et al 2005 Peripheral neuropathies, 4th edn. WB Saunders, London

Echaniz-Laguna A, Guiraud Chaumeil C, Tranchant C et al 2002 Homozygous exon 7 deletion of the SMN centromeric gene (SMN2): a potential susceptibility factor for adult-onset lower motor neuron disease. Journal of Neurology 249:290–293

Edström L, Thornell LE, Eriksson L 1980 A new type of hereditary distal myopathy with characteristic sarcoplasmic bodies and intermediate (skeletin) filaments. Journal of the Neurological Sciences 47:171–190

Edwards RHT 1971 Percutaneous needle-biopsy of skeletal muscle in diagnosis and research. Lancet ii:593–595

Edwards RHT, Maunder C, Lewis PD et al 1973 Percutaneous needle biopsy in the diagnosis of muscle diseases. Lancet ii:1070–1071

Edwards RHT, Round JM, Jones DA 1983 Needle biopsy of skeletal muscle: a review of 10 years' experience. Muscle and Nerve 6:676–683

Emery AEH 1977 Muscle histology and creatine kinase levels in the foetus in Duchenne muscular dystrophy. Nature (London) 266:472–473

Emery AEH 1980 Duchenne muscular dystrophy: genetic aspects, carrier detection and antenatal diagnosis. British Medical Bulletin 36:117–122

Emery AE 1989 Emery–Dreifuss muscular dystrophy and other related disorders. British Medical Bulletin 45:722–787

Emery AE 1991 Population frequencies of inherited neuromuscular diseases – a world survey. Neuromuscular Disorders 1:19–29

Emery AEH 1993 Duchenne muscular dystrophy. Oxford University Press, Oxford

Emery AEH, Dreifuss FE 1966 Unusual type of benign X-linked muscular dystrophy. Journal of Neurology, Neurosurgery and Psychiatry 29:338–342

Emery AEH, Emery MLH 1995 The history of a genetic disease: Duchenne muscular dystrophy or Meryon's disease. Royal Society of Medicine Press, London

Emser W, Schimrigk K 1977 Myxedema myopathy: a case report. European Neurology 16:286–291

Emslie-Smith AM, Engel AG 1990 Microvascular changes in early and advanced dermatomyositis: a quantitative study. Annals of Neurology 27:343–356

Eng GD, Epstein BS, Engel WK et al 1978 Malignant hyperthermia and central core disease in a child with congenital dislocating hips. Archives of Neurology (Chicago) 35:189–197

Engel AG 1966 Electron microscopic observations in thyrotoxic and corticosteroid-induced myopathies. Mayo Clinic Proceedings 41:797–808

Engel AG 1970 Evolution and content of vacuoles in primary hypokalemic periodic paralysis. Mayo Clinic Proceedings 45: 774–814

Engel AG 1972 Neuromuscular manifestations of Graves' disease. Mayo Clinic Proceedings 47:919–925

Engel AG, Angelini C 1973 Carnitine deficiency of human skeletal muscle with associated lipid storage myopathy: a new syndrome. Science 179:899–902

Engel AG, Arahata K 1984 Monoclonal antibody analysis of mononuclear cells in myopathies. II. Phenotypes of autoinvasive cells in polymyositis and inclusion body myositis. Annals of Neurology 16:209–215

Engel AG, Biesecker G 1982 Complement activation in muscle fiber necrosis: demonstration of the membrane attack complex of complement in necrotic fibers. Annals of Neurology 12:289–296

Engel AG, Hohlfeld R 2004 Acquired Autoimmune Myasthenia Gravis. In: Engel AG, Franzini-Armstrong C (eds) Myology, 3rd edn. McGrath-Hill, New York, pp 1755–1790

Engel AG, Gomez MR, Groover RV 1971 Multicore disease. Mayo Clinic Proceedings 10:666–681

Engel AG, Angelini C, Gomez MR 1972 Fingerprint body myopathy. Mayo Clinic Proceedings 47:377–388

Engel AG, Tsujihata M, Lindstrom JM, Lennon VA 1976 The motor end plate in myasthenia gravis and in experimental autoimmune myasthenia gravis. A quantitative ultrastructural study. Annals of the New York Academy of Sciences 274:60–79

Engel AG, Lambert EH, Howard FM 1977 Immune complexes (IgG and C3) at the motor end-plate in myasthenia gravis. Ultrastructural and light microscopic localization and electrophysiologic correlations. Mayo Clinic Proceedings 52:267–280

Engel AG, Rebouche CJ, Wilson DM et al 1981 Primary systemic carnitine deficiency. II. Renal handling of carnitine. Neurology 31:819–825

Engel AG, Ohno K, Sine SM 2003 Congenital myasthenic syndromes: A diverse array of molecular targets. Journal of Neurocytology 32:1017–1037

Engel AG, Ohno K, Sine S 2004 Congenital myasthenic syndromes. In: Engel AG, Franzini-Armstrong C (eds) Myology, 3rd edn. McGrath-Hill, New York, pp 1801–1844

Engel WK 1961 Muscle target fibres, a newly recognized sign of denervation. Nature (London) 191:389–390

Engel WK 1967 Focal myopathic changes produced by electromyographic and hypodermic needles. Archives of Neurology (Chicago) 16:509–511

Engel WK 1971 'Ragged-red fibers' in ophthalmoplegia syndromes and their differential diagnosis. Abstracts of the IInd International Congress on Muscle Diseases, November 1971, Perth, Australia, ICS No 237. Excerpta Medica, Amsterdam

Engel WK, Cunningham GC 1963 Rapid examination of muscle tissue. An improved trichrome method for fresh-frozen biopsy sections. Neurology 13:919–923

Engel WK, Foster JM, Hughes BP et al 1961 Central core disease – an investigation of a rare muscle cell abnormality. Brain 84:167–185

Engel WK, Brooke MH, Nelson PG 1966 Histochemical studies of denervated or tenotomized cat muscle. Illustrating difficulties in relating experimental animal conditions to human neuromuscular diseases. Annals of the New York Academy of Sciences 138:160–185

Engel WK, Bishop DW, Cunningham GG 1970a Tubular aggregates in type II muscle fibers: ultrastructural and histochemical correlation. Journal of Ultrastructural Research 31:507–525

Engel WK, Vick NA, Glueck CJ et al 1970b A skeletal muscle disorder associated with intermittent symptoms and a possible defect of lipid metabolism. New England Journal of Medicine 282:697–704

England SB, Nicholson LV, Johnson MA et al 1990 Very mild muscular dystrophy associated with the deletion of 46% of dystrophin. Nature 11:180–182

Eränkö O, Palkama A 1961 Improved localization of phosphorylase by the use of polyvinyl pyrrolidine and high substrate concentration. Journal of Histochemistry and Cytochemistry 9:585

Erb WH 1884 Ueber die 'juvenile form' der progressiven Muskelatrophie, ihri Beziehungen zur sogennanten Pseudohypertrophie der Muskeln. Deutsche Archiv für Klinische Medizin 34:467

Ervasti JM, Campbell KP 1991 Membrane organization of the dystrophin–glycoprotein complex. Cell 66:1121–1131

Ervasti JM, Campbell KP 1993 A role for the dystrophin–glycoprotein complex as a transmembrane linker between laminin and actin. Journal of Cell Biology 122: 809–823

Evans M, Rees A 2002a The myotoxicity of statins. Current Opinion in Lipidology 13:415–420

Evans M, Rees A 2002b Effects of HMG-CoA reductase inhibitors on skeletal muscle; all statins the same? Drug Safety 25:649–663

Fananapazir L, Dalakas MC, Cyran F et al 1993 Missense mutations in the beta-myosin heavy-chain gene cause central core disease in hypertrophic cardiomyopathy. Proceedings of the National Academy of Sciences of the United States of America 90:3993–3997

Fanin M, Angelini C 2002 Muscle pathology in dysferlin deficiency. Neuropathology and Applied Neurobiology 28:461–470

Fanin M, Danieli GA, Vitiello L et al 1992 Prevalence of dystrophin positive fibers in 85 Duchenne muscular dystrophy patients. Neuromuscular Disorders 2:41–45

Fardeau M, Tomé FM, Derambure S 1976 Familial fingerprint body myopathy. Archives of Neurology 33:724–725

Fardeau M, Godet-Guillain J, Tomé FMS et al 1978a Congenital neuromuscular disorders: a critical review. In: Aguayo AJ, Karpati G (eds) Current Topics in Nerve and Muscle Research. Excerpta Medica, Amsterdam, p 164

Fardeau M, Godet-Guillain J, Tomé FM et al 1978b A new familial muscular disorder demonstrated by the intra-sarcoplasmic accumulation of a granulo-filamentous material which is dense on electron microscopy (author's translation) Revue Neurologique (Paris) 134: 411–425 (French)

Fardeau M, Matsumura K, Tome FM et al 1993 Deficiency of the 50 kDa dystrophin associated glycoprotein (adhalin) in severe autosomal recessive muscular dystrophies in children native from European countries. Contes Rendus de l'Academie des Sciences. Serie III 316:799–804

Farkas-Bargeton E, Dibler M F, Arsénio-Nunes ML et al 1977 Etude de la maturation histochimique, quantitative et ultrastructurale du muscle foetal humain. Journal of the Neurological Sciences 31:245–258

Fenichel GM, Sul YC, Kilroy AW, Blouin R 1982 An autosomal-dominant dystrophy with humeropelvic distribution and cardiomyopathy. Neurology 32:1399–1401

Ferlini A, Sewry C, Melis MA et al 1999 X-linked dilated cardiomyopathy and the dystrophin gene. Neuromuscular Disorders 9:339–346

Fernandez C, Figarella-Branger D, Alla P et al 2002 Colchicine myopathy: a vacuolar myopathy with selective type I muscle fiber involvement. An immunohistochemical and electron microscopic study of two cases. Acta Neuropathologica (Berlin) 103:100–106

Ferreiro A, Estournet B, Chateau D et al 2000 Multi-minicore disease – searching for boundaries: phenotype analysis of 38 cases. Annals of Neurology 48, 745–757

Ferreiro A, Fardeau M 2002 80th ENMC International Workshop on Multi-Minicore Disease: 1st International MmD Workshop. 12–13 May 2000, Soestduinen, The Netherlands. Neuromuscular Disorders 12:60–68

Ferreiro A, Monnier N, Romero NB et al 2002a A recessive form of central core disease, transiently presenting as multi-minicore disease, is associated with a homozygous mutation in the ryanodine receptor type 1 gene. Annals of Neurology 51:750–759

Ferreiro A, Quijano-Roy S, Pichereau C et al 2002b Mutations of the selenoprotein N gene, which is implicated in rigid spine muscular dystrophy, cause the classical phenotype of multi-minicore disease: reassessing the nosology of early-onset myopathies. American Journal of Human Genetics 71:739–749

Ferreiro A, Ceuterick-de Groote C, Marks JJ et al 2004 Desmin-related myopathy with Mallory body-like inclusions caused by mutations of the selenoprotein N gene. Annals of Neurology 55:676–686

Fidzianska A 1976 Morphological differences between the atrophied small muscle fibres in amyotrophic lateral sclerosis and

Werdnig-Hoffman disease. Acta Neuropathologica 17:321–327

Fidzianska A, Badurska B, Ryniewicz B et al 1981 'Cap disease': new congenital myopathy. Neurology 31:1113–1120

Fidzianska A, Goebel HH, Osborn M et al 1983 Mallory body-like inclusions in a hereditary congenital neuromuscular disease. Muscle and Nerve 6:195–200

Fidzianska A, Toniolo D, Hausmanowa-Petrusewicz I 1998 Ultrastructural abnormality of sarcolemmal nuclei in Emery–Dreifuss muscular dystrophy (EDMD). Journal of Neurological Sciences 159:88–93

Figarella-Branger D, Nedelec J, Pellisier JF et al 1990 Expression of various isoforms of neural cell adhesive molecules and their highly polysialylated counterparts in diseased human muscles. Journal of the Neurological Sciences 98:21–36

Filipe MI, Lake B 1990 Histochemistry in pathology, 2nd edn. Churchill Livingstone, Edinburgh

Forbes GB 1953 Glycogen storage disease. Report of a case with abnormal glycogen structure in liver and skeletal muscle. Journal of Paediatrics 42:645–653

Frame B, Heinze EG, Block MA et al 1968 Myopathy in primary hyperparathyroidism. Observations in three patients. Annals of Internal Medicine 68:1022–1027

Frosk P, Greenberg CR, Tennese AA et al 2005 The most common mutation in FKRP causing limb girdle muscular dystrophy type 2I (LGMD2I) may have occurred only once and is present in Hutterites and other populations. Human Mutation 25:38–44

Fujii Otsu K, Zorzato F et al 1991 Identification of a mutation in porcine ryanodine receptor associated with malignant hyperthermia. Science 253:448–451

Fukunaga H, Engel AG, Lang B, Newsom-Davis J, Vincent A 1983 Passive transfer of Lambert-Eaton myasthenic syndrome with IgG from man to mouse depletes the presynaptic membrane active zones. Proceedings of the National Academy of Sciences of the United States of America 80:7636–7640

Fukuyama Y, Kawazura M, Haruna H 1960 A peculiar form of congenital progressive muscular dystrophy: report of fifteen cases. Pediatria Universitatis Tokio 4:5–8

Gache Y, Chavanas S, Lacour JP et al 1996 Defective expression of plectin/HD1 in epidermolysis bullosa simplex with muscular dystrophy. Journal of Clinical Investigation 97:2289–2298

Gambelli S, Dotti MT, Malandrini A et al 2004 Mitochondrial alterations in muscle biopsies of patients on statin therapy. Journal of Submicroscopic Cytology and Pathology 36:85–89

Gangopadhyay SB, Sherratt TG, Heckmatt JZ et al 1992 Dystrophin in frame shift deletion patients with Becker muscular dystrophy. American Journal of Human Genetics 51:562–570

Gerull B, Gramlich M, Atherton J et al 2002 Mutations of TTN, encoding the giant muscle filament titin, cause familial dilated cardiomyopathy. Nature Genetics 30:201–204

Glass IA, Nicholson LV, Watkiss E et al 1992 Investigation of a female manifesting Becker muscular dystrophy. Journal of Medical Genetics 29:578–582

Gnecchi-Ruscone R, Taylor J, Mercuri E et al 1999 Cardiomyopathy in Duchenne, Becker, and sarcoglycanopathies: a role for coronary dysfunction? Muscle Nerve 22:1549–1556

Gobbi P, Sewry C, Dunn M et al 1998 Dystrophin and sarcoglycan expression in dilated cardiomyopathies: a large population study. Neuromuscular Disorders 8:243

Godlewski HG 1963 Are active and inactive phosphorylase histochemically distinguishable? Journal of Histochemistry and Cytochemistry 11:108–112

Goebel H 2002 Rare myopathies of childhood. In: Karpati G (ed) Structural and molecular basis of skeletal muscle diseases. ISN Neuropathology Press, pp 287–289

Goebel HH, Anderson JR 1999 Structural congenital myopathies (excluding nemaline myopathy, myotubular myopathy, and desminopathies): 56th European Neuromuscular Center (ENMC) sponsored international workshop. Neuromuscular Disorders 9:50–57

Goebel HH, Borchert A 2002 Protein surplus myopathies and other rare congenital myopathies. Seminars in Paediatric Neurology 9:160–170

Goebel HH, Muller J, Gillen HW et al 1978 Autosomal dominant 'spheroid body myopathy'. Muscle and Nerve 1: 14–26

Goebel HH, Schloon H, Lenard HG 1981 Congenital myopathy with cytoplasmic bodies. Neuropediatrics 12:166–180

Goebel HH, Anderson JR, Hubner C et al 1997 Congenital myopathy with excess of thin myofilaments. Neuromuscular Disorders 7:160–168

Goebel HH, Brockmann K, Bönnemann CG et al 2004 Actin-related myopathy without any missense mutation in the ACTA1 gene. Journal of Child Neurology 19:149–153

Goldberg LR, Hausmanowa-Petrusewicz I, Fidzianska A et al 1998 A dystrophin missense mutation showing persistence of dystrophin and dystrophin-associated proteins yet a severe phenotype. Annals of Neurology 44:971–976

Goldfarb LG, Park KY, Cervenakova L et al 1998 Missense mutations in desmin associated with familial cardiac and skeletal myopathy. Nature Genetics 19: 402–403

Gosztonyi G, Naschold U, Grozdanovic Z et al 2001 Expression of Leu-19 (CD56, N-CAM) and nitric oxide synthase (NOS) 1 in denervated and reinnervated human skeletal muscle. Microscopy Research Technique 55:187–197

Gowers WR 1879 Pseudohypertrophic muscular paralysis. A clinical lecture. J&A Churchill, London

Greenberg SA, Pinkus JL, Pinkus GS et al 2005 Interferon-alpha/beta-mediated innate immune mechanisms in dermatomyositis. Annals of Neurology 57:664–678

Greenfield JG, Shy GM, Alvord EC et al 1957 An atlas of muscle pathology in neuromuscular diseases. Edinburgh: Livingstone

Greenfield JG, Cornman T, Shy GM 1958 The prognostic value of the muscle biopsy in the floppy infant. Brain 81:461–484

Gregorio CC, Granzier H, Sorimachi H et al 1999 Muscle assembly: a titanic achievement? Current Opinion in Cell Biology 11:181–225

Grewal PK, Holzfeind PJ, Bittner RE et al 2001 Mutant glycosyltransferase and altered glycosylation of alpha-dystroglycan in the myodystrophy mouse. Nature Genetics 28:151–154

Grohmann K, Schuelke M, Dires A et al 2001 Mutations in the gene encoding immunoglobulin mu-binding protein 2 cause spinal muscular atrophy with respiratory distress type 1. Nature Genetics 29:75–77

Gronert GA, Thompson RL, Onofrio BM 1980 Human malignant hyperthermia: awake episodes and correction by dantrolene. Anaesthesia and Analgesia 59:277–278

Gubitz AK, Feng W, Dreyfuss G 2004 The SMN complex. Experimental Cell Research 296:51–56

Guerard MJ, Sewry CA, Dubowitz V 1985 Lobulated fibers in neuromuscular diseases. Journal of the Neurological Sciences 69:345–356

Guibaud P, Carrier H, Mathieu M et al 1978 Familial congenital muscular dystrophy caused by phosphofructokinase deficiency. Archives of Francaises de Pediatrie 35:1105–1115

Guis S, Mattei JP, Liote F 2003 Drug-induced and toxic myopathies. Best Practice Research in Clinical Rheumatology 17:877–907

Gullberg D, Tiger CF, Velling T 1999 Laminins during muscle development and in muscular dystrophies. Cell and Molecular Life Sciences 56:442–460

Gurnett CA, Bodnar JA, Neil J, Connolly AM 2004 Congenital myasthenic syndrome: presentation, electrodiagnosis, and muscle biopsy. Journal of Child Neurology 19:175–182

Hackman P, Vihola A, Havavuori H et al 2002 Tibial muscular dystrophy is titinopathy caused by mutations in TTN, the gene encoding the giant skeletal-muscle protein titin. American Journal of Human Genetics 71:492–500

Hackman JP, Vihola AK, Udd AB 2003 The role of titin in muscular disorders. Annals of Medicine 35:434–441

Hale DE, Barshaw ML, Coates PM et al 1985 Long-chain acyl-coenzyme A dehydrogenase deficiency: an inherited cause of nonketotic hypoglycaemia. Pediatric Research 19:666–671

Hale DE, Stanley CA, Coates P 1990 The long-chain acyl-CoA dehydrogenase deficiency. In: Tanaka K, Coates PM (eds) Fatty Acid Oxidation: Clinical, Biochemical and Molecular Aspects. Alan R Liss, New York, pp 303–311

Haliloglu G, Topaloglu H 2004 Glycosylation defects in muscular dystrophies.

Current Opinion in Neurology 17: 521–527

Haller RG, Henriksson KG, Jorfeldt L et al 1991 Deficiency of skeletal muscle succinate dehydrogenase and aconitase: pathophysiology of exercise in a novel human muscle oxidative defect. Journal of Clinical Investigation 88:1197–1206

Haltia M, Leivo I, Somer H et al 1997 Muscle-eye-brain disease: a neuropathological study. Annals of Neurology 41:173–180

Han F, Lang AE, Racacho L et al 2003 Mutations in the epsilon-sarcoglycan gene found to be uncommon in seven myoclonus-dystonia families. Neurology 61:244–246

Hantai D, Richard P, Koenig J et al 2004 Congenital myasthenic syndromes. Current Opinion in Neurology 17:539–551

Harriman DG 1988 Malignant hyperthermia myopathy – a critical review. British Journal of Anaesthesia 60:309–316

Harriman DGF 1982 The pathology of malignant hyperpyrexia. In: Mastaglia FL, Walton J (eds) Skeletal muscle pathology. Churchill Livingstone, Edinburgh, pp 575–591

Hart Z, Chang CH 1988 A newborn infant with respiratory distress and stridulous breathing. Journal of Pediatrics 113: 150–155

Hatefi Y 1985 The mitochondrial electron transport and oxidative phosphorylation system. Annual Review of Biochemistry 54:1015–1069

Hauser MA, Horrigan SK, Salmikangas P et al 2000 Myotilin is mutated in limb girdle muscular dystrophy 1A. Human Molecular Genetics 9:2141–2147

Havard CWH 1972 Clinical endocrinology: endocrine exophthalmos. British Medical Journal 1:360–363

Havard CWH, Campbell EDR, Ross HB et al 1963 Electromyographic and histological findings in the muscles of patients with thyrotoxicosis. Quarterly Journal of Medicine 32:145–163

Hayashi YK, Engvall E, Arikawa-Hirasawa E et al 1993 Abnormal localization of laminin subunits in muscular dystrophies. Journal of Neurological Science 119:53–64

Hayashi YK, Chou FL, Engvall E et al 1998 Mutations in the integrin alpha7 gene cause congenital myopathy. Nature Genetics 19:94–97

Hayashi YK, Ogawa M, Tagawa K et al 2001 Selective deficiency of alpha-dystroglycan in Fukuyama-type congenital muscular dystrophy. Neurology 57:115–121

He Y, Jones KJ, Vignier N et al 2001 Congenital muscular dystrophy with primary partial laminin alpha2 chain deficiency: molecular study. Neurology 57:1319–1322

Heckmatt JZ, Leeman S, Dubowitz V 1982 Ultrasound imaging in the diagnosis of muscle disease. Journal of Paediatrics 101:656–660

Heckmatt JZ, Moosa A, Hutson C et al 1984 Diagnostic needle muscle biopsy: a practical and reliable alternative to open biopsy. Archives of Disease in Childhood 59:528–532

Heckmatt JZ, Sewry CA, Hodes D et al 1985 Congenital centronuclear (myotubular) myopathy. A clinical, pathological and genetic study in eight children. Brain 108:941–964

Helbling-Leclerc A, Zhang X, Topaloglu H et al 1995 Mutations in the laminin alpha 2-chain gene (LAMA2) cause merosin-deficient congenital muscular dystrophy. Nature Genetics 11:216–218

Helliwell TR, Ellis JM, Mountford RC et al 1992a A truncated dystrophin lacking the C-terminal domain is localized at the muscle membrane. American Journal of Human Genetics 50:508–514

Helliwell TR, Nguyen thi Man, Morris GE et al 1992b The dystrophin-related protein, utrophin, is expressed on the sarcolemma of regenerating human skeletal muscle fibres in dystrophies and inflammatory myopathies. Neuromuscular Disorders 2:177–184

Helliwell TR, Green AR, Green A et al 1994 Hereditary distal myopathy with granulo-filamentous cytoplasmic inclusions containing desmin, dystrophin and vimentin. Journal of Neurological Sciences 124:174–187

Helliwell TR, Ellis IH, Appleton RE 1998 Myotubular myopathy: morphological, immunohistochemical and clinical variation. Neuromuscular Disorders 8:152–161

Henriksson KG 1979 'Semi-open' muscle biopsy technique: a simple outpatient procedure. Acta Neurologica Scandinavica 59:317–323

Herman GE, Finegold M, Zhao W et al 1999 Medical complications in long-term survivors with X-linked myotubular myopathy. Journal of Pediatriatrics 134:206–214

Herrmann R, Straub V, Blank M et al 2000 Dissociation of the dystroglycan complex in caveolin-3-deficiency in limb girdle muscular dystrophy. Human Molecular Genetics 9:2335–2340

Hers HG 1959 Etudes enzymatiques sur fragments hēpatiques: application ē la classification des glycogenoses. Revue Internationale ā Hāpatologie 9:35–55

Hill CL, Zhang Y, Sigurgeirsson B et al 2001 Frequency of specific cancer types in dermatomyositis and polymyositis: a population-based study. Lancet 357:96–100

Hillaire D, Leclerc A, Faure S et al 1994 Localization of merosin-negative congenital muscular dystrophy to chromosome 6q2 by homozygosity mapping. Human Molecular Genetics 3:1657–1661

Hilton-Jones D 2001 Inflammatory muscle diseases. Current Opinion in Neurology 14:591–596

Hirano M, Ott BR, Raps EC et al 1992 Acute quadriplegic myopathy: a complication of treatment with steroids, nondepolarizing blocking agents, or both. Neurology 42:2082–2087

Ho M, Brown RH 2002 Caveolinopathies. In: Karpati G (ed) Structural and molecular basis of skeletal muscle. ISN Neuropathology Press, Basel, pp 33–36

Hodges BL, Hayashi YK, Nonaka I et al 1997 Altered expression of the alpha7beta1 integrin in human and murine muscular dystrophies. Journal of Cell Science 110:2873–2881

Hoffman EP, Brown RH, Kunkel LM 1987 Dystrophin: the protein product of the Duchenne muscular dystrophy locus. Cell 51:919–928

Hoffman EP, Pegaro E 2002 Heparin sulfate proteoglycan (perlecan) deficiency. Schwartz–Jampel syndrome. In: Karpati G (ed) Structural and molecular basis of skeletal muscle. ISN Neuropathology Press, Basel, pp 43–44

Hogan K 1998 The anesthetic myopathies and malignant hyperthermias. Current Opinion in Neurology 11:469–476

Holt IJ, Harding AE, Perry RKH et al 1990 A new mitochondrial disease associated with mitochondrial DNA heteroplasmy. American Journal of Human Genetics 46:428–433

Hoppel CL, Tomec RJ 1972 Carnitine palmityl transferase: location of two enzymatic activities in rat liver mitochondria. Journal of Biological Chemistry 247:832–841

Huizing M, Rakocevic G, Sparks SE et al 2004 Hypoglycosylation of alpha-dystroglycan in patients with hereditary IBM due to GNE mutations. Molecular Genetics and Metabolism 81:196–202

Ikezoe K, Furuya H, Ohyagi Y et al 2003 Dysferlin expression in tubular aggregates: their possible relationship to endoplasmic reticulum stress. Acta Neuropathologica (Berlin) 105:603–609

Ilkovski B, Nowak KJ, Domazetovska A et al 2004 Evidence for a dominant-negative effect in ACTA1 nemaline myopathy caused by abnormal folding, aggregation and altered polymerization of mutant actin isoforms. Human Molecular Genetics 13:1727–1743

Illingworth B, Cori GT 1952 Structures of glycogens and amylopectins III. Normal and abnormal human glycogen. Journal of Biological Chemistry 199:653–660

Illingworth B, Cori GT 1956 Amylo-1,6-glucosidase in muscle tissue in generalized glycogen storage disease. Journal of Biological Chemistry 218:123–129

Ionescu V, Radu H, Nicolescu P 1975 Identification of Duchenne muscular dystrophy carriers. Archives of Pathology 99:436–441

Isaacs H, Heffron JJA, Badenhorst M 1975 Central core disease: a correlated genetic, histochemical, ultrastructural and biochemical study. Journal of Neurology, Neurosurgery and Psychiatry 38:1177–1186

Isenberg DA 1983 Immunoglobulin deposition in skeletal muscle in primary muscle disease. Quarterly Journal of Medicine 207:297–310

Ishibashi-Ueda H, Imakita M, Yutani C et al 1990 Congenital nemaline myopathy with dilated cardiomyopathy autopsy study. Human Pathology 21:77–82

Ishii H, Hayashi YK, Nonaka L et al 1997 Electron microscopic examination of basal lamina in Fukuyama congenital muscular dystrophy. Neuromuscular Disorders 7: 191–197

Ishikawa H, Sugie K, Murayama K et al 2002 Ullrich disease: collagen VI deficiency: EM suggests a new basis for muscular weakness. Neurology 59:920–923

Ishikawa H, Sugie K, Murayame K et al 2004 Ullrich disease due to deficiency of collagen VI in the sarcolemma. Neurology 62:620–623

Itoh-Satoh M, Hayashi T, Nishi H 2002 Titin mutations as the molecular basis for dilated cardiomyopathy. Biochemical and Biophysical Research Communications 291:385–393

Izumo S, Nadal-Ginard B, Mahdavi V 1986 All members of the MHC multigene family respond to thyroid hormone in a highly tissue-specific manner. Science 231:597–600

Jakubiec-Puka A, Kordowska J, Catani C et al 1990 Myosin heavy chain isoform composition in striated muscle after denervation and self-reinnervation. European Journal Biochemistry 193:623–628

Jenis EH, Lindquist RR, Lister RC 1969 New congenital myopathy with crystalline intranuclear inclusions. Archives of Neurology (Chicago) 20:281–282

Jerusalem F, Angelini C, Engel AG et al 1973 Mitochondrial-lipid-glycogen (MLG) disease of muscle. Archives of Neurology (Chicago) 29:162–169

Jerusalem F, Ludin H, Bischoff A et al 1979 Cytoplasmic body neuromyopathy presenting as respiratory failure and weight loss. Journal of the Neurological Sciences 41:1–9

Jimenez-Mallebrera C, Torelli S, Brown SC et al 2003a Profound skeletal muscle depletion of alpha-dystroglycan in Walker–Warburg syndrome. European Journal of Paediatric Neurology 7:129–137

Jimenez-Mallebrera C, Brown SC, Sewry CA, Muntoni F 2005 Congenital muscular dystrophy: cellular and molecular aspects. Cellular and Molecular Life Sciences 62:809–823

Jobsis GJ, Keizers H, Vreijling JP et al 1996 Type VI collagen mutations in Bethlem myopathy, an autosomal dominant myopathy with contractures. Nature Genetics 14:113–115

Jockusch BM, Veldman H, Griffiths GW et al 1980 Immunofluorescence microscopy of a myopathy. α-Actinin is a major constituent of nemaline rods. Experimental Cell Research 127:409–420

Johnson MA, Polgar J, Weightman D et al 1973 Data on the distribution of fibre types in thirty-six human muscles. An autopsy study. Journal of Neurological Sciences 18:111–129

Johnston JJ, Kelley RI, Crawford TO et al 2000 A novel nemaline myopathy in the Amish caused by a mutation in troponin T1. American Journal of Human Genetics 67:814–821

Jungbluth H, Sewry C, Brown SC et al 2000 Minicore myopathy in children – A clinical and histopathological study of 19 cases. Neuromuscular Disorders 10:264–273

Jungbluth H, Sewry CA, Brown SC et al 2001 Mild phenotype of nemaline myopathy with sleep hypoventilation due to a mutation in the skeletal muscle alpha-actin (ACTA1) gene. Neuromuscular Disorders 11:35–40

Jungbluth H, Muller CR, Halliger-Keller B et al 2002 Autosomal recessive inheritance of RYR1 mutations in a congenital myopathy with cores. Neurology 59:284–287

Jungbluth H, Sewry CA, Buj-Bello A et al 2003 Early and severe presentation of X-linked myotubular myopathy in a girl with skewed X-inactivation. Neuromuscular Disorders 13:55–59

Jungbluth H, Davis MR, Muller C et al 2004a Magnetic resonance imaging of muscle in congenital myopathies associated with RYR1 mutations. Neuromuscular Disorders 14:785–790

Jungbluth H, Sewry CA, Councell S et al 2004b Magnetic resonance imaging of muscle in nemaline myopathy. Neuromuscular Disorders 14:779–784

Jungbluth H, Beggs A, Bonnemann C et al 2004c 111th ENMC International Workshop on Multi-minicore Disease. 2nd International MmD Workshop, 9–11 November 2002, Naarden, The Netherlands. Neuromuscular Disorders 14:754–766

Jurkat-Rott K, McCarthy T, Lehmann-Horn F 2000 Genetics and pathogenesis of malignant hyperthermia. Muscle and Nerve 23:4–17

Jurkat-Rott K, Müller-Höcker J, Pongratz D, Lehmann-Horn F 2002 Chloride and sodium channel myotonias. In: Karpati G (ed) Structural and molecular basis of skeletal muscle diseases. ISN Neuropathology Press, Basel, pp 90–94

Kaindl AM, Ruschendorf F, Krause S et al 2004 Missense mutations of ACTA1 cause dominant congenital myopathy with cores. Journal of Medical Genetics 41:842–848

Kalimo H, Savontaus ML, Lang H et al 1988 X-linked myopathy with excessive autophagy: a new hereditary muscle disease. Annals of Neurology 23:258–265

Kanagawa M, Saito F, Kenz S et al 2004. Molecular recognition by LARGE is essential for expression of functional dystroglycan. Cell 117:953–964

Karpati G, Hilton-Jones D, Griggs RS (eds) 2001 Disorders of voluntary muscle, 7th edn. Cambridge University Press, Cambridge

Karpati G 2002 Myosin heavy chain depletion syndrome. In: Karpati G (ed) Structural and molecular basis of skeletal muscle diseases. ISN Neuropathology Press, Basel, pp 83–84

Karpati G, Carpenter S, Engel AG et al 1975 The syndrome of systemic carnitine deficiency. Neurology 25:16–24

Karpati G, Pouliot Y, Carpenter S 1988 Expression of immunoreactive major histocompatibility complex products in human skeletal muscles. Annals of Neurology 23:64–72

Karpati G, Sinnreich M 2004 A clever road from myopathology to genes: the myotilin story Neurology 62:1248–1249

Kearns TP, Sayre GP 1958 Retinitis pigmentosa external ophthalmoplegia and complete heart block. Archives of Ophthalmology 60:280–289

Kennard C, Swash M, Huson RA 1980 Myopathy due to epsilon aminocaproic acid. Muscle and Nerve 3:202–206

Kennedy WR, Alter M, Sung JH 1968 Progressive proximal spinal and bulbar muscular atrophy of late onset. A sex-linked recessive trait. Neurology (Minneapolis) 18:671–680

Khaleeli AA, Gohil K, McPhail G et al 1983 Muscle morphology and metabolism in hypothyroid myopathy: effects of treatment. Journal of Clinical Pathology 36:519–526

Khan MA 1995 Effects of myotoxins on skeletal muscle fibres. Progress in Neurobiology 46:541–560

Kim DS, Hayashi YK, Matsumoto H et al 2004 POMT1 mutation results in defective glycosylation and loss of laminin-binding activity in alpha-DG. Neurology 62:1009–1011

King JO, Denborough MA 1973a Malignant hyperpyrexia in Australia and New Zealand. Medical Journal of Australia 1:525–528

King JO, Denborough MA 1973b Anesthetic induced malignant hyperpyrexia in children. Journal of Pediatrics 83:37–40

King RHM 1999 Atlas of peripheral nerve pathology. Arnold, London

Kingler W, Lechmann-Horn F, Jurkat-Rou K 2005 Complications of anaesthesia in neuromuscular disorders. Neuromuscular Disorders 15:195–206

Kingston HM, Sarfarazi M, Thomas NS et al 1984 Localisation of the Becker muscular dystrophy gene on the short arm of the X chromosome by linkage to cloned DNA sequences. Human Genetics 67:6–17

Kirschner J, Jausser I, Zou Y et al 2005 Ullrich congenital muscular dystrophy: connective tissue abnormalities in the skin support overlap with Ehlers–Danlos syndromes. American Journal of Medical Genetics 30:296–301

Kissel P, Schmitt J, Due M et al 1970 Myasthenia and thyrotoxicosis. In: Walton JN, Canal N, Scarlato G (eds) Muscle diseases. ICS No 199. Excerpta Medica, Amsterdam, p 464

Kobayashi H, Baumbach L, Matise TC et al 1995 A gene for a severe lethal form of X-linked arthrogryposis (X-linked infantile spinal muscular atrophy) maps to human chromosome Xp11.3-q11.2. Human Molecular Genetics 4:1213–1216

Koenig M, Hoffman EP, Bertelson CJ et al 1987 Complete cloning of the Duchenne muscular dystrophy (DMD) cDNA and preliminary genomic organization of the DMD gene in normal and affected individuals. Cell 50:509–517

Kubisch C, Schoser BG, von During M et al 2003 Homozygous mutations in caveolin-3 cause a severe form of rippling muscle disease. Annals of Neurology 53:512–520

La Spada AR, Wilson EM, Lubahn DB et al 1991 Androgen receptor gene mutation in X-linked spinal and bulbar muscular atrophy. Nature 352:77–79

Laing NG, Wilton SD, Akkari PA et al 1995 A mutation in the alpha tropomyosin gene TPM3 associated with autosomal dominant nemaline myopathy. Nature Genetics 9:75–79

Laing NG, Clarke NF, Dye DE et al 2004 Actin mutations are one cause of congenital fibre type disproportion. Annals of Neurology 56:689–694

Laing NG, Ceuterick-de Groote C, Dye DE et al 2005 Myosin storage myopathy: slow skeletal myosin (MYH7) mutation in two isolated cases. Neurology 64:527–529

Lake BD, Wilson J 1975 Zebra body myopathy: clinical, histochemical and ultrastructural studies. Journal of the Neurological Sciences 24:437–446

Lamande SR, Bateman JF, Hutchinson W et al 1998a Reduced collagen VI causes Bethlem myopathy: a heterozygous COL6A1 nonsense mutation results in mRNA decay and functional haploinsufficiency. Human Molecular Genetics 7:981–989

Lamande SR, Sigala E, Pan TC et al 1998b The role of the alpha3(VI) chain in collagen VI assembly. Expression of an alpha3(VI) chain lacking N-terminal modules N10-N7 restores collagen VI assembly, secretion, and matrix deposition in an alpha3(VI)-deficient cell line. Journal of Biological Chemistry 273:7423–7430

Lammens M, Moerman P, Fryns JP et al 1997 Fetal akinesia sequence caused by nemaline myopathy. Neuropediatrics 28:116–119

Lamont PJ, Dubowitz V, Landon DN et al 1998 Fifty year follow-up of a patient with central core disease shows slow but definite progression. Neuromuscular Disorders 8:385–391

Lampe AK, Bushby KM 2005 Collagen VI related muscle disorders. J Med Genet 42:673–685

Lampe AK, Dunn DM, von Niederhausem AC et al 2005 Automated genomic sequence analysis of the three collagen VI genes: applications to Ullrich congenital muscular dystrophy and Bethlem myopathy. Journal of Medical Genetics 42:108–120

Lane RJM 1996a Toxic and drug-induced myopathies. In: Lane RJM (ed) Handbook of muscle disease. Marcel Dekker, New York, pp 391–405

Lane RJM 1996b HIV-related myopathies. In: Lane RJM (ed) Handbook of muscle disease. Marcel Dekker, New York, pp 623–627

Lane RJM, Mastaglia FL 1978 Drug-induced myopathies in man. Lancet 2:562–565

Lane RJM, Phillips M 2003 Rhabdomyolysis. British Medical Journal 327:115–116

Lane RJM, Radoff FM 1981 Alcohol and serum creatine kinase levels. Annals of Neurology 10:581–582

Lane RJM, McLelland NJ, Martin AM et al 1979 Epsilon aminocaproic acid myopathy. Postgraduate Medical Journal 55:282–285

Lane RJM, McLean KA, Moss J et al 1993 Myopathy in HIV infection: the role of zidovudine and the significance of tubuloreticular inclusions. Neuropathology and Applied Neurobiology 19:406–413

Lang B, Vincent A 2002 The Lambert–Eaton myasthenic syndrome. In: Karpati G (ed) Structural and molecular basis of skeletal muscle diseases. ISN Neuropathology Press, Basel, pp 166–169

Laporte J, Biancalana V, Tanner SM et al 2000 MTM1 mutations in X-linked myotubular myopathy. Human Mutations 15:393–409

Laporte J, Kress W, Mandel JL 2001 Diagnosis of X-linked myotubular myopathy by detection of myotubularin. Annals of Neurology 50:42–46

Larsson NG, Holme E, Kristiansson B et al 1990 Progressive increase of the mutated mitochondrial DNA fraction in Kearns–Sayre syndrome. Pediatric Research 28:131–136

Layzer RB, Rowland LP, Ranney HM 1967 Muscle phosphofructokinase deficiency. Archives of Neurology (Chicago) 17:512–523

Layzer RB, Havel RJ, McIlroy MB 1980 Partial deficiency of carnitine palmityltransferase: physiologic and biochemical consequences. Neurology 30:627–633

Levitt RC, Olckers A, Meyers S et al 1992 Evidence for the localization of a malignant hyperthermia susceptibility locus (MHS2) to human chromosome 17q. Genomics 14:562–566

Lewis PD 1972 Neuromuscular involvement in pituitary gigantism. British Medical Journal 1:499–500

Lewis PD, Pallis C, Pearse AGE 1971 'Myopathy' with tubular aggregates. Journal of the Neurological Sciences 13:381–388

Libby RT, Champliaud MF, Claudepierre T et al 2000 Laminin expression in adult and developing retinae: evidence of two novel CNS laminins. Journal of the Neurosciences 20:6517–6528

Lim LE, Campbell KP 1998 The sarcoglycan complex in limb-girdle muscular dystrophy. Current Opinion in Neurology 11:443–452

Liu J, Aoki M, Illa I et al 1998 Dysferlin, a novel skeletal muscle gene, is mutated in Miyoshi myopathy and limb girdle muscular dystrophy. Nature Genetics 20:31–36

Loehr JP, Goodman WI, Frerman FE 1990 Glutaric acidemia type II: Heterogeneity of clinical and biochemical phenotypes. Pediatric Research 27:311–315

Lojda Z, Gossrau R, Schiebler TH 1979 Enzyme histochemistry: A laboratory manual. Springer Verlag, Berlin

Loke J, MacLennan DH 1998 Malignant hyperthermia and central core disease: disorders of Ca^{2+} release channels. American Journal of Medicine 104:470–486

Lombes A, Mendell JR, Nakase H et al 1989 Myoclonic epilepsy and ragged-red fibers with cytochrome c oxidase deficiency: neuropathology, biochemistry, and molecular genetics. Annals of Neurology 26:20–33

Longman C, Brockington M, Torelli S et al 2003 Mutations in the human LARGE gene cause MDC1D, a novel form of congenital muscular dystrophy with severe mental retardation and abnormal glycosylation of alpha-dystroglycan. Human Molecular Genetics 12:2853–2861

Lovitt S, Marden FA, Gundogdu B et al 2004 MRI in myopathy. Neurology Clinic 22:509–538

Lu QL, Morris GE, Wilson SD et al 2000 Massive idiosyncratic exon skipping corrects the nonsense mutation in dystrophic mouse muscle and produces functional revertant fibers by clonal expansion. Journal of Cell Biology 6:985–996

Luft R, Ikkos D, Palmieri G et al 1962 A case of severe hypermetabolism of nonthyroid origin with a defect in the maintenance of mitochondrial respiratory control: a correlated clinical, biochemical, and morphological study. Journal of Clinical Investigation 41:1776–1804

Lundberg PO, Osterman PO, Stålberg E 1970 Neuromuscular signs and symptoms in acromegaly. In: Walton JN, Canal N, Scarlato G (eds) Muscle Diseases. ICS No 199. Excerpta Medica, Amsterdam, p 531

Luu JY, Bockus D, Remington F et al 1989 Tubuloreticular structures and cylindrical confronting cisternae: a review. Human Pathology 20:617–627

Macdonald RD, Engel AG 1969 The cytoplasmic body: another structural anomaly of the Z disc. Acta Neuropathologica (Berlin) 14:99–107

Machuca-Tzili L, Brook D, Hilton-Hones D 2005 Clinical and molecular aspects of the myotonic dystrophies: A review. Muscle and Nerve 32:1–318

Magee KR, Shy GM 1956 A new congenital non-progressive myopathy. Brain 79:610–621

Mair WGP, Tomé FMS 1972 Atlas of the ultrastructure of diseased human muscle. Churchill Livingstone, Edinburgh

Mallette IE, Patten BM, Engel WK 1975 Neuromuscular disease in secondary hyperparathyroidism. Annals of Internal Medicine 82: 474–483

Mandel JL, Laporte J, Buj-Bello A, Sewry C, Wallgren-Pettersson C 2002 X-linked myotubular myopathy. In: Karpati G (ed) Structural and molecular basis of skeletal muscle diseases. ISN Neuropathology Press, Basel, pp 124–129

Manilal S, Nguyen TM, Sewry CA et al 1996 The Emery–Dreifuss muscular dystrophy protein, emerin, is a nuclear membrane protein. Human Molecular Genetics 5:801–808

Manilal S, Sewry CA, Nguyen thi Man et al 1997 Diagnosis of X-linked Emery–Dreifuss muscular dystrophy by protein analysis of leukocytes and skin. Neuromuscular Disorders 7:63–66

Manilal S, Recan D, Sewry CA et al 1998 Mutations in Emery–Dreifuss muscular dystrophy and their effects on emerin protein expression. Human Molecular Genetics 7:855–864

Manilal S, Sewry CA, Pereboev A et al 1999 Distribution of emerin and lamins in the heart and implications for Emery–Dreifuss muscular dystrophy. Human Molecular Genetics 8:353–359

Mankodi A, Logigian E, Callahan L et al 2000 Myotonic dystrophy in transgenic mice expressing an expanded CUG repeat. Science 289:1769–1773

Manta P, Terzis G, Papadimitriou C et al 2004 Emerin expression in tubular aggregates. Acta Neuropathologica (Berlin) 107:546–552

Manya H, Sakai K, Kobayashi K et al 2003 Loss-of-function of an N-acetylglucosaminyltransferase, POMGnT1, in muscle-eye-brain disease. Biochemistry Biophysics and Research Communications 306:93–97

Manzur AY, Sewry CA, Ziprin J et al 1998 A severe clinical and pathological variant of central core disease with possible autosomal recessive inheritance. Neuromuscular Disorders 8:467–473

Marston SB, Redwood CS 2003 Modulation of thin filament activation by breakdown or isoform switching of thin filament proteins: physiological and pathological implications. Circulation Research 93:1170–1178

Martin JE, Mather K, Swash M et al 1991 Expression of heat shock protein epitopes in tubular aggregates. Muscle and Nerve 14:219–225

Martinsson T, Oldford A, Darin N et al 2000 Autosomal dominant myopathy: missense mutation (Glu-706 Lys) in the myosin heavy chain IIa gene. Proceedings of the National Academy of Sciences of the United States of America 97:14614–14619

Mastaglia FL 1973 Pathological changes in skeletal muscle in acromegaly. Acta Neuropathologica (Berlin) 23:273–286

Mastaglia FL, Barwick DD, Hall R 1970 Myopathy in acromegaly Lancet ii:907–909

Mathieu J, Lapointe G, Brassard A et al 1997 A pilot study on upper esophageal sphincter dilatation for the treatment of dysphagia in patients with oculopharyngeal muscular dystrophy. Neuromuscular Disorders 7:S100–104

Matsuda C, Kayashi YK, Ogawa M et al 2001 The sarcolemmal proteins dysferlin and caveolin-3 interact in skeletal muscle. Human Molecular Genetics 10:1761–1766

Matsumura K, Nonaka I, Campbell KP 1993 Abnormal expression of dystrophin-associated proteins in Fukuyama-type congenital muscular dystrophy. Lancet 341:521–522

Maunder-Sewry CA, Dubowitz V 1981 Needle muscle biopsy for carrier detection in Duchenne muscular dystrophy Part 1.

Journal of the Neurological Sciences 49:305–324

Mayer U 2003 Integrins: redundant or important players in skeletal muscle? Journal of Biology Chemistry 278:14587–14590

McCarthy TV, Quane KA, Lynch PJ 2000 Ryanodine receptor mutations in malignant hyperthermia and central core disease. Human Mutation 15:410–417

McConchie SM, Coakley J, Edwards RH et al 1990 Molecular heterogeneity in McArdle's disease. Biochimica et Biophysica Acta 1096:26–32

McDouall RM, Dunn MJ, Dubowitz V 1989 Expression of class I and II MHC antigens in neuromuscular diseases. Journal of the Neurological Sciences 89:213–226

McEntagart M, Parsons G, Buj-Bello A et al 2002 Genotype–phenotype correlations in X-linked myotubular myopathy. Neuromuscular Disorders 12:939–946

McFadzean AJS, Yeung R 1967 Periodic paralysis complicating thyrotoxicosis in Chinese. British Medical Journal 1:451–455

McLennan 1992 Malignant hyperthermia. Science 25:789–794

McNally EM, de Sa Moreira E, Duggan DJ et al 1998 Caveolin-3 in muscular dystrophy. Human Molecular Genetics 7:871–877

McShane MA, Hammans SR, Sweeney M et al 1991 Pearson syndrome and mitochondrial encephalopathy in a patient with a deletion of mtDNA. American Journal of Human Genetics 48:39–42

Meinehofer MC, Askanas V, Proux-Daegelen D et al 1977 Muscle-type phosphorylase activity present in muscle cells cultured from three patients with myophosphorylase deficiency. Archives of Neurology (Chicago) 34:779–781

Meltzer HY, Kuncl RW, Click J et al 1976 Incidence of Z band streaming and myofibrillar disruption in skeletal muscle from healthy young people. Neurology 26:853–857

Mendell JR, Sahenk Z, Gales T et al 1991 Amyloid filaments in inclusion body myositis. Novel findings provide insight into nature of filaments. Archives of Neurology 48:1229–1234

Meola G 2000 Myotonic dystrophies. Current Opinion in Neurology 13:519–525

Meola G, Moxley RT 2004 Myotonic dystrophy type 2 and related myotonic disorders. Journal of Neurology 251:1173–1182

Mercuri C, Counsell S, Allsop J et al 2001 Selective muscle involvement on magnetic resonance imaging in autosomal dominant Emery–Dreifuss muscular dystrophy. Neuropediatrics 33:10–14

Mercuri E, Yuva Y, Brown SC et al 2002 Collagen VI involvement in Ullrich syndrome: a clinical, genetic, and immunohistochemical study. Neurology 14:1354–1359

Mercuri E, Brockington M, Straub V et al 2003 Phenotypic spectrum associated with mutations in the fukutin-related protein gene. Annals of Neurology 53:537–542

Mercuri E, Jungbluth H, Muntoni F 2005 Muscle imaging in clinical practice: diagnostic value of muscle magnetic resonance imaging in inherited neuromuscular disorders. Current Opinion in Neurology 5:526–537

Meredith C, Herrmann R, Parry C et al 2004 Mutations in the slow skeletal muscle fiber myosin heavy chain (MYH7) cause Laing early-onset distal myopathy (MPD1). American Journal of Human Genetics 75:703–708

Merlini L, Villanova M, Sabatelli P et al 1999 Decreased expression of laminin β1 in chromosome 21-linked Bethlem myopathy. Neuromuscular Disorders 9:326–329

Meryon E 1852 On granular and fatty degeneration of the voluntary muscles. Medico-Chirurgical Transactions 35:73

Mian L, Dickson DW, Spiro AJ 1997 Abnormal expression of laminin β1 chain in skeletal muscle of adult-onset limb-girdle muscular dystrophy. Archives of Neurology 54:1457–1461

Michel RN, Dunn SE, Chin ER 2004 Calcineurin and skeletal muscle growth. Proceedings of the Nutrition Society 63:341–349

Michele DE, Campbell KP 2003 Dystrophin-glycoprotein complex: post-translational processing and dystroglycan function. Journal of Biological Chemistry 278:15457–15460

Midroni G, Bilbao JM 1995 Diagnosis of peripheral neuropathology. Butterworth-Heinemann, Boston

Miller RG, Layzer RB, Mellenthin MA et al 1985 Emery–Dreifuss muscular dystrophy with autosomal dominant transmission. Neurology 35:1230–1233

Miller FW 1993 Myositis-specific autoantibodies. Touchstones for understanding the inflammatory myopathies. JAMA 270:1846–1849

Miller G, Heckmatt JZ, Dubowitz V 1983 Drug treatment of juvenile dermatomyositis. Archives of Disease in Childhood 58:445–450

Millevoi S, Trombitas K, Kolmerer B et al 1998 Characterization of nebulette and nebulin and emerging concepts of their role for vertebrate Z-discs. Journal of Molecular Biology 282:111–123

Millikan CG, Haines SF 1953 The thyroid gland in relation to neuromuscular disease. Archives of Internal Medicine 82:5–39

Minetti C, Bado M, Broda P et al 2002 Impairment of caveolae formation and T-system disorganization in human muscular dystrophy with caveolin-3 deficiency. American Journal of Pathology 160:265–270

Minetti C, Bado M, Morreale G et al 1996 Disruption of muscle basal lamina in congenital muscular dystrophy with merosin deficiency. Neurology 46:1354–1358

Minetti C, Sotgia F, Bruno C et al 1998 Mutations in the caveolin-3 gene cause autosomal dominant limb-girdle muscular dystrophy. Nature Genetics 18:365–368

Mirabella M, Alvarez RB, Bilak M et al 1996 Difference in expression of phosphorylated tau epitopes between sporadic inclusion-body myositis and hereditary inclusion-body myopathies. Journal of Neuropathology and Experimental Neurology 55:774–786

Mitchell G, Heffron JJ 1982 Porcine stress syndromes. Advances in Food Research 28:167–230

Mogensen J, Klausen IC, Pedersen AK et al 1999 Alpha-cardiac actin is a novel, disease gene in familial hypertrophic cardiomyopathy. Journal of Clinical Investigations 103:R39–43

Mokri B, Engel AG 1975 Duchenne dystrophy: electron microscopic findings pointing to a basic or early abnormality in the plasma membrane of the muscle fiber. Neurology 25:1111–1120

Monnier N, Romero NB, Lerale J et al 2000 An autosomal dominant congenital myopathy with cores and rods is associated with a neomutation in the RYR1 gene encoding the skeletal muscle ryanodine receptor. Human Molecular Genetics 9:2599–2608

Monnier N, Romero NB, Lerale J et al 2001 Familial and sporadic forms of central core disease are associated with mutations in the C-terminal domain of the skeletal muscle ryanodine receptor. Human Molecular Genetics 10:2581–2592

Monnier N, Ferreiro A, Marty I et al 2003 A homozygous splicing mutation causing a depletion of skeletal muscle RYR1 is associated with multi-minicore disease congenital myopathy with ophthalmoplegia. Human Molecular Genetics 12:1171–1178

Moosa A, Dubowitz V 1971 Slow nerve conduction velocity in cretins. Archives of Disease in Childhood 46:852–854

Moosmann B, Behl C 2004 Selenoprotein synthesis and side-effects of statins. Lancet 363:892–894

Moreira ES, Vainzof M, Marie SK et al 1997 The seventh form of autosomal recessive limb-girdle muscular dystrophy is mapped to 17q11-12. American Journal of Human Genetics 61:151–159

Moreira ES, Wiltshire TJ, Gaulkner G et al 2000 Limb girdle muscular dystrophy type 2G is caused by mutations in the gene encoding the sarcomeric protein telethonin. Nature Genetics 24:163–166

Morgan BP, Sewry CA, Siddle K et al 1984 Immunolocalization of complement component C9 on necrotic and non-necrotic muscle fibres in myositis using monoclonal antibodies: a primary role of complement in autoimmune cell damage. Immunology 52:181–188.

Morgan-Hughes JA 1992 Mitochondrial myopathies. In: Mastaglia FL, Walton J (eds) Skeletal muscle pathology. Churchill Livingstone, Edinburgh, pp 367–424

Morgan-Hughes JA 2001 Tubular aggregates in skeletal muscle: their functional significance and mechanisms of pathogenesis. Current Opinion in Neurology 11:439–442

Morisawa Y, Fujieda M, Murakami N et al 1998 Lysosomal glycogen storage disease with normal acid maltase with early fatal outcome. Journal of Neurological Sciences 160:175–179

Mostacciuolo ML, Miorin M, Martinello F et al 1996 Genetic epidemiology of congenital muscular dystrophy in a sample from north-east Italy. Human Genetics 97:277–279

Mounkes L, Kozliv S, Burke B et al 2003 The laminopathies: nuclear structure meets disease. Current Opinion in Genetics and Development 13:223–230

Mounkes LC, Stewart CL 2004 Aging and nuclear organisation: lamins and progeria. Current Opinion in Cell Biology 16:322–327

Mukuno K 1969 Electron microscopic studies on human extraocular muscles under pathologic conditions. I. Rod formation in normal and diseased muscles (polymyositis and ocular myasthenia). Japanese Journal of Ophthalmology 13:35–51

Müller R, Kugelberg E 1959 Myopathy in Cushing's syndrome. Journal of Neurology, Neurosurgery and Psychiatry 22:314–319

Muller-Felber W, Schlotter B, Topfer M et al 1999 Phenotypic variability in two brothers with sarcotubular myopathy. Neurology 246:408–411

Muller-Hocker J, Schafer S, Mendel B et al 2000 Nemaline cardiomyopathy in a young adult: an ultraimmunohistochemical study and review of the literature. Ultrastructural Pathology 24:407–416

Mullin BR, Levinson RE, Friedman A et al 1977 Delayed hypersensitivity in Graves' disease and exophthalmos: identification of thyroglobulins in normal human orbital muscle. Endocrinology 100:351–366

Munoz-Marmol AM, Strasser G, Isamat M et al 1998 A dysfunctional desmin mutation in a patient with severe generalized myopathy. Proceedings of the National Academy of Sciences of the United States of America 95:11312–11317

Munsat T, Davies KE 1992 Report on International SMA Consortium Meeting held in Bonn, Germany, June 1992. Neuromuscular Disorders 2:423–428

Munsat TL 1991 Workshop report: International collaboration. Neuromuscular Disorders 1:81

Muntoni F 2005 Walker–Warburg syndrome and limb girdle muscular dystrophy; two sides of the same coin. Neuromuscular Disorders 15:269–270

Muntoni F, Guicheney P 2002 85th ENMC International Workshop on Congenital Muscular Dystrophy, 6th international CMD workshop, 1st workshop of the MYO-CLUSTER project GENRE, 27–28th October

2000, Naarden, The Netherlands. Neuromuscular Disorders 12:69–78

Muntoni F, Sewry CA 1998 Congenital muscular dystrophy: from rags to riches. Neurology 51:14–16

Muntoni F, Sewry CA 2003 Central core disease: new findings in an old disease. Brain 126:2339–2340

Muntoni F, Voit T 2004 The congenital muscular dystrophies in 2004: a century of exciting progress. Neuromuscular Disorders 14:635–649

Muntoni F, Gobbi P, Sewry C et al 1994a Deletions in the 5′ region of dystrophin and resulting phenotypes. Journal of Medical Genetics 31:843–847

Muntoni F, Catani G, Mateddu A et al 1994b Familial cardiomyopathy, mental retardation and myopathy associated with desmin-type intermediate filaments. Neuromuscular Disorders 4:233–241

Muntoni F, Sewry C, Wilson L et al 1995a Prenatal diagnosis in congenital muscular dystrophy. Lancet 345:591

Muntoni F, Wilson L, Marrosu G et al 1995b A mutation in the dystrophin gene selectively affecting dystrophin expression in the heart. Journal of Clinical Investigations 96:693–699

Muntoni F, Lichtarowicz-Krynska EJ, Sewry CA et al 1998 Early presentation of X-linked Emery–Dreifuss muscular dystrophy resembling limb-girdle muscular dystrophy. Neuromuscular Disorders 8:72–76

Muntoni F, Goodwin F, Sewry C et al 1999 Clinical spectrum and diagnostic difficulties of infantile ponto-cerebellar hypoplasia type 1. Neuropediatrics 30:243–248

Muntoni F, Brockington M, Blake DJ et al 2002a Defective glycosylation in muscular dystrophy. Lancet 360:1419–1421

Muntoni F, Bertini E, Bönnemann C et al 2002b 98th ENMC International Workshop on Congenital Muscular Dystrophy (CMD), 7th workshop of the international consortium on CMD, 2nd workshop of the MYO-CLUSTER project GENRE, 26–28th October 2001, Naarden, The Netherlands. Neuromuscular Disorders 12:889–896

Muntoni F, Valero de Bernabe B, Bittner R et al 2003 114th International Workshop on Congenital Muscular Dystrophy (CMD), 8th workshop of the international consortium on CMD, 3rd workshop of the MYO-CLUSTER project GENRE, 17–19 January, Naarden, The Netherlands. Neuromuscular Disorders 13:579–588

Muntoni F, Brockington M, Torelli S, Brown SC 2004 Defective glycosylation in congenital muscular dystrophies. Current Opinion in Neurology 17:205–209

Nagano A, Arahata K 2000 Nuclear envelope proteins and associated diseases. Current Opinion in Neurology 13:533–539

Nagulesparen M, Trickey R, Davies MJ et al 1976 Muscle changes in acromegaly. British Medical Journal 2:914–915

Nakahara K, Kuriyama M, Sonoda Y et al 1998 Myopathy induced by HMG-CoA reductase inhibitors in rabbits: a pathological, electrophysiological, and biochemical study. Toxicology and Applied Pharmacology 152:99–106

Naom I, Sewry C, D'Alessandro M et al 1997 Prenatal diagnosis of merosin congenital muscular dystrophy: the role of linkage and immunocytochemical analysis. Neuromuscular Disorders 7:176–179

Navarro CL, De Sandre-Giovannoli A, Bernard R et al 2004 Lamin A and ZMPSTE24 (FACE-1) defects cause nuclear disorganization and identify restrictive dermopathy as a lethal neonatal laminopathy. Human Molecular Genetics 13:2493–2503

Naylor EW, Mosovich LL, Guthrie R et al 1980 Intermittent non-ketotic dicarboxylic aciduria in two siblings with hypoglycaemia: an apparent defect in beta-oxidation of fatty acids. Journal of Inherited Metabolic Diseases 3:19–24

Neerunjun JS, Dubowitz V 1977 Regeneration of muscles transplanted between normal and dystrophic mice: a quantitative study of early transplants. Journal of Anatomy 124:459–467

Neville H, Brooke MH 1973 Central core fibers: structured and unstructured. In: Kakulas B (ed) Basic research in mycology. Proceedings of International Congress on Muscle Diseases, Perth, Australia, November 1971, Part 1. ICS No. 294. Excerpta Medica, Amsterdam, pp 497–511

Neville HE 1979 Ultrastructural changes in diseases of human skeletal muscle. In: Vinken PJ, Bruyn GW (eds) Handbook of clinical neurology, Vol 40. Diseases of

Muscle, Part 1. Amsterdam, North-Holland, pp 63–123

Neville H, Maunder-Sewry CA, McDougall J et al 1979 Chloroquine-induced cytosomes with curvilinear profiles in muscle. Muscle and Nerve 2:376–381

Neville HE, Ringel SP, Guggenheim MA et al 1983 Ultrastructural and histochemical abnormalities of skeletal muscle in patients with chronic vitamin E deficiency. Neurology 33:483–488

Nguyen HT, Gubis RM, Wydro RM et al 1982 Sarcomeric myosin heavy chain is coded by a highly conserved multigene family. Proceedings of the National Academy of Sciences of the United States of America 79:5230–5240

Nicholson LV, Johnson MA, Bushby KM et al 1993 Integrated study of 100 patients with Xp21 linked muscular dystrophy using clinical, genetic, immunochemical, and histopathological data. Part 2. Correlations within individual patients. Journal of Medical Genetics 30:737–744

Nicholson LV, Johnson MA, Bushby KM et al 1993b Integrated study of 100 patients with Xp21 linked muscular dystrophy using clinical, genetic, immunochemical, and histopathological data. Part 3. Differential diagnosis and prognosis. Journal of Medical Genetics 30:745–751

Nicole S, Davoine CS, Topaloglu H et al 2000 Perlecan, the major proteoglycan of basement membranes, is altered in patients with Schwartz–Jampel syndrome (chondrodystropic myotonia). Nature Genetics 26:480–483

Nigro V, Okazaki Y, Belsito A et al 1997 Identification of the Syrian hamster cardiomyopathy gene. Human Molecular Genetics 6:601–607

Nishino I, Spinazzola A, Hirano M 1999 Thymidine phosphorylase gene mutations in MNGIE, a human mitochondrial disorder. Science 283:689–692

Nishino L, Fu J, Tanji K et al 2000 Primary LAMP-2 deficiency causes X-linked vacuolar cardiomyopathy and myopathy (Danon disease). Nature 406:906–910

Nomizu S, Person DA, Saito C et al 1992 A unique case of reducing body myopathy. Muscle and Nerve 15:463–466

Nonaka I, Koga Y, Shikura K et al 1988 Muscle pathology in cytochrome c oxidase deficiency. Acta Neuropathologica 77:152–160

Nonaka I, Noguchi S, Nishino I 2005 Distal myopathy with rimmed vacuoles and hereditary inclusion body myopathy. Current Neurology and Neuroscience Reports 5:61–65

Norris FH, Panner BJ 1966 Hypothyroid myopathy. Archives of Neurology (Chicago) 14:574–589

North K 2004 Congenital myopathies. In: Engel AG, Franzini-Armstrong C (eds) Myology, 3rd edn. McGrath-Hill, New York, pp 1473–1533

North KN, Beggs AH 1996 Deficiency of a skeletal muscle isoform of alpha-actinin (alpha-actinin-3) in merosin-positive congenital muscular dystrophy. Neuromuscular Disorders 6:229–235

North KN, Laing NG, Wallgren-Pettersson C et al and the ENMC International Consortium on Nemaline Myopathy 1997 Nemaline myopathy: current concepts. Journal of Medical Genetics 34:705–713

North KN, Yang N, Wattanasirichaigoon D et al 1999 A common nonsense mutation results in α-actinin-3 deficiency in the general population. Nature Genetics 21:353–354

Nowak KJ, Wattanasirichaigoon D, Goebel HH et al 1999 Mutations in the skeletal muscle alpha-actin gene in patients with actin myopathy and nemaline myopathy. Nature Genetics 23:208–212

Odermatt A, Taschner PE, Khanna VK et al 1996 Mutations in the gene-encoding SERCA1, the fast-twitch skeletal muscle sarcoplasmic reticulum Ca^{2+} ATPase, are associated with Brody disease. Nature Genetics 14:191–194

Odermatt A, Taschner PE, Scherer SW et al 1997 Characterization of the gene encoding human sarcolipin (SLN), a proteolipid associated with SERCA1: absence of structural mutations in five patients with Brody disease. Genomics 45:541–553

Odermatt A, Becker S, Khanna VK et al 1998 Sarcolipin regulates the activity of SERCA1, the fast-twitch skeletal muscle sarcoplasmic reticulum Ca2+-ATPase. Journal of Biological Chemistry 273:12360–12369

Ognibene A, Sabatelli P, Petrini S et al 1999 Nuclear changes in a case of X-linked Emery–Dreifuss muscular dystrophy. Muscle Nerve 22:864–869

Okinaka S, Shizume K, Watanabe A et al 1957 The association of periodic paralysis and hyperthyroidism in Japan. Journal of Clinical Endocrinology 17:1454–1459

Oldfors A, Fyhr IM 2001 Inclusion body myositis: genetic factors, aberrant protein expression, and autoimmunity. Current Opinion in Rheumatology 13:469–475

Olson TM, Michels VV, Thibodeau SN et al 1998 Actin mutations in dilated cardiomyopathy, a heritable form of heart failure. Science 280:750–752

Onengut S, Ugur SA, Karasoy H et al 2004 Identification of a locus for an autosomal recessive hyaline body myopathy at chromosome 3p22.2–p21.32. Neuromuscular Disorders 14:4–9

Ording H, Brancadoro V, Cozzolino S et al 1997 In vitro contracture test for diagnosis of malignant hyperthermia following the protocol of the European MH Group: results of testing patients surviving fulminant MH and unrelated low-risk subjects. The European Malignant Hyperthermia Group. Acta Anaesthesiologica Scandinavica 41:955–966

Osawa E, Noguchi S, Mizuno Y et al 1998 From dystrophinopathy to sarcoglycanopathy: evolution of a concept of muscular dystrophy. Muscle and Nerve 21:421–438

Osborn M, Goebel HH 1983 The cytoplasmic bodies in a congenital myopathy can be stained with antibodies to desmin, the muscle-specific intermediate filament protein. Acta Neuropathologica (Berlin) 62:149–152

Padberg G 2002 Large telomeric deletion disease, facioscapulohumeral muscular dystrophy. In: Karpati G (ed) Structural and molecular basis of skeletal muscle diseases. ISN Neuropathology Press, Basel, pp 119–122

Padykula HA, Hermann E 1955 The specificity of the histochemical method for adenosine triphosphate. Journal of Histochemistry and Cytochemistry 3:170–195

Palace J, Vincent A, Beeson D 2001 Myasthenia gravis: diagnostic and management dilemmas. Current Opinion in Neurology 14:583–589

Pan TC, Zhang RZ, Sudano DG et al 2003 New molecular mechanism for Ullrich congenital muscular dystrophy: a heterozygous in-frame deletion in the COL6A1 gene causes a severe phenotype. American Journal of Human Genetics 73:355–369

Papadopoulou LC, Sue CM, Davidson MM et al 1999 Fatal infantile cardioencephalomyopathy with COX deficiency and mutations in SCO2, a COX assembly gene. Nature Genetics 23:333–337

Pardo JV, D'Angelo Siliciano J, Craig SW 1983 A vinculin-containing cortical lattice in skeletal muscle: transverse lattice elements ('costameres') mark sites of attachment between myofibrils and sarcolemma. Proceedings of the National Academy of Sciences of the United States of America 80:1008–1012

Payne CM, Curless RG 1976 Concentric laminated bodies – ultrastructural demonstration of fibre type specificity. Journal of the Neurological Sciences, 29:311–322

Pearse AG, Johnson M 1970 Histochemistry in the study of normal and diseased muscle with special reference to myopathy with tubular aggregates. In: Walton J N, Canal N, Scarlato G (eds) Muscle diseases. ICS No. 199. Excerpta Medica, Amsterdam, pp 25–32

Pearse AGE 1968 Histochemistry: theoretical and applied, 3rd edn. Churchill, London, Vol 1

Pearse AGE 1972 Histochemistry: theoretical and applied, 3rd edn. Churchill, London, Vol 2

Pearson CM, Rimer DG, Mommaerts WF 1961 A metabolic myopathy due to absence of muscle phosphorylase. American Journal of Medicine 30:502–517

Pearson HA, Lobel JS, Kocoshis SA et al 1979 A new syndrome of refractory sideroblastic anemia with vacuolization of marrow precursors and exocrine pancreatic dysfunction. Journal of Pediatrics 95:976–984

Pegoraro E, Mancias P, Swerdlow SH et al 1996 Congenital muscular dystrophy with primary laminin alpha2 (merosin) deficiency presenting as inflammatory myopathy. Annals of Neurology 40:782–791

Pelin K, Hilpela P, Donner K et al 1999 Mutations in the nebulin gene associated with autosomal recessive nemaline myopathy. Proceedings of the National Academy of Sciences of the United States of America 96:2305–2310

Pepe G, de Visser M, Bertini E et al 2000 Bethlem myopathy 86th ENMC International Workshop, 10–11 November 2000, Naarden, The Netherlands Neuromuscular Disorders 12:296–305

Perkoff GT, Silber R, Tyler FH et al 1959 Studies in disorders of muscle. XII. Myopathy due to the administration of therapeutic amounts of 17-hydroxycortico-steroids. American Journal of Medicine 26:891–898

Perng MD, Wen SF, van den IJssel P 2004 Desmin aggregates and αB-crystallin. Molecular Biology of the Cell 15:2335–2346

Pette D, Staron RS 1997 Mammalian skeletal muscle fiber type transitions. International Review of Cytology 170:143–223

Pette D, Staron RS 2000 Myosin isoforms, muscle fiber types, and transitions. Microscopy Research and Technique 50:500–509

Pette D, Staron RS 2001 Transitions of muscle fiber phenotypic profiles. Histochemistry and Cell Biology 11:359–372

Pette D, Vrbova G 1999 What does chronic electrical stimulation teach us about muscle plasticity? Muscle and Nerve 22:666–677

Philpot J, Sewry C, Pennock J et al 1995 Clinical phenotype in congenital muscular dystrophy correlation with expression of merosin in skeletal muscle. Neuromuscular Disorders 5:301–305

Philpot J, Cowan F, Pennock J et al 1999 Merosin-deficient congenital muscular dystrophy: the spectrum of brain involvement on magnetic resonance imaging. Neuromuscular Disorders 9:81–85

Piccolo F, Moore SA, Ford GC et al 2000 Intracellular accumulation and reduced sarcolemmal expression of dysferlin in limb-girdle muscular dystrophies. Annals of Neurology 48:902–912

Piccolo F, Moore SA, Mathews KD et al 2002 Limb-girdle muscular dystrophies. Advances in Neurology 88:273–291

Pichiecchio A, Uggetti C, Ravaglia S et al 2004 Muscle MRI in adult-onset acid maltase deficiency. Neuromuscular Disorders 14:51–55

Pickett JBE, Layers RB, Levin SR et al 1975 Neuromuscular complications of acromegaly. Neurology 25:638–645

Plaster NM, Tawil R, Tristani-Firouzi M et al 2001 Mutations in Kir2.1 cause the developmental and episodic electrical phenotypes of Andersen's syndrome. Cell 105:511–519

Pleasure DE, Walsh GO, Engel WK 1970 Atrophy of skeletal muscle in patients with Cushing's syndrome. Archives of Neurology (Chicago) 22:118–125

Poon E, Cowman EV, Newey SE et al 2002 Association of syncoilin and desmin: linking intermediate filament proteins to the dystrophin-associated protein complex. Journal of Biological Chemistry 277:3433–3439

Poppe M, Cree L, Bourke J et al 2003 The phenotype of limb-girdle muscular dystrophy type 2I. Neurology 60:1246–1251

Porter GA, Dmytrenko GM, Winkelmann JC et al 1992 Dystrophin co-localizes with β-spectrin in distinct subsarcolemma domains in mammalian skeletal muscle. Journal of Cell Biology 117:997–1005

Pourmand R, Azzarelli B 1994 Adult-onset of nemaline myopathy, associated with cores and abnormal mitochondria. Muscle and Nerve 17:1218–1220

Prick MJJ, Gabreels FJM, Trijbels JMF et al 1983 Progressive poliodystrophy (Alpers' disease) with a defect in cytochrome aa$_3$ in muscle: A report of two unrelated patients. Clinical Neurology and Neurosurgery 85:57–70

Prince FP, Hikida RS, Hagerman FC et al 1981 A morphometric analysis of human muscle fibers with relation to fiber types and adaptations to exercise. Journal of the Neurological Sciences 49:165–179

Prineas JW, Mason AS, Henson RA 1965 Myopathy in metabolic bone disease. British Medical Journal 5441:1034–1036

Prineas J, Hall R, Barwick DD et al 1968 Myopathy associated with pigmentation following adrenalectomy for Cushing's syndrome. Quarterly Journal of Medicine 37:63–77

Quane KA, Healy JM, Keating KE et al 1993 Mutations in the ryanodine receptor gene in central core disease and malignant hyperthermia. Nature Genetics 5:51–55

Raffaele Di Barletta M, Ricci E, Galluzzi G et al 2000 Different mutations in the LMNA gene cause autosomal dominant and autosomal recessive Emery–Dreifuss muscular dystrophy. American Journal of Human Genetics 66:1407–1412

Rajendram R, Mantle D, Peters TJ 2003 The importance of alcohol-induced muscle disease. Journal of Muscle Research and Cell Motility 24:55–63

Ramsay ID 1966 Muscle dysfunction in hyperthyroidism. Lancet ii:931–934

Ratinov G, Baker WP, Swainman KE 1965 McArdle's syndrome with previously unreported electrocardiographic and serum enzyme abnormalities. Annals of Internal Medicine 62:328–334

Rebouche CJ, Engel AG 1981 Primary systemic carnitine deficiency: 1. Carnitine biosynthesis. Neurology 31:813–818

Rebouche CJ, Engel AG 1983 Carnitine metabolism and deficiency syndromes. Mayo Clinic Proceedings 58:533–540

Resnick JS, Dorman JD, Engel WK 1969 Thyrotoxic periodic paralysis. American Journal of Medicine 47:831–836

Richard I, Broux O, Allamand V et al 1995 Mutations in the proteolytic enzyme calpain 3 cause limb-girdle muscle dystrophy type 2A. Cell 81:27–40

Richard P, Charron P, Carrier L et al 2003 Hypertrophic cardiomyopathy: distribution of disease genes, spectrum of mutations, and implications for a molecular diagnosis strategy. Circulation 107:2171–2174

Riemersma S, Vincent A, Beeson D et al 1996 Association of arthrogryposis multiplex congenita with maternal antibodies inhibiting fetal acetylcholine receptor function. Journal of Clinical Investigation 98:2358–2363

Riggs JE, Schochet SS, Fakadej AV et al 1984 Mitochondrial encephalomyopathy with decreased succinate-cytochrome c reductase activity. Neurology 34:48–53

Ringel SP, Neville HE, Duster MC et al 1978 A new congenital neuromuscular disease with trilaminar fibers. Neurology 28:282–289

Roe CR, Coates PM 1989 Acyl-CoA dehydrogenase deficiencies. In: Scriver CR et al (eds) The metabolic basis of inherited disease. McGraw Hill, New York, pp 889–914

Rogers M, Sewry CA, UPadhyaya M 2004 Histological, immunocytochemical, molecular and ultrastructural characteristics of FSHD muscle. In: Upadhyaya M and Cooper N (eds) FSHD facioscapulohumeral muscular dystrophy: clinical medicine and molecular cell biology. BIOS Scientific Publishers, London, pp 275–298

Rohkman R, Boxler K, Ricker K et al 1983 A dominantly inherited myopathy with excessive tubular aggregates. Neurology 33:331–336

Romero NB, Nivoche Y, Lunardi J 1993 Malignant hyperthermia and central core disease: analysis of two families with heterogeneous clinical expression. Neuromuscular Disorders 3:547–551

Romero NB, Monnier N, Viollet L et al 2003 Dominant and recessive central core disease associated with RYR1 mutations and fetal akinesia. Brain 126:2341–2349

Romi F, Gilhus NE, Aarli JA 2005 Myasthenia gravis: clinical, immunological, and therapeutic advances. Acta Neurologica Scandinavica 111:134–141

Rose M, Griggs R 2002 Endocrine disorders and myotrophic molecules. In: Karpati G (ed) Structural and molecular basis of skeletal muscle diseases. ISN Neuropathology Press, Basel, pp 260–264

Rotig A, Cormier V, Blanche S et al 1990 Pearson's marrow-pancreas syndrome: A multisystem mitochondrial disorder in infancy. Journal of Clinical Investigation 86:1601–1608

Round JM, Matthews Y, Jones DA 1980 A quick simple and reliable method for ATPase in human muscle preparations. Histochemical Journal 12:707–709

Sabatelli P, Squarzoni S, Petrini S et al 1998 Oral exfoliative cytology for the non-invasive diagnosis in Emery–Dreifuss muscular dystrophy patients and carriers. Neuromuscular Disorders 8:67–71

Sabatelli P, Bonaldo P, Lattanzi G et al 2001 Collagen VI deficiency affects the organization of fibronectin in the extracellular matrix of cultured fibroblasts. Matrix Biology 20:475–486

Sabatelli P, Columbaro M, Mura I et al 2003 Extracellular matrix and nuclear abnormalities in skeletal muscle of a patient with Walker-Warburg syndrome caused by POMT1 mutation. Biochimica et Biophysica Acta 20:57–62

Sahgal V, Sahgal S 1977 A new congenital myopathy. A morphological, cytochemical and histochemical study. Acta Neuropathologica (Berlin) 37:225–230

Saito Y, Murayama S, Kawai M et al 1999 Breached cerebral glia limitans–basal lamina complex in Fukuyama-type congenital muscular dystrophy. Acta Neuropathologica 98:330–336

Samaha FJ, Quinlan JG 1996 Myalgia and cramps: dystrophinopathy with wide-ranging laboratory findings. Journal of Child Neurology 11:21–24

Sambrook MA, Heron JR, Aber GM 1972 Myopathy in association with primary hyperaldosteronism. Journal of Neurology, Neurosurgery and Psychiatry 35:202–207

Sanes JR 2003 The basement membrane/basal lamina of skeletal muscle. Journal of Biological Chemistry 78:12601–12604

Sanes JR, Lichtman JW 2001 Induction, assembly, maturation and maintenance of a postsynaptic apparatus. Nature Reviews Neuroscience 2: 791–805

Sanoudou D, Beggs AH 2001 Clinical and genetic heterogeneity in nemaline myopathy – a disease of skeletal muscle thin filaments. Trends in Molecular Medicine 7:362–368

Sansone V, Griggs RC, Meola G et al 1997 Andersen's syndrome: a distinct periodic paralysis. Annals of Neurology 42:305–312

Santavouri P, Leisti J, Kruss S 1977 Muscle, eye, and brain disease: a new syndrome. Neuropediatrie 8b (suppl.):553

Santavuori P, Somer H, Sainio K 1989 Muscle-eye-brain disease (MEB). Brain Development 11:147–153

Sarnat HB 1990 Myotubular myopathy: arrest of morphogenesis of myofibres associated with persistence of fetal vimentin and desmin. Four cases compared with fetal and neonatal muscle. Canadian Journal of Neurological Sciences 17:109–123

Sasaki T, Shikura K, Sugai K et al 1989 Muscle histochemistry in myotubular (centronuclear) myopathy. Brain Development 11:26–32

Sato K, Imai F, Hatayama I et al 1977 Characterization of glycogen phosphorylase isoenzymes present in cultured skeletal muscle from patients with McArdle's disease. Biochemical and Biophysical Research Communications 78:663–668

Sato T, Walker DL, Peters HA et al 1971 Chronic polymyositis and myxovirus-like inclusions. Electron microscopic and viral studies. Archives of Neurology (Chicago) 24:409–418

Scacheri PC, Hoffman EP, Fratkin JD et al 2001 A novel ryanodine receptor gene mutation causing both cores and rods in congenital myopathy. Neurology 55:1689–1696

Schapira AHV, Cooper JM, Morgan-Hughes JA et al 1990 Mitochondrial myopathy with a defect of mitochondrial protein transport. New England Journal of Medicine 323:37–42

Schiaffino S, Hanzlikova V, Pierobon S 1970 Relations between structure and function in rat skeletal muscle fibers. Journal of Cell Biology 47:107–119

Schmalbruch H 1975 Segmental fibre breakdown and defects of the plasmalemma in diseased human muscles. Acta Neuropathologica (Berlin) 33:129–141

Schmid R, Mahler R 1959 Chronic progressive myopathy with myoglobinuria. Demonstration of a glycogenolytic defect in the muscle. Journal of Clinical Investigation 38:2044–2058

Schnell C, Kan A, North KN 2000 'An artefact gone awry': identification of the first case of nemaline myopathy by Dr RDK Reye. Neuromuscular Disorders 10:307–312

Schochet SS Jr, McCormick WF 1973 Polymyositis with intranuclear inclusions. Archives of Neurology (Chicago) 28:280–283

Schollmeyer JV, Goll D, Stromer MH et al 1974 Studies on the composition of the Z disk. Journal of Cell Biology 63:303

Schoser BG, Schneider-Gold C, Kress W et al 2004 Muscle pathology in 57 patients with myotonic dystrophy type 2. Muscle and Nerve 29:275–281

Schoser BG, Frosk P, Engel AG et al 2005 Commonality of TRIM32 mutation in causing sarcotubular myopathy and LGMD2H. Annals of Neurology 57:591–595

Schotland DL, DiMauro S, Bonilla E et al 1976 Neuromuscular disorder associated with a defect in mitochondrial energy supply. Archives of Neurology 33:475–479

Schott GD, Wills MR 1975 Myopathy and hypophosphataemic osteomalacia presenting in adult life. Journal of Neurosurgery and Psychiatry 38:297–304

Schröder R, Goebel H 2002 Plectin deficiency. In: Karpati G (ed) Structural and molecular basis of skeletal muscle diseases. ISN Neuropathology Press, Basel, pp 78–80

Schröder R, Reimann J, Salmikangas P et al 2003 Beyond LGMD1A: myotilin is a component of central core lesions and nemaline rods. Neuromuscular Disorders 13:451–455

Segura-Totten M, Wilson KL 2004 BAF: roles in chromatin, nuclear structure and retrovirus integration. Trends in Cell Biology 14:261–266

Seidman JG, Seidman C 2001 The genetic basis for cardiomyopathy: from mutation identification to mechanistic paradigms. Cell 104:557–567

Seitelberger F, Wanko T, Gavin MA 1961 The muscle fiber in central core disease. Histochemical and electron microscopic observations. Acta Neuropathologica (Berlin) 1:223–237

Selcen D, Engel AG 2003 Myofibrillar myopathy caused by novel dominant negative alpha B-crystallin mutations. Annals of Neurology 54:804–810

Selcen D, Engel AG 2004 Mutations in myotilin cause myofibrillar myopathy. Neurology 62:1363–1371

Selcen D, Engel AG 2005 Mutations in ZASP define a novel form of muscular dystrophy in humans. Annals of Neurology 57:269–276

Selcen D, Stilling G, Engel AG 2001 The earliest pathologic alterations in dysferlinopathy. Neurology 56:1472–1482

Selcen D, Fukudu T, Shen XM et al 2004 Are MuSK antibodies the primary cause of myasthenic symptoms. Neurology 62:1363–1371

Selcen D, Ohno K, Engel AG 2004 Myofibrillar myopathy: clinical, morphological and genetic studies in 63 patients. Brain 127:439–451

Senderek J, Bergmann C, Weber S et al 2003 Mutation of the SBF2 gene, encoding a novel member of the myotubularin family, in Charcot–Marie–Tooth neuropathy type 4B2/11p15. Humun Molecular Genetics 12:349–356

Sengers RCA, Fischer JC, Trijbels JMF et al 1983 A mitochondrial myopathy with a defective respiratory chain and carnitine deficiency. European Journal of Pediatrics 240:332–337

Serratrice G, Monges A, Roux H et al 1969 Myopathic forms of phosphofructokinase deficit. Revue Neurologique 120:271–277

Serratrice G, Pellissier JF, Cros D 1978 Les atteintes musculaires des osteomalacies etude clinique, histoenzymologique et ultrastructurale de 10 cas. Revue du Rhumatisme 45:621–630

Servidei S, Bertin E, Dionisi-Vici C et al 1988 Benign infantile mitochondrial myopathy due to reversible cytochrome c oxidase deficiency: A third case. Clinical Neuropathology 7:209–210

Sewry CA 1989 Contribution of immunocytochemistry to the pathogenesis of spinal muscular atrophy. In: Merlini L, Granata C, Dubowitz V (eds) Current concepts in childhood spinal muscular atrophy, Springer-Verlag, Vienna, pp 57–68

Sewry CA 1998 The role of immunocytochemistry in congenital myopathies. Neuromuscular Disorders 8:394–400

Sewry CA 2002 Marinesco–Sjögren syndrome. In: Karpati G (ed) Structural and molecular basis of skeletal muscle diseases. ISN Neuropathology Press, Basel, pp 277–278

Sewry CA, Dubowitz V 2001 Histochemistry and immunocytochemistry of muscle in health and disease. In: Karpati G, Hilton-Jones D, Griggs RS (eds) Disorders of voluntary muscle, 7th edn. Cambridge University Press, Cambridge, pp 251–282

Sewry CA, Muntoni F 1999 Inherited disorders of the extracellular matrix. Current Opinion in Neurology 12:519–526

Sewry CA, Qui Lu 2001 Immunological reagents and amplification systems. In: Bushby K, Anderson LVB (eds) Methods in molecular medicine – the muscular dystrophies. Humana Press Totowa, pp. 325–328

Sewry CA, Dubowitz V, Abraha A et al 1987 Immunocytochemical localisation of complement components C8 and C9 in human diseased muscle; the role of complement in muscle fibre damage. Journal of the Neurological Sciences 81:141–153

Sewry CA, Voit T, Dubowitz V 1988 Myopathy with unique ultrastructural feature in Marinesco–Sjögren syndrome. Annals of Neurology 24:576–580

Sewry CA, Clerk A, Heckmatt JZ et al 1991 Dystrophin abnormalities in polymyositis and dermatomyositis. Neuromuscular Disorders 1:333–339

Sewry CA, Wilson LA, Dux L et al 1992 Experimental regeneration in canine muscular dystrophy. 1. Immunocytochemical evaluation of dystrophin and β-spectrin expression. Neuromuscular Disorders 2:331–342

Sewry CA, Sansome A, Clerk A et al 1993 Manifesting carriers of Xp21 muscular dystrophy; lack of correlation between dystrophin expression and clinical weakness. Neuromuscular Disorders 3:141–148

Sewry CA, Muntoni F, Sansome A et al 1994a Sarcolemmal expression of utrophin in diverse neuromuscular disorders. Muscle and Nerve 1:S103

Sewry CA, Matsumura K, Campbell KP et al 1994b Expression of dystrophin-associated glycoprotein and utrophin in carriers of Duchenne muscular dystrophy. Neuromuscular Disorders 4:401–409

Sewry CA, Sansome A, Matsumura K et al 1994c Deficiency of the 50 kDa dystrophin-associated glycoprotein and abnormal expression of utrophin in two south Asian cousins with variable expression of severe childhood autosomal recessive muscular dystrophy. Neuromuscular Disorders 4:121–129

Sewry CA, Chevallay M, Tomé FMS 1995 Expression of laminin subunits in human fetal skeletal muscle. The Histochemical Journal 27:497–504

Sewry CA, Philpot J, Sorokin L et al 1996 Diagnosis of merosin (laminin a2)-deficient congenital muscular dystrophy by skin biopsy. Lancet 347:582–584

Sewry CA, D'Alessandro M, Wilson LA et al 1997a Expression of laminin chains in skin in merosin-deficient congenital muscular dystrophy. Neuropediatrics 28:217–222

Sewry CA, Naom I, D'Alessandro M et al 1997b Variable phenotype in merosin-deficient congenital muscular dystrophy and differential immunolabelling of two fragments of the laminin α2 chain. Neuromuscular Disorders 7:169–175

Sewry CA, Brown SC, Mercuri E et al 2001a Skeletal muscle pathology in autosomal dominant Emery–Dreifuss muscular dystrophy with lamin A/C mutations. Neuropathology Applied Neurobiology 27:281–290

Sewry CA, Brown SC, Pelin K et al 2001b Abnormalities in the expression of nebulin in chromosome-2 linked nemaline myopathy. Neuromuscular Disorders 11:146–153

Sewry CA, Muller C, Davis M et al 2002 The spectrum of pathology in central core disease. Neuromuscular Disorders 12:930–938

Sewry CA, Jimenez-Mallebrera C, Feng L, Quinlivan R, Muntoni F 2005a Over-expression of utrophin in patients with limb-girdle muscular dystrophies. Neuromuscular Disorders 15:717

Sewry CA, Nowak KJ, Ehmsen JT, Davies KE 2005b A and B utrophin in human muscle and sarcolemmal A-utrophin associated with tumours. Neuromuscular Disorders 15:779–785

Sher J, Shafiq SA, Schutta HS 1979 Acute myopathy with selective lysis of myosin filaments. Neurology 29:100–106

Sher JH, Rimalovski AB, Athanassiades TJ et al 1967 Familial centronuclear myopathy: a clinical and pathological study. Neurology 17:727–742

Shimizu H, Masunaga T, Kurihara Y et al 1999 Expression of plectin and HD1 epitopes in patients with epidermolysis bullosa simplex associated with muscular dystrophy. Archives of Dermatological Research 291:531–537

Shorer Z, Philpot J, Muntoni F et al 1995 Demyelinating peripheral neuropathy in merosin-deficient congenital muscular dystrophy. Journal of Child Neurology 10:472–475

Shoubridge EA 2001 Skeletal muscle pathology in autosomal dominant Emery–Dreifuss muscular dystrophy with lamin A/C mutations. American Journal of Medical Genetics 106:46–52

Shy GM, Engel WK, Somers JE et al 1963 Nemaline myopathy. A new congenital myopathy. Brain 86:793-810

Sigurgeirsson B, Lindelof B, Edhag O et al 1992 Risk of cancer in patients with dermatomyositis or polymyositis. A population-based study. New England Journal of Medicine 326:363–367

Silan F, Yoshioka M, Kobayashi K et al 2003 A new mutation of the Fukutin gene in a non-Japanese patient. Annals of Neurology 53:392–396

Silver S, Osserman KE 1957 Hyperthyroidism and myasthenia gravis. Journal of the Mount Sinai Hospital 24:1214–1220

Simon LT, Horoupian DS, Dorfman LJ et al 1990 Polyneuropathy, ophthalmoplegia, leukoencephalopathy, and intestinal pseudo-obstruction: POLIP syndrome. Annals of Neurology 28:349–360

Simpson JA 1968 The correlations between myasthenia gravis and disorders of the thyroid gland. In: Research Committee of the Muscular Dystrophy Group of Great Britain (ed) Research in muscular dystrophy, proceedings of fourth symposium. Pitman Medical, London, p 31

Sjöström M, Squire JM 1977 Cryoultramicrotomy and myofibrillar fine structure: a review. Journal of Microscopy 111:239–278

Sjöström M, Kidman S, Henriksson Larsen K et al 1982 Z- and M-band appearance in different histochemically defined types of human skeletal muscle fibers. Journal of Histochemistry and Cytochemistry 30:1–11

Skaria JB, Katiyar B, Srivastara T et al 1975 Myopathy and neuropathy associated with osteomalacia. Acta Neurologica Scandinavica 51:37–58

Skordis LA, Dunckley MG, Burglen L et al 2001 Characterisation of novel point mutations in the survival motor neuron gene SMN, in three patients with SMA. Human Genetics 108:356–357

Skyllouriotis ML, Marx M, Skyllouriotis P et al 1999 Nemaline myopathy and cardiomyopathy. Pediatric Neurology 20:319–321

Smith FJ, Eady RA, Leigh IM et al 1996 Plectin deficiency results in muscular dystrophy with epidermolysis bullosa. Nature Genetics 13:450–457

Smith R, Stern G 1967 Myopathy, osteomalacia and hyperparathyroidism. Brain 90:593–602

Sorimachi H, Kinbara K, Kimura S et al 1995 Muscle-specific calpain p94, responsible for limb-girdle muscular dystrophy type 2A, associates with connectin, through IS2, a p94-specific sequence. Journal of Biological Chemistry 270:31158–31162

Soussi-Yanicostas N, Ben Hamida C, Bejaoui K et al 1992 Evolution of muscle specific proteins in Werdnig–Hoffman's disease. Journal of Neurological Sciences 109:111–120

Sparrow JC, Nowak KJ, Durling HJ et al 2003 Muscle disease caused by mutations in the skeletal muscle alpha-actin gene (ACTA1). Neuromuscular Disorders 13:519–531

Speer MC, Yamaoka LH, Gilchrist JH et al 1992 Confirmation of genetic heterogeneity in limb-girdle muscular dystrophy linkage to an autosomal dominant form to chromosome 5q. American Journal of Human Genetics 50:1211–1217

Speer MC, Tandan R, Rao PN et al 1996 Evidence for locus heterogeneity in the Bethlem myopathy and linkage to 2q37. Human Molecular Genetics 5:1043–1046

Sperl W, Ruitenbeek W, Trijbels JMF 1988 Mitochondrial myopathy with lactic acidemia, Fanconi–DeToni–Debre syndrome and a disturbed succinate: cytochrome c oxido-reductase activity. European Journal of Pediatrics 147:418–421

Spinazzola A, Marti R, Nishino I et al 2002 Altered thymidine metabolism due to defects of thymidine phosphorylase. Journal of Biological Chemistry 277:4128–4132

Spiro AJ, Shy GM, Gonatas NK 1966 Myotubular myopathy. Persistence of fetal muscle in an adolescent boy. Archives of Neurology 14:1–14

Squier M, Chalk C, Hilton-Jones D et al 1991 Type 2 fiber predominance in Lambert–Eaton myasthenic syndrome. Muscle and Nerve 14:625–632

Stanley CA, Hale DE, Coates PM et al 1983 Medium-chain acyl-CoA dehydrogenase deficiency in children with non-ketotic hypoglycemia and low carnitine levels. Pediatric Research 17:877–884

Stephens HR, Duance VC, Dunn MJ et al 1982. Collagen types in neuromuscular diseases. Journal of the Neurological Sciences 53:45–62

Straub V, Campbell KP 1997 Muscular dystrophies and the dystrophin–glycoprotein complex. Current Opinion in Neurology 10:168–175

Straub V, Ettinger AJ, Durbeej M et al 2003 ε-Sarcoglycan replaces α-sarcoglycan in smooth muscle to form a unique dystrophin–glycoprotein complex. The Journal of Biological Chemistry 274:27989–27996

Stromer MH 1995 Immunocytochemistry of the muscle cell cytoskeleton. Microscopy Research and Technique 31:95–105

Sunada Y, Saito F, Higuchi I et al 2002 Deficiency of a 180-kDa extracellular matrix protein in Fukuyama type congenital muscular dystrophy skeletal muscle. Neuromuscular Disorders 12:117–120

Sung SS, Brassington AM, Grannatt K et al 2003 Mutations in genes encoding fast-twitch contractile proteins cause distal arthrogryposis syndromes. American Journal of Human Genetics 72:681–690

Suomalainen A, Kaukonen J 2001 Diseases caused by nuclear genes affecting mtDNA stability. American Journal of Medical Genetics 196:53–61

Swash M 1992 Pathology of the muscle spindle. In: Mastaglia FL, Lord Walton of Detchant (eds) Skeletal muscle pathology, 2nd edn. Churchill Livingstone, Edinburgh, pp 665–697

Tajsharghi H, Thornell LE, Darin N et al 2002 Myosin heavy chain IIa gene mutation E706K is pathogenic and its expression increases with age. Neurology 58:780–786

Tajsharghi H, Thornell LE, Lindberg C et al 2003 Myosin storage myopathy associated with a heterozygous missense mutation in MYH7. Annals of Neurology 54:494–500

Takada F, Vander-Woude DL, Tong HQ et al 2001 Myozenin: an alpha-actinin- and gamma-filamin-binding protein of skeletal muscle Z lines. Proceedings of the National Academy of Sciences of the United States of America 98:1595–1600

Takeuchi T 1962 Histochemical differentiation of phosphorylase a, phosphorylase b and phosphorylase-kinase. Journal of Histochemistry and Cytochemistry 10: 688

Takeuchi T, Kuriaki H 1955 Histochemical detection of phosphorylase in animal tissue. Journal of Histochemistry and Cytochemistry 3:153–160

Tang TT, Sedmak GV, Siegesmund KA et al 1975 Chronic myopathy associated with Coxsackie virus Type A9: a combined electron microscopical and viral isolation study. New England Journal of Medicine 292:608–611

Tanner SM, Orstavik KH, Kristiansen M et al 1999 Skewed X-inactivation in a manifesting carrier of X-linked myotubular myopathy and in her non-manifesting carrier mother. Human Genetics 104:249–253

Taratuto 2002 Congenital myopathies and related disorders. Current Opinion in Neurology 15:553–561

Tarui S, Okuso G, Ikura Y et al 1965 Phosphofructokinase deficiency in skeletal muscle. A new type of glycogenosis. Biochemical and Biophysical Research Communications 19:517–523

Tarui S, Kono N, Nasu T et al 1969 Enzymatic basis for coexistence of myopathy and hemolytic disease in inherited muscle phosphofructokinase deficiency. Biochemical and Biophysical Research Communications 34:77–83

Tarui S, Kono N, Kuwajima M et al 1978 Type VII glycogenosis (muscle and erythrocyte phosphofructokinase deficiency). Monographs in Human Genetics 9:42–47

Tawil R, Griggs RC 2001 Facioscapulohumeral muscular dystrophy. In: Karpati G, Hilton-Jones D, Griggs RC (eds) Disorders of voluntary muscle, 7th edn. Cambridge University Press, Cambridge, pp 464–470

Taylor J, Muntoni F, Dubowitz V et al 1997a Abnormal expression of utrophin in Duchenne and Becker muscular dystrophy is age-related. Neuropathology & Applied Neurobiology 23:399–405

Taylor J, Muntoni F, Dubowitz V et al 1997b Early onset autosomal dominant myopathy; a role for laminin β1? Neuromuscular Disorders 7:211–216

Tein I, De Vivo DC, Hale DE et al 1991 Short-chain L-3-hydroxyacyl-CoA dehydrogenase deficiency in muscle: a new cause for recurrent myoglobinuria and encephalopathy. Annals of Neurology 30:415–419

Telerman-Toppet N, Gerard JM, Coërs C 1973 Central core disease: a study of clinically unaffected muscle. Journal of the Neurological Sciences 19:207–233

Tews DS 2001 Role of nitric oxide and nitric oxide synthases in experimental models of denervation and reinnervation. Microscopy Research Technique 55:181–186

Thanh Le Thiet, Nguyen Thi Man, Hori S et al 1995 Characterization of genetic deletions in Becker muscular dystrophy using monoclonal antibodies against a deletion-prone region of dystrophin. American Journal of Medical Genetics 58:177–186

Thanvi BR, Lo TC 2004 Update on myasthenia gravis. Postgraduate Medical Journal 80:690–700

Thompson LV 2002 Skeletal muscle adaptations with age, inactivity, and therapeutic exercise. Journal of Orthopaedic and Sports Physical Therapy 32:44–57

Thompson HM, Cao H, Chen J et al 2004 Dynamin 2 binds gamma-tubulin and participates in centrosome cohesion. Nature Cell Biology 6:335–342

Thornell LE, Edström L, Eriksson A et al 1980 The distribution of intermediate filament protein (Skeletin) in normal and diseased human skeletal muscle. Journal of the Neurological Sciences 47:153–170

Thornton C 2002 The myotonic dystrophies. In: Karpati G (ed) Structural and molecular basis of skeletal muscle diseases. ISN Neuropathology Press, Basel, pp 108–114

Tiger CF, Champliaud MF, Pedrosa-Domellof F et al 1997 Presence of laminin alpha5 chain and lack of laminin alpha1 chain during human muscle development and in muscular dystrophies. Journal of Biological Chemistry 272:28590–28595

Tilgen N, Zorzato F, Halliger-Keller B et al 2001 Identification of four novel mutations in the C-terminal membrane spanning domain of the ryanodine receptor 1: association with central core disease and alteration of calcium homeostasis. Human Molecular Genetics 10:2879–2887

Tiranti V, Hoertnagel K, Carrozzo R et al 1998 Mutations of SURF-1 in Leigh disease associated with cytochrome c oxidase deficiency. American Journal of Human Genetics 63:1609–1621

Toda T, Segawa M, Nomura Y et al 1994 Localization of a gene for Fukuyama type congenital muscular dystrophy to chromosome 9q31-33. Nature Genetics 5:283–286

Tomé FMS, Fardeau M 1980 Nuclear inclusions in oculopharyngeal dystrophy. Acta Neuropathologica (Berlin) 49:85–87

Tomé FM, Evangelista T, Leclerc A et al 1994 Congenital muscular dystrophy with merosin deficiency. Comptes Rendus de l'Academie des Sciences. Serie III, Sciences de la Vie 317:351–357

Tomé FMS, Fardeau M, Lebon P et al 1981 Inclusion body myositis. Acta Neuropathologica, Supplement (Berlin) 7:287–291

Toop J, Emery AEH 1974. Muscle histology in fetuses at risk for Duchenne muscular dystrophy. Clinical Genetics 5:230–233

Topaloglu H, Muntoni F, Dubowitz V et al 1996 Expression of HLA class I antigens in skeletal muscle is a diagnostic marker in juvenile dermatomyositis. Journal of Child Neurology 12:60–63

Torelli S, Brown SC, Jimenez-Mallebrera C et al 2004 Absence of neuronal nitric oxide synthase (nNOS) as a pathological marker for the diagnosis of Becker muscular dystrophy with rod domain deletions. Neuropathology and Applied Neurobiology 30:540–545

Towbin JA 1998 The role of cytoskeletal proteins in cardiomyopathies. Current Opinion in Cell Biology 10:131–139

Tritschler HJ, Bonilla E, Lombes A et al 1991 Differential diagnosis of fatal and benign cytochrome c oxidase-deficient myopathies of infancy: an immunohistochemical approach. Neurology 41:300–305

Tupler R, Gabellini D 2004 Molecular basis of facioscapulohumeral muscular dystrophy. Cellular and Molecular Life Sciences 61:557–566

Turnbull DM, Bartlett K, Stevens D et al 1984 Short-chain acyl-CoA dehydrogenase deficiency associated with a lipid-storage myopathy and secondary carnitine deficiency. New England Journal of Medicine 311:1232–1236

Turnbull DM, Shepherd IM, Ashworth B et al 1988a Lipid storage myopathy associated with low acyl-CoA dehydrogenase activities. Brain 111:815–828

Turnbull DM, Bartlett K, Eyre JA et al 1988b Lipid storage myopathy due to glutaric aciduria type II: treatment of a potentially fatal myopathy. Developmental Medicine and Child Neurology 30:667–672

Tyni T, Pihko H 1999 Long-chain 3-hydroxyacyl-CoA dehydrogenase deficiency. Acta Paediatrica 88:237–345

Ucar M, Mjorndal T, Dahlqvist R 2000 HMG-CoA reductase inhibitors and myotoxicity. Drug Safety 22:441–457

Udd B, Vihola A, Sarparanta J et al 2005 Titinopathies and extension of the M-line mutation phenotype beyond distal myopathy and LGMD2J. Neurology 64:636–642

Upadhyaya M, Cooper ND 2004 Introduction and Overview of FSHD. In: FSHD facioscapulohumeral muscular dystrophy: clinical medicine and molecular cell biology. BIOS Scientific Publishers, London, pp 1–16

Usuki F, Takenaga S, Higuchi I 1994 Morphologic findings in biopsied skeletal muscle and cultured fibroblasts from a female patient with Danon's disease (lysosomal glycogen storage disease without acid maltase deficiency). Journal of the Neurological Sciences 127:54–60

Vachon PH, Xu H, Liu L et al 1997 Integrins (alpha7beta1) in muscle function and survival. Disrupted expression in merosin-deficient congenital muscular dystrophy. Journal of Clinical Investigation 100:1870–1881

Vainzof M, Passos-Bueno MR, Canovas M et al 1996 The sarcoglycan complex in the six autosomal recessive limb-girdle (AR-LGMD) muscular dystrophies. Human Molecular Genetics 5:1963–1969

Vainzof M, Costa CS, Marie SK et al 1997 Deficiency of alpha-actinin-3 (ACTN3) occurs in different forms of muscular dystrophy. Neuropaediatrics 28:223–228

Vainzof M, Anderson LV, McNally EM et al 2001 Dysferlin protein analysis in limb-girdle muscular dystrophies. Journal of Molecular Neurosciences 17:71–80

Vainzof M, Richard P, Herrmann R et al 2005 Pre-natal diagnosis in laminin α2 chain (merosin)-deficient congenital muscular dystrophy: A collective experience of five international centres. Neuromuscular Disorders 15:588–594

Valnot I, Osmond S, Gigarel N et al 2000a Mutations of the SCO1 gene in mitochondrial cytochrome c oxidase deficiency with neonatal-onset hepatic failure and encephalopathy. American Journal of Medical Genetics 67:1104–1109

Valnot I, von Kleist-Retzow JC, Barrientos A et al 2000b A mutation in the human heme A: farnesyltransferase gene (COX10) causes cytochrome c oxidase deficiency. Human Molecular Genetics 9:1245–1249

van der Kooi AJ, Bonne G, Eymard B et al 2002 Lamin A/C mutations with lipodystrophy, cardiac abnormalities, and muscular dystrophy. Neurology 59:620–623

van der Maarel SM, Frants RR 2005 The D4Z4 repeat-mediated pathogenesis of facioscapulohumeral muscular dystrophy. American Journal of Human Genetics 76:375–386

van Reeuwijk J, Janssen M, van den Elzen C et al 2005 POMT2 mutations cause alpha-dystroglycan hypoglycosylation and Walker–Warburg syndrome. Journal of Medical Genetics 42:907–912

Verloes A, Massin M, Lombet J et al 1997 Nosology of lysosomal glycogen storage diseases without in vitro acid maltase deficiency. Delineation of a neonatal form. American Journal of Human Genetics 72:135–142

Vicale CT 1949 The diagnostic features of a muscular syndrome resulting from hyperparathyroidism, osteomalacia owing to renal tubular acidosis, and perhaps to related disorders of calcium metabolism. Transactions of the American Neurological Association 74:143–147

Vicart P, Caron A, Guicheney P et al 1998 A missense mutation in the alphaB-crystallin chaperone gene causes a desmin related myopathy. Nature Genetics 20:92–95

Vihola A, Bassez G, Meola G 2003 Histopathological differences of myotonic dystrophy type 1 (DM1) and PROMM/DM2. Neurology 60:1854–1857

Villanova M, Louboutin JP, Chateau D et al 1995 X-linked vacuolated myopathy: complement membrane attack complex on surface membrane of injured muscle fibres. Annals of Neurology 37:637–645

Vincent A, Rothwell P 2004 Myasthenia gravis. Autoimmunity 37:317–319

Voit T, Tomé FMS 2004 The congenital muscular dystrophies. In: Engel AG, Franzini-Armstrong C (eds) Myology, 3rd edn. McGrath-Hill, New York, pp 1203–1238

Voit T, Sewry CA, Meyer K et al 1995 Preserved merosin M-chain (or laminin-alpha 2) expression in skeletal muscle distinguishes Walker–Warburg syndrome from Fukuyama muscular dystrophy and merosin-deficient congenital muscular dystrophy. Neuropediatrics 26:148–155

Vorgerd M, van der Ven PF, Bruchertseifer V et al 2005 A mutation in the dimerization domain of filamin C causes a novel type of autosomal dominant myofibrillar myopathy. American Journal of Human Genetics 77:297–304

Waclawik AJ, Lindal S, Engel AG 1993 Experimental lovastatin myopathy. Journal of Neuropathology and Experimental Neurology, 52:542–549

Wallgren-Pettersson C 2000 Report of the 72nd ENMC International Workshop on Myotubular Myopathy, Hilversum, The Netherlands, 1–3 October 1999. Neuromuscular Disorders 10:521–525

Wallgren-Petterson C, Laing N 2000 Report of the 70th ENMC International Workshop: Nemaline myopathy 11–13 June 1999, Naarden, The Netherlands. Neuromuscular Disorders 10:299–306

Wallgren-Pettersson C, Thomas N 1994 Report on the 20th ENMC sponsored international workshop: myotubular/centronuclear myopathy. Neuromuscular Disorders 4: 71–74

Wallgren-Pettersson C, Avela K, Marchand S et al 1995 A gene for autosomal recessive nemaline myopathy assigned to chromosome 2q by linkage analysis. Neuromuscular Disorders 5:441–443

Wallgren-Pettersson C, Pelin K, Hilpela P et al 1999 Clinical and genetic heterogeneity in autosomal recessive nemaline myopathy. Neuromuscular Disorders 9:564–572

Wallgren-Petterson C, Laing N 2001 83rd ENMC International Workshop. 4th Workshop on nemaline myopathy 22–24 September 2000, Naarden, The Netherlands. Neuromuscular Disorders, 11:89–595

Wallgren-Pettersson C, Donner K, Sewry C et al 2002 Mutations in the nebulin gene can cause severe congenital nemaline myopathy. Neuromuscular Disorders 12:674–679

Wallgren-Pettersson C, Laing NG 2003 109th ENMC International Workshop, 5th Workshop on Nemaline Myopathy, 11–13 October 2002, Naarden, The Netherlands. Neuromuscular Disorders 13:501–507

Wallgren-Pettersson C, Pelin K, Nowak KJ et al 2004 Genotype–phenotype correlations in nemaline myopathy caused by mutations in the genes for nebulin and skeletal muscle alpha-actin. Neuromuscular Disorders 18:461–470

Walsh FS, Moore SE 1985 Expression of cell adhesion molecule, N-CAM, in diseases of a human skeletal muscle. Neuroscience Letters 59:73–78

Walter MC, Braun C, Vorgerd M et al 2003 Variable reduction of caveolin-3 in patients with LGMD2B/MM. Journal of Neurology 250:1431–1438

Wanders RJ, Vreken P, den Boer ME et al 1999 Disorders of mitochondrial fatty acyl-CoA beta-oxidation. Journal of Inherited Metabolic Diseases 22:442–487

Wedel DJ 1992 Malignant hyperthermia and neuromuscular disease. Neuromuscular Disorders 1992 2:157–164

Weiler T, Greenberg CR, Zelinski T et al 1998 A gene for autosomal recessive limb-girdle muscular dystrophy in Manitoba Hutterites maps to chromosome region 9q31–q33: evidence for another limb-girdle muscular dystrophy locus. American Journal of Human Genetics 63:140–147

Weir AP, Burton EA, Harrod G, Davies KE 2002 A- and B-utrophin have different expression patterns and are differentially up-regulated in mdx muscle. Journal of Biological Chemistry 277:45285–45290

Wewer UM, Durkin ME, Zhang X et al 1995 Laminin beta 2 chain and adhalin deficiency in the skeletal muscle of Walker–Warburg syndrome (cerebro-ocular dysplasia-muscular dystrophy). Neurology 45:2099–2101

Wewer UM, Thornell LE, Loechel F et al 1997 Extrasynaptic location of laminin beta 2 chain in developing and adult human skeletal muscle. American Journal of Pathology 151:621–631

Whalen RG, Sell SM, Butler-Browne GS et al 1981 Three myosin heavy chain isozymes appear sequentially in rat muscle development. Nature 292:805–809

Wheeler MT, Zarnegar S, McNally EM 2002 Zeta-sarcoglycan, a novel component of the sarcoglycan complex, is reduced in muscular dystrophy. Human Molecular Genetics 11:2147–2154

Williams RS 1959 Triamcinolone myopathy. Lancet i:698–701

Williamson RA, Henry MD, Daniels KJ et al 1997 Dystroglycan is essential for early embryonic development: disruption of Reichert's membrane in Dag1-null mice. Human Molecular Genetics 6:831–841

Willner JH, DiMauro S, Eastwood A et al 1979 Muscle carnitine deficiency: genetic heterogeneity. Journal of the Neurological Sciences 41:235–246

Wilson KL 2000 The nuclear envelope, muscular dystrophy and gene expression. Trends in Cell Biology 10: 125–129

Wilson LA, Dux L, Cooper BJ et al 1994 Experimental regeneration in canine muscular dystrophy; 2. Expression of myosin heavy chain isoforms. Neuromuscular Disorders 4:25–37

Wood D, Zeviani M, Prelle A 1987 Is nebulin the defective gene product in Duchenne muscular dystrophy? New England Journal of Medicine 316:107–108

Wullner U 2003 Genes implicated in the pathogenesis of spinocerebellar ataxias. Drugs Today 39:927–937

Yamaguchi M, Robson RM, Stromer MH et al 1978 Actin filaments form the backbone of nemaline myopathy rods. Nature (London) 271:265–267

Yamaguchi M, Robson RM, Stromer MH et al 1982 Nemaline myopathy rod bodies: structure and composition. Journal of the Neurological Sciences 56:35–56

Yamaguchi S, Orii T, Suzuki Y et al 1991 Newly identified forms of electron transfer flavoprotein deficiency in two patients with glutaric aciduria type II. Pediatric Research 29:60–63

Yamamoto T, Shibata N, Kanazawa M et al 1997 Early ultrastructural changes in the central nervous system in Fukuyama congenital muscular dystrophy. Ultrastructural Pathology 21:355–360

Yamamoto T, Kato Y, Kawaguchi M et al 2004 Expression and localization of fukutin, POMGnT1, and POMT1 in the central nervous system: consideration for functions of fukutin. Medical Electron Microscopy 37:200–207

Yarom R, Reches A 1980 Thick filament degeneration in a case of acute quadriplegia. Journal of the Neurological Sciences 45:13–22

Yarom R, Shapira Y 1977 Myosin degeneration in congenital myopathy. Archives of Neurology (Chicago) 34:114–115

Yoshida M, Ozawa E 1990 Glycoprotein complex anchoring dystrophin to sarcolemma. Journal of Biochemistry (Tokyo) 108:748–752

Yoshida A, Kobayashi K, Manya H et al 2001 Muscular dystrophy and neuronal migration disorder caused by mutations in a glycosyltransferase, POMGnT1. Developmental Cell 1:717–724

Zeviani M, Van Dyke DH, Servidei S et al 1986 Myopathy and fatal cardiopathy due to cytochrome c oxidase deficiency. Archives of Neurology 43:1198–1202

Zeviani M, Peterson P, Servidei S et al 1987 Benign reversible muscle cytochrome c oxidase deficiency: A second case. Neurology 37:64–67

Zhang W, Vajsar J, Cao P et al 2003 Enzymatic diagnostic test for muscle-eye-brain type congenital muscular dystrophy using commercially available reagents. Clinical Biochemistry 36:339–344

Zhu Z, Yao J, Johns T et al 1998 SURF1 encoding a factor involved in the biogenesis of cytochrome c oxidase, is mutated in Leigh syndrome. Nature Genetics 20:337–343

Zimprich A, Grabowski M, Asmus F et al 2001 Mutations in the gene encoding epsilon-sarcoglycan cause myoclonus-dystonia syndrome. Nature Genetics 29:66–69

Zuk JA, Feltcher A 1988 Skeletal muscle expression of class II histocompatibility antigens (HLA-DR) in polymyositis and other muscle diseases with an inflammatory infiltrate. Journal of Clinical Pathology 41:410–414

Glossary of genetic terms

Alternative splicing: If there are multiple exons and introns in a gene, then by choosing different splice donor/acceptor sites, different portions of the primary transcript, containing different exons, are retained in the mature transcript. By this process a single gene can give rise to multiple mature RNA transcripts, coding for proteins with variable structural elements.

Deletion: Deletions of all or part of the coding regions of the gene will delete the corresponding sequence from the protein product, or the entire product, depending on the size of the deletion. Deletions in the promotor or other non-coding regions may still impair the production of an mRNA transcript, and hence block protein production.

Exons: Exons are regions of those portions of the DNA within the gene that are transcribed into mature transcripts. They can be coding (i.e. determining a protein sequence) or non-coding (regions at either end of the RNA which regulate the translation of the transcript).

Frameshift mutation: The sequence of nucleotide triplets follows 'in frame' from the start codon (e.g. AUG,GAC,GCA). Deletion or insertion of a single nucleotide in the coding sequence alters the triplet sequence in which the codons are 'read' and shifts the reading frame (e.g. deletion of the fifth nucleotide in the above example would give AUG,GCG,CA etc.). This changes the amino acid sequence coded from this point. The shift in frame may also introduce premature 'stop' codons which will terminate the synthesis of the protein, or produce a longer protein by preventing the normal 'in-frame' stop codon from being recognized.

Genetic heterogeneity: Refers to the presence of more than one separate gene for an individual disease.

Introns: Introns are the regions of DNA within the gene that separate the exons. They do not (normally) code for protein sequence, but may contain regulatory elements that determine the efficiency of expression of the gene, or affect the choice of the exons included in the mature transcript.

Linkage: This expresses the association of a gene for a disease with DNA markers which are located close to it.

LOD score: This represents the logarithm of the odds for linkage and indicates the statistical support for linkage versus non-linkage between two loci. A lod score of 3 or greater, which corresponds to a p value of 0.05, has conventionally been accepted as statistical evidence for linkage and a lod score of -2 or less as evidence against linkage.

Missense mutations: These are point mutations in the coding sequence that result in the substitution of one amino acid for another in the final protein, but since the frame is unaffected, the rest of the protein sequence will be normal. The effect depends entirely on the importance of that amino acid in the protein structure, and can vary from no effect to a completely inactive protein.

Nonsense mutations: These are point mutations which produce a stop codon which terminates translation. A frameshift mutation may also introduce a stop codon downstream from the mutation site.

Point mutation: Point mutation is the alteration of a single nucleotide in the DNA to another nucleotide. Depending on the nucleotide mutated, the result may range from no effect at all, since most amino acids are coded for by more than one combination of nucleotides, to a complete block of product synthesis.

Promoter: This is a regulatory region of DNA in a gene which precedes the start of the coding sequence, and which, by interacting with a variety of protein factors, determines when, where, and how much expression of the gene should occur.

Splice mutation: A point mutation at the splice donor or acceptor sites will prevent normal splicing of the primary RNA transcript, resulting in an altered mature transcript. This may not be translatable, may be translated lacking one or more exons, or may create a new exon which includes intronic DNA, which could also be translated into protein. A point mutation may create a new alternative splice donor or acceptor site, resulting again in a defective mature transcript, or one with a different coding region.

Splicing: Splicing is the process by which the primary RNA transcript is cut, sequences corresponding to introns are removed, and the cut ends joined together so that the exons are then contiguous in the mature transcript. The places at which the splicing begins and ends are termed the splice donor and splice acceptor sites.

Transcription: Transcription is the process of copying a DNA sequence into a complementary RNA sequence, known as the primary transcript. This may then be edited by a process of splicing (see above) to form the mature mRNA used for translation into protein.

Translation: Translation is the synthesis of a protein product by assembling single amino acids into a polypeptide, the sequence of which is determined by the RNA sequence in the coding portion of the mature transcript. The amino acids are specified by triplets of nucleotides called codons.

APPENDIX 2

Useful websites

National Library of Medicine: Pubmed
http://www4.ncbi.nlm.nih.gov/PubMed/

Online Mendelian Inheritance in Man
http://www.ncbi.nlm.nih.gov/entrez/query.fcgi?db=OMIM&cmd

Neuromuscular Disorders, **official Journal of the WMS**
http://www.elsevier.com/wps/find/journaldescription.cws_home/973/description#description

World Muscle Society
http://www.worldmusclesociety.org
With access to the gene tables published in *Neuromuscular Disorders*

Child Neurology Home Page
http://waisman.wisc.edu/child-neuro/index.html

Leiden Muscular Dystrophy pages
http://www.dmd.nl/

Neuromuscular Disease Center, Washington University School of Medicine, St. Louis, MO
http://www.neuro.wustl.edu/neuromuscular

MuscleNet (Italy)
http://telethon.bio.unipd.it

Mutation Database of Inherited Peripheral Neuropathies
http://www.molgen.ua.ac.be/CMTMutations/

Nijmegen Center for Mitochondrial Disorders
http://go.to/ncmd

The European Neuromuscular Centre
http://www.enmc.org

Dutch Neuromuscular Centre
http://www.isno.nl

German Muscular Dystrophy Network
http://www.md-net.org/

Antibody Resource Page
http://www.antibodyresource.com/

Index